T0304706

Rehabilitation Engineering

Rehabilitation Science in Practice Series

Series Editors

Marcia J. Scherer
Institute for Matching Person & Technology, Webster, New York, USA

Dave Muller
University of Suffolk, UK

Everyday Technologies in Healthcare
Christopher M. Hayre, Dave Muller, Marcia Scherer

Enhancing Healthcare and Rehabilitation: The Impact of Qualitative Research
Christopher M. Hayre and Dave Muller

Neurological Rehabilitation: Spasticity and Contractures in Clinical Practice and Research
Anand D. Pandyan, Hermie J. Hermens, Bernard A. Conway

Quality of Life Technology Handbook
Richard Schulz

Computer Systems Experiences of Users with and Without Disabilities: An Evaluation Guide for Professionals
Simone Borsci, Masaaki Kurosu, Stefano Federici, Maria Laura Mele

Assistive Technology Assessment Handbook – 2nd Edition
Stefano Federici, Marcia Scherer

Ambient Assisted Living
Nuno M. Garcia, Joel Jose P.C. Rodrigues

Rehabilitation Engineering: Principles and Practice
Alex Mihailidis and Roger Smith

Principles and Practice For more information about this series, please visit: https://www.crcpress.com/Rehabilitation-Science-in-Practice-Series/book-series/CRCPRESERIN

Rehabilitation Engineering

Principles and Practice

Edited by
Alex Mihailidis and Roger Smith

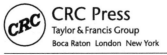

CRC Press
Taylor & Francis Group
Boca Raton London New York

CRC Press is an imprint of the
Taylor & Francis Group, an **informa** business

MATLAB® is a trademark of The MathWorks, Inc. and is used with permission. The MathWorks does not warrant the accuracy of the text or exercises in this book. This book's use or discussion of MATLAB® software or related products does not constitute endorsement or sponsorship by The MathWorks of a particular pedagogical approach or particular use of the MATLAB® software.

First edition published 2023
by CRC Press
6000 Broken Sound Parkway NW, Suite 300, Boca Raton, FL 33487-2742

and by CRC Press
4 Park Square, Milton Park, Abingdon, Oxon, OX14 4RN

CRC Press is an imprint of Taylor & Francis Group, LLC

ISBN: 978-1-138-19826-5 (hbk)
ISBN: 978-1-032-35482-8 (pbk)
ISBN: 978-1-315-27048-7 (ebk)

DOI: 10.1201/b21964

Typeset in Times
by Deanta Global Publishing Services, Chennai, India

Access the companion website: www.routledge.com/9781138198265

Contents

SECTION I   INTRODUCTION AND OVERVIEW

Contents _____

Contents _____

Preface

Rehabilitation engineering is an interdisciplinary specialty that relies on a thorough understanding of the human mind and body, technology, design principles, and technical design methods. Additionally, one key content area that makes this technical design field unique is its understanding of aging and disability.

Much like a human factors engineer or ergonomist, a rehabilitation engineering professional focuses on improving the functional interaction between the human being and technology. Much like a biomedical engineer, technology that helps a human improve their health, safety, function, and quality of life through life sciences is the goal. Much like core engineering specialties like electrical and electronics, mechanical, civil, industrial, and software engineering, the rehabilitation engineering professional must be technically competent. However, unique to this rehabilitation engineering specialty, the professional must also be able to effectively understand and relate to other rehabilitation professionals such as occupational and physical therapists, recreation therapists, speech language pathologists, social workers, psychologists, physiatrists, nurses, and educators.

A good rehabilitation engineering practitioner integrates these areas of skill and knowledge and participates as part of the rehabilitation, health, and educational team seamlessly and efficiently.

Rehabilitation engineering, however, is an elusive area of study and practice. It is relatively a young profession and area of study. Only a few universities have specific instructional programs specific to rehabilitation engineering practice. While there are many reasons for the sparse distribution of rehabilitation engineering training programs, three reasons jump out: (1) rehabilitation engineering practice is not directly funded by major third-party funding sources in healthcare or education; (2) in recent years, related specialty areas have emerged that have developed their own conferences and communities, which include specialties such as software accessibility and rehabilitation robotics; and (3) perhaps the main challenge of rehabilitation engineering education is that it is daunting. Because rehabilitation engineering depends heavily on so many underlying disciplines in the physical, biological, social, health, educational, and technical sciences, broad-based instruction is required. Coalescing a competent highly interdisciplinary instructional team is a challenge. This textbook has accepted this challenge and is intended to facilitate the education of the rehabilitation engineer.

The purpose of this textbook is to bridge the reader from their core technical training and closer to the specialty of rehabilitation engineering. As editors of this textbook, we think that this resource can serve as a core textbook in rehabilitation engineering elective courses in biomedical engineering and human factors programs, or even in architecture, art and design programs, or other design-oriented programs.

Rehabilitation engineering may be seen as an "add-on" to the design professions. Biomedical engineers, human factors engineers, architects, software developers, medical device designers, and health-related device inventors of all types will benefit from the information in this text.

The timing is right with the current emphasis on entrepreneurial programming throughout North America, Europe, Asia, and the rest of the world. As healthy aging is becoming more dominant worldwide, as the launch of the WHO assistive technology initiative in 2018 increases globally and entrepreneurial competition grows across nations and regions, the need for competent rehabilitation engineers becomes more pressing each day.

The chapters in this text prepare learners to understand the scope of rehabilitation engineering and the depth of the many specialties related to rehabilitation engineering. These chapters highlight the breadth of disability, the scope of functional areas rehabilitation engineers address, and the foundational underpinnings of rehabilitation and technology.

The chapters in the text can be read in order as the textbook was designed as a single document with a sequence of concepts. However, the chapters are not interdependent. Each is prepared to stand alone and can be taken as an individual treatise of its respective core content in rehabilitation engineering. The learning objectives of each chapter aim to orient the reader and the instructor. Additional readings are also available and listed with most chapters.

Importantly, the text not only teaches core concepts of accessibility and universal design but also serves as a model. Each of the more than 125 illustrations has accompanying equivalent text descriptions (EqTDs). These are for readers who use screen readers and cannot see illustrations as sighted people do, or for other readers who may be challenged to understand the content of an illustration. These

EqTDs have multiple levels of descriptions and exemplify how one modality of information is insufficient for readers that may bring an impairment or impairments to the reading task. Please note where the EqTDs are located that describe each illustration.

The editors of this textbook bring not only their interdisciplinary scholarly wisdom and rehabilitation and technology perspectives on practice through their engineering and rehabilitation work backgrounds, but they are also both past presidents of RESNA, the globally recognized Rehabilitation Engineering and Assistive Technology Society of North America. They tapped the extraordinary wisdom of some of their premier colleagues in assistive technology and engineering. We heartily thank each of them for helping to create a textbook to represent the field.

We would be remiss if we did not point out the key historical context of the release of this textbook. Globally, the World Health Organization launched a major assistive technology initiative in 2018 to bring technology and disability together— not just for highly resourced countries. Also, the manufacturing powerhouse of China launched the Belt and Road Initiative to address the technology supply for people with disabilities, starting with the large population of China and then globally. In 2019, assistive technology and rehabilitation organizations worldwide pulled together and created GAATO, the Global Alliance of Assistive Technology Organizations. These major international efforts indicate more robust attention to assistive technology and rehabilitation engineering for the future. We hope that this textbook can be part of the educational solution for bringing technology to all the people in the world who need it.

Alex Mihailidis, Ph.D., P.Eng, RESNA Fellow
Professor
Department of Occupational Science and Occupational Therapy
Barbara G. Stymiest Research Chair in Rehabilitation Technology – KITE
Research Institute and University of Toronto
Scientific Director of the AGE-WELL Network of Centres of Excellence
University of Toronto

Roger Smith, Ph.D., OT, FAOTA, RESNA Fellow
Professor
Programs in Occupational Therapy, Science, and Technology
Department of Rehabilitation Sciences and Technology
Director, Rehabilitation Research Design and Disability (R2D2) Center
University of Wisconsin-Milwaukee

MATLAB® is a registered trademark of The MathWorks, Inc. For product information, please contact:

The MathWorks, Inc.
3 Apple Hill Drive
Natick, MA 01760-2098 USA
Tel: 508 647 7000
Fax: 508-647-7001
E-mail: info@mathworks.com
Web: www.mathworks.com

Editors

Alex Mihailidis, Ph.D., P.Eng, is the Barbara G. Stymiest Research Chair in Rehabilitation Technology at the University of Toronto (U of T) and Toronto Rehabilitation Institute. He is also the Scientific Director for the AGE-WELL Network for Centres of Excellence, which focuses on the development of new technologies and services for older adults. He is an Associate Professor in the Department of Occupational Science and Occupational Therapy (U of T) and the Institute of Biomaterials and Biomedical Engineering (U of T), with a cross appointment in the Department of Computer Science (U of T). He has been conducting research in the field of pervasive computing and intelligent systems in health for the past 15 years. He has published over 150 journal papers, conference papers, and abstracts in the field. He is also highly active in the rehabilitation engineering profession, currently as Immediate Past-President for RESNA (Rehabilitation Engineering and Assistive Technology Society of North America). He was named a Fellow of RESNA in 2014.

Roger Smith, MD, Ph.D., is Director of the Rehabilitation Research Design and Disability Center at the University of Wisconsin-Milwaukee. His research has focused on the measurement of interventions for people with disabilities and populations of all ages, particularly in the domains and outcomes of assistive technologies and training and accessible environments. Dr. Smith has also taught courses at the graduate level in assistive technologies and rehabilitation.

Contributor biographies are included in the online supplementary material of this book.

Section I
Introduction and overview

Chapter 1 History of rehabilitation engineering

Gerald Weisman and
Gerry Dickerson

Contents

1.1 Chapter overview

The term "rehabilitation engineering" was first defined as "To improve the quality of life of the physically handicapped through a total approach to rehabilitation, combining medicine, engineering, and related sciences" (Reswick 2002, 11–16). "Assistive technology" is the product of rehabilitation engineering. First legally defined in 1988, (ATRC 2018) in the Technology-Related Assistance Act of 1988, "assistive technology device" means any item, piece of equipment, or product system, whether acquired commercially off the shelf, modified, or customized,

DOI: 10.1201/b21964-2

that is used to increase, maintain, or improve functional capabilities of individuals with disabilities."

Assistive technology distinguishes us from the rest of the animal kingdom. It is one factor that makes us uniquely human. There are several obvious anatomical differences between us and other mammals, such as our large brain and our unusual ability to walk on our hind legs, freeing our forelimbs to develop a high degree of manipulative ability. The most apparent product of our brains and hands is technology. While the technology of our ancestors changed very little for more than two million years, there has been tremendous growth during the last 200 thousand years. Technology, in modern terms, is only a few hundred years old. The growth of technology is consistent with the growth of scientific discoveries. Humans have created assistive technology to feed themselves, to provide shelter, to get around, to communicate with one another, and to find recreation in the world around them. Assistive technology has extended the abilities of humans in all these pursuits, and new technologies continue to expand our abilities, opportunities, and horizons.

There is no difference between these uses of assistive technology and its use by people with disabilities. In either case, technology extends abilities and allows people to accomplish what they would not otherwise be able to do. We could not fly without airplanes, and someone with quadriplegia couldn't go down the road without a wheelchair. Telephones allow us to speak to people halfway around the world, while a telecommunications device for the deaf (TDD) enables a person who is deaf or hearing-impaired to use the telephone. Tractors and plows enable a farmer to till 40 acres in a single day and if that farmer is paraplegic a lift will allow them to get onto the tractor.

This chapter will explore the history of the field of rehabilitation engineering and the fruits of those efforts in the development of assistive technology devices. The earliest examples of devices to aid in the independence of people with disabilities and functional limitations will be explored, as well as the evolution of these devices. Many devices and technologies first developed for use by people with disabilities have evolved to become mainstream consumer products. Conversely, many consumer goods have become important assistive technologies for people with functional limitations.

The social and environmental factors that have contributed to the development and growth of the field will be identified. The professionalism of the field, and the political and legal frameworks that have contributed to building the field, will be explored.

1.1.1 History of engineering

Necessity is the mother of invention is a well-known proverb that best describes the fundamental nature of engineering. The practice of engineering originated in ancient times. The history of engineering has been described as composed of four eras by Auyang (2006):

- **Prescientific revolution:** The prehistory of modern engineering features ancient master builders and Renaissance engineers such as Leonardo da Vinci.
- **Industrial revolution:** From the 18th through early 19th century, civil and mechanical engineers changed from practical artists to scientific professionals.
- **Second industrial revolution:** In the century before World War II, chemical, electrical, and other science-based engineering branches developed electricity, telecommunications, cars, airplanes, and mass production.
- **Information revolution:** As engineering science matured after the war, microelectronics, computers, and telecommunications jointly produced information technology.

The origin of the word "engineering" comes from medieval Latin ingeniator, from ingeniare, to "contrive, devise" and "engine" from Latin ingenium "talent, device." The engineer thus creates new and clever devices. Imhotep, the engineer and architect of the Pyramid of Djoser, a step pyramid at Saqqara in Egypt during the time period of 2630–2611 BC, is considered one of the first engineers.

At the time, and before the industrial revolution, engineering was primarily a craft in which trial and error was the predominant practice. While some recording of practice took place, it was not until the Renaissance that technical drawings became common. The notebooks of Leonardo da Vinci are excellent examples of the recording of his inventions.

The Industrial Revolution, from the 18th through the early 19th centuries, brought the adoption of the scientific approach to solving practical problems and designing products. Universities were established to teach the new scientific methods augmenting and replacing the traditional apprenticeship. Information about new inventions and practices was more readily available and more widely shared through publications and professional organizations.

Engineering also benefited from the creation of a method to record the development and design of inventions. Gaspard Monge of Mezieres (En.wikipedia. org 2018b) invented descriptive geometry and thus created a way to represent three-dimensional objects in two dimensions. He developed his orthographic projection drawing techniques while working as a draftsman for French military fortifications around 1765. Because his work involved military fortifications, it was kept secret until 1794. Technical drawing was further advanced around 1799 by Marc Isambard Brunel (En.wikipedia.org 2018d). Brunel designed and developed metal machines to mass produce blocks or pulleys for the British navy. While the processes for mass producing the blocks were a significant contribution to the practice of engineering, his greater contribution was the development of the drawings of the machines.

Technology and the practice of engineering progressed from the Industrial Revolution through the Second Industrial Revolution and most recently through the Information Revolution. The development and use of electricity and mass production characterized the Second Industrial Revolution. Advances in physics and chemistry spurred the growth of electrical and chemical engineering. Engineering schools and curricula became well established and graduate programs were created. World War II and the subsequent Cold War and Space Race created an environment where research and development expanded, creating all kinds of new technologies and thus establishing the Information Revolution. Graduate engineering schools became well established (Creatingtechnology.org 2018).

1.1.2 Biomedical engineering

Biomedical engineering has been an interdisciplinary activity among the medical, biological, and engineering fields for hundreds of years. It was not until the 1960s that biomedical engineering became a field in its own right. The Biomedical Engineering Society was incorporated in 1968 and had 171 founding members. By 2018, the society had more than 7000 members.

According to the Biomedical Engineering Society (Bmes.org 2018), "A biomedical engineer uses traditional engineering expertise to analyze and solve problems in biology and medicine providing an overall enhancement of health care."

The field of biomedical engineering has grown significantly since the 1960s. Many engineering disciplines have become involved with biomedical technology. Figure 1.1 illustrates the many specialties that have come to define the breadth of biomedical engineering (Enderle and Bronzino 2012).

Figure 1.2 illustrates a classification of engineering in medicine presented by James B. Reswick (The University of Tennessee, Knoxville 1977).

Reswick describes the "bioengineer" as someone who is typically trained to teach, perform, and lead research in the medical and biological fields emphasizing the engineering aspects. Except in the context of the research being performed, the bioengineer is rarely concerned with the direct care of patients. According to Reswick, the medical engineer applies "engineering in a direct way which improves patient care in the long run and often is directed to the specific problem of a particular patient." The medical engineer works closely with physicians and other medical and healthcare professionals. The clinical engineer focuses primarily on the equipment and technology used for therapy and diagnosis in the healthcare environment.

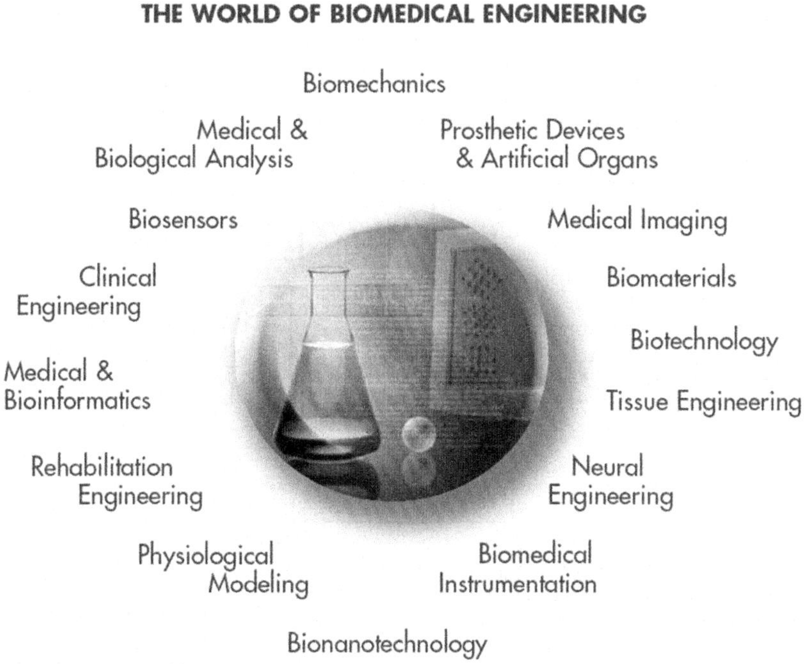

THE WORLD OF BIOMEDICAL ENGINEERING

Biomechanics

Medical & Biological Analysis

Prosthetic Devices & Artificial Organs

Biosensors

Medical Imaging

Clinical Engineering

Biomaterials

Biotechnology

Medical & Bioinformatics

Tissue Engineering

Rehabilitation Engineering

Neural Engineering

Physiological Modeling

Biomedical Instrumentation

Bionanotechnology

Figure 1.1 The world of biomedical engineering (after Enderle and Bronzino 2012).

It was primarily in the 1960s that the problems of medical technology causing injuries to patients were identified as an issue to be addressed. Of particular concern was the electrical safety of patients in hospitals. Activists such as Ralph Nader raised the issue of patient safety. Nader stated, "at least 1,200 Americans are electrocuted annually during routine diagnostic and therapeutic procedures" (Nader 1971, 98). Questions of legal rights and responsibilities were raised if a hospital patient was injured as a result of equipment failure. Which healthcare professional should bear the responsibility—the physician, the nurse, or the clinical engineer? Issues of training in the use of sophisticated medical equipment were also raised.

The issues around medical technology and equipment led to the development of certification programs for clinical engineers. The Association for the Advancement of Medical Instrumentation (AAMI) formed the International Certification Commission for Clinical Engineers. The first certifications for clinical engineers were awarded at the AAMI meeting in Atlanta in 1976. The certification process has gone through a number of changes over the years since. The AAMI suspended its program in 1999. Starting in 2002, clinical engineers can be certified under the Clinical Engineering Certification under

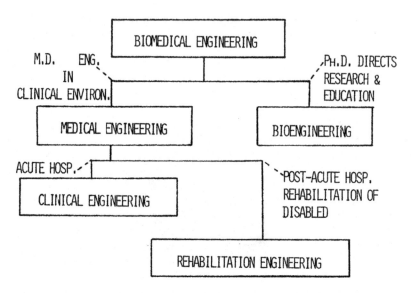

Figure 1.2 Engineering in medicine classification (after Reswick, The University of Tennessee, Knoxville 1977).

the sponsorship of the American College of Clinical Engineering under the administration of the Healthcare Technology Certification Commission and the United States and Canadian Board of Examiners for Certification in Clinical Engineering.

Reswick (The University of Tennessee, Knoxville 1977) goes on to describe the rehabilitation engineer as, "involved with patients on a continuing and active basis. He is concerned both with the development of new devices and the advancement of science as it relates to the rehabilitation of disabled persons." It is important to note Reswick's description is primarily concerned with those working within a medical model. However, his description also applies to those rehabilitation engineers working in various other models, i.e., vocational or independent living.

1.2 Assistive technology

The development of devices to aid people with disabilities is clearly one of the results of rehabilitation engineering practice. Assistive technology devices have been made since ancient times. The simplest and oldest assistive technologies are the walking stick and under-arm crutch. Illustrations of such devices appear in Egyptian hieroglyphs as early as 3000 BC.

1.2.1 Prosthetics

Prostheses are devices used to primarily replace missing or non-functional body parts. The earliest known prosthesis is suspected to be an artificial toe made of wood and leather found on an Egyptian mummy (Figure 1.3). Found on a mummy of a 50–60-year-old woman in 2000 near the ancient city of Thebes, the prosthesis dates from 950–710 BC. While the Egyptians were known to replace certain body parts of corpses in order to make them viable in the afterlife, a biomechanical study by Finch et al. (2012) suggests the toe prosthesis was probably functional during the woman's life.

An artificial lower leg, known as the "Roman Capua Leg" was found in a grave attached to a skeleton in Capua, Italy. The prosthesis was made of bronze and is dated to 300 BC (Broughttolife.sciencemuseum.org.uk 2018).

German mercenary knight Götz von Berlichingen was known as a Robin Hood in 16th-century Bavaria. It was during a battle around 1504 that a cannonball took Berlichingen's hand. He commissioned an artist to fabricate an iron hand. The iron prostheses (Figure 1.4) sported hinged fingers to enable Berlichingen to continue battling with his sword (Atlas Obscura 2018).

Modern amputation surgery and prosthetics probably began with Ambroise Paré, a French army barber/surgeon. He advanced the techniques of amputation and prosthetics. His contributions to prosthetics include "an above-knee device that was a kneeling peg leg and foot prosthesis that had a fixed position, adjustable harness, knee lock control and other engineering features that are used in today's devices" (Amputee-coalition.org 2018).

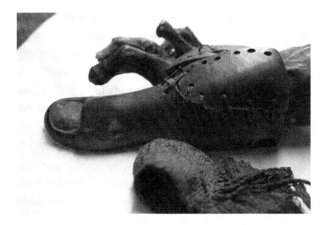

Figure 1.3 Egyptian toe (Choi, 2007).

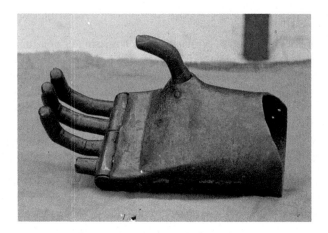

Figure 1.4 Iron hand prostheses (Atlas Obscura, 2018).

The first non-locking below-knee prosthesis was introduced in 1696 by Pieter Andriaanszoon Verduyn (Figure 1.5), which allowed for knee movement (Nya mcenterforhistory.org 2018).

Upper-limb prosthetics were significantly advanced by Peter Baliff in 1818 when he invented a prosthesis that was powered by the user's opposite shoulder (Figure 1.6). Through a series of leather straps, the device enabled the user to power and control the fingers of the prosthesis. Powered prostheses continued to evolve with electric motors and control mechanisms using myoelectric signals (Zuo and Olson 2014).

Advances in prosthetics, particularly lower-limb prosthetics, followed advances in the surgical techniques of amputation. Gaseous anesthesia developed in the 1840s enabled doctors to perform longer and more detailed amputation surgeries, allowing for better preparation of the stump for interfacing with the prostheses (Garden 2018).

Upper- and lower-limb prosthetics continued to advance, particularly in response to the needs of soldiers disabled through wars in the 19th and 20th centuries. The latest developments in lower-extremity prosthetics include inventions by amputees themselves. The Cheetah Flex-Foot was developed by Van Phillips in 1984 after a waterskiing accident. The Cheetah Flex-Foot is a radical design that provides flexibility and the ability to store energy. The prosthesis (Figure 1.7) has become a favorite of athletes (Vlaskamp, Soede, and Gelderblom 2011). Hugh Herr, a double amputee, developed the first commercially available prosthetic foot to mimic the function of the real human foot. According to the Medical Center Orthotics and Prosthetics website, the distributor of the iWalk BiOM (Figure 1.8),

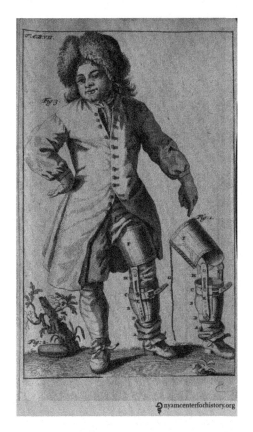

Figure 1.5 Verduyn prosthesis (Nyamcenterforhistory.org 2018).

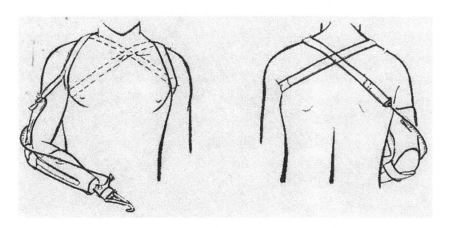

Figure 1.6 Body-powered prosthesis (Upperlimbprosthetics.info 2018).

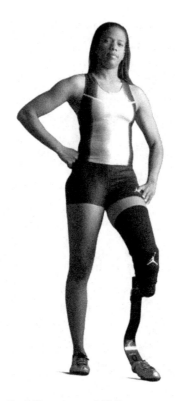

Figure 1.7 Cheetah Flex-Foot (Ossur.com 2018).

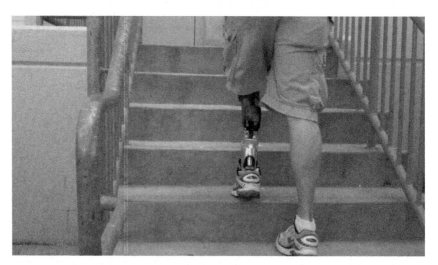

Figure 1.8 iWalk BiOM (Business Insider 2018).

By using robotics to replicate the calf muscles and Achilles tendon, the iWalk BiOM feels and functions like no other foot/ankle prosthesis. With each step, the iWalk BiOM provides a powered push-off which propels the wearer forward. It is the only prosthesis in the world that does not depend on the wearer's energy. With the iWalk BiOM, users will experience natural walking mechanics and increased stability, mobility, and confidence.

(MCOP Prosthetics 2018)

1.2.2 Technology for vision impairments

Eyeglasses, specifically reading glasses, first appeared in Italy between 1268 and 1300 AD. According to the Zenni Optical website (Surrence 2013),

The first illustrations of someone wearing this style of eyeglasses are in a series of mid-14th-century paintings by Tommaso da Modena, who featured monks using monocles and wearing these early pince-nez (French for "pinch nose") style eyeglasses to read and copy manuscripts.

Before personal computers became available, typewriters were ubiquitous. The typewriter was one of the first examples of advances in technology first inspired by the needs of people with disabilities that ultimately became generally useful and available to the general population. Pellegrino Turri built the first typewriter around 1808 in order to help his blind friend, Countess Carolina Fantoni da Fivizzono, to write legibly.

In response to a request by Napoleon for a code that soldiers could use to communicate silently and without light, Army Captain Charles Barbier de la Sierra developed a system, known as "night writing," that used 12 raised dots (Vlaskamp, Soede, and Gelderblom 2011). Barbier taught his system to blind students at the Royal Institution for Blind Youth in Paris, France. One of those students, Louis Braille, was interested in the method. Braille, born January 4, 1809, was blinded by an accident in his father's shop in 1812. He was 10 years old when he met Barbier and then modified the code by reducing the number of dots to six. Braille published his first book in Braille in 1829. An example of a Braille page is presented in Figure 1.9.

Braille's system of writing required a slate and stylus to punch holes in the paper in order to raise the dots. The writer punches each dot one at a time. Needless to say, this process was slow and inefficient. The first successful mechanical Braille writer was invented by Frank H. Hall, the superintendent of the Illinois Institution for the Education of the Blind (see Figure 1.10). From a Brief History of the Illinois Institution for the Education of the Blind 1849–1893:

Under the direction of the Superintendent, a machine for writing Braille has been constructed by which a pupil can write many times as fast as he could write with a "stylus and tablet," with the further advantage of having what he has written in a convenient position to be read. With these machines, the pupils solve their problems in algebra and write their letters and school exercises.

(Antiquetypewriters 2018)

While Braille significantly increased the literacy of blind individuals, those with visual impairments are challenged by printed materials. Samuel Genensky became visually impaired soon after birth. He was determined to live his life as

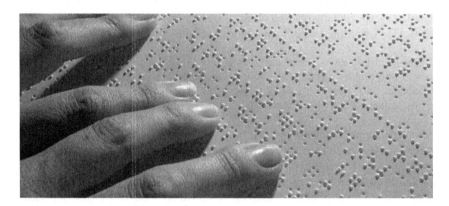

Figure 1.9 Braille page (Blind Foundation 2018).

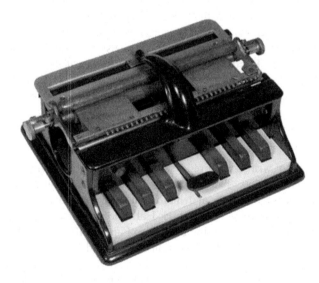

Figure 1.10 Hall Braille writer (Antiquetypewriters.com 2018).

a partially sighted person and not as a blind person. While at Perkins School for the Blind,

> one teacher told him, "Why don't you act like a well-behaved blind child?" to which he replied, "Because I am not blind." He remarked later that this retort had significant importance in his life because by it he permanently placed himself in the camp of the sighted and not in the camp of the blind, and at that point, he determined to make it in life "using everything [he] had going for [him] including [his] none-too impressive residual vision."

(En.wikipedia.org 2018e)

While working at the RAND corporation in 1968, Genensky and colleague Paul Baran developed the first practical and user-friendly closed-circuit TV (CCTV) magnifier system (see Figure 1.11) (Vlaskamp, Soede, and Gelderblom 2011).

Reading printed materials by blind and visually impaired people was significantly advanced by Ray Kurzweil who invented the first machine to read printed material using computer-generated speech in 1977. The Kurzweil reading machine was revolutionary in advancing three new technologies that have since become commonplace. The machine included "omni-font character recognition (OCR), the CCD (Charge Coupled Device) flat-bed scanner, and text-to-speech synthesis" (Figure 1.12) (Vlaskamp, Soede, and Gelderblom 2011).

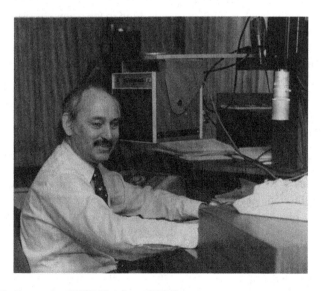

Figure 1.11 Genensky CCTV (Cclvi.org 2018).

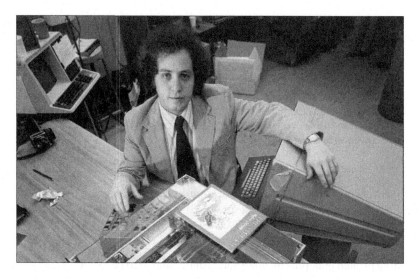

Figure 1.12 Kurzweil reading machine (https://www.gettyimages.com/detail/news-photo/raymond-kurzweil-of-cambridge-massachusetts-is-shown-with-news-photo/515406792?#raymond-kurzweil-of-cambridge-massachusetts-is-shown-with-the-he-picture-id515406792).

1.2.3 Technology for hearing impairments

Assistive technology for the hearing-impaired began in the 13th century with animal horns being used to amplify sounds. Man-made trumpets, primarily made from tin, were first developed in the 17th century. While Alexander Graham Bell is best known for inventing the telephone, it was his interest in helping deaf and hearing-impaired people that contributed significantly to the development of assistive technology. Bell's mother was profoundly deaf, and Bell was a teacher of the deaf in Boston. In 1874, Bell began to formulate the design of his device. He stated, "If I could make a current of electricity vary in intensity precisely as the air varies in density during the production of sound, I should be able to transmit speech telegraphically" (Bell 2018). He hoped this device would help people with hearing impairments to speak. His telephone was patented in 1876 and 1877.

Vacuum tubes used in the fabrication of microphones and amplifiers contributed to the development of wearable hearing aids. Probably the earliest wearable vacuum tube hearing aid made in the United States was Arthur Wengel's "Stanleyphone," available in 1937 and 1938 (Sandlin 2000). The Aurex hearing aid (Figure 1.13) developed by Walter Huth was the first to use American-made vacuum tubes. Around 1952, hearing aids became smaller and more energy efficient with the advent of the transistor. The microelectronic/digital era, beginning in the late 1960s, resulted in size reductions and the increased performance of

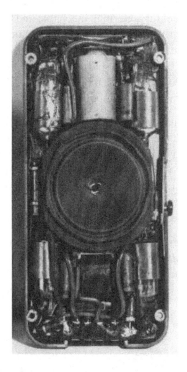

Figure 1.13 Aurex vacuum tube hearing aid (Sandlin, 2000).

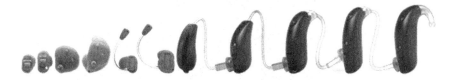

Figure 1.14 Belltone hearing aids (Beltone.com 2018).

hearing aids. Starting around 1988, the programming of hearing aids became available, making the device better tuned to the specific audiogram of the user (Sandlin 2000) (Figure 1.14).

1.2.4 Technology for mobility impairments

For those people with mobility impairments, wheeled chairs became a solution for transporting the individual and ultimately for the person to have independent mobility. Wheeled furniture and wheeled carts, common in the 4th and 5th centuries BC, were used for people with disabilities. Self-propelled chairs were first reported in the 17th century. German mechanic and inventor Johann Hautsch made rolling chairs in Nürnberg (Encyclopedia Britannica 2018). Wheelchair use became prominent in the United States after the Civil War, when chairs were typically made of wood (Figure 1.15). In fact, the first US patent for a wheelchair was awarded to Sarah Potter on December 25, 1894. The wooden chair had a fixed frame, and push-rims for self-propulsion.

The modern era of manual wheelchairs began in 1932 when mechanical engineer Harry Jennings built the first tubular steel wheelchair for his disabled friend Herbert Everest (Figure 1.16). The wheelchair was capable of folding by using a cross frame. The folding wheelchair was capable of being transported in a vehicle, making the outside community more readily available to the person with a disability. They founded the Everest & Jennings (E&J) wheelchair company, which dominated the wheelchair market through the 1980s.

The typical E&J steel manual wheelchair weighed approximately 55 pounds. Modifications to these wheelchairs, particularly for sports, e.g., wheelchair basketball, generally involved reducing weight and modifying the wheels by mounting them at an angle and installing wheel guards to protect the spokes.

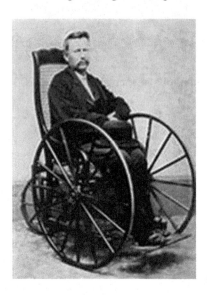

Figure 1.15 Civil War wheelchair (https://www.bing.com/images/search?view =detailV2&ccid=suMAcA5L&id=9FDAAA26E2BB497B1E7B91F35C797E4 CD3374DD0&thid=OIP.suMAcA5LFmZ9jFrGUIxCmwHaKO&mediaurl=https %3a%2f%2fs-media-cache-ak0.pinimg.com%2f236x%2f12%2ff1%2f70%2f1 2f170412a810cb02ad4d9064e56c840.jpg&exph=276&expw=200&q=Old +Wheelchairs+From+the+1800&simid=608018877235528118&selectedIndex =15&ajaxhist=0).

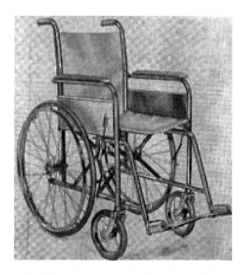

Figure 1.16 E&J 1932 wheelchair.

The wheelchair was revolutionized with the introduction of the Quickie wheelchair in 1979. Marilyn Hamilton was an avid hang glider enthusiast when in 1978 an accident left her with paraplegia. Using her knowledge of hang-gliding technology Hamilton, along with Jim Okamoto and Don Helsman, created an ultralightweight wheelchair. Their chair featured adjustability, high performance, and bolt-on accessories (Marilynhamilton.com 2018). At a time when almost all wheelchairs were manufactured with chrome-plated steel, the Quickie significantly changed the aesthetics of wheelchairs by introducing colors to their materials (Figure 1.17).

In response to a request from Canadian World War II disabled veteran, John Counsell, the Canadian National Research Council (NRC) created a project to create the first electric wheelchair to be mass produced. George Klein, a mechanical engineer at the NRC, developed an electric wheelchair with "a unique package of technologies including the joystick, tighter turning systems and separate wheel drives that are still features of electric wheelchairs today" (U of T Engineering News 2018). Klein and the NRC shared the design of the wheelchair, patent free, with manufacturers in order to facilitate the manufacture and distribution of the wheelchair. Klein was a pioneer in what has come to be known as participatory action research, wherein consumers and end-users of the technology are collaborators in the process of its development.

Electric or powered wheelchairs evolved with the separation of the drive components and the seating systems first developed by Fortress in the early 1980s (Figure 1.18).

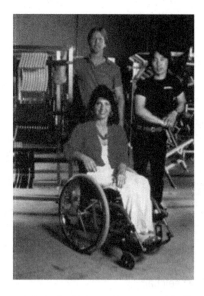

Figure 1.17 Hamilton and Quickie (Stimdesigns.com 2018).

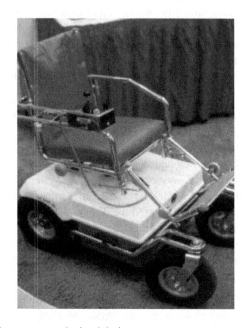

Figure 1.18 Fortress-powered wheelchair.

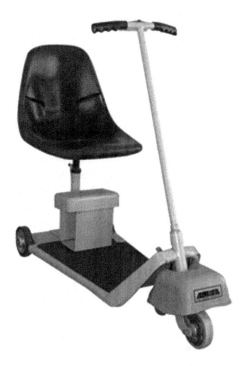

Figure 1.19 Amigo mobility scooter (Myamigo.com 2018).

The form factor of the powered wheelchair changed with the design and development of the mobility scooter by Allan Thieme. Thieme, a plumber, invented the first mobility scooter in 1968 for a family member with mobility impairments due to multiple sclerosis. The "Amigo," or "friendly wheelchair" became the first product of Amigo Mobility International, Inc. in Bridgeport, Michigan, and the beginnings of the "scooter" industry (Figure 1.19).

1.2.5 Technology for communication impairments

Communication is a fundamental and critical human need. Augmentative and alternative communication (AAC) technology meets the needs of people with disabilities with communication impairments. Simple language boards with displays of pictures, icons, or traditional orthography serve as an effective means of communication. Communication technology and language boards in particular were advanced with the use of Bliss Symbols. Charles Bliss, a survivor of Dachau and Buchenwald concentration camps became a refugee in Shanghai and Sydney from 1942 to 1949. Inspired by Chinese characters, he "wanted to create an easy-to-learn international auxiliary language to allow communication between different linguistic communities" (En.wikipedia.org 2018a). Bliss Symbols "consists of several hundred basic symbols, each representing a concept, which can be composed together to generate new symbols" and concepts (Vlaskamp, Soede, and Gelderblom 2011). The application of Bliss Symbols (Figure 1.20) to augmentative communication was pioneered by Shirley McNaughton in 1971 at the Ontario Crippled Children's Centre, Ontario, Canada (now Holland Bloorview Kids Rehabilitation Hospital).

It was at about the same time, in 1971, that AAC systems progressed from simple language boards to electronic devices. Rick Foulds, a student at Tufts University in Massachusetts, and Gregg Vanderheiden at the University of Wisconsin developed electronic communication devices to respond to the needs of children with communication limitations. Foulds developed the Tufts Interactive Communicator (TIC; Figure 1.21), a device that used scanning input to display letters on a screen and on a printer. The letters on the TIC were arranged in order of frequency of use, so the most frequently used letters could be selected in the least amount of time. Subsequent devices incorporated letter prediction by dynamically changing the display of letters to be scanned. The Auto Monitoring Communication Board (AutoCom; Figure 1.22) was a direct selection device developed by Vanderheiden at the Trace Center at the University of Wisconsin. The AutoCom was a user-programmable device, where the user could develop their own vocabulary. The AutoCom was commercialized by Telesensory Systems and the Prentke Romich Company (Vanderheiden 2003).

Notable augmentative communication devices developed and available in the 1970s include the Handivoice (Figure 1.23) and the Canon Communicator (Figure 1.24). The Canon Communicator was a small portable device that was printed out on a small paper tape. It was notable for being the first device developed and commercialized by a major manufacturer. The Handivoice was one of the first available devices that utilized computer-generated speech (Vanderheiden 2003).

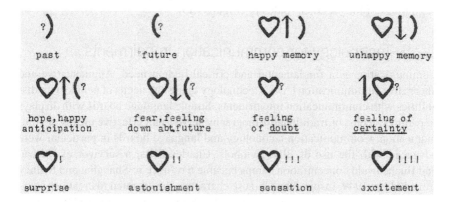

Figure 1.20 Bliss Symbols (Idsgn.org 2018).

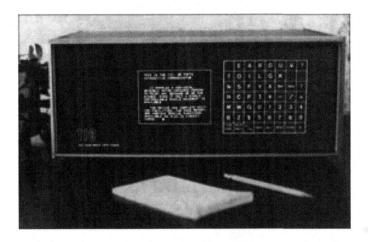

Figure 1.21 Tufts Interactive Communicator (TIC) (Rehab.research.va.gov 2018).

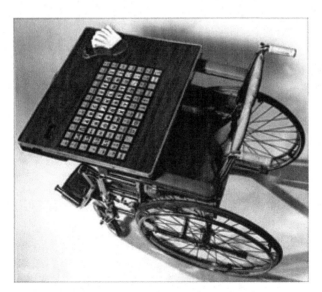

Figure 1.22 Auto monitoring communication board (AutoCom) (Rehab.research.va. gov 2018).

1.2.6 Computer technology

The introduction of the Apple II personal computer (see Figure 1.25) to the world by Steve Wozniak and Steve Jobs in 1977 promised a level playing field for people with disabilities. People with disabilities would have the ability to use the computer to compensate for functional limitations in communication and

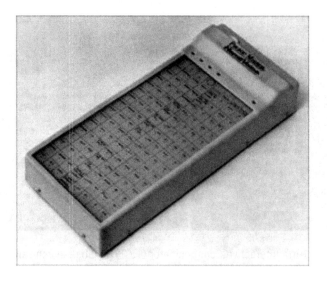

Figure 1.23 Handivoice (Rehab.research.va.gov 2018).

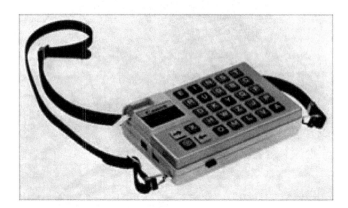

Figure 1.24 Canon Communicator (Rehab.research.va.gov 2018).

access to tools that would enhance their productivity. While the graphic display and user-friendly design of the Apple II were touted as a revolution in computer design, it also presented challenges to people with certain functional limitations. Specialized programs were being developed for people with disabilities to run on the Apple II. Many of these programs could be accessed by adaptive control systems, i.e., scanning, coding, etc. However, people with disabilities could not access the standard programs being used to increase productivity, such as word processors and Visicalc, an interactive visible calculator. Unlike present-day

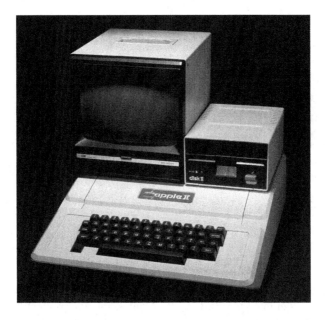

Figure 1.25 Apple II computer (http://americanhistory.si.edu/collections/search/object/nmah_334638).

computers, the Apple II computer could only run one program at a time. Access to the Apple II took a significant leap with the introduction of the adaptive firmware card (AFC) (Figure 1.26) by Paul Schwejda and Judy McDonald. The AFC enabled transparent access to the computer. It was a keyboard emulator that generated text as if it was coming from the keyboard with one or two switches. The AFC could be accessed by scanning or coded input (e.g., Morse Code). Schwejda and Vanderheiden published an article in *Byte* magazine in September 1982 (Schwejda and Vanderheiden 1982) describing the AFC, including all the technical details of the AFC and a schematic.

1.3 The beginning of modern rehabilitation engineering

The development of assistive technologies and devices for people with disabilities have mostly come as a result of disease, injury, and warfare. Ancient and medieval societies saw disabilities as a consequence of hunting and war, and in some cases, occupational accidents. Through the middle of the 20th century, disabled soldiers were primarily as a result of amputations. The US Civil War between the Union northern states and the southern Confederate states produced as many as 30,000 amputations on the Union side alone. James Edward Hanger, a Confederate soldier, became the first amputee of the Civil War when a cannonball

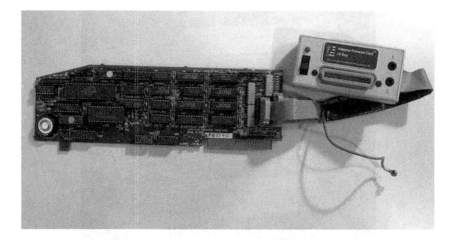

Figure 1.26 Adaptive Firmware Card

tore through his leg at the Battle of Philippi. In 1861, Hanger fashioned an artificial leg and was granted patents from the Confederate government. He was later granted a US patent in 1891. The prosthetics company Hanger started in 1861 is now a US$1 Billion+ company providing prosthetics and orthotics around the world (Hanger.com 2018).

Amputations continued to be a predominant cause of disability in warfare through World War II. The development of penicillin by Alexander Fleming in 1928 significantly increased the survivability of battlefield injuries, particularly amputations (American Chemical Society 2018). In 1945, at about the same time the Battle of the Bulge was being waged in the Ardennes, Surgeon General Norman T. Kirk, an orthopedic surgeon, asked the United States National Research Council of the National Academy of Sciences to convene of meeting of experts at Northwestern University in Chicago with the aim of recommending the best artificial limbs for veterans. The attendees of the meeting included doctors, engineers, and prosthetists. The consensus of those in attendance was that the design of prosthetics required further research and development. Dudley Childress described this meeting as the beginning of modern research on prosthetics and the beginnings of the field of rehabilitation engineering (Childress 2003). Soon after the meeting a Committee on Prosthetic Devices was formed under the National Research Council. The Committee ultimately evolved into the Committee on Prosthetics Research and Development (CPRD) initially directed by Brig. General F. S. Strong Jr and ultimately by A. Bennet Wilson Jr (Childress 2003). According to Hays (2010), "NRC committees reviewed proposals for contracts in support of prosthetics research, held meetings to review state-of-the-art prosthetics and advise on new directions, and interacted directly with contractors." Funds supporting contracts came from the Office of Scientific Research and Development (OSRD) and the War Department from 1945 to 1947; after that, the US Veterans' Administration (VA, now known as the Department of Veterans Affairs) provided the funding. Public Law 729, 80th Congress, June 19, 1948, formally authorized VA research in the fields of prosthetics and sensory devices and provided a budget of US$1 million per year. The law required VA to "make available the results of such research so as to benefit all disabled people." The budget remained flat until 1962, when the US$1 million funding ceiling was lifted by Public Law 87–572, which authorized "such funds as were necessary" for the program.

Soon after the passage of Public Law 729 and the initial funding of research for prosthetics and sensory aids, the VA created the Prosthetics and Sensory Aids Service. The Service, based at the VA Central Office in Washington, DC, administered contracts for research as well as intramural research. Augustus Thorndike was the initial director, followed in 1955, by Robert E. Stewart who served as director until 1973.

Stewart directed the establishment of the VA Prosthetics Center (VAPC) in 1956. The VAPC combined clinical services and research in prosthetics and sensory aids. At the time, Eugene Murphy was Assistant Director of Research operating out of the VA Regional Office in New York. Murphy supervised the intramural research program at the VAPC and was responsible for coordinating the contract research program. Anthony Staros soon became the director of the VAPC. As described by Hays (2010),

> While the VAPC carried out a variety of practical projects, primarily to improve upper and lower limb prostheses, it became increasingly involved in the evaluation of devices developed by others. It established a network of VA Prosthetics Service units at VA hospitals willing and able to evaluate new devices. In some cases, when the new device was clearly beneficial, it would be adopted in VA for general clinical use. The VAPC also played an active role in prosthetics education.

Disease was a major contributor to the development of assistive technology devices and rehabilitation engineering. Poliomyelitis (polio) infections were known as far back as ancient times. However, it was the outbreak of 1952, the worst in the history of the United States, that contributed most significantly to the development of rehabilitation engineering. There were approximately 57,628 cases of polio reported, of which 3145 died and 21,269 were left with mild to disabling paralysis (En.wikipedia.org 2018c). The vaccine developed by Jonas Salk in 1955 and modified to an oral vaccine by Albert Sabin put an end to the polio epidemic. Many people who survived polio in the 1950s matured to become strong advocates and were at the leading edge of the disability rights and universal design movements of the late 1960s and 1970s.

The late 1950s and early 1960s saw another outbreak of disabling conditions caused by the use of thalidomide. Prescribed primarily as a sedative or hypnotic, thalidomide was also prescribed to pregnant women to combat nausea and morning sickness. The drug caused malformations of the eyes, ears, and deafness, defects of the heart and kidneys, and most significantly, phocomelia (malformation of the limbs) in the unborn children of the pregnant women. There were approximately 10,000 cases of phocomelia throughout the world. Only 50% of the children survived, mostly in Europe and Canada. The US Food and Drug Administration (FDA) refused to approve the drug, thus limiting the impact in the United States (En.wikipedia.org 2018f). Canada responded to the needs of the children affected by thalidomide by creating centers that would provide technology to meet the needs of the children affected by thalidomide. These centers included:

- Manitoba Rehabilitation Hospital, Winnipeg, Manitoba.
- Ontario Crippled Children's Centre (now called the Holland Bloorview Kids Rehabilitation Hospital), Toronto, Ontario.
- Rehabilitation Institute of Montreal, Montreal, Quebec.

These centers recruited teams of prosthetists, orthotists, and technicians to provide clinical services and conduct research and development. Engineers were recruited to lead the research and development activities at these centers, including James Foorte, Colin McLaurin, and Andre Lippay respectively. The centers contributed to the development of assistive technologies by creating new prostheses, seating systems, and manual and powered mobility devices (Hobson 2002).

The CPRD, as described above, coordinated projects researching prosthetics and sensory aids throughout the 1960s. In a report entitled "Rehabilitation Engineering: A Plan for Continued Progress," published in 1971 the CPRD listed research the committee was coordinating along with other projects in sensory aids totaling 103 projects. The term "rehabilitation engineering" was first identified in this report. The preface of the report stated:

> In 1966, at the request of the then Vocational Rehabilitation Administration, CPRD developed a set of recommendations for research in orthotics and prosthetics for the next five-year period or so. This report seems to have been useful to the sponsors of research and to those planning work during the past four years. Most of the recommendations made in the report have been acted upon. Thus, it seems appropriate at this time to develop a new set of recommendations for the next five to ten years. Sensory aids for the blind and deaf are included as a logical extension to prosthetics and orthotics, and, with the addition of structural internal prostheses, the whole area can be known as rehabilitation engineering.

The CPRD was chaired at the time by Colin McLaurin with A. Bennet Wilson acting as the Executive Director.

It was in this 1971 report the CPRD determined their program and the field had matured to such a degree that "certain centers of excellence could and should be established to carry out integrated programs of research, development, evaluation, and education in rehabilitation engineering" (National Research Council (US) Committee on Prosthetics Research and Development and National Academy 1971). Their recommendation for centers included having "strong teaching affiliations with medical and engineering schools and have available a substantial patient load." They suggested,

> At least half-a-dozen rehabilitation engineering centers are needed in the near future and they probably should be spread across the country on some sort of a geographical basis. The objectives of rehabilitation engineering centers should be:
>
> 1. To improve the quality of life of the physically handicapped through a total approach to rehabilitation, combining medicine, engineering, and related science. (This thus becomes the first definition of the term "rehabilitation engineering.")
> 2. To perform research and development in pioneering areas wherein a center has developed unique capabilities.
> 3. To collaborate with laboratories and industry to carry new devices and techniques through all phases of research, development, and clinical evaluation to active production and patient use.
> 4. To make available new devices and techniques to all patients referred to the center.
> 5. To educate others to provide these devices and techniques to patients throughout the nation.
> 6. To cooperate with other centers in fitting and evaluating their developments whenever the need is indicated.
> 7. To provide an environment for education of physicians, engineers, and other technical persons in related life and physical sciences.
> 8. To communicate effectively with other centers through recognized means and cooperative effort.

Soon after this report was released, the US Department of Health, Education, and Welfare funded the first two Rehabilitation Engineering Centers in 1971. The two centers were at Rancho Los Amigos Medical Center in Downey, California, and Moss Rehabilitation Hospital in Philadelphia, Pennsylvania. Three more centers were established the following year at Texas Institute for Rehabilitation and Research in Houston, Texas, Northwestern University and the Rehabilitation Institute of Chicago in Chicago, Illinois, and Children's Hospital Center in Boston, Massachusetts (Hobson 2002).

The passage of the Rehabilitation Act of 1973 (PL93–112) was a watershed moment for the civil rights of people with disabilities in the United States, as well as the advancement of rehabilitation engineering. Section 504 of the Rehabilitation Act was the first time the law extended civil rights to people with disabilities. It prohibited discrimination against people with disabilities in programs that were funded by the federal government. The law became a model for the Americans with Disabilities Act passed in 1990.

The Rehabilitation Act of 1973 also contributed significantly to ensuring electronic and information technology would be accessible and useable by people with disabilities. Instead of simply regulating the design of the technology, the law stated that the federal government would only purchase technology that was accessible. Market pressures and the desire to sell their products to the federal government ensured manufacturers would make their products accessible to people with disabilities. Section 508 of the Rehabilitation Act of 1973 establishes requirements for electronic and information technology developed, maintained, procured, or used by the federal government. It requires federal electronic and information technology to be accessible to people with disabilities, including employees and members of the public.

Most importantly in the context of rehabilitation engineering, the Rehabilitation Act of 1973 established the Rehabilitation Engineering Research Centers. Section 202(b)2 states:

> Establishment and support of rehabilitation engineering research centers to (a) develop innovative methods of applying advanced medical technology, scientific achievement, and psychological and social knowledge to solve rehabilitation problems through, planning and conducting research, including cooperative research with public and private agencies and organizations, designed to produce new scientific knowledge, equipment, and devices suitable for solving problems in the rehabilitation of handicapped individuals and for reducing environmental barriers and to (b) cooperate with state agencies designated pursuant to Section 101 in developing systems of information exchange and coordination to promote the prompt utilization of engineering and other scientific research to assist in solving problems in the rehabilitation of handicapped individuals.

(GovTrack.us 1973)

Twelve Rehabilitation Engineering Research Centers (RERCs) were soon established by the Rehabilitation Services Administration of the US Department of Health, Education, and Welfare in response to the requirements of the Rehabilitation Act of 1973 (Rehabilitation Services Administration, US Department of Health, Education, and Welfare, and the Veterans Administration 1978). These centers are included in Table 1.1.

1.4 Rehabilitation engineering service delivery

As the Rehabilitation Services Administration (RSA) and the VA took on the responsibilities of managing and coordinating the rehabilitation engineering programs,

Table 1.1 Rehabilitation Engineering Research Centers (RERCs)

Organization	Location	Director	Core Area
Rancho Los Amigos Hospital	Downey, CA	James B. Reswick	Functional Electrical Stimulation of Paralyzed Nerves and Muscles
Krusen Research Center, Moss Rehabilitation Hospital	Philadelphia, PA	A. Bennett Wilson, Jr	Locomotion and Mobility
Children's Hospital Medical Center	Boston, MA	William Berenberg	Neuromuscular Control Using Sensory Feedback Systems
Texas Institute for Rehabilitation and Research	Houston, TX	William A. Spencer	Effects of Pressure on Tissue
Northwestern University	Chicago, IL	Clinton L. Compere	Internal Total Joint Replacement
University of Iowa, Orthopedics Department, Dill Children's Hospital	Iowa City, IA	Carroll B. Larson	Low Back Pain
Smith-Kettlewell Institute of Visual Sciences	San Francisco, CA	Lawrence A. Scadden	Sensory Aids for Blind and Deaf
University of Tennessee, Department of Orthopedic Surgery	Memphis, TN	Robert E. Tooms	Mobility Systems for Severely Disabled
Case Western Reserve University, School of Medicine	Cleveland, OH	Charles H. Herndon	Upper Extremity Functional Electrical Stimulation
Cerebral Palsy Research Foundation of Kansas	Wichita, KS	John. F. Jonas	Vocational Aspects of Rehabilitation
University of Michigan, College of Engineering	Ann Arbor, MI	J. Raymond Pearson	Automotive Transportation for the Handicapped
University of Virginia, School of Medicine	Charlottesville, VA	Warren G. Stamp	Spinal Cord Injury

including the Rehabilitation Engineering Research Centers established by the Rehabilitation Act of 1973, the Committee on Prosthetics Research and Development was disbanded in 1976. It was between 1973 and 1977 that a series of 12 state-of-the-art workshops in rehabilitation engineering were held on various topics. A summary meeting, chaired by Colin McLaurin, was held in Washington, DC on May 12–13, 1977 resulting in a report entitled "Rehabilitation Engineering: A Plan for Continued Progress II" (Rehabilitation Services Administration, US Department of Health, Education, and Welfare, and the Veterans Administration 1978).

With the passage of the Rehabilitation Act of 1973 and the establishment of the RERC program and centers, rehabilitation engineering research was maturing. The 12 workshops and the May 1977 meeting resulted in recommendations regarding the service delivery of rehabilitation engineering. Additionally, recommendations were made regarding knowledge gaps and recommended research, evaluation of devices, education and information transfer, service delivery, and the formation of a national organization (Rehabilitation Services Administration, US Department of Health, Education, and Welfare, and the Veterans Administration 1978).

It was during this time, and at these workshops, that a consensus on the problems of delivering rehabilitation engineering services and the role of the rehabilitation engineer in service delivery was formulated. During the conference on "Delivery of Rehabilitation Engineering Services in the State of California" held in Pomona, California on January 16–18, 1977 recommendations were made in a number of areas related to delivering rehabilitation engineering services including information, education, costs for services and equipment, research and development, standards for services and standardization of parts and components, testing and evaluation, production and distribution, prescriptions, service and repair, and rehabilitation engineers. It was noted during the workshop,

> There is a confusion regarding who is the clinical engineer and who is the research engineer. The problem, as the group saw it, is primarily from the clinical side. The research problems seem to be pretty well in hand, but there are not enough clinical engineers and enough knowledge regarding them. The technology is available, but it does not get to the patients.
>
> **(State of California, Health and Welfare Agency,**
> **Department of Rehabilitation 1977)**

A series of projects were conducted during the 1970s and early 1980s to demonstrate the feasibility and efficacy of delivering rehabilitation engineering services within a medical model (The University of Tennessee Crippled Children's Hospital School, Rehabilitation Engineering Program 1976) as well as a vocational rehabilitation model (University of Tennessee Rehabilitation Engineering Program 1978).

Rehabilitation engineering service delivery took a significant leap forward with the passage of the 1986 amendments to the Rehabilitation Act. The amendments required state vocational rehabilitation agencies to "describe how rehabilitation engineering services will be provided to assist an increasing number of individuals with handicaps." This required the state agencies to modify their state plans to include rehabilitation engineering services. Additionally, the amendments defined rehabilitation engineering by including,

> The term rehabilitation engineering means the systematic application of technologies, engineering technologies, or scientific principles to meet the needs and address the barriers confronted by individuals with handicaps in areas which include education, rehabilitation, employment, transportation, independent living, and recreation.

(GovTrack.us 1986)

Recognizing the increasing importance of addressing the delivery of services, RESNA (see Section 1.6 below) coordinated an invitational symposium at Petit Jean State Park, Arkansas, on September 19–23, 1987 resulting in a book entitled *Rehabilitation Technology Service Delivery: A Practical Guide*. Gerry Warren, the President of RESNA at the time wrote in the forward of the book,

> This publication represents the cornerstone of a new era in rehab engineering and technology. We have surpassed the eras that focused on producing new technology, defining consumer needs, and technology transfer. We are coming to grips with what we know now to be a pivotal aspect of using technology to meet the needs of disabled people. We have solidly entered the era of service delivery.

(Perlman and Enders 1987)

Seven models of service delivery were identified in the RESNA guide (Perlman and Enders 1987):

- Durable medical equipment (DME) supplier.
- Department within a comprehensive rehabilitation program.
- Technology service delivery center in a university.
- State agency-based program.
- The private rehabilitation engineering/technology firm.
- Local affiliate of a national nonprofit disability organization.
- Miscellaneous types of programs, including volunteer groups and information/resource centers.

Through the middle and end of the 1980s, discussions were held regarding the terminology of rehabilitation engineering. As described above, the beginnings of the field involved a large number of engineers. It soon became apparent there

33

were many more individuals involved in providing technology to people with disabilities. It seemed the use of the term, engineering, was limiting. The passage of the "Technology-Related Assistance for Individuals with Disabilities Act of 1988" (Tech Act) contributed to the discussions of how to define the technology devices and services used by people with disabilities. The Tech Act recognized a "substantial number of assistive technology devices" existed, however people "do not have access to the assistive technology devices and assistive technology services that such individuals need to allow such individuals to function in society commensurate with their abilities." The Tech Act was designed as a systems-change act to develop "consumer-responsive state-wide program(s) of technology-related assistance for individuals of all ages with disabilities." The state-wide programs were meant to provide information about assistive technology devices and services, funding, increased capacity, and increased coordination. Most importantly, the Tech Act legally defined the terms "assistive technology device" and "assistive technology service" for the first time. The definitions in the Tech Act include:

(1) ASSISTIVE TECHNOLOGY DEVICE—The term "assistive technology device" means any item, piece of equipment, or product system, whether acquired commercially off the shelf, modified, or customized, that is used to increase, maintain, or improve functional capabilities of individuals with disabilities.

(2) ASSISTIVE TECHNOLOGY SERVICE—The term "assistive technology service" means any service that directly assists an individual with a disability in the selection, acquisition, or use of an assistive technology device. Such term includes—

(A) the evaluation of the needs of an individual with a disability, including a functional evaluation of the individual in the individual's customary environment;

(B) purchasing, leasing, or otherwise providing for the acquisition of assistive technology devices by individuals with disabilities;

(C) selecting, designing, fitting, customizing, adapting, applying, maintaining, repairing, or replacing assistive technology devices;

(D) coordinating and using other therapies, interventions, or services with assistive technology devices, such as those associated with existing education and rehabilitation plans and programs;

(E) training or technical assistance for an individual with disabilities, or, where appropriate, the family of an individual with disabilities; and

(F) training or technical assistance for professionals (including individuals providing education and rehabilitation services), employers, or other individuals who provide services to, employ, or are otherwise substantially involved in the major life functions of individuals with disabilities.

(GovTrack.us 1988)

1.5 Rehabilitation engineering affects the complex rehabilitation technology market

The impact of rehabilitation engineering, on the commercial complex rehabilitation technology (CRT) marketplace, will probably never be fully appreciated for its impact.

There are countless instances where rehabilitation engineering changed the CRT landscape and the lives of persons with disabilities. Described below are a few of the first instances of technology transfer to the commercial CRT market from both research and clinical rehabilitation engineering programs.

Starting back in the mid-1960s, before the term rehabilitation engineering had been coined, physicians, clinicians, and engineers at Goldwater Hospital, located on Roosevelt Island in New York City, removed the cross brace of an E&J manual wheelchair with recline, rigidized the frame, and added a rack to support a ventilator and a battery (Figure 1.27). This gave consumers residing at Goldwater the ability not only for movement within the hospital, but also excursions into "Island Town."

Following the success of this intervention, the frame rigidizing was done to an E&J powered wheelchair frame which, along with new drive control interventions, allowed ventilator-dependent residents of Goldwater Hospital independent mobility within the community. Around the same time, The Rehabilitation Institute

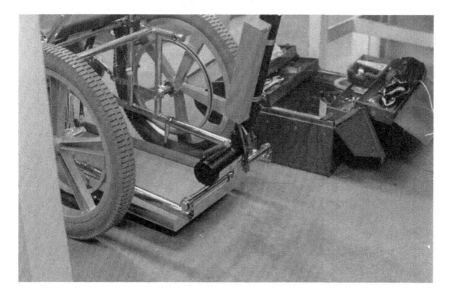

Figure 1.27 View of Goldwater frame (Dickerson).

of Chicago (RIC; Illinois, United States) was developing "Quad Systems" that included power-independent recline and sip-and-puff interfaces that allowed people with high-level spinal cord injuries, including those requiring respiratory support, full, independent control of their powered chairs' direction and the added benefit of postural change utilizing the power recline.

The MED Group (a group of independent equipment suppliers) was located in Chicago and members of that group realized the impact of these technologies and successfully executed a technology transfer of the sip-and-puff control, power-recline E&J wheelchair (Figure 1.28).

The MED Group also brought to the commercial marketplace what became known as the MED Micro-Dec, which was also developed at RIC. The Micro-Dec was a compact, portable Environmental Control Unit that was one of the first to utilize X-10 control modules.

Other significant contributions to the seating and wheeled mobility world came from a technology transfer agreement between the MED Group and the University of Tennessee-Rehabilitation Engineering Program (UT-REP). The Molded Plastic Inserts (MPI) pediatric seating system and the Spherical Thoracic Supports were developed at UT-REP under the leadership of Doug Hobson and Elaine Trefler.

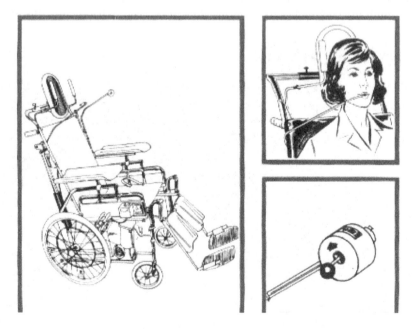

Figure 1.28 MED catalogue circa 1980 (Dickerson).

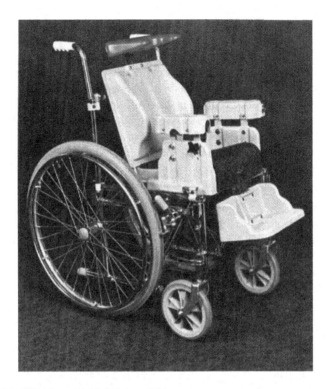

Figure 1.29 MPI circa 1980 (Dickerson).

The MPI was a modular component seating system that consisted of four sizes of seats and five sizes of backs, along with accessories including armrests, headrests, trays, and footrests. The seats and backs were constructed using acrylonitrile butadiene styrene (ABS) plastic with only a moderate polyethylene seat pad. While successful at UT-REP, the commercial launch was problematic at first as parents and clinicians struggled to embrace the solid plastic shells. The modularity and ease of cleaning and growth, combined with the success of the early adaptors, made the MPI a very successful commercial product that was developed by rehabilitation engineers (Figure 1.29).

Also developed at UT-REP around the same time, were the spherical thoracic support pads. These unique supports were also technology transferred to the MED Group and remain a product today, available from Otto Bock.

1.6 Rehabilitation engineering finds a home

In addition to the conference on "Delivery of Rehabilitation Engineering Services in the State of California" held in Pomona, California, another meeting was held on

November 3–5, 1977 at the University of Tennessee in Knoxville, on "Rehabilitation Engineering Education" (The University of Tennessee, Knoxville 1977). Recommendations from these conferences foreshadowed a number of important activities in the growth and development of the rehabilitation engineering field. A recommendation at the California meeting suggested, "There should be a meeting of rehabilitation engineers scheduled in the near future, so that the field could begin to interchange information and also start a self-policing and regulating effort" (State of California, Health and Welfare Agency, Department of Rehabilitation 1977). Joe Traub of the Rehabilitation Services Administration and Tony Staros of the VA organized just such meetings called the Interagency Conferences on Rehabilitation Engineering. The first meeting was held in Washington, DC in 1978.

Additionally, recommendations at the California and Tennessee meetings suggested an organization of rehabilitation engineers be formed. The recommendation from the California meeting suggested, "An organization for rehabilitation engineers should be established—for the exchange of information and ideas" (State of California, Health and Welfare Agency, Department of Rehabilitation 1977). As Doug Hobson recollected,

> At the 1978 (Interagency) meeting, Staros, Traub, McLaurin, Reswick, and Hobson met to formulate a concept for a multidisciplinary society on rehabilitation engineering that would function independently from government. It was to provide the forum for information sharing and rehabilitation technology development and application that had been so effective within the CPRD model. In 1979, the concept of a new society, along with founding bylaws, was presented to a multidisciplinary forum (at the Interagency conference) of about 250 people. The concept was accepted, and the Rehabilitation Engineering Society of North America (RESNA) was born, with Jim Reswick as its founding President. Colin McClaurin was RESNA's second president, and the rest is recorded history.
>
> **(Hobson 2002, 17)**

Figures 1.30 and 1.31 illustrate the founding documents of RESNA.

RESNA, now known as the Rehabilitation Engineering and Assistive Technology Society of North America, became the professional home for professionals and consumers with an interest in rehabilitation engineering and assistive technology, primarily in North America. RESNA is a worldwide leader in the development and maintenance of assistive technology device standards, the certification of assistive technology professionals and the accreditation of education programs for assistive technology.

1.7 Summary and conclusions

Technology extends abilities and allows people to accomplish what they would not otherwise be able to do. Assistive technology enhances the abilities and

THE REHABILITATION ENGINEERING SOCIETY
OF NORTH AMERICA
What It Is — Whom It Is For — What It May Become

The Rehabilitation Engineering Society of North America (RESNA) represents a joining together of persons who participate in the development and delivery of technology to people with disabilities. The goal of RESNA is to improve the quality of life of handicapped persons in all possible ways; from recognition of their needs, through design, development, evaluation, and production of devices both internal and external, and modification of housing and transportation environments, to enhancing the effectiveness of the delivery system to meet the needs of the disabled wherever they may be.

RESNA and the Rehabilitation Engineering Delivery System

The Rehabilitation Engineering Delivery System is complex and many faceted. It involves many kinds of professionals and institutions and includes, most importantly, the person with disability and his/her family. To be successful, all components of this system must function effectively both as individual units and as an interconnected network.

RESNA in its structure will mirror the Rehabilitation Engineering Delivery System. As a society it will be concerned with the total problem of making technology available to persons with disabilities. Some of its task groups will provide professional forums for experts concerned with their own role in the delivery process, while other committees will reflect the system as a whole and the interaction of its components. The professionals in the Rehabilitation Engineering Delivery System may be listed as follows:

1. *Consumers* - Persons with disabilities and their families who need the benefits of technology.
2. *Practitioners* - Physicians and allied health professionals including counselors who recognize the potential of a disabled person and who prescribe the specific Rehabilitation Engineering devices, provide service, and/or arrange for home and work modifications.
3. *Administrators* - Directors and staff of federal, state, and local agencies (public and private) that have health, social, and vocational responsibilities for persons with disabilities.
4. *Manufacturers and Distributors* - Members of firms and institutions that make equipment and services available to the handicapped, including builders.
5. *Operators* - Members of companies that provide transportation, hotels, restaurants, recreation facilities that are accessible to persons with disabilities.
6. *Authorizers and Providers* - Health agencies (e.g., Medicare) and insurance companies that must authorize purchase of equipment and services and provide third party payment.
7. *Inventors and Designers* - Rehabilitation engineers and others who design and develop implants, assistive equipment, vehicles and housing to meet the needs of persons with disabilities.
8. *Researchers* - Medical, Engineering, Allied Health, Social, Psychological, Vocational, and other professionals who conduct research activities, the result of which lead to better understanding of the needs of persons with disabilities and how better to solve their problems.
9. *Educators* - University and college professionals who train rehabilitation engineers, allied health persons, designers, architects and technicians, for service to the disabled.
10. *Legislators* - Politicians and staff personnel at federal, state, and local levels who pass and oversee legislation that concerns the application of technology to persons with disabilities.

This list above, in many ways defines the Rehabilitation Engineering Society of North America. First, it describes the persons who are eligible for membership. Their credentials, activities, and interests vary widely, but the one thing they share in common is a deep concern for making the benefits of technology available to persons with disability. Thus, Rehabilitation Engineering — the application of science and technology to improving the quality of life of persons with disabilities — is the rallying point of RESNA. Each of the person-types represented has an equal responsibility in the overall delivery process. The process starts with the needs of the disabled person and ends when his/her needs are met. Each person plays a unique role and the system itself will not work if any part does not function effectively. RESNA is concerned with the entire system, and to be effective it must build its membership with all persons in the system.

Secondly, the above list essentially defines elements of the Rehabilitation Engineering delivery system. A basic concept in systems theory is that the inter-relationship between the components of the system is as important as

Figure 1.30 RESNA founding document.

are the elements themselves. While the parts of the system are easily recognized, the inter-relationships or connections are difficult to define. In fact, most of the barriers to the delivery of Rehabilitation Engineering services are found in the connections or lack thereof between the elements of the system. A major goal of RESNA is to deal with these interactions and find ways to remove the barriers that inhibit the overall system from functioning effectively. For example, one of the major barriers is the lack of information and a system to make information available to the many persons within the delivery system. Many factors are affected by the lack of information or access to it, including definition of needs, research priorities, legislation, funding, availability of devices with associated indications for applicability and training. This is an area in which RESNA can and will contribute.

As one looks at the Rehabilitation Engineering Delivery System as a whole, and at the same time examines the activities and problems associated with his/her individual specialty, he/she cannot help but identify many action areas wherein RESNA can be effective. These range from national planning and funding support at the highest federal levels to the specific application of technology for one person with a disability, wherever he/she may be. The list will be long and important. As the Society becomes organized into sub-task groups and committees, action plans will evolve to cover the needs. As of this time, no one group, including ourselves, is in a position to draw the blueprint for the Society. It will become clearer when the membership itself organizes itself to deal with the issues it believes most important and of manageable size. But we do have a vision of what our society might be in three or four years.

RESNA in Three Years

- We see a membership of many thousands of persons who know why they wish to join together and who freely give of their energies and time in activities that they find enjoyable and rewarding, rallying around the concept of improving the quality of life of their fellowman through the appiciation of technology.
- We see a forum of resource persons and activities to which all of the constituencies — government, researchers, manufacturers, practitioners, and disabled persons themselves — can turn for professional help in planning, evaluations, state-of-the-art studies, peer reviews or whatever the particular need may be.
- We see Annual Meetings that are attended by thousands of persons following the precedent and continuing the momentum already established by the Intergency Conference on Rehabilitation Engineering. Exhibits, technical papers, workshops, teaching sessions and, above all, personal contacts, will confirm the reality of the common and individual interests of the members of the society.
- We see organization into subgroups, some comprised of members from all elements in the Rehabilitation Engineering Delivery System that deal with national and international needs, while other sub-groups will be formed around the individual professional expertise of the membership to deal with the needs of their professions.
- We see expanding publication activity that in some forms will appeal to the entire membership at large, and in other forms, provide high quality professional journal space for scientific and other professional articles.
- We see an executive office, staffed with professionals who carry on many kinds of projects requiring full time attention, including workshops, evaluation studies, peer review, special studies, contracted assistance to public and private agencies as well as manufacturers for information and services vital to planning, marketing, and setting of priorities.
- We see professional Rehabilitation Engineering subgroups that are particularly concerned with accreditation and certification of rehabilitation engineers by state and local institutions as the Rehabilitation Engineer becomes a recognized professional in the health service delivery system. Accreditation is directly related to training and thus RESNA will have an impact on new Rehabilitation Engineering University Programs.
- We see RESNA as a member of an international federation of similar societies emerging in nations throughout the world and maintaining an active involvement on the international scene.

These are some of the visions we have. While visionary at this point, we believe they are realizable because they are founded on sound concepts and because the people who can make the society all of these things — and much more — exist in North America, are concerned about the potential of technology for the disabled person and are ready and willing to join together in action groups that will have the power to bring about change.

We cannot offer you now a perfect "slot" in a developed organization. But we can offer you the opportunity to join with your colleagues in a personally rewarding activity that will benefit millions of persons with disabilities. Will you join us?

The Founding Committee of RESNA
James B. Reswick
Anthony Staros
Joseph Traub
Colin McLaurin
Douglas Hobson

Figure 1.31 RESNA founding document.

opportunities for people with disabilities to lead more independent lives. The history of assistive technology and rehabilitation engineering provides lessons in the invention and development of devices and technology that aid people with disabilities. A central tenet of the development of assistive technology is the involvement of people with disabilities in defining the needs and problems and substantially being involved in the design process.

Many devices and technologies first developed for use by people with disabilities have evolved to become mainstream consumer products. Conversely, many consumer goods have become important assistive technologies for people with functional limitations.

The history of assistive technology describes the many kinds of devices that have been developed and used by people with disabilities. Prosthetics, technologies for visual impairment, hearing impairments, and communication, as well as mobility and computer technologies, are only some of the categories of devices that enhance the abilities of people with disabilities.

Public policies, including the passage of laws, have contributed to the advancement of the development and provision of assistive technology. These laws include the funding for research, development, and delivery of assistive technology.

The need for assistive technology and advances in engineering have led to the development of the professional practice of biomedical engineering and, specifically, rehabilitation engineering. In addition to the creation of university-based academic programs, professional organizations have been established in order to provide information, training, and networking for assistive technology and rehabilitation engineering professionals.

1.8 Discussion questions

1. How would you explain the growth of biomedical and rehabilitation engineering?
2. Considering the evolution of prosthetic development, discuss what you see as the future of prosthetics.
3. Discuss the importance of consumer-centered design and its role in the development of assistive technology.
4. Discuss how certain current mainstream technologies can benefit people with disabilities.
5. Discuss how professional organizations such as RESNA can advance the field of rehabilitation engineering and assistive technology.

Bibliography

American Chemical Society. "Discovery and Development of Penicillin." https://www.acs.org/content/acs/en/education/whatischemistry/landmarks/flemingpenicillin.html.

Amputee-coalition.org. "A Brief History of Prosthetics." https://www.amputee-coalition.org/resources/a-brief-history-of-prosthetics/.

Antiquetypewriters. "Antique Typewriters - The Martin Howard Collection: Hall Braille-Writer 1." Accessed 4/23, 2018, http://www.antiquetypewriters.com/collection/typewriter.asp?Hall%20Braille-writer%201#.WwWpIUxFyP8.

Atlas Obscura. "Object of Intrigue: The Prosthetic Iron Hand of a 16th-Century Knight." Accessed 4/30, 2018, https://www.atlasobscura.com/articles/object-of-intrigue-the-prosthetic-iron-hand-of-a-16thcentury-knight.

ATRC. "The Tech Act – ATRC." Accessed 4/19, 2018, http://www.atrc.org/the-tech-act/.

Auyang, Sunny Y. 2006. *Engineering—An Endless Frontier*. Cambridge, MA: Harvard University Press.

Bell, A. "Alexander Graham Bell – Inventions – HISTORY.Com." Accessed 4/23, 2018, https://www.history.com/topics/inventions/alexander-graham-bell.

Bmes.org. "Bmes." Accessed 3/30, 2018, https://www.bmes.org/history.

Broughttolife.sciencemuseum.org.uk. "Copy of Roman Artificial Leg, London, England, 1905–1915." Accessed 4/22, 2018, http://broughttolife.sciencemuseum.org.uk/broughttolife/objects/display?id=91684.

Childress, Dudley S. 2003. "Development of Rehabilitation Engineering Over the Years: As I See It." *Journal of Rehabilitation Research and Development* 39 (6; Supp): 1–10.

Creatingtechnology.org. "History of Engineering." Accessed 3/29, 2018, http://www.creating-technology.org/history.htm#1.

En.wikipedia.org. "Blissymbols." Accessed 4/28, 2018, https://en.wikipedia.org/wiki/Blissymbols.

———. "Gaspard Monge." Accessed 3/29, 2018, https://en.wikipedia.org/wiki/Gaspard_Monge.

———. "History of Poliomyelitis." Accessed 5/3, 2018, https://en.wikipedia.org/wiki/History_of_poliomyelitis.

———. "Marc Isambard Brunel." Accessed 3/29, 2018, https://en.wikipedia.org/wiki/Marc_Isambard_Brunel.

———. "Samuel Genensky." Accessed 4/30, 2018, https://en.wikipedia.org/wiki/Samuel_Genensky.

———. "Thalidomide." Accessed 5/3, 2018, https://en.wikipedia.org/wiki/Thalidomide.

Encyclopedia Britannica. "History of the Wheelchair." Accessed 4/26, 2018, https://www.britannica.com/topic/history-of-the-wheelchair-1971423.

Enderle, John, and Joseph Bronzino. 2012. *Introduction to Biomedical Engineering*. 3rd ed. Amsterdam: Elsevier/Academic Press.

Finch, Jacqueline Louise, Glyn Harvey Heath, Ann Rosalie David, and Jai Kulkarni. 2012. "Biomechanical Assessment of Two Artificial Big Toe Restorations from Ancient Egypt and their Significance to the History of Prosthetics." *JPO: Journal of Prosthetics and Orthotics* 24 (4): 181–191.

Garden, H. "How Prosthetic Limbs Work." Accessed 4/30, 2018, https://science.howstuffworks.com/prosthetic-limb1.htm.

GovTrack.us. "Rehabilitation Act (1973 - H.R. 8070)." Accessed 5/2, 2018, https://www.govtrack.us/congress/bills/93/hr8070.

———. "Rehabilitation Act Amendments of 1986 (1986 - H.R. 4021)." Accessed 5/2, 2018, https://www.govtrack.us/congress/bills/99/hr4021.

———. "Technology-Related Assistance for Individuals with Disabilities Act of 1988 (1988 - S. 2561)." Accessed 5/2, 2018, https://www.govtrack.us/congress/bills/100/s2561.

Hanger.com. "The J.E. Hanger Story - Hanger, Inc." Accessed 5/3, 2018, http://www.hanger.com/history/Pages/The-J.E.-Hanger-Story.aspx.

Hays, M. 2010. *A Historical Look at the Department of Veterans Affairs Research and Development Program*. Baltimore, MD: VA R&D Communications. https://www.research.va.gov/pubs/docs/ORD-85yrHistory.pdf.

Hobson, Douglas A. 2002. "Reflections on Rehabilitation Engineering History: Are There Lessons to Be Learned?" *Journal of Rehabilitation Research and Development* 39 (6) Supplement: 17.

Marilynhamilton.com. "Marilyn Hamilton : Envision : Conceive, Believe, Achieve : If You Can't Stand Up Stand Out." Last modified 2018, accessed 4/28, 2018, http://www.marilynhamilton.com/Introduction_Envision.html.

MCOP Prosthetics. "iWalk BiOM Foot/Ankle Prosthesis." *MCOP Prosthetics*. Last modified 2018, accessed 4/30, 2018, https://mcopro.com/prosthetics/technology/iwalk-biom/.

Nader, R. 1971. "Ralph Nader's Most Shocking Exposé." *Ladies Home Journal* 88: 98.

National Research Council (US) Committee on Prosthetics Research and Development and of Sciences National Academy. 1971. *Rehabilitation Engineering: A Plan for Continued Progress*. Washington, DC: National Academy of Sciences.

Nyamcenterforhistory.org. "Pieter Adriaanszoon Verduyn | Books, Health and History." Last modified 2018, accessed 4/30, 2018.

Perlman, L., and A. Enders. 1987. *Rehabilitation Technology Service Delivery: A Practical Guide*. Washington, DC: RESNA, Association for the Advancement of Rehabilitation Technology. https://files.eric.ed.gov/fulltext/ED313816.pdf.

Rehabilitation Services Administration, U.S. Department of Health, Education, and Welfare, and the Veterans Administration. 1978. *Rehabilitation Engineering: A Plan for Continued Progress II*. Washington, DC: Rehabilitation Engineering Center, University of Virginia. https://web.stanford.edu/group/resna/History/RehabilitationEngineering-1978.pdf.

Reswick, James B. 2002. "How and When Did the Rehabilitation Engineering Center Program Come into Being?" *Journal of Rehabilitation Research and Development* 39 (6) Supplement: 11–16. https://pdfs.semanticscholar.org/4de2/f32b6a5f1580f683a71d60341a2596b05112.pdf.

Sandlin, Robert E. 2000. *Textbook of Hearing Aid Amplification*. San Diego, CA: Plural Publishing, Cengage Learning.

Schwejda, P., and G. Vanderheiden. 1982. "Adaptive-Firmware Card for the Apple II." *Adaptive-Firmware Card for the Apple-Ii* 7 (9): 276.

State of California, Health and Welfare Agency, Department of Rehabilitation. 1977. *Development of a Model Rehabilitation Engineering Delivery System in California--A Beginning*. Sacramento, CA: State of California, Health and Welfare Agency, Department of Rehabilitation.

Surrence, M. "The History of Eyeglasses | Zenni Optical." Accessed 4/22, 2018, https://www.zennioptical.com/blog/history-eyeglasses/.

The University of Tennessee Crippled Children's Hospital School, Rehabilitation Engineering Program. 1976. *Activities Report*, September 1974–June 1976. Knoxville, TN: University of Tennessee.

The University of Tennessee, Knoxville. 1977. *Report of the Workshop on Rehabilitation Engineering Education*. Knoxville, TN: The University of Tennessee.

U of T Engineering News. "The Maker: George Klein and the First Electric Wheelchair - U of T Engineering News." Accessed 4/28, 2018, https://news.engineering.utoronto.ca/maker-george-klein-first-electric-wheelchair/.

University of Tennessee Rehabilitation Engineering Program. 1978. *An Approach to a Rehabilitation Engineering Service Delivery System for Vocational Rehabilitation Clients, the Results of a Two Year Demonstration Project, October 1, 1976–September 30, 1978.* Knoxville, TN: University of Tennessee.

Vanderheiden, Gregg C. 2003. "A Journey through Early Augmentative Communication and Computer Access." *Journal of Rehabilitation Research and Development* 39 (6; SUPP): 39–53.

Vlaskamp, Frank, Thijs Soede, and Gert Jan Gelderblom. 2011. *History of Assistive Technology: 5000 Years of Technology Development for Human Needs.* Heerlen, Netherlands: Zuyd Univ.

Zuo, Kevin J., and Jaret L. Olson. 2014. "The Evolution of Functional Hand Replacement: From Iron Prostheses to Hand Transplantation." *Plastic Surgery* 22 (1): 44–51.

Chapter 2 Assistive technology

L. Alvarez, A. Cook and J. Polgar

Contents

DOI: 10.1201/b21964-3

2.1 Chapter overview

Assistive technology (AT) can be broadly defined as including a range of "devices, services, strategies, and practices that are conceived and applied to ameliorate the problems faced by individuals who have disabilities" (Cook and Polgar 2014). By thinking about AT as extending beyond a device, rehabilitation engineers will be ideally positioned to consider the range of factors, needs and solutions that can most benefit AT users. This chapter provides an overview of the conceptual underpinnings of AT development, research, services (practice) and education. In addition, the chapter will expose students to a range of factors that impact the relation between human, activity, AT and environment. The chapter will explore AT that supports different functions and the participation of individuals in different activities including (Figure 2.1) mobility (e.g., using a wheelchair to navigate

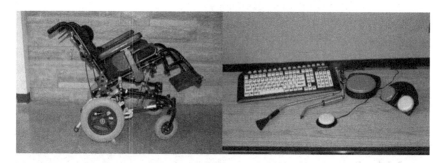

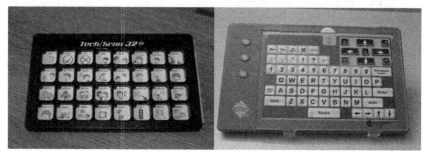

Figure 2.1 Examples of assistive technology devices that support activities such as mobility, control of the environment, communication and cognition (Courtesy of Janice Polgar).

the environment), manipulation and control of the environment (e.g., using a switch or adapted keyboard to access a computer), communication and cognition (e.g., using a picture-based augmentative and alternative communication device that supplements speech).

Finally, the chapter invites readers to reflect upon the ethical tensions facing AT as a field of practice, and to consider the implications of their role in the design, development and implementation of AT.

2.2 Theoretical models and frameworks: Structuring assistive technology reasoning

Theoretical models allow members of a discipline to establish a common ground upon which to further develop inquiry, practice and reflection. Historically, models and frameworks have been developed to simplify and explain a phenomenon (Duncan 2006). This can be seen in several engineering disciplines where abstraction and approximation of the most relevant properties of an object can serve the design, modeling and development processes (Seeler 2014). However, AT lives in the intersection between engineering and the health sciences and humanities. AT seeks to reduce the disabling influence that environments can have on an individual (Cook and Polgar 2014). Thus, the complex nature of this human activity–environment–technology interaction requires models and frameworks that can comprehensively address the different factors that influence such interaction. The following section provides a description of how such models can serve the needs of AT practitioners, including rehabilitation engineers, in research and development, practice and education.

2.2.1 Informing research and development

Models have served science for generations. From the Hodgkin–Huxley model of the neuron that led to our understanding of nerve condition and intracellular interaction, to the physical models used by Watson and Crick to untangle the mystery of DNA, models have informed research. Now they are also informing research and development in AT.

Models inform the AT research and development process in several ways. One of the most important is the use of models to characterize the assistive device system in terms of the intended use, the contexts of use, the characteristics of the user and the characteristics of the technology used. One such model is the human activity assistive technology (HAAT) model. Models like HAAT describe the interrelationships that exist in the application of ATs. They are useful at various stages of the research and development cycle. Models can help place raw data from surveys, focus groups and other data collection activities into a meaningful

47

relationship, enabling development of device characteristics. This in turn can help define specifications for development of innovative technology-based approaches to user needs.

Comprehensive models like the HAAT can also provide a framework for the evaluation of prototype devices to determine their ability to meet the needs of people with disabilities. Factors relating to user characteristics can be separated from those related to environmental, social, cultural and institutional contexts that influence successful device use. AT models also support the evaluation of competing technologies for effectiveness, efficiency and efficacy.

2.2.2 Informing practice

Evidence-based practice (EBP) has become a paramount element of healthcare policy, funding and implementation, including rehabilitation settings. In its most fundamental form, EBP seeks to elicit conscious, explicit and judicious use of current best evidence to guide decision making regarding the care and strategies around an individual's health (Sackett et al. 1996). AT practitioners, including rehabilitation engineers, face an important commitment to advance EBP in AT. By doing so, practitioners can integrate rigorous evidence into practice and demonstrate the impact of AT use and improve funding. Models and frameworks can also allow AT practitioners to develop a practice that is client-centered, and that systematically assesses and considers the match between human, technology, activity and context.

Client-centered AT is one that recognizes the client, not as a recipient of AT, but as an active partner and primary stakeholder in the AT process (Cook and Polgar 2014). AT practitioners must utilize an AT model or framework that reflects the primary role of the user, and that supports the considerations regarding the client's needs and skills. By using a model that emphasizes the individual and not just the technology capabilities or potential, practitioners can ensure that the resulting match serves the client's priorities and is sustainable over time. Moreover, client-centered models allow users, practitioners and other stakeholders, to plan for, explain and predict successful outcomes (Giesbrecht 2013).

2.2.3 Informing education

Application of AT models in education prioritizes acquisition of reasoning processes that develop technology most likely to enable function over acquisition of knowledge of technology alone. Comprehensive models such as HAAT (Section 2.3.1) and comprehensive assistive technology (CAT) (Section 2.3.3) inform curricular content in terms of depth and breadth of knowledge, professional reasoning and research (as described in Section 2.2.1). The rapid pace of complex technology development requires students to gain competence in professional reasoning, using a process that guides thinking in the development and application of technology. As students become more competent reasoners, they make increasingly complex connections among ideas and use these in sophisticated ways to inform thinking and practice in AT design and application. AT models provide a systematic approach to increase professional reasoning and expand the depth and breadth of knowledge related to AT. Similar to practice above, development of technology that is beneficial to the user requires knowledge about the person, their needs, preferences and abilities, the activities in which they need and want to engage and the contexts in which they will be engaging in these activities. Models like HAAT, matching person and technology (MPT) and CAT provide a systematic way of learning and reasoning around these aspects, influencing the likelihood that new and existing technology will be accepted and used.

2.3 Assistive technology: Models and frameworks

2.3.1 The HAAT model

The HAAT model describes a person (human) doing something (activity) in a context with the use of AT (see Figure 2.2) (Cook and Polgar 2014; Cook and Polgar 2012). The elements of the person, the activity, context and AT comprise a system that is transactional in nature and that enables performance and participation in needed and desired daily activities.

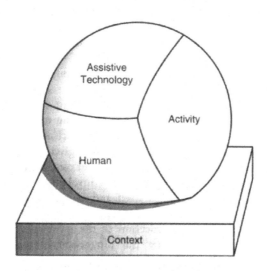

Figure 2.2 The HAAT model. This figure was published in Cook and Polgar (2015, 41).

2.3.1.1 Human Understanding the person guides AT development and selection by clarifying what the client can do and what personal skills and abilities the technology needs to augment or replace. In service delivery, consideration is given to the client's cognitive, sensory and physical abilities, as well as to the meaning that the activity holds, including whether it is important for them to perform the activity on their own or with assistance (Cook and Polgar 2014).

2.3.1.2 Activity Activity (or occupation) includes areas of self-care, instrumental activities of daily living, productivity and leisure as well as manipulation, cognition, mobility and communication that support these daily activities. Further, when understanding the activity, considerations of timing (how long, how frequent), location (where the activity occurs) and whether it is a solitary or joint activity, provide a greater depth of understanding of how the occupation is performed and thus, what the technology needs to do in order to support it (Cook and Polgar 2014).

2.3.1.3 Context The context in which the person engages in activities is comprised of physical, social, cultural and institutional elements. Physical aspects include the built or natural environment as well as physical aspects of heat, light and sound that affect the performance or use of technology (e.g., LED screens are difficult to see in high light situations). The presence of others in the context in which the technology is used, and their knowledge of and/or willingness to support the use of the technology influence the possibilities for its use to support activity engagement. Cultural aspects of inclusion of persons with disabilities or others (e.g., older adults, women) in community activities and the degree to which independence and autonomy are valued will affect access and use of technology. Finally, institutional aspects of funding, regulations and legislation affect who has access to technology and the conditions under which technology is accessed and used (Cook and Polgar 2014).

2.3.1.4 Assistive technology AT includes devices and strategies in the continuum of low to high complexity. Low technology is simple, often easy to obtain, like a mouth stick or head pointer. High technology is more complex and more difficult to obtain, such as an alternative and augmentative communication device. The HAAT model differentiates between hard and soft technologies. Hard technologies include the physical device, whereas soft technologies incorporate decision-making around device selection and different means of instruction on device use (Cook and Polgar 2014). The human/technology interface (HTI) is another necessary consideration in device design and selection. HTI influences how the user inputs and receives information from the device. Understanding the user's sensory, physical and cognitive abilities is important to determine what HTI they will be able to use.

2.3.2 The SETT framework

The student, environments, tasks, tools (SETT) framework (Zabala 2002) is a tool designed to help collaborative teams create student-centered, environmentally useful, task-focused systems that foster educational success for students with disabilities. The SETT framework gathers information about the student, the customary environments in which the student spends time and the required tasks the students need to carry out to be successful participants in the teaching/learning process.

SETT guides practitioners through a series of questions associated with students, environments, tasks and tools intended to guide the development of an AT plan for a specific student. The following are some of the questions in each category that guide AT decision-making: (1) Student questions: What does the student need to do? What are the student's special needs? What are the student's current abilities? (2) Environment questions: What materials and devices are available? What resources are available? (3) Task questions: How can activities be modified to meet student needs? How can tech support the student's participation in the activities? (4) Tools questions: What strategies might be used to increase student performance? What no-tech, low-tech and high-tech options should be considered? How might tools be tried with students in environments where they will be used?

2.3.3 The CAT model

The CAT model (Hersh and Johnson 2008a; Hersh and Johnson 2008b) was developed to (1) identify accessibility barriers, (2) analyze existing AT systems, (3) design and develop new AT systems and (4) evaluate outcomes (Hersh and Johnson 2008b). The model is described as an extension of an earlier HAAT model (Cook and Hussey 2002) and draws on aspects of the International Classification of Functioning, Disability and Health (ICF) (WHO 2001) and the Matching Person and Technology model (Scherer and Glueckauf 2005).

The model is hierarchical, involving three levels (attributes, components and factors). The highest level (attributes) comprises the elements of an AT system, including person (characteristics, social aspects and attitudes), context (social and cultural), activity and AT (Hersh and Johnson 2008a). Activity includes fundamental activities (e.g., communication, mobility, etc.) and contextual activities (e.g., activities of daily living, employment, leisure/recreational and educational activities). Finally, AT is divided into activity specification, design issues, system technology issues and end-user issues (Hersh and Johnson 2008b).

2.3.4 The MPT model

The MPT model (Scherer 2002) involves the AT user in a collaborative process to identify technology that can best support the user's needs, health and wellness.

This ecological model incorporates three primary elements: the milieu (or context), the person and the AT. Like the HAAT and the CAT, each of these elements is comprised of several different variables. The milieu includes social, cultural, physical and attitudinal aspects of the context in which the individual will use the AT. Person aspects include temperament, personality and preferences for technology as well as experience and predisposition to technology use (inclusive of all technology, not just assistive technology). Salient aspects of the technology include a blend of practical aspects such as cost and availability, device performance and aesthetic aspects of comfort and appearance (Corradi, Scherer and Lo Presti 2012).

This model has been operationalized through several evidence-based assessments, most of which involve a comparison of self and collaborator reports on device attributes, use, need and contextual aspects. This comparison yields a technology recommendation that balances the client needs and preferences with the contextual support/constraints. A key premise is that this user-driven process will result in technology that is accepted and used for maximum benefit across key settings. An application process is described that begins with understanding the person and their needs, incorporates the assessment and its analysis, includes device recommendation and concludes with follow-up and re-assessment with MPT measures to evaluate the process outcome (Corradi, Scherer and Lo Presti 2012).

More details on the MPT are provided in Chapter 4.

2.3.5 Theoretical career path

Developed by Gitlin (1998), the theoretical career path describes the AT user as involved in a "user career." As such, the user progresses through a path involving four stages of expertise in AT use including novice, early, experienced and expert user. At each step, the path considers the needs and factors that may influence the individual's mastering of the AT device. For example, a novice user is described as an individual likely to be in hospital who has a need for a device, device instruction and for determining environmental fit. An expert user, on the other hand, is an individual who has been at home for one or more years and has mastered the use of the device.

The theoretical career path has been used as a model to inform decision making and research (Fok 2011). The model provides a structured way of outlining the trajectory of use of an AT device considering the influential factors and the needs of the user at each stage. However, the complexity of AT use (e.g., multiple device use), as well as the personal factors (e.g., cultural background) may limit the scope of the model (Demers et al. 2008). As such, engineers and other practitioners are encouraged to use complementary perspectives that account for the complex interactions between human, activity, technology and environment.

2.3.6 The HETI model

Developed by Smith (Smith 1991), the human environment/technology (HETI) model focuses on the relationship between the human and the technology. Using an engineering framework, the model considers the input, processing and output elements required for successful use. The AT user receives an input from the environment, which is then processed and used to inform the appropriate motor output. This, in turn, results in an input to the AT device, which must be capable of processing the information and subsequently producing an output which is appropriate for the user.

The HETI model has been applied to inform the assessment and intervention approach to various types of assistive technologies, including computer access (Hoppestad 2004) and powered mobility (Field 1999). By considering the in-depth interaction between the person and technology, this model provides rehabilitation engineers with tools to consider, develop, design and implement client-centered assistive technology solutions.

2.4 Assistive technology: The human

Development of successful AT solutions requires an understanding of the user's needs, preferences and cultural, social and other environmental backgrounds (Mihailidis and Polgar 2016). Use of a client-centered process by rehabilitation engineers supports acquisition of this understanding. But what exactly does it mean to practice in a client-centered manner? This section provides an overview of the important factors that rehabilitation engineers must consider when designing or developing AT.

2.4.1 Needs and wants

At the center of the AT process are the needs and preferences of the user. Guiding questions that can help identify such needs and wants include:

- What does the user want to do?
- How is that activity meaningful/important to the user?
- What are the demands of that activity that AT may be able to bridge?
- How can AT enable participation in what the client wants and needs to do?
- What characteristics or features of the AT would suit the clients' preferences?

The user's need to perform a meaningful activity determines whether an AT device is the best approach, and that drives the selection and implementation of the device. For example, a client may wish to access their computer to engage in work-related activities, or to communicate with family and friends. The demands of these two scenarios may require two different AT solutions, which are informed by the meaning the client ascribes to each activity.

Personal meaning is derived from a user's previous experiences, the sense of competence, accomplishment, challenge and emotional engagement with a certain activity (Cook and Polgar 2014). Thus, personal meaning is fluid, dynamic and may change over time. As part of an interdisciplinary team, rehabilitation engineers ensure timely engagement of the user in the service or development processes and consider the meaning the user attributes to certain activities. User involvement informs the selection of AT, or the design and customization of available options that can be useful in the desired context. By partnering with users as primary stakeholders of the AT process, practitioners can ensure that the AT solutions are satisfactory to the user, increasing the likelihood of long-term use.

2.4.2 Body structures and functions

In order to perform an activity and participate in a meaningful occupation, the activity and environmental demands must match the person's skills (Townsend and Polatajko 2013). AT provides one means by which a match between the user's skills and activity engagement can be achieved. Critical to that process is the identification of the different motor, cognitive and sensory functions and emotional state of the user as they affect activity performance. The ICF (WHO 2001) provides a standardized framework that describes human functioning in the context of health and disability. Used across multiple settings and populations by both healthcare professionals and government agencies, the ICF can assist rehabilitation engineers in considering the body functions that influence activity performance and AT use.

The ICF defines body functions as "physiological functions of body systems (including psychological functions)" (WHO 2001). These include: mental functions (i.e., functions that allow an individual to be alert and responsive to the environment, to communicate with others, to process and analyze information, to learn, reason and organize their behavior); sensory (i.e., those pertaining to all forms of sensation, such as seeing, hearing, tasting, touching or pain); voice and speech (functions that involve the production of sounds and speech); respiratory functions (i.e., respiration and exercise tolerance); neuromusculoskeletal and movement-related functions (i.e., movement and mobility), among others (WHO 2001). Evaluation of the user's function (existing and future) in relevant categories of the ICF is necessary to determine implications for AT use. For example, an individual who has experienced a change in voice functions may not benefit from voice-activated technologies. Alternately, identification of reliable movements is useful for determination of how the user will access/control the AT.

2.4.3 Habits and roles

In addition to considering the person's wants, needs and body functions, client-centered AT requires careful consideration of a person's habits and roles. Habits are "behavior patterns operating below conscious awareness that are acquired through context-dependent repetition" (Fritz and Cutchin 2016, 92–98). For example, an older adult may be accustomed to picking up and reading the newspaper every morning, while a younger adult may check the news online upon arrival at work. Habits influence AT design and selection because they may impact how a person wishes to use their AT device, or the ways in which she or he will incorporate it in their daily routines. Successful use of AT may require individuals to become aware of and modify their habits. For example, an older adult with vision loss will need to adapt their occupation of newspaper reading if they can no longer read print and use an auditory means to learn news.

Roles, on the other hand, comprise "a set of socially agreed upon expectations, functions or obligations … that a person assumes and which become part of that person's social identity" (Reed 2005, 567–626). Examples of roles include parent, student, employee, etc. Roles are dependent on cultural expectations and socially constructed norms. Understanding a user's roles is necessary, given that using an AT solution to perform an activity may differ from one role to another. For example, a user may need to read a lengthy technical document at work and provide feedback, which will require a word processor that is easily accessible. The same user may also need to read a story to a child, which requires an intelligible voice output. Activities associated with different roles require different AT solutions.

2.4.4 Technology acceptance

Technology acceptance refers to an individual's favorable reception, approval and intention to use a new technology (Arning and Ziefle 2007). An adequate and thorough consideration of client factors can increase the likelihood of improved user satisfaction and the identification of an AT solution that meets the needs of the user. The MPT suite of assessments is designed to maximize the likelihood of device acceptance and use (Corradi, Scherer and Lo Presti 2012).

A growing body of literature identifies client factors as primary determinants of technology abandonment among AT users. In 1993, for example, Phillips and Zhao (1993) reported that out of 227 AT users with disabilities, 29.3% had completely abandoned the use of their device. More recently, Cruz and Emmel (Cruz et al. 2016) found that 37% of participants in their sample (n = 91) who reported abandoning the use of their AT device, did so because they "did not like it." Barriers to AT acceptance include habits and routines, the perceived matching of devices to the age, gender and lifestyle of the user and the attitudes of the user's family and friends towards the device (Corradi, Scherer and Lo Presti 2012; Ravneberg

2012). Thus, rehabilitation engineers must partner with users to address the client factors that can lead to long-term adoption and use of the device.

2.5 Assistive technology: The activity

2.5.1 Mobility

According to the ICF (WHO 2001), mobility is the process of moving from one place to another, including very localized moving (e.g., from sitting to standing), as well as moving over greater distances (e.g., within a neighborhood and beyond). Several conditions (including neurological, cardiopulmonary, musculoskeletal, etc.) can impair mobility.

AT for localized mobility involves equipment such as transfer/sliding boards, lifts, grab bars or rails. Simpler items that support mobility over longer distances include canes, crutches and walkers. As mobility needs increase, users require greater AT support in the form of wheelchairs (manual and powered) or scooters (see Chapter 12 for more details). Given the great variability among intended use, preferences and biomechanical considerations, wheelchairs are among the most complex mobility ATs. Considerations regarding wheelchairs include type (e.g., manual vs powered); use setting (e.g., indoors vs smooth terrain); degree of adjustability (e.g., options for stability vs mobility of propulsion); complexity (e.g., addition of features such as tilt and recline) and seating (i.e., systems that provide postural support, maintain tissue integrity and provide comfort) (Cook and Polgar 2014). In addition, powered wheelchairs require careful consideration of controllers. Depending on the user's ability to reliably control body parts, the chair can be operated via a joystick, or through an array of mechanical, pneumatic or proximity switches. Smart wheelchairs are still in the developmental phase at this time. These chairs provide different levels of autonomy for key functions such as navigation and collision avoidance. Ultimately, these chairs may be fully autonomous in all wheelchair functions; however, in the short term, it is likely that most will require at least some action on the part of the user to navigate and avoid collisions.

Other devices that support mobility include safe transportation mobility aids (e.g., child car seats, docking systems that secure the wheelchair to the vehicle), vehicle modifications (e.g., left-foot accelerator) and orientation aids for people with low vision (e.g., long canes with which the user detects obstacles in the forward path of travel).

2.5.2 Manipulation and control of the environment

Manipulation refers to those activities that we normally accomplish using the fingers and hands. Gross motor manipulation includes reaching, grasp/release, lifting, carrying and coordination of pushing, pulling, throwing/catching (WHO 2001). Fine motor manipulation includes pinch, point and dexterity of finger movements for computer entry, joystick control and switch-activated AT. Handwriting, food preparation, eating, using door handles and elevator buttons and appliance control depend on manipulation. Manipulation can be limited by conditions that affect range of motion, strength, cause pain or result in deformities, including musculoskeletal (e.g., osteoporosis, fracture and amputation) and neuromuscular (e.g., cerebral palsy, spinal cord injury, stroke, traumatic brain injury, amyotrophic lateral sclerosis) conditions. People who experience these conditions can benefit from manipulative aids.

Manipulative aids are either alternative (a different method) or augmentative (assistance). Devices can be either specific purpose, designed for one task, or general purpose, for two or more tasks. Turning pages in a book can be done with a mouth stick (general purpose) or an electronic page-turner (specific purpose). A robotic arm is a general-purpose manipulative aid. A hand splint is a general-purpose aid that can be used to hold a fork for eating or a pen for writing. Mainstream tools or appliances can also be fitted with enlarged, ergonomically designed or telescoping handles (e.g., utensils). High-tech manipulation devices include electronic aids to daily living (EADLs) that control appliances, entertainment electronics and doors and windows (Cook and Polgar 2014). The high cost of these devices is not generally publicly funded.

2.5.3 Communication

Augmentative and alternative communication (AAC) is a form of AT that supports people who have complex communication needs (CCN) across their lifespan. AAC strategies include high-tech solutions such as speech-generating devices (SGDs), which are devices or apps that produce digitally recorded or synthesized speech output. People with CCN who obtain SGDs can live independently, develop social relationships and be active members of their communities (Bryen, Cohen and Carey 2004; Collier 2005). AAC also includes low-tech solutions, such as unaided or body-based communication. These strategies require only the person's own body, such as pointing and other gestures, pantomime, facial expressions, eye-gaze and manual signing or finger spelling. Users may also benefit from aided AAC including a pen or pencil, a letter or picture communication board, a computer, a cellphone or an SGD.

Estimates indicate that approximately two million people in the United States, and between 0.3% and 1.0% of the total world population of school-aged children have a need for AAC (Beukelman and Mirenda 2012). Infants, toddlers and preschoolers with CCN require AAC for development of language, communication and literacy. Individuals who acquire disabilities later in life need AAC for work, relationships, social networks and independence.

2.5.4 Cognition

The ICF (WHO 2001) refers to cognitive functions as including general and specific mental functions. Relevant to AT, the general classification includes orientation—to time, to place, to self and to objects. AT has more application when considering the classification of specific mental functions: Memory, attention, perception, knowledge acquisition, organization and application, higher level or executive functions of planning, time management and concept formation. Cognition can be impaired through a congenital disability such as an intellectual impairment (e.g., Down syndrome), or through an acquired disability (e.g., traumatic brain injury, dementia). As a result, users with varying needs and skills may benefit from cognitive AT throughout their life span.

AT options to support cognitive functions have exploded recently. They involve low technology such as paper-based day planners, and complex electronic devices such as computers, smartphones and robotic technologies. Smart technology has the benefit of being highly customizable. It can be programmed to provide a simple sequence of pictures to guide an individual with an intellectual impairment through the completion of a desired task. Alternately, it can be very complex, requiring multiple steps and explicit sequences of actions for successful use; GPS navigation system programming is an example of a complex system.

2.6 Ethical tensions in assistive technology: Challenges and opportunities

By supporting people with disabilities to participate in the activities they want and need to do, AT can have important positive impacts on a person's autonomy and social participation. However, the development, implementation and monitoring of AT also result in complex ethical considerations that rehabilitation engineers must acknowledge and be equipped to address. AT can also support the independence and participation of older adults who may experience age-related impairments. A fast-growing segment of the world's population, older adults increasingly face needs that can be supported by the use of AT including but not limited to mobility, cognition, social interactions and health management. Such growing demand for targeted user-centered design, development and implementation expands the opportunities and challenges that AT practitioners will face. For example, privacy has already emerged as a determinant of home healthcare robot adoption for older adults, highlighting emerging tensions between safety and privacy in AT for older adults (Alaiad, Zhou and Koru 2014).

The following sections provide an overview of the most prominent principle-based AT ethical issues and considerations. Although not exhaustive, these sections are meant to elicit reflection among student rehabilitation engineers and professionals regarding ethical tensions in AT (see Chapter 8 for more details). Overall, partnering effectively and proactively with the user and other stakeholders (e.g., healthcare professionals, family, caregivers, etc.) provides a suitable environment and opportunity to discuss and consider the ethical tensions and implications of any AT decision.

2.6.1 Autonomy

The principle of autonomy refers to a person's right to self-determination, and to be free from privacy risks and unnecessary constraints (Alvarez and Cook 2017). In its most basic form, this principle requires AT practitioners to provide thorough and comprehensive information regarding the available options, features and limitations of the technology, and equip users to make informed decisions. Rehabilitation engineers have a mandate to ensure that adequate information regarding privacy concerns is available to the user and other stakeholders. For example, monitoring technologies for individuals with Alzheimer's disease may support a person's safety but may be invasive of a person's privacy. The issues in this scenario are complicated even further when considering that the user may be unable or unwilling to provide informed consent.

2.6.2 Fidelity

In the context of healthcare, users expect to be treated with respect by a loyal, trustworthy professional who is both competent and follows regulations and procedures (Purtilo 2005). Such notions comprise fidelity and extend to professionals involved in the AT process. A rehabilitation engineer may encounter fidelity-related ethical tensions when there is a conflict between what they think the technology can offer, what the funding agency is willing to provide, and what the user wants. In addition, conflicts of interest may compromise the engineer's fidelity when the interests of industries, manufacturers and funding agencies are at odds. Such ethical tensions require a responsible adherence to the professional code of ethics, and transparency with the client and other stakeholders.

2.6.3 Beneficence and non-maleficence

As primary stakeholders in the AT process, rehabilitation engineers have a mandate to strive for the good of the user (beneficence) and avoid doing harm (non-maleficence). Specifically, the rehabilitation engineer will need to develop AT devices that will put the user first at all times. An example of a problematic area includes robotics (Alvarez and Cook 2017). When programming a companion robot or a driverless vehicle, rehabilitation engineers will face important dilemmas pertaining to the safety of devices, which are incapable moral reasoning. As such, engineers must engage in critical reflection and discussions regarding the ethical implications of emerging technologies.

2.6.4 Justice

As a principle for ethical consideration, justice is "the moral obligation to act on the basis of fair adjudication between competing claims" (Gillon 1994, 184–188). Fair adjudication involves considerations of price, affordability, access and opportunity. Rehabilitation engineers face important questions regarding the need for capital that can support AT innovations, while ensuring accessibility and affordability of the finished product, especially for marginalized populations.

2.6.5 Stigma

Although AT can increase a person's ability to participate in social contexts, the use of AT can result in users being perceived as "less able" or "weak" (Alvarez and Cook 2017). Rehabilitation engineers can reduce opportunities for stigma by partnering with stakeholders and involving users and caregivers in the design and development process, and considering aesthetic and environmental factors in their developments.

2.7 Future vision

Rapid advancements in technological innovations open a future of possibilities for AT. Robots that can reduce social isolation, automated vehicles that can increase the community mobility of medically unfit drivers and SGDs with improved speech output are but some of the examples of what the future of AT seems to hold. But, if people are to remain at the center of what drives AT, "a human doing an activity in context" (Cook and Polgar 2014), then rehabilitation engineers and other AT practitioners must work towards a future beyond technical advancements. Ultimately, the future of AT must be defined by increased autonomy, self-determination, access, opportunity and participation for people with disabilities. AT practitioners must partner with users and stakeholders (policymakers, funding agencies, governments and regulatory agencies) to ensure that AT is characterized by equity and client-centered practice. Universal access and the use of mainstream technologies may offer opportunities toward the pursuit of this goal.

2.8 Discussion questions

1. What is the role of the rehabilitation engineer in an interdisciplinary AT team?
2. What considerations must the rehabilitation engineer integrate when practicing in an AT setting)? How do these considerations differ from other rehabilitation engineering settings?

3. What are some examples of integrating client-centered practice in rehabilitation engineering? How can target users be involved in the research and design process?
4. How do AT models influence AT design, development, delivery and evaluation?
5. What is the responsibility of rehabilitation engineers in regard to AT ethical tensions?

Bibliography

Alaiad, A., L. Zhou, and G. Koru. 2014. "An Exploratory Study of Home Healthcare Robots Adoption Applying the UTAUT Model." *International Journal of Healthcare Information Systems and Informatics (IJHISI)* 9 (4): 44–59.

Alvarez, L. and A. Cook. 2017. "Ethical and Social Implications of the Use of Robots in Rehabilitation Practice." In *Robotic Assistive Technologies: Principles and Practice*, edited by P. Encarnao and A. Cook, 333–358. Boca Raton, FL: CRC Press.

Arning, K. and M. Ziefle. 2007. "Barriers of Information Access in Small Screen Device Applications: The Relevance of User Characteristics for a Transgenerational Design." In *Universal Access in Ambient Intelligence Environments*, edited by C. Stephanidis and M. Pieper, 117–136. Heidelberg, Germany: Springer.

Beukelman, D. R. and P. Mirenda. 2012. *Augmentative & Alternative Communication: Supporting Children & Adults with Complex Communication Needs*. Baltimore, MD: Brookes Publishing Co.

Bryen, D. N., K. Cohen, and A. Carey. 2004. "Augmentative Communication Employment Training and Supports (ACETS): Some Employment-Related Outcomes." *The Journal of Rehabilitation* 70 (1): 10–18.

Collier, B. 2005. "When I Grow Up...Supporting Youth Who Use Augmentative Communication for Adulthood."

Cook, A. and S. Hussey. 2002. *Assistive Technology: Principles and Practice*. St. Louis, MO: Mosby.

Cook, A. and J. Polgar. 2012. *Essentials of Assistive Technologies*. St. Louis, MO: Elsevier Mosby.

———. 2014. *Assistive Technologies: Principles and Practice*. St. Louis, MO: Elsevier Mosby.

———. 2015. "Activity, Human, and Context: The Human Doing an Activity in Context." In *Assistive Technologies: Principles & Practices*. 4th ed., 41. St. Louis, MO: Mosby Elsevier.

Corradi, F., M. J. Scherer, and A. Lo Presti. 2012. "Measuring the Assistive Technology Match." In *Assistive Technology Assessment Handbook*, edited by S. Federici and M. J. Scherer, 53–69. London, UK: CRC Press.

Cruz, D. M., M. G. Emmel, M. G. Manzini, and P. V. Braga Mendes. 2016. "Assistive Technology Accessibility and Abandonment: Challenges for Occupational Therapists." *The Open Journal of Occupational Therapy* 4 (1). https://doi.org/10.15453/2168-6408.1166

Demers, L., M. J. Fuhrer, J. W. Jutai, M. J. Scherer, I. Pervieux, and F. DeRuyter. 2008. "Tracking Mobility-Related Assistive Technology in an Outcomes Study." *Assistive Technology* 20 (2): 73–83.

Duncan, E. A. S. 2006. *Foundations for Practice in Occupational Therapy*. London, UK: Elsevier Churchill Livingstone.

Field, D. 1999. "Powered Mobility: A Literature Review Illustrating the Importance of a Multifaceted Approach." *Assistive Technology* 11 (1): 20–33.

Fok, D. 2011. "Development and Testing of a Low Vision Product Selection Instrument (Lv-Psi): A Mixed-Methods Approach." University of Western Ontario.

Fritz, H. and M. P. Cutchin. 2016. "Integrating the Science of Habit: Opportunities for Occupational Therapy." *OTJR (Thorofare NJ)* 36 (2): 92–98.

Giesbrecht, E. 2013. "Application of the Human Activity Assistive Technology Model for Occupational Therapy Research." *Aust Occup Ther J* 60 (4): 230–240.

Gillon, R. 1994. "Medical Ethics: Four Principles Plus Attention to Scope." *BMJ (Clinical Research Ed.)* 309 (6948): 184–188.

Gitlin, L. N. 1998. "From Hospital to Home: Individual Variations in Experience with Assistive Devices among Older Adults." In *Designing and Using Assistive Technology*, edited by D. B. Gray, L. A. Quatrano and M. L. Lieberman, 109–122. Baltimore, MD: Paul H. Brookes.

Hersh, M. and M. Johnson. 2008a. "On Modelling Assistive Technology Systems – Part I: Modelling Framework." *Technology and Disability* 20 (3): 193–215.

———. 2008b. "On Modelling Assistive Technology Systems Part 2: Applications of the Comprehensive Assistive Technology Model." *Technology and Disability* 20 (4): 251–270.

Hoppestad, B. S. 2004. "Essential Elements for Assessment of Persons with Severe Neurological Impairments for Computer Access Using Assistive Technology Devices: A Delphi Study." University of Tennessee. http://trace.tennessee.edu/cgi/viewcontent.cgi?article=3771&context=utk_graddiss.

Mihailidis, A. and J. M. Polgar. 2016. "Occupational Therapy and Engineering: Being Better Together." *Can J Occup Ther* 83 (2): 68–69.

Phillips, B. and H. Zhao. 1993. "Predictors of Assistive Technology Abandonment." *Assistive Technology* 5 (1): 36–45.

Purtilo, R. 2005. *Ethical Dimensions in the Health Professions*. Philadelphia, PA: Elsevier Saunders.

Ravneberg, B. 2012. "Usability and Abandonment of Assistive Technology." *Journal of Assistive Technologies* 6 (4): 259–269.

Reed, K. L. 2005. "An Annotated History of the Concepts Used in Occupational Therapy." *Occupational Therapy: Performance, Participation, and Well-Being*, edited by C. Christiansen, C. Manville Baum, and J. Bass-Haugen, 567–626. New Jersey: Slack, Thorofare, NJ.

Sackett, D. L., W. M. Rosenberg, J. A. Gray, R. B. Haynes, and W. S. Richardson. 1996. "Evidence Based Medicine: What it is and What it isn't." *BMJ* 312 (7023): 71–72.

Scherer, M. J. 2002. *Assistive Technology: Matching Device and Consumer for Successful Rehabilitation*. Washington, DC: American Psychological Association.

Scherer, M. J. and R. Glueckauf. 2005. "Assessing the Benefits of Assistive Technologies for Activities and Participation." *Rehabilitation Psychology* 50 (2): 132–141.

Seeler, K. A. 2014. *System Dynamics: An Introduction for Mechanical Engineers*. New York: Springer.

Smith, R. O. 1991. "Technological Approaches to Performance Enhancement." In *Occupational Therapy: Overcoming Human Performance Deficits*, edited by C. Baum and C. Christiansen, 747–786. Thorofare, NJ: Slack.

Townsend, E. and H. Polatajko. 2013. *Enabling Occupation II: Advancing an Occupational Therapy Vision for Health, Well-Being and Justice through Occupation*. Ottawa, ON: Canadian Association of Occupational Therapists.

WHO. 2001. *World Health Organization: International Classification of Functioning, Disability and Health: ICF*. Geneva. Switzerland: World Health Organization.

Zabala, J. S. 2002. *Resources for Assistive Technology in Education: About the SETT Framework*. Vol. 2019. Alberta.

Chapter 3 Key human anatomy and physiology principles as they relate to rehabilitation engineering

Qussai Obiedat, Bhagwant S. Sindhu, and Ying-Chih Wang

Contents

3.1 Chapter overview

For rehabilitation engineers and assistive technology practitioners, it is critical to have basic knowledge of human body systems. Human body systems are one of the many factors that impact the ability of an individual to function, which includes body functions, activities, and participation (WHO 2001). In 2001, the World Health Organization (WHO) published the International Classification of Functioning, Disability, and Health (ICF) – its present approach to classify disability and function (WHO 2001). As described in more detail in this chapter, the ICF provides an interactive model of disability by defining disability as "the outcome of dynamic interaction between health conditions (diseases, disorders, injuries, etc.) and contextual environment" (Hurst 2003; Kearney and Pryor 2004). The ICF has a total of four components: (a) body functions and structures, (b) activities and participation, (c) environmental factors, and (d) personal factors. These four components interact with each other indicating a multi-directional perspective of human health. At a cellular level, the ICF uses the term "body function" to describe physiological and psychological functions of the body systems and "body structure" as the anatomic parts of the body. Problems in the body structure or function may result in an impairment. Further, the ICF defines an activity as "execution of a task in a uniform environment" and participation as "involvement in a life situation in the current environment of the individual." Although the ICF describes activity and participation as separate entities, the ICF classifies them together as it can be difficult to distinguish the two factors in the context of physical, social, and attitudinal world (WHO 2001). Furthermore, the ICF incorporates the social approaches of disablement by including environmental factors (Bickenbach et al. 1999). Environmental factors constitute the physical, social, and attitudinal environment in which the individual lives. These factors focus on the individual and the society. In contrast to environmental factors, personal factors indicate the background of an individual, including gender, race, and age (WHO 2001). Overall, the ICF emphasizes the complex interaction between the health status of an individual and the various contextual factors, which include environmental and personal factors (Hurst 2003; Kearney and Pryor 2004). Therefore, knowledge and understanding of various body systems and how they interact with other components of the ICF can assist rehabilitation engineers and assistive technology practitioners in developing solutions that will not only be accepted by the individual but also enhance their performance and participation (Baum et al. 2010).

The purpose of this chapter is to provide a brief introduction to key concepts of human body systems as they relate to rehabilitation engineering. Major human body systems include integumentary, muscular, skeletal, circulatory, nervous, lymphatic, respiratory, endocrine, digestive, urinary, and reproductive systems. In this chapter, we will briefly review musculoskeletal, integumentary, nervous, cardiovascular, and respiratory systems as they are commonly affected among individuals receiving rehabilitation services. The different systems in our body are interconnected and function as a unit. Consequently, an injury to one system may affect other systems as well, resulting in multiple impairments. Table 3.1 lists some examples of common disorders that may affect different body systems with some sample interventions. For a comprehensive review of human anatomy and physiology, please refer to textbooks written for rehabilitation professionals such as physical and occupational therapists. Rehabilitation professionals typically complete five or more university-level courses to gain a comprehensive understanding of concepts related to human body systems, including human anatomy, physiology, neuroscience, and kinesiology.

64

Table 3.1 Exemplars of Disorders Affecting Individuals Receiving Rehabilitation Services, with Brief Descriptions of Affected Body Systems, Related Symptoms, Functional Limitations, and Typical Rehabilitation Interventions

Disorders	Affected Systems	Example of Related Symptoms	Example of Functional Limitations	Sample Intervention
Arthritis	Musculoskeletal	Joint pain Range of motion (ROM) restriction	Inability to write	Splinting/Orthotics
Stroke	Nervous Musculoskeletal	Hemiplegia	Inability to speak	Augmentative and Alternative Communication (AAC) device
Burns	Integumentary Musculoskeletal Nervous	ROM restriction Loss of sensation	Inability to reach	Workspace modification
Traumatic brain injury (TBI)	Nervous Musculoskeletal	Hand tremor	Inability to hold tools or utensils	Weighted or stabilizing hand grips
Spinal cord injury (SCI)	Nervous Integumentary Musculoskeletal Cardiovascular Respiratory	Quadriplegia/Paraplegia	Inability to walk	Wheelchair

3.2 Musculoskeletal system

The musculoskeletal system in the human body consists of bones and muscles, as well as cartilage, ligaments, joints, and other connective tissues that support and connect different body organs and tissues together. This system is responsible for providing the human body shape, support, stability, as well as movement (Lippert 2006). The scientific study of human movement is termed kinesiology. Kinesiology is a general umbrella term that combines the fields of anatomy, physiology, physics, and geometry, and links them to human movement. Therefore, kinesiology uses principles of mechanics, musculoskeletal anatomy, and neuromuscular physiology. In contrast, biomechanics is the study of mechanical principles that are related directly to the study of the human body, especially studying internal and external forces exerted on the skeleton (Hamill, Knutzen, and Derrick 2015). The emphasis of this section of this chapter is to provide a fundamental understanding of the human muscles and skeleton, including joints.

Before we describe the components of the human musculoskeletal system, it is essential to understand the terminology commonly used to describe the location of a body structure and its position relative to other structures, as well as to describe different body movements. This terminology is essential for rehabilitation engineers to be able to communicate effectively with rehabilitation and medical professionals.

As the human body is constantly moving, the relationship between various body parts to each other is continuously changing. Thus, we need an arbitrary position to act as a starting frame from which the location of different body structures or movements can be described. Two arbitrary positions are used to fulfill this need and are called anatomical and fundamental positions. The anatomical position portrays the human body in an upright standing position, with eyes facing forward and feet close together pointing forward, arms by the sides with the hands facing forward (Figure 3.1). In contrast, the fundamental position portrays the body in the same position as the anatomical position except for the hands facing the sides of the body (Lippert 2006) (Figure 3.1). In both positions, specific terms are used to describe the location of one body structure and its relative position to another. Table 3.2 summarizes some of the commonly used terms with examples for describing the location of body structures.

In addition, there are specific terms that are used to describe the movements of different body parts. Generally, flexion is a term used to describe the bending movement of one bone on another, causing a decrease in the joint angle. Extension is the straightening movement that causes an increase of the joint angle, and usually returns the body part to the anatomical position after it has been flexed. The

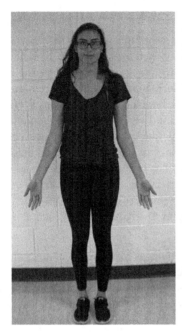 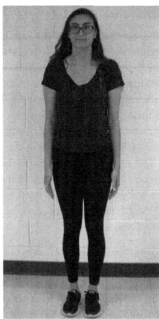

Figure 3.1 Anatomical position. Fundamental position (courtesy of Qussai Obiedat, 2019).

Table 3.2 Commonly Used Terms Describing Anatomical Location

Term	Description	Example
Superior	Above a body structure	Eyes are superior to the nose
Inferior	Below a body structure	The nose is inferior to the eyes
Anterior	To the front of the body	Sternum is anterior to the scapula
Posterior	To the back of the body	The scapula is posterior to the sternum
Medial	Toward the body midline	The sternum is medial to the ribs
Lateral	Away from the body midline	The shoulders are lateral to the spinal column
Proximal	Toward the origin	The hip is proximal to the knee
Distal	Away from the origin	The elbow is distal to the shoulder

continuation of extension beyond the anatomical position is known as hyperextension. Abduction is the movement of a body part away from the body midline, and the reversed movement is known as adduction (Lippert 2006). Movements associated with specific joints are described in the following subsection on the muscular system.

3.2.1 Skeletal system

The human skeleton provides a rigid framework that supports the body and gives it shape, while skeletal muscles that are attached to bones move the skeleton. The skeleton also protects some internal organs, contains and protects the red bone marrow which is responsible for blood formation, and stores excess calcium in the body (Scanlon and Sanders 2007). The human skeleton contains a total of 206 bones, and they are grouped into two main divisions: axial skeleton and appendicular skeleton. The axial skeleton forms the axis of the body and consists of approximately 80 bones including the bones of the skull, vertebral column, and rib cage. The appendicular skeleton attaches to the axial skeleton and contains the 126 bones of the extremities (Lippert 2006). There are four bone types in the human body: 1) long bones such as the humerus, 2) short bones such as wrist carpals, 3) flat bones such as scapula, and 4) irregular bones such as vertebrae (Scanlon and Sanders 2007).

A joint is described as the area where two bones meet or articulate (Scanlon and Sanders 2007). The human body includes several types of joints, and the amount of motion allowed in each type varies. Some joints allow a wide range of motion, such as the shoulder joint, while others allow for very limited motion, such as the acromioclavicular joint. In addition, some joints may allow motion around more than one axis, while other joints move around a single axis. This is known as degrees of freedom of a joint. For example, the hip joint has three degrees of freedom while the elbow joint has only one degree of freedom. Besides allowing motion, joints also help to bear the weight of the body and provide stability to the body (Lippert 2006). In any joint in the body, movement occurs in a plane and around an axis. There are three planes of motion and three axes. Planes of motion are arbitrarily fixed planes of reference that divide the body, and each of these planes is perpendicular to the other two planes. The axis of motion is a straight line that runs through the center of a joint around which a part rotates (Lippert 2006). Table 3.3 illustrate the three planes and axes, and the motions occurring in each (Figures 3.2.1 to 3.2.6).

Studying the healthy structure and function of the skeletal system is essential for understanding normal body movements, and how a pathology or an injury affects a specific movement. Disorders affecting the skeletal system may interrupt the normal mechanics of body movements. Some of these interruptions are temporary, such as those resulting from fractures, while other interruptions could have a lasting effect, such as joint arthritis or deformities. Rehabilitation engineers should have a working knowledge of these different conditions and the way they affect body movements in order to accommodate the disturbed status of the body when designing or implementing any related technology or solution. For example, lordosis, kyphosis, and scoliosis are types of spine deformities, which occur when the natural curvatures of the spine are misaligned or exaggerated in certain areas.

Table 3.3 Illustration of Planes of Motion and Axes of Rotation

Plane	Description	Plane Figure	Axis	Description	Axis Figure	Motion
Sagittal	Perpendicular to the ground and passes through the body from front to back, dividing it into left and right	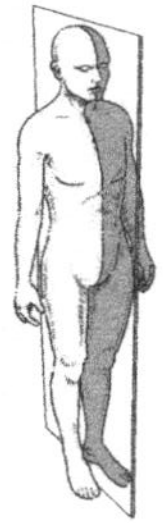 Figure 3.2.1 Sagittal plane.	Frontal	Runs through a joint from side to side	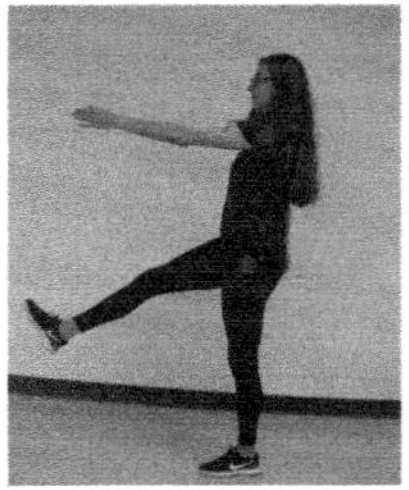 Figure 3.2.2 Frontal axis (courtesy of Qussai Obiedat, 2019).	Flexion/Extension
Frontal (coronal)	Perpendicular to the ground and passes through the body side to side, dividing it into front and back	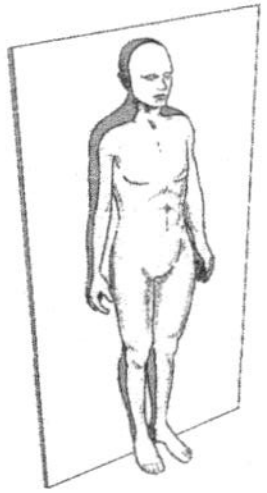 Figure 3.2.3 Frontal (coronal) plane.	Sagittal	Runs through a joint from front to back	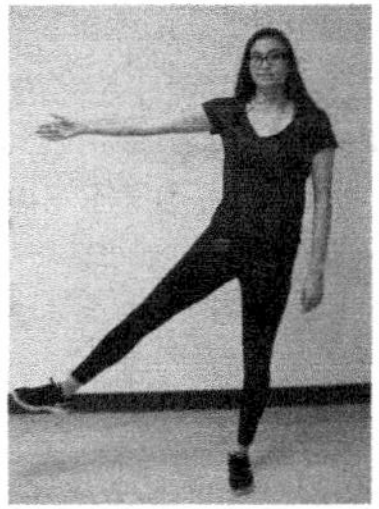 Figure 3.2.4 Sagittal axis (courtesy of Qussai Obiedat, 2019).	Abduction/adduction Radial/ulnar deviation Eversion/inversion

(Continued)

69

Table 3.3 (Continued) Illustration of Planes of Motion and Axes of Rotation

Plane	Description	Plane Figure	Axis	Description	Axis Figure	Motion
Transverse (horizontal)	Parallel to the ground and passes the body through horizontally, dividing it into top and bottom	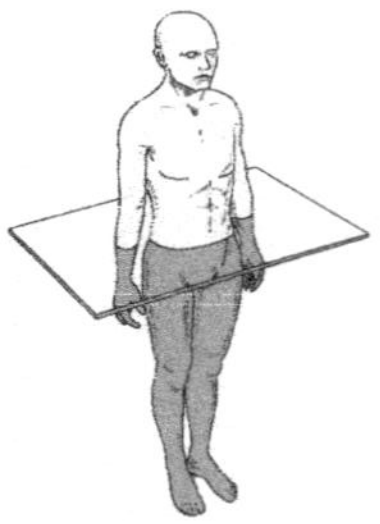 Figure 3.2.5 Transverse (horizontal) plane.	Vertical (longitudinal)	Runs through a joint from top to bottom	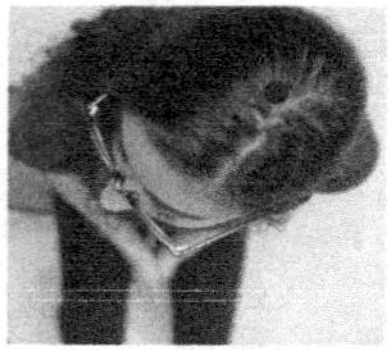 Figure 3.2.6 Vertical (longitudinal) axis (courtesy of Qussai Obiedat, 2019).	Medial/lateral rotation Supination/ pronation Right/left rotation Horizontal abduction/ adduction

Source: Courtesy of Qussai Obiedat, 2019

Typically, the manifestation of these deformities is unique and different for each individual. For example, an individual with muscular dystrophy, who has a co-occurring spinal deformity, using a powered wheelchair may require a customized seating and positioning solution in order to prevent the progression of the deformity and to maximize functional abilities.

3.2.2 Muscular system

The human body contains more than 600 skeletal muscles. Most of these muscles are attached to the skeleton, while a few are attached to the undersurface of the skin, such as palmaris longus in the upper limb. The primary function of skeletal muscles is to move the skeleton. In addition, muscles protect internal organs, as well as produce heat, when contracting, to help maintain body temperature (Scanlon and Sanders 2007). Generally, each skeletal muscle crosses at least one joint and has at least two tendons that attach both ends of a muscle into two different sites, the origin and insertion. The origin is the less movable or stationary attachment of the muscle, and the insertion is the more movable attachment (Lippert 2006). Typically, when a muscle contracts, the muscle shortens, moving the joint and bringing the insertion closer to the origin. Thus, muscles can only provide a pulling force and cannot generate a pushing force, and when they relax, they exert no force. However, muscle contraction does not always involve motion (Lippert 2006).

Skeletal muscles produce three types of contractions: (1) isometric, (2) isotonic, and (3) isokinetic. First, during an isometric contraction, a muscle generates a force to hold a joint in its position without any change in the muscle length or motion in the joint (Lippert 2006). For example, when holding a dumbbell in a hand while maintaining the elbow flexed at a 90-degree angle, the biceps brachii muscle, which is one of the elbow flexor muscles, is in isometric contraction. Second, during an isotonic contraction, the muscle's length and joint angle change. For example, when holding a dumbbell in your hand and flexing the elbow to bring it up toward the shoulder, the biceps brachii muscle is in isotonic contraction. The isotonic contraction is further subdivided into two phases: concentric and eccentric contractions. During a concentric contraction, a muscle shortens, bringing the origin and insertion of that muscle closer to each other. Therefore, the earlier example of moving the dumbbell toward the shoulder is an example of isotonic concentric contraction. In contrast, during an eccentric contraction, a muscle lengthens to move the origin and insertion away from each other while controlling the speed of the movement. For example, after bringing the dumbbell toward your shoulder, as in a concentric contraction, when you try to extend your elbow to move the dumbbell back down slowly, the biceps brachii muscle is eccentrically contracting. Last, an isokinetic contraction is less common and requires use of special equipment (Lippert 2006). During an isokinetic contraction, both muscle length and joint angle change, but this change happens under constant speed or velocity while the resistance to the motion varies, which is regulated by special equipment. In contrast to isokinetic contraction, an isotonic contraction involves constant resistance while the motion speed varies. Therefore, in isokinetic contraction, the machine is preset to maintain a constant speed no matter how hard a person pushes, while the resistance will vary. For example, the harder the person pushes, the machine will give more resistance, and if the person does not push as hard, the machine will generate less resistance (Lippert 2006). Several studies have shown that isokinetic exercises can lead to better strength gains in both young and old individuals, and thus can be used as an intervention for individuals with musculoskeletal injuries undergoing rehabilitation (Gault and Willems 2013; Symons et al. 2005; Hortobaágyi and DeVita 2000; Roig et al. 2009).

To understand how movement occurs around any joint, we have to understand the different roles that muscles assume during a certain joint motion. The role of a muscle during a joint motion depends on several variables, such as the type of joint, direction of motion, and the amount of resistance to the motion. Changes in these variables will cause a change in the muscle's role. The different roles are agonist, antagonist, stabilizer, or neutralizer (Lippert 2006). An agonist is a muscle or group of muscles that is directly responsible for causing the motion. It is also known as the prime mover. Some muscles assist in a particular motion but are not as effective as the prime mover, those are referred to as assisting movers. In order to determine whether a muscle is a prime or an assisting mover, several factors must be considered including the muscle's size, the muscle's angle of pull, leverage, and the muscle's contractile potential (Lippert 2006). These factors will be discussed later in this chapter. An antagonist performs the exact opposite motion of the agonist for the same motion, which indicates that for the motion to occur, the antagonist should be relaxed when the agonist is working. In cases when both the agonist and the antagonist are working at the same time it will result in a co-contraction, which usually occurs when we try to perform a movement that needs to be accurate and precise. A stabilizer or a fixator is responsible for providing support or stabilizing body structures surrounding the joint in which the motion is taking place to allow the agonist to work more efficiently. Finally, a neutralizer is responsible for preventing unwanted motion, typically in muscles that can perform more than one action (Lippert 2006). In order to further understand these different roles, let us consider the following example. When performing a dumbbell biceps curls exercise (Figure 3.3), the agonist role is assumed by the biceps, and the triceps will act as the antagonist. The biceps brachii is responsible for both elbow flexion as well as forearm supination, and since only elbow flexion movement is desired in this exercise, the pronator teres muscle (pronates the forearm) will act as a neutralizer to counteract the supination of the forearm. Several muscles will act as stabilizers, including the deltoid muscle (stabilize shoulder) and trunk muscles.

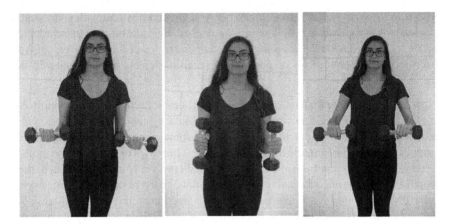

Figure 3.3 Dumbbell biceps curls exercise (courtesy of Qussai Obiedat, 2019).

During motion, both prime and assisting movers work together to perform a particular function, and those muscles are usually referred to as synergistic muscles. The biceps brachii is responsible for elbow flexion, but it is not the only muscle. The brachioradialis and brachialis are also responsible for the same motion. The role of prime mover will depend on the angle of pull of each muscle when performing the motion. In the biceps curls example, the biceps brachii will act as the prime mover when performing the exercise while the hand is palm-up. When the hand is thumb-up, the brachioradialis takes over to become the prime mover, while the brachialis will become the prime mover when the hand is palm-down (Scanlon and Sanders 2007). Another thing to consider when thinking about muscles' angle of pull is that our body contains several pulleys. Pulleys are formed from bone prominences in the body and are responsible for changing the direction or the angle of pull, and the amount of force generated by the contracted muscles. For example, the patella (kneecap) acts as a pulley for the tendons of the quadriceps muscle. It changes the direction of pull to perform a knee extension and improves the mechanical advantage of the quadriceps muscle (Lippert 2006).

Another factor to consider is how many joints a muscle crosses in the body. Single-joint muscles are those that span only one joint, while multi-joint muscles span two or more joints. The importance of this factor is that the force magnitude and joint range of motion (ROM) will vary depending on the relative position of each joint in the multi-joint muscles. For example, try to make a fist and flex your wrist, note the ROM of your wrist. Now flex your wrist while your hand is open. You will notice that the ROM increased. The reason for this increase is due to the length of the extensor digitorum muscle. The extensor digitorum spans over the wrist and the finger joints and is responsible for the extensions of the fingers and assists in the wrist extension as well. When you are making a fist with your hand, the tendons of the extensor digitorum are stretched, thus minimizing the available ROM for wrist flexion. Major joints in the upper and lower limbs, movements in each joint, and the muscles responsible for each movement are summarized in Table 3.4.

Now, it is essential to understand how we control muscle contractions and movements in our body. All movements are controlled by the central nervous system (CNS), which includes the brain and the spinal cord. The brain generates impulses to stimulate muscle contractions. These impulses originate in the motor cortex of the CNS and transmit down the spinal cord via spinal tracts. Then, the impulses travel through the nerves (motor neurons) of the peripheral nervous system (PNS) until they reach the neuromuscular junction at the designated muscle. Here, the impulses will spread in both directions along the muscle fibers, causing the muscle to contract.

There are two strategies that a muscle uses to increase muscular force output: recruitment coding and rate coding. Recruitment coding means "sequence of motor unit activation." Muscles produce higher forces by following the size principle. That is, smaller motor units are recruited first, and successively larger motor units are recruited as the force requirement increases (Astrand and Rodahl 1977; Milner-Brown, Stein, and Yemm 1973a; Edgerton 1978). Rate coding means "frequency of motor neuron firing" which represents how frequently the motor units are activated by the nervous system. As the firing rate of the motor unit increases, it produces an increasing amount of muscular force (Astrand and Rodahl 1977; Milner-Brown, Stein, and Yemm 1973a; Milner-Brown, Stein, and Yemm 1973b; Edgerton 1978).

It is important to keep in mind that body movements for performing daily activities typically happen as a combination of movements from different body joints and segments. Movement restrictions in one joint will result in several functional limitations. Several pathologies, conditions, and injuries can affect the musculoskeletal system and result in movement and functional limitations. We need to understand the underlying pathology/condition in order to understand the limitations of people with disabilities for designing interventions. For example, scapular movement limitations will restrict upper limb upward reaching by about a third that could require modifications of workspaces, tools, or Activities of Daily Living (ADL) equipment, while the loss of pronation and supination would prevent dexterous hand motions such as placing items or typing on a keyboard. Another factor that we need to keep in mind is that people with disabilities usually develop compensatory strategies to overcome movement limitations. For example, in the case of having forward reaching limitations due to upper extremities problems, they usually tend to use trunk movements to extend their reach.

74

Table 3.4 Major Joints in Upper and Lower Limbs, Movements and Muscles Responsible for Each Movement (Lippert 2006)

Joint	Movement	Muscle(s)	Joint	Movement	Muscle(s)
Shoulder	Flexion	Anterior deltoid Coracobrachialis Pectoralis major-clavicular Biceps	**Wrist**	Radial deviation	Flexor carpi radialis Extensor carpi-radialis longus
	Extension	Latissimus dorsi Teres major Posterior deltoid Triceps-long head		Ulnar deviation	Flexor carpi ulnaris Extensor carpi ulnaris
	Abduction	Supraspinatus Middle deltoid	**Hip**	Flexion	Psoas major Sartorius Iliacus
	Adduction	Latissimus dorsi Teres major Pectoralis major		Extension	Gluteus maximus Hamstrings
	Internal rotation	Subscapularis Teres major Latissimus dorsi Pectoralis major Anterior deltoid		Abduction	Gluteus Medius Sartorius
	External rotation	Infraspinatus Teres minor Posterior deltoid		Adduction	Gracilis Pectineus Adductor brevis Adductor longus Adductor magnus

(Continued)

Table 3.4 (Continued) Major Joints in Upper and Lower Limbs, Movements and Muscles Responsible for Each Movement (Lippert 2006)

Joint	Movement	Muscle(s)	Joint	Movement	Muscle(s)
	Horizontal abduction	Posterior deltoid		Medial rotation	Gluteus minimus
	Horizontal adduction	Pectoralis major		Lateral rotation	Sartorius
		Anterior deltoid			Gemellus inferior
					Gemellus superior
					Obturator externus
					Obturator infernus
					Quadratus femoris
					Piriformis
Elbow	Flexion	Biceps	Knee	Flexion	Hamstrings
		Brachioradialis			
		Brachialis			
	Extension	Triceps		Extension	Quadriceps
Radioulnar	Supination	Supinator	Ankle	Dorsiflexion	Tibialis anterior
		Biceps			Extensor digitorum longus
					Extensor hallucis longus
	Pronation	Pronator teres		Plantarflexion	Gastrocnemius
		Pronator quadratus			Soleus
Wrist	Flexion	Flexor carpi radialis		Eversion	Peroneus longus
		Palmaris longus			Peroneus Brevis
		Flexor carpi ulnaris			Tertius
	Extension	Extensor carpi-radialis longus		Inversion	Tibialis anterior,
		Extensor carpi-radialis brevis			Tibialis posterior
		Extensor carpi ulnaris			

3.3 Integumentary system

The integumentary system comprises skin and its appendages. Skin is the largest organ and covers the entire surface of the body. Skin is composed of three primary layers: the epidermis, the dermis, and the subcutaneous tissue. The epidermis is the outermost layer of the skin, contains no blood vessels, serves as a barrier to infection, and helps the skin to regulate body temperature (Costanzo 2014; Hall 2015). The main cell types that make up the epidermis are keratinocytes (barrier function), melanocytes (cells producing pigment for skin color and protection from the UV light), Langerhans cells (antigen-presenting immune cells), and Merkel cells (receptors for light touch sensation). The epidermis is further subdivided into the following strata: corneum, lucidum, granulosum, spinosum, and basal layers. The basal cell layer has column-shaped basal cells that divide and push older cells toward the surface of the skin. As the cells move up through the skin, they differentiate and become filled with keratin, flatten and eventually die, and are sloughed off. The dermis is the layer of skin beneath the epidermis and harbors many nerve endings that provide the sense of touch and temperature. The dermis is structurally divided into two areas: a superficial layer of the papillary region composed of loose areolar connective tissue, and a deeper layer of the reticular region composed of dense irregular connective tissue. These structures and protein fibers give the dermis its properties of strength, extensibility, and elasticity. Several essential sensory receptors such as the Meissner's corpuscle (dynamic touch), the Pacinian corpuscle (pressure), the Ruffini corpuscle (stretch of skin), and a number of free nerve-ending types (pain) are in the dermis. The subcutaneous tissue, also called the hypodermis, consists primarily of loose connective tissue and lobules of fat (Costanzo 2014; Hall 2015).

Rehabilitation professionals provide services to individuals whose integumentary system may be directly injured, such as from burns, or may be affected by secondary complications, such as pressure sores post paralysis. Burns are examples of an injury that can affect the integumentary system and result in several complications. For example, joint contractures or loss of ROM could result from burns, as the burnt skin loses its elasticity due to the formation of scar tissue. Orthotics and pressure garments are some intervention examples that are commonly used by rehabilitation personnel for controlling such complications. In addition, individuals living with paralysis are at elevated risk of developing skin problems (e.g., pressure ulcers) due to limited mobility coupled with impaired sensation, and can be a devastating complication (e.g., wound healing, infections, difficulties in self-care). Pressure ulcers, for instance, could range from minor skin redness (mild) to deep craters that infect muscle and bone underneath the skin. The process may begin with an abrasion to the skin (sliding in the bed), a bump or fall that damages the skin, or prolonged and unrelieved pressure on the bony prominences, which in turn compresses a blood vessel supplying the skin with nutrients and oxygen. When skin is starved of blood for too long, tissue dies, resulting in the formation of a pressure sore, also known as a decubitus ulcer (Pendleton and Schultz-Krohn 2017). Thus, rehabilitation engineers should keep in mind such skin complications when designing and fabricating rehabilitation technologies, such as wheelchair seats, and include some features that can reduce and eliminate pressure on immobilized skin.

Currently, there are a variety of tissue-engineered artificial skins grown in a laboratory and are composed of dermis and epidermis. Alternatively, there are efforts in pursuing approaches for inducing regeneration in skin or accelerating wound closure (Bello, Falabella, and Eaglstein 2001).

3.4 Respiratory and cardiovascular systems

The respiratory system consists of the nose, nasal cavity, pharynx, larynx, trachea, bronchi and their subdivisions, and lungs, as well as associated muscles and blood vessels. A primary function of the respiratory system is respiration, which includes exhaling carbon dioxide and inhaling oxygen via the respiratory system. Other functions of the respiratory system include regulation of blood pH and assisting with voice production and olfaction (OpenStax College 2013; Putte, Regan, and Russo 2015).

The cardiovascular system primarily consists of blood, the heart, and all the associated blood vessels. A major function of the cardiovascular system is to work with the respiratory system to allow blood to transport carbon dioxide and oxygen. Other major functions of blood include transporting nutrients and body waste, as well as forming a component of the immune system. The heart functions as a pump to push blood to various organs including muscles, brain, and lungs. Generally, arteries are blood vessels that carry oxygenated blood away from the heart. Likewise, veins are blood vessels that carry deoxygenated blood toward the heart. For example, vertebral arteries travel away from the heart, up through the neck, to carry oxygenated blood to the brain. An exception to this rule is that the pulmonary artery carries deoxygenated blood away from the heart to the lungs and the pulmonary vein carries oxygenated blood from the lungs to the heart. A blockage of blood supply to an organ may result in cell death due to lack of oxygen and nutrients as well as due to an inability to remove waste products. For example, with regards to brain tissue, a sudden loss of blood supply to a region of the brain is described as ischemia. Further, a sustained ischemic condition results in necrosis (cell death) of an area of the brain and is described as an infarct. Furthermore, an infarct that presents with local neurological deficits is described as a stroke (Lundy-Ekman 2013).

The cardiovascular and respiratory systems are also referred together as the cardiopulmonary system as they work together to complete the function of respiration. A compromised cardiopulmonary system has been shown to contribute to reduced physical activity in individuals with neuromuscular disease (McDonald 2002).

When compared with conditioned individuals, poorly conditioned able-bodied individuals may have associated impairment in the cardiopulmonary system, including lower peak oxygen consumption, ventilation, stroke volume, heart rate and cardiac output, and higher heart rate and oxygen consumption at submaximal workloads (Carroll et al. 1979; Dean and Ross 1991; McDonald 2002; Sanjak et al. 1987; Sockolov et al. 1977; Wright et al. 1996). Approximately three-fourths of individuals post stroke exhibit a cardiac disease (Roth 1993; Roth 1994), which contributes to their disability (Gresham et al. 1979; Stoller et al. 2012). Consequently, individuals with stroke may benefit from cardiovascular exercise, especially to improve peak oxygen intake and walking distance, when included in their rehabilitation program (Stoller et al. 2012).

Besides paralysis, individuals experiencing an SCI are commonly affected by a range of autonomic dysregulations, including cardiovascular dysfunction. Generally, those with cervical or high-thoracic SCIs have lower resting arterial pressure than that of able-bodied individuals. Also, respiratory function is reduced to 55–59% of the predicted values for able-bodied individuals (Haisma et al. 2006). Additionally, there are several secondary complications after an SCI. For example, blood pooling in legs and/or feet, due to the paralysis of the lower limb muscles which acts as a pump to increase the venous blood return to the heart.

3.5 Nervous system

The nervous system is a complex network of neurons and associated supporting cells, which carry messages from the brain and spinal cord to various parts of the body, and vice versa. Overall, the nervous system includes both the CNS which comprises the brain and the spinal cord, and the PNS which consists of 12 pairs of cranial nerves and 31 pairs of spinal nerves, and their associated ganglia. The brain is like a computer that receives information from various parts of the body and relays messages to different body parts to control their functions. The cranial nerves and spinal nerves are like wires and cables that transmit impulses along the length of the nerve cell in the form of an electrical signal, like power lines (Lundy-Ekman 2013).

When a stimulus occurs, the **sensory neurons** receive signals through sensory receptors, detect internal or external stimuli, and generate electrical impulses. Touch, pressure, temperature, pain sensation from the skin, muscle spindles embedded in muscles, joint proprioception around joint capsules, and senses of vision, auditory, and olfactory signals are examples of the sensory receptors in the body. Signals from multiple sources travel to the thalamus via ascending pathways in the spinal cord and are further relayed to specific areas of the cerebral cortex for interpretation and integration. The thalamus is the principal relay station for all sensory input, except olfaction, to the cerebral cortex from the spinal cord, brain stem, cerebellum, and other parts of the cerebrum. The primary auditory cortex interprets characteristics of sound and hearing. The primary visual cortex receives inputs concerning shape, color, and movement. The primary olfactory area receives impulses for smell. If an action is required, the primary motor cortex, the region of the cerebral cortex involved in the planning, control, and execution of voluntary movements, transmits nerve impulses to the muscles via motor neurons (i.e., descending pathways) and makes muscles move (e.g., drinking a cup of tea, shooting a basketball, dancing). While performing a sequence of movements, the brain continues to receive feedback such as perception of movement and spatial orientation from the head and body. Besides the motor cortex, the cerebellum and the basal ganglia make essential and distinct contributions to motor control. The cerebellum reduces movement errors by detecting differences between intended and actual movements and modulates movements via its projections to the upper motor neurons. In contrast, inputs to the basal ganglia facilitate proper initiation of movement and prevent unwanted movements by tonic inhibition (Lundy-Ekman 2013).

Damage to a sensory nerve may lead to inability to detect external stimuli such as touch, pressure, or temperature sensation. If damage occurs to a motor neuron that connects the brain to an effector muscle, an individual may lose the control to move a single or a group of muscles innervated by that nerve. Damage somewhere in the ascending/sensory or descending/motor pathways will interrupt the transmission of the signals. Damage to the cerebellum may lead to a variety of motor control problems including (but not limited to) loss of coordination of motor movement, undershoot or overshoot of intended position with the hand, arm, leg, or eye (dysmetria), inability to perform rapid alternating movements (adiadochokinesia), and staggering, wide-based walking (ataxic gait). Loss of dopamine-secreting cells in the basal ganglia may lead to Parkinson's disease, a slowly progressive neurologic disorder, and is characterized by rigidity or stiffness in movements, slowness of movement, and inability to initiate movement. Accumulating Huntingtin protein in the brain, especially in cells in the basal ganglia, may gradually lead to Huntington's disease, characterized by involuntary movements (chorea), unsteady gait, and slurred speech (Lundy-Ekman 2013).

Physiologically, neural signals or electrical impulses are transmitted by the so-called action potentials that occur when the membrane potential rises and falls as ions enter and flow out of the axon membrane. An action potential begins with depolarization, during which the cell undergoes a shift in electric charge distribution in which the Na^+ channels open and Na^+ begins to enter the nerve cell resulting in less negative charge inside the cell. Then the K^+ channels open, K^+ begins to leave the cell. The Na^+ channels become refractory, no more Na^+ enters the cell. K^+ continues to leave the cell, and then gradually closes (i.e., repolarization). Lastly, the Na^+/K^+ pump restores the resting membrane potential to the original state (Lundy-Ekman 2013).

If electrical impulses travel along the neural membrane without any insulation, the axonal conduction velocity may travel at merely 2–10 m/s, the speed at which an electrochemical impulse propagates down a neural pathway. Amazingly, some neurons conduct at speed of 80–120 m/s. Such a high conduct velocity cannot be achieved by a passive flow of ions alone. To increase the conduction velocity of action potentials, the nerve fibers are further insulated with the fat-like substance forming a sheath around the nerve fibers, a process called **myelination**. The presence of myelin prevents the local current from leaking across the internodal membrane. The result is a greatly enhanced velocity of action potential conduction. The propagation of action potentials along myelinated axons from one node of Ranvier to the next node is called the saltatory conduction. As such, damage to the myelin has a significant impact on the nerve conduction velocity and the results could be devastating. For example, individuals may suffer from immune system attacks and damage to the protective myelin sheath causing communication problems between the brain and the rest of the body. Multiple sclerosis (MS) damages the myelination of the CNS, resulting in widely varying central nerve symptoms. Guillain-Barre syndrome (GBS) damages the myelination of the PNS, causing muscle weakness, reflex loss, and numbness or tingling in parts of the body. GBS can lead to temporary total body paralysis for weeks, which makes the follow-up rehabilitation a lengthy process to recondition the muscles (Lundy-Ekman 2013).

The nervous system does not have the capacity to store glucose. In order for the nervous system to maintain its electrical activity, it requires a regular supply of oxygen and glucose. The brain receives both oxygen and glucose via the blood. Thus, any interruption to the blood flow to the brain may result in compromised neurological function due to damage to nervous tissue, which commonly manifests as a cerebrovascular accident (CVA) or stroke. A CVA may be caused due to a blockage in a blood vessel (ischemic) or due to rupture of a blood vessel (hemorrhagic). The extent of impaired neurological function depends on the region of the nervous system impacted by either the ischemia or hemorrhage (Lundy-Ekman 2013; OpenStax College 2013).

The nervous system is the control center of the human body. Any disruption in its function will manifest in several functional limitations. The severity of the limitations will generally depend on the location of the disorder/injury and the size of the damage. CNS disorders can be caused by trauma, which is commonly referred to as traumatic brain injury (TBI), and symptoms can vary widely from paralysis to mood disorders, depending on the site of the injury. Several diagnostic technologies have been developed to assess the nervous system non-invasively. A magnetoencephalography (MEG) scan is an imaging technique that identifies brain activity and measures weak magnetic fields produced in the brain, while electroencephalography (EEG) measures the neuronal electrical currents outside the human head (Hari et al. 2018). Functional magnetic resonance imaging (fMRI) is another imaging technique that uses blood flow differences in the brain to provide in vivo images of neuronal activity (Dutta, Woo, and Krummel 2012). All of these techniques can be used to provide millisecond-accurate information about neuronal currents supporting human brain function.

When a person attempts to move their body and muscles contract, an electromyography (EMG) measurement can be used to detect and record the electrical activity in muscles as a byproduct of contraction. An EMG is the summation of action potentials from the muscle fibers under the electrodes placed on the skin. The more muscles that contract, the greater the amount of action potentials recorded and the greater the EMG reading. Rehabilitation engineers developing an EMG-based orthosis system or exoskeleton technology for neuromotor rehabilitation now use such signals. For example, Yoshiyuki Sankai, professor of the Graduate School of Systems & Information Engineering at the University of Tsukuba, has developed the Hybrid Assistive Limb (HAL) powered exoskeleton in helping disabled and elderly people walk and is further modified for construction and other uses. Cyberdyne's HAL robot suit registers these EMG biosignals through a sensor attached to the skin of the wearer. Based on the signals obtained, the Cybernic Voluntary Control (CVC) analyzes the data, and the power unit moves the joint to support and amplify the wearer's motion (Sankai 2010). Alternatively, other devices were developed to apply artificial electrical stimulation in a precise sequence to activate the muscles. The NESS H200 Wireless Hand Rehabilitation System (Bioness Inc.) stimulates the appropriate nerves and muscles of the forearm and hand and helps the muscles to relearn, to respond to signals for movement (Mikołajewska and Mikołajewski 2012).

3.6 Future developments

Technologies are being developed that are likely to change how human anatomy, neuroscience, and biomechanics will be taught in the future. Currently, human body specimens and human body models are commonly used to facilitate the learning of concepts covered in this chapter. However, the use of human body specimens is expensive. Increasingly, student learning is being facilitated using alternative methods such as the use of computer software. In future, it appears that instructors teaching human anatomy, physiology, biomechanics, and neuroscience will use a combination of methods to facilitate student learning including dissection/prosection, interactive multimedia, and imaging (Sugand, Abrahams, and Khurana 2010). Recent developments in hologram technologies make it possible to see a representation of a human body in 3D. For example, the newly developed HoloLens by Microsoft® enables students to navigate through the layers of skin, muscle, blood vessels, and organs to the skeleton. Students are able to enlarge, turn, or rotate any of the structures to view how the different body structures are interrelated. In future, we are likely to see greater adoption of resources such as HoloLens for teaching human anatomy, neuroscience, and biomechanics.

From an interventions perspective, technological advancements in fabrication and prototyping will open several avenues for providing custom design AT products. 3D printing is one example, in which individual anthropometric measurements can be factored in the design to provide a proper fit between the individual and end product.

Case study

John is a 65-year-old male who has had a stroke (cerebrovascular accident) eight months ago. John was diagnosed with a hemorrhagic stroke due to rupture in the middle cerebral artery (MCA) which affected the right hemisphere of his brain. The MCA is the largest cerebral artery and is the vessel most commonly affected by strokes. John has a history of hypertension and led a sedentary lifestyle before the stroke. He used to work as a manager in an import/export business and was a workaholic. After the stroke, John became hemiplegic and suffers from hypertonia (spasticity) in his left side. The stroke caused several major problems including deficits in both gross and fine motor movements, impaired language ability, impaired balance, and fatigue.

John started receiving rehabilitation services right after his stroke including physical therapy (PT), occupational therapy (OT), and speech language pathology (SLP). His main concerns were to be independent again in ambulation, ADLs, communication, driving, and to play golf as he decided to retire. The following are some examples of the assistive technologies that John started to use over the course of his recovery:

Communication: AAC device
Ambulation: wheelchair, tripod cane
Eating: rocker knife, plate guard, non-slip mat
Driving: car modifications including steering knob and extended handles
Dressing: dressing stick
Pathing: grab bars, shower bench

Bibliography

Astrand, P. O. and K. Rodahl, eds. 1977. *Textbook of Work Physiology*, edited by P. O. Astrand and K. Rodahl. 2nd ed. New York: McGraw-Hill.

Baum, C., C. Barrows, J. D. Bass-Haugen, D. Chasanoff, L. Dale, G. Jenkins, P. Kramer, et al. 2010. "Blueprint for Entry-Level Education." *The American Journal of Occupational Therapy: Official Publication of the American Occupational Therapy Association* 64 (1): 186–194.

Bello, Ysabel M., Anna F. Falabella, and William H. Eaglstein. 2001. "Tissue-Engineered Skin." *American Journal of Clinical Dermatology* 2 (5): 305–313.

Bickenbach, Jerome E., Somnath Chatterji, Elizabeth M. Badley, and T. Bedirhan Üstün. 1999. "Models of Disablement, Universalism and the International Classification of Impairments, Disabilities and Handicaps." *Social Science & Medicine* 48 (9): 1173–1187.

Carroll, James E., James M. Hagberg, Michael H. Brooke, and Jack B. Shumate. 1979. "Bicycle Ergometry and Gas Exchange Measurements in Neuromuscular Diseases." *Archives of Neurology* 36 (8): 457–461.

Costanzo, LS. 2014. *Physiology*. 5th ed. Philadelphia, PA: Saunders.

Dean, Elizabeth and Jocelyn Ross. 1991. "Effect of Modified Aerobic Training on Movement Energetics in Polio Survivors." *Orthopedics* 14 (11): 1243–1246.

Dutta, Sanjeev, Russell K. Woo, and Thomas M. Krummel. 2012. "Chapter 4 - Advanced and Emerging Surgical Technologies and the Process of Innovation." In *Pediatric Surgery*, 7th ed., edited by Arnold G. Coran. Philadelphia, PA: Mosby. https://doi.org/10.1016/B978-0-323-07255-7.00004-0.

Edgerton, V. R. 1978. "Mammalian Muscle Fiber Types and Their Adaptability." *American Zoologist* 18 (1): 113–125.

Gault, M. L. and M. E. Willems. 2013. "Aging, Functional Capacity and Eccentric Exercise Training." *Aging and Disease* 4 (6): 351–363.

Gresham, G. E., T. F. Phillips, P. A. Wolf, P. M. McNamara, W. B. Kannel, and T. R. Dawber. 1979. "Epidemiologic Profile of Long-Term Stroke Disability: The Framingham Study." *Archives of Physical Medicine and Rehabilitation* 60 (11): 487–491.

Haisma, J. A., L. H. V. Van der Woude, H. J. Stam, M. P. Bergen, T. A. R. Sluis, and J. B. J. Bussmann. 2006. "Physical Capacity in Wheelchair-Dependent Persons with a Spinal Cord Injury: A Critical Review of the Literature." *Spinal Cord* 44 (11): 642.

Hall, John E. 2015. *Guyton and Hall Textbook of Medical Physiology*. 13th ed. Philadelphia, PA: Saunders.

Hamill, J., K. Knutzen, and T. R. Derrick. 2015. *Biomechanical Basis of Human Movement*. 4th ed. Philadelphia, PA: Wolters Kluwer Health.

Hari, Riitta, Sylvain Baillet, Gareth Barnes, Richard Burgess, Nina Forss, Joachim Gross, Matti Hämäläinen, Ole Jensen, Ryusuke Kakigi, and François Mauguière. 2018. "IFCN-Endorsed Practical Guidelines for Clinical Magnetoencephalography (MEG)." *Clinical Neurophysiology* 129 (8): 1720–1747.

Hortobaágyi, Tibor and Paul DeVita. 2000. "Favorable Neuromuscular and Cardiovascular Responses to 7 Days of Exercise with an Eccentric Overload in Elderly Women." *The Journals of Gerontology Series A: Biological Sciences and Medical Sciences* 55 (8): B401–B410.

Hurst, Rachel. 2003. "The International Disability Rights Movement and the ICF." *Disability and Rehabilitation* 25 (11–12): 572–576.

Kearney, Penelope M. and Julie Pryor. 2004. "The International Classification of Functioning, Disability and Health (ICF) and Nursing." *Journal of Advanced Nursing* 46 (2): 162–170.

Lippert, L. S. 2006. *Clinical Kinesiology and Anatomy*, 4th ed. Philadelphia, PA: F.A. Davis.

Lundy-Ekman, L. 2013. *Neuroscience: Fundamentals for Rehabilitation*. Philadelphia, PA: Elsevier Health Sciences.

McDonald, C. M. 2002. "Physical Activity, Health Impairments, and Disability in Neuromuscular Disease." *American Journal of Physical Medicine & Rehabilitation* 81 (11 Suppl): S108–S120.

Mikołajewska, Emilia and Dariusz Mikołajewski. 2012. "Neuroprostheses for Increasing Disabled Patients' Mobility and Control." *Advances in Clinical and Experimental Medicine* 21 (2): 263–272.

Milner-Brown, H. S., R. B. Stein, and R. Yemm. 1973a. "The Orderly Recruitment of Human Motor Units during Voluntary Isometric Contractions." *The Journal of Physiology* 230 (2): 359–370.

———. 1973b. "Changes in Firing Rate of Human Motor Units during Linearly Changing Voluntary Contractions." *The Journal of Physiology* 230 (2): 371–390.

OpenStax College. 2013. "Chapter 22: The Respiratory System." In *Anatomy & Physiology*, 981. Houston, TX: OpenStax College.

Pendleton, Heidi McHugh and Winifred Schultz-Krohn. 2017. *Pedretti's Occupational Therapy-E-Book: Practice Skills for Physical Dysfunction*. Philadelphia, PA: Elsevier Health Sciences.

Putte, C. V., J. Regan, and A. Russo. 2015. "Respiratory System." In *Seeley's Essentials of Anatomy & Physiology*, edited by C. VanPutte, J. Regan and A. Russo, 9th ed., 412. New York: McGraw-Hill.

Roig, M., K. O'Brien, G. Kirk, R. Murray, P. McKinnon, B. Shadgan, and W. D. Reid. 2009. "The Effects of Eccentric Versus Concentric Resistance Training on Muscle Strength and Mass in Healthy Adults: A Systematic Review with Meta-Analysis." *British Journal of Sports Medicine* 43 (8): 556–568.

Roth, Elliot J. 1993. "Heart Disease in Patients with Stroke: Incidence, Impact, and Implications for Rehabilitation Part 1: Classification and Prevalence." *Archives of Physical Medicine and Rehabilitation* 74 (7): 752–760.

———. 1994. "Heart Disease in Patients with Stroke. Part II: Impact and Implications for Rehabilitation." *Archives of Physical Medicine and Rehabilitation* 75 (1): 94–101.

Sanjak, M., D. Paulson, R. Sufit, W. Reddan, D. Beaulieu, L. Erickson, A. Shug, and B. R. Brooks. 1987. "Physiologic and Metabolic Response to Progressive and Prolonged Exercise in Amyotrophic Lateral Sclerosis." *Neurology* 37 (7): 1217–1220.

Sankai, Yoshiyuki. 2010. "HAL: Hybrid Assistive Limb Based on Cybernics." In *Robotics Research*, 25–34. New York: Springer.

Scanlon, V. C. and T. Sanders. 2007. *Essentials of Anatomy and Physiology*, 5th ed. Philadelphia, PA: F.A. Davis.

Sockolov, R., B. Irwin, R. H. Dressendorfer, and E. M. Bernauer. 1977. "Exercise Performance in 6-to-11-Year-Old Boys with Duchenne Muscular Dystrophy." *Archives of Physical Medicine and Rehabilitation* 58 (5): 195–201.

Stoller, Oliver, Eling D. de Bruin, Ruud H. Knols, and Kenneth J. Hunt. 2012. "Effects of Cardiovascular Exercise Early after Stroke: Systematic Review and Meta-Analysis." *BMC Neurology* 12 (1): 45.

Sugand, Kapil, Peter Abrahams, and Ashish Khurana. 2010. "The Anatomy of Anatomy: A Review for its Modernization." *Anatomical Sciences Education* 3 (2): 83–93.

Symons, T. Brock, Anthony A. Vandervoort, Charles L. Rice, Tom J. Overend, and Greg D. Marsh. 2005. "Effects of Maximal Isometric and Isokinetic Resistance Training on Strength and Functional Mobility in Older Adults." *The Journals of Gerontology Series A: Biological Sciences and Medical Sciences* 60 (6): 777–781.

WHO. 2001. *World Health Organization: International Classification of Functioning, Disability and Health: ICF.* Geneva, Switzerland: World Health Organization.

Wright, Nancy C., David D. Kilmer, Megan A. McCrory, Susan G. Aitkens, Bryan J. Holcomb, and Edmund M. Bernauer. 1996. "Aerobic Walking in Slowly Progressive Neuromuscular Disease: Effect of a 12-Week Program." *Archives of Physical Medicine and Rehabilitation* 77 (1): 64–69.

Chapter 4 Psychosocial and cultural aspects of rehabilitation engineering interventions

Marcia Scherer and
Malcolm MacLachlan

Contents

DOI: 10.1201/b21964-5

4.1 Overview

In June 2017, a colleague in Australia posted this on the Australian Rehabilitation and Assistive Technology Association (ARATA) listserv under the subject: The stuff you find in filing cabinets – ARATA 1997 conference:

> Here's a bit of fun. It's the conference program from ARATA's conference in Canberra 20 years ago!
>
> It's fascinating looking at some of the paper titles – they could pop up in next year's conference as the subject material evolves and updates, but the topics remain relevant.

The post attracted considerable agreement. A reading of the attached pdf of the conference program made it clear that while devices and products and systems have certainly evolved, supports for their selection and use have not always kept pace. Following are just a few of the topics with timeless themes.

4.1.1 Communication

- Communication Always ... Technology Sometimes
- Perceptions of Conversation Success by Augmented Communicators and the Co-Workers

4.1.2 Service delivery

- Finding the Answers: A Problem-Solving Framework in Action
- To Whom is the Prescriber Responsible?
- What do Customers Really Want? A Survey of Customers and What They Look for in a Supplier
- Benefits and Costs of Using Assistive Technology: An Analysis of the Literature

4.1.3 Special groups

- Factors Influencing the Introduction of Assistive Technology to People with Motor Neuron Disease

What makes these topics so timeless is the fact that they heavily involve fundamental but highly variable human and personal elements. Many voices have come together to express the need for more attention being given to the personal, social, and cultural aspects of technology assessment, selection, and training for use. For example, the National Academies of Sciences, Engineering, and Medicine issued a report on *The Promise of Assistive Technology to Enhance Activity and Work Participation* (2017) and stated:

maximal user performance requires that individuals receive the appropriate devices for their needs, proper fitting of and training in the use of the devices, and appropriate follow-up care. Even [then], assistive products and technologies may not fully mitigate the effects of impairments or associated activity limitations. The committee emphasizes that environmental, societal, and personal factors are as important in determining individuals' overall functioning with respect to employment.

By personal factors, they mean what can and also what cannot be changed. Examples provided include ethnic, cultural, and language barriers; age; socioeconomic status; insurance coverage; education; and previous work and life experiences.

4.2 Defining personal factors

The World Health Organization's International Classification of Functioning, Disability and Health (ICF) (World Health Organization 2001) (as previously introduced in Chapter 2) is a member of the World Health Organization's Family of International Classifications (WHO–FIC) designed to provide a common worldwide language of disease and disability [http://www.who.int/classifications/]. WHO–FIC consists of:

- International Classification of Diseases (ICD), which as the name implies, classifies diseases and other health problems
- International Classification of Health Interventions (ICHI), which is a common tool for reporting and analyzing the distribution and evolution of health interventions
- International Classification of Functioning, Disability, and Health (ICF), which measures health and disability at both individual and population levels

The ICF (World Health Organization 2001), considers personal factors to be an important component of the framework and, while left deliberately nebulous in definition, include gender, age, coping styles, social background, education, profession, past and current experience, overall behavior pattern, character, and other factors that influence how disability is experienced by the individual (see Figure 4.1). The WHO has proposed a taxonomical development of personal factors and there have been efforts to identify examples of personal factors in the relevant literature (Geyh et al. 2011).

The ICF **applies to all people worldwide regardless of age, gender, ethnicity or race, and health condition.** This universality means health and disability are each continuums within dimensions of functioning and each person has

Interactions between the components of ICF

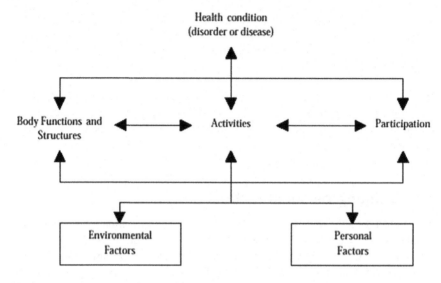

Figure 4.1 Diagram of the International Classification of Functioning, Disability, and Health (ICF) framework (World Health Organization 2001a).

a particular pattern of functioning. According to the WHO/ESCAP *Training Manual on Disability Statistics* (World Health Organization 2008):

> The core of ICF's concept of disability are the facts that disability is multidimensional and the product of an interaction between an individual's certain conditions and his or her physical, social, and attitudinal barriers. The bio-psychosocial model embedded in the ICF broadens the perspective of disability and allows medical, individual, social, and environmental influences on functioning and disability to be examined. Structurally, the ICF is based on three levels of functioning (body functions and structures, activities, and participation) with parallel levels of disability (impairments, activity limitations, and participation restrictions). Human functioning is understood as a continuum of health states and every human being exhibits one or another degree of functioning in each domain, at the body, person and society levels. In the ICF language, contextual factors (environmental factors and personal factors) also constitute disability. Environmental factors include availability of assistive devices, family and community support, supportive services and policies and attitudes of different people. Personal factors include health conditions (diseases, disorders and injuries). ICF conceptualizes disability, not solely as a problem that resides in the individual, but as a health experience that occurs in a context.

(World Health Organization 2008)

ESCAP goes on to further describe the two fundamental components of this context: environmental factors and personal factors. Environmental factors are all of the physical, social, and attitudinal features that together characterize the environment in which a person lives, from climate and terrain to architectural characteristics and legal and social structures. Personal factors include gender, age, coping styles, social background, education, profession, past and current experience, overall behavior pattern, character, and other factors that influence how disability is experienced by the individual. Personal factors are not currently classified in the ICF but users may incorporate them in their applications of the classification. Disability policy depends crucially on whether improving outcomes is a matter of investing in changes to the person's capacity levels, by means of medical or rehabilitative interventions, or investing in accessibility, accommodation and other environmental changes (World Health Organization 2008).

The ICF does not view disability as being defined merely by what occurs in the components of body functions and body structures. Rather, it is defined by the entire lived experience of having restrictions in and barriers to performing activities and to participation. The need to address the individual's unique and individualized lived experience is well recognized.

> People with the same impairments experience different kinds and degrees of incapacity and vastly different restrictions on what actually happens in their lives ... The converse is also true: people can experience the same restrictions in what they can do in their day-to-day lives even though they have different impairments. At the level of actual performance, the contrast is even greater. Impairments as diverse as missing limbs and anxiety can both attract stigma and discrimination that may limit a person's participation in work.
>
> **(World Health Organization 2008)**

Support from appropriately selected technologies can make it possible to pursue employment, education, and involvement in community life. Yet, individuals' views of the value of assistive technology (AT) in accomplishing these objectives, and their predisposition to use one or more, vary considerably.

The matching person and technology (MPT) model focuses on three primary areas that were found to most differentiate technology users and non-users (Scherer 1986): (a) personal and psychosocial characteristics, needs, and preferences; (b) milieu/environmental factors; and (c) functions and features of the technology being evaluated. The need for an AT to enhance a person's functioning (perform an activity and participate in life roles) is assumed. For example, for a person with paralysis below the waist, there are few options for mobility other than a wheelchair. The MPT model was initially presented in 1989 (Scherer and McKee 1989). The influences on technology use and non-use as conceptualized in the MPT model have been used by several other AT researchers and authors (e.g.,

American Medical Association 1996; Craddock and McCormack 2002; Lasker and Bedrosian 2001; Zapf and Rough 2002; Zapf et al. 2016) for a version for use with a special education population; and a version translated for use in AT centers in Italy (Federici et al. 2003).

Elements within each of the three primary components – the **person, the milieu or environments of use, and the technology** – can contribute either a positive or a negative influence on technology selection and use. Too many negative influences will reduce the chance of technology adoption and use. In fact, the technology itself may appear perfect for a given need, but if it doesn't meet the person's priorities or preferences or does not receive the needed environmental support, that perfect technology may go unused, or it may be used inappropriately and cause frustration and expense for those involved.

The model in Figure 4.2 emerged from research exploring the differences between technology users and non-users (Scherer 1993) and the elements have since been confirmed by numerous studies as they were summarized in many systematic reviews of AT adoption, use or rejection (e.g., Baxter et al. 2012; Dirks

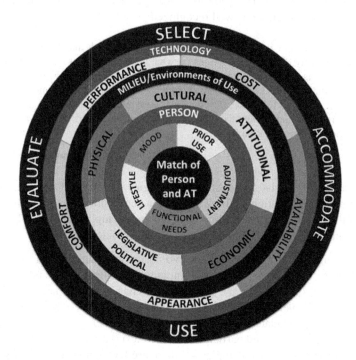

Figure 4.2 Matching person and technology (MPT) model. The target or goal is the most appropriate match of person and technology having considered the various influences known to impact that match (Institute for Matching Person & Technology, 1995 http://matchingpersonandtechnology.com).

and Bühler 2018; Tuazon, Jahan, and Jutai 2019; Wessels et al. 2003; Wielandt et al. 2006). More recently, position papers from the Global Research, Innovation, and Education in Assistive Technology (GREAT) summit [http://www.who.int/phi/implementation/assistive_technology/great_summit/en/] articulate the need for a more informed approach to AT selection and to achieving a good match of a person (individual with a disability and/or caregiver) and most appropriate AT and/or other supports and strategies.

4.3 Importance of personal factors in the successful use of assistive technologies

Each unique individual has a set of personal characteristics, background experiences, and expectations which guide behaviors and preferences. Personal preferences, in turn, guide the selection of a solution as well as the choice to use or not use an assistive solution, under what circumstances, and in which settings or environments. There are, indeed, many personal factors that impact decision making. Due to limitations of space, only some are included in the layer labeled **Person** (Figure 4.3).

Working with an individual to select the most appropriate support begins with the establishment of a partnership where strengths, limitations/needs, and goals are explored. Then, four key questions to ask consumers are:

1. What tasks (physical, mental, sensory, verbal, etc.) do you find to be the most difficult or frustrating for you to perform?

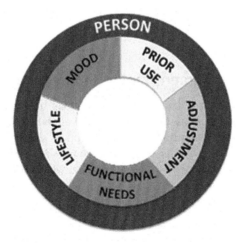

Figure 4.3 MPT model person component (Scherer 2002).

2. What most stands in your way of performing them?
3. What have you used that has worked well for you?
4. What have you used that has NOT worked well for you?

As noted earlier, cognitive changes, ways of coping with challenges, underlying personality and personal factors, and mood state can each be a facilitator to the use of AT or serve as a barrier to AT adoption and use. Mood state, in particular (presence of depression, anxiety), can affect a person's engagement in rehabilitation and expectations of benefit from rehabilitation interventions. Mood can also alter perceptions of self, energy, and receptivity to new and alternate ways of doing things. It can generally be said, however, that the more an individual needs or would benefit from an AT, the higher the probability that it will be tried and used. But the desire to use support may be weak. This is why a personalized, user-centered approach is so crucial.

To achieve a user-focused support selection process, the provider should first allow time to establish rapport and build a trusting relationship with the user. Key questions that can be asked should focus on the individual as a unique person. Examples include the following.

4.3.1 Desire for Support

- What are the person's priorities?
- Does the person perceive a discrepancy between the current and desired situation?
- Does the person prefer to have someone else help them because they desire that interpersonal contact?
- How much will the use of the support affect typical routines? How much does that matter to the person?

4.4 Milieu/environment factors influencing use

Self-concept, expectations, and personal aspirations of an individual may be shaped by social interactions that control the availability of positive personal regard, resources, and opportunities. Social support systems have a profound influence on how people with disabilities interpret their experiences and evaluate their options and alternatives, and they even affect what options and alternatives are presented in the first place.

Moving outward from the center of the circle and beyond the characteristics of the person, considerations related to the characteristics and requirements of the environment(s)/milieu of use and their impact on the individual become crucial (Figure 4.4).

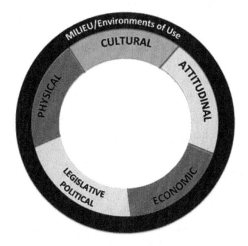

Figure 4.4 MPT model milieu component (Scherer 2002).

The word **milieu** is used because it connotes the ICF concept that our environment is not just a built one consisting of physical objects, but a place comprised of people who have a variety of attitudes and values. As we have discussed, attitudinal and cultural factors are important, as well as characteristic of the individual's built or physical environment. Within the ICF, the interface with the "built environment" for a person with disabilities or an older person with diminished physical or cognitive function is part of environmental factors. Resolving the environmental issues is a critical element in promoting independence. Mann, Ottenbacher, Fraas et al. (1999) reported that making minor modifications to the residences of frail elderly people produced more independence and allowed individuals to remain more functional in their homes, rather than being institutionalized. This resulted in a slower rate of decline of the person's activities and reduced costs due to fewer nursing home placements.

Culture determines personal perspectives, values and beliefs, biases, and is a part of one's milieu. People with disabilities vary in their desire for, or acceptance of, AT vs personal assistance vs help from family members. Often, this is an outcome of one's culture and expectations as well as available resources. Family members may resent the use or presence of an AT in the home. It may also be that they cannot take on the financial burden of obtaining the most appropriate supports. Financial limitations are a primary reason for individuals not getting the supports they need and want. For example, the public school that Ryan attended did not meet his educational and social needs but in order to go to a school that had the appropriate resources, his family would have to pay private fees.

To use a truly idiographic, person-centered approach requires understanding such influences and pressures, level of program/professional trust, as well as language differences (a person who is deaf may require a sign language interpreter, a Native American may only communicate in his or her native language). Changes in the traditional family structure, in the cultural backgrounds, and in the linguistic heritages of families necessitate the need to develop skills in working with families from diverse backgrounds and understanding their perspectives regarding the selection and use of technology.

Sample considerations regarding the characteristics and requirements of the milieu/environments include key contextual factors.

4.4.1 Personal attitudes

- Do caregivers and the family have expectations and desires for the person different from those of the individual? Professionals?
- What are the predispositions of relevant others (employers, co-workers, teachers, etc.) to using a technology with this particular person?

4.4.2 Personal physical context

- Are all of the necessary physical supports in place for this person to access and use the planned technology?
- If assistance is required for the use of the technology, is it available?
- Do room settings need to be reorganized?
  - Is adequate space available in the room?
  - Is the lighting sufficient?
  - Will the person need to be near an electrical outlet?
  - Will the person require extra table/desk space for a device?
  - Will the person have clear access within the room?
- Will the person have physical access to all work, social, and lavatory facilities?
- If the device needs to be portable, is it sufficiently easy for the person to move and carry?

4.4.3 Legislative/political context

- Are the people in settings where AT will be used familiar with all of the relevant legislation related to technology use?
- Have additional supportive/advocacy resources in the community been identified?

4.4.4 Economic context

- What are the repair record and maintenance requirements of the technology and how much do repairs or regular maintenance typically cost?

- Will the vendor provide services at the person's home or work location? At what cost?
- How often are upgrades available and how much do they cost?
- Does funding exist to appropriately provide the device and ongoing support?
- Is a plan in place to upgrade or replace technologies that are no longer suitable?
- Have additional supports and assistance been considered and are they available if needed?

4.4.5 Cultural context

- Within the person's familial culture, what have been their experiences and opportunities?
- Will the family encourage and support the use of technology? Sometimes caregivers and family members are primary users of these technologies. It's important to assess their perspectives as well as those of the persons.
- Will associates (co-workers, friends, etc.) encourage and support use?

We have so far considered the link between person and technology. The CIDIO™ INITIATIVE is an educational framework that seeks to produce a more holistic approach to engineering by placing technology–human interaction in the broader context of culture, then society, and then environment. This chapter will now address engineering and, in particular, AT from the cultural perspective.

4.5 Culture and assistive technology: how culture impacts use and reflects good (or bad)

The social model of disability understands disability to be the experience someone has of their society, not a personal attribute that they own. As such, society transforms some impairments, but not others, into disabilities. A visual impairment corrected by readily available and accessible eyeglasses may not have any disabling effects. On the other hand, a wheelchair user who cannot access her school classroom because there is no access ramp, **becomes** disabled, by the lack of access. The physical, the psychological, and the social environment are the mediators of ability or disability, not the impairment.

Cultures and people "make each other up"; cultures provide their adherents with guidelines for living; ways of understanding what is good or bad, acceptable or unacceptable, frightening or reassuring. However, some aspects of being human are socially and culturally understood as being problematic across just about all cultures, and impairment is one of these (MacLachlan 2006). So too is how people see and use assistive products. A study by Kaye, Yeager, and Reed (2008) explored disparities in the use of assistive products. Their sample was of almost 2,000 adult assistive product users registered with the California Independent Living Centers. They reported that technology use was influenced by a number of demographic factors, including race/ethnicity, education, income, and type and severity of disability.

Kaye et al. (2008) classified the technological sophistication of products as follows. **High-tech** products were digitally based, such as computer hardware or software, or a communication device. **Medium-tech** products were those with electronic or motorized equipment (for example, a powered wheelchair, scooter, or hearing aid). **Low-tech** products were non-motorized, non-electronic products, such as a magnifier, cane, or oxygen tank. One can argue with this classification in terms of the sophistication of technology versus the type of technology; and, as the authors note, these categories are not necessarily mutually exclusive. However, our interest here is to establish any relationship between different categories of technology use and ethnicity.

Kaye et al. (2008) found that groups they categorized as "African American" and "Latino/Hispanic" both reported a lower percentage of current AT users (57.8 and 61.2 % respectively) compared to "White non-Latino" respondents (72.4%). The number of products people used also varied with "African American" and "Latino/Hispanic" respondents reporting using fewer products (an average of 1.4 and 1.5 respectively) compared to "White non-Latino" respondents (an average of 2.3 products). Perhaps most intriguing and concerning from an engineering perspective is that the type of technology used also appeared to systematically vary in terms of ethnicity.

- For "**Low-tech**" products, usage rates were "White non-Latino" (57.9), "Latino/Hispanic" (46.7%), and "African American" (45%)
- For "**Medium-tech**" products, usage rates were: "White non-Latino" (40.5%), "Latino/Hispanic" (28.2%), and "African American" (28%)
- For "**High-tech**" products, usage rates were: "White non-Latino" (23.1%), "Latino/Hispanic" (11.3%), and "African American" (12.8%)

All of the findings reported above in terms of ethnicity reflect statistically significant differences between the "White non-Latino" group and the other two ethnic groups (at a level of $p < 0.01$). This patterning of assistive products used by this particular grouping of ethnicities (we recognize that there may be other and better ways to categorize ethnic differences) is concerning. It may be that it reflects different attitudes to assistive products within these groups, different attitudes regarding assistive products towards these groups by practitioners, or intervening variables such as different purchasing power, awareness, or geographic accessibility, associated with membership of these ethnic groupings.

More recently published was Orellano-Colon et al.'s (2017) work, which actually draws on the US National Health Interview Survey, conducted some years before – in 2009. In this survey rather different results were found. Using the categories of "African Americans" and "European Americans" they reported that proportionately more "African Americans" (10%) as compared to "European Americans" (7.5%) used some type of AT. Furthermore, having some type of physical impairment was a significantly stronger predictor of AT use among "African Americans" (odds ratio = 222.49) than among "European Americans" (odds ratio = 50.77, p < 0.001). More generally these researchers concluded that "the predictive strength of AT usage based on disability types and other demographic variables differed by races". So, while this research also suggests that AT use is patterned by ethnic group categorization, it suggests a different patterning in a national health survey than in a state-based survey of independent living centers (from California). While the results are different (and both may be valid), they concur on the relevance of race/ethnicity/culture to AT use.

Hopefully the reader has picked up on the confusing and inconsistent terminology in this area. Race, ethnicity, and culture are often conflated and confusingly used in an interchangeable manner. While a discussion of these terms is beyond our scope here; in general, "race" refers to biological and particularly genetic-related differences, "ethnicity" to notions of identity or belongingness, and "culture" to broader societal constructions and understandings (MacLachlan 2006). However, with many more people now able to be categorized as having an "inter-racial marriage", or coming from a "mixed ethnic background", or living in a "multicultural" society, such categories are both more confusing and more important, especially if they pattern the extent of access to, or use of, AT.

Generally, "culture" is used as a term to capture variations that may arrise related to race/ethnicity/culture. A useful review of the literature on the intersection between culture, disability, and AT is presented by Ripat and Woodgate (2011) who conclude that "Understanding how an individual's culturally defined identity is shaped as an AT user, and the meaning the AT holds to that person and family, is essential to providing culturally appropriate AT services" (Ripat and Woodgate 2011). However, they also, and importantly stress that the providers belong to a culture too, as well as to a "professional culture", which is framed by their professional experiences and outlook. This means that both AT users and providers are potentially ethnocentric, and in quite different and perhaps intersecting ways. While we suggest that "culture" is a useful broad term to use, it is also important to recognize that it incorporates the idea of sub-cultures and sub-identities. Ripat and Woodgate (2011) also highlight that some AT users may strongly identify with a "disability culture", constituted from shared experiences, beliefs, and values. A disability sub-culture – for instance Deaf/deaf culture – may reject the idea of AT to "correct" an impairment, seeing Deafness instead as a different and equally valid form of being in the world, and therefore giving deaf a capital "D", in the same way as the identity of being Black, or of being American, deserve to be capitalized.

Ripat and Woodgate (2011) conclude that "there is a paucity of knowledge about the intersection of AT and culture, and that this intersection requires further research. Embarking on this investigation is mandatory if we seek to meet the needs of the culturally diverse individuals who use AT".

Culture is, however, an amalgam; it is constituted of many identities and people may have multiple identities. For instance, a person who uses a prosthetic limb may well see themself as "disabled", but also as a woman, a mother, a refugee, a rural dweller, a doctor, a wife, a housekeeper. All these sorts of identities are valued in different ways in different cultures, and they are often arranged in a distinctive hierarchy of dominance (influence or importance) within any one culture, with often many cultures constituting a larger society. Thus, cultural identity intersects with other types of identity, but it also provides guidelines for how we interpret these identities, and their **intersectionality**. Therefore, a black refugee woman who uses a wheelchair may have a very different experience in the United States to a Native American using a wheelchair, or a white Anglo American.

While surveys of different technologies can certainly find, for instance, that satisfaction with prosthetic devices (Pezzin et al. 2004) including specific concerns regarding mechanical and comfort features (Østlie et al. 2012) may be mediated by ethnicity and gender, it is probably not helpful to make sweeping generalizations about what different ethnic groups think or feel about different technologies. Nobody is "just" an ethnic group, and our emphasis on matching the person and technology also embraces the recognition of complex individual differences and intersectionalities, at least at the attitudinal level.

While we have already argued for the importance of intersectionality, it is also very important to stress that those factors that may influence different attitudes towards AT are also often associated with people's access to them, such as age (Nihei et al. 2019). In different societies displaced people, rural dwellers, girls, or others, may be discriminated against. Those groupings that are more marginalized by mainstream society may have no, or less, access to the resources, personnel, and services that are required to give them an equal opportunity, to others closer to central social concerns. Addressing such problems will also require action at the policy level, where it will be important for those potential AT users most marginalized to have involvement in the process of producing new policy and service delivery models (Amin et al. 2011; Huss and MacLachlan 2016). One issue that is strongly related to culture and resonates at each of these levels is stigma.

4.6 Culture and stigma

The UNCRPD and the *World Report on Disability* (World Health Organization 2011) have highlighted stigma as the greatest barrier for people with disabilities becoming fully included in society. Goffman (1963) described stigma as "the process by which the reaction of others spoils normal identity". Stigma affects those with disabilities and their careers and may discourage people from seeking the services they require (Green 2003). Household survey data from 13 low-income countries indicates clearly that in those countries where there is greater stigma toward people with disabilities, the schooling of children with a disability suffers significantly (Filmer 2008). MacLachlan, Mannan, and McVeigh (2016) argue that the belief that misfortune is somehow "motivated" or "meaningful" may allow others a sense of protection from its frightening apparent randomness. Thus, disability and impairment may be attributed to retribution for wrongdoing, the actions of malevolent spirits (possibly sent by other people), and many other factors, including the will of God.

Research in high-income contexts has shown that a person with a disability may be seen to be "contagious", with others seeking to avoid their company or place themselves further away from someone with a disability, than someone without a disability (MacLachlan et al. 2012). Research in low-income contexts has found that many parents refuse to take children with disabilities on public transport, while some parents disown them entirely. Perceived differences between stigmatized and dominant groups can lead to the social exclusion of people with disability, marginalizing them, and reducing their power and resources within society (Link and Phelan 2001; Wazakili et al. 2011).

It is of course understandable for people to have a negative attitude towards factors that they feel somehow limit the potential for another person to fully participate in society. Stigma operates by transferring that negative attitude from the impairment to the individual who experiences the impairment and often disability. In most cultures, this leads others to reject or distance themselves from people with impairment, thus making it more difficult for them to be experienced by other people as different, **but equivalent**, human beings. Instead, those with impairments are often "othered" and feared, leading those around them to "move away" from them, both physically and psychologically.

Embodiment is a term used to express the identification of an abstract idea with a physical object: an athletic woman may embody the ideas of health and vitality, an overweight man may embody the idea of indulgence or a lack of self-control. Importantly, what a physical representation embodies is culturally determined; it is not necessarily correct, or fair, but rather expresses a prevailing view, a cultural norm, which may indeed discriminate against those who violate the culture's norms of what is "right", "acceptable", or "normal" (MacLachlan 2004).

Assistive technologies therefore have a crucial role to play, not just in providing functional opportunities by helping users overcome activity limitations, but also by signaling the embodiment of positive characteristics, rather than negative ones. While technologies have the potential to enable and therefore counter stigmatizing views of people with disability, in many cases they may not have this effect. Technologies can be seen to embody ability, or to embody disability. Individual and societal attitudes to enabling technologies can be negative. People may "see" the technology – the prosthetic arm, the wheelchair, the Zimmer frame – to represent the person, rather than supporting them, and so diminish the agency and dignity of the person. Technology design may be clunky or ugly, heightening rather than lessening stigma.

Stigma is a defining challenge for social inclusion (Cobigo et al. 2012) as it is channeled through cultural constructions and norms, as well as social structures (institutions, rules, policies, laws) (MacLachlan, Mannan, and McVeigh 2016). Stigma does not only relate to how society "sees" people with impairment, it can also be internalized as self-stigma, where individuals develop a negative view of themselves, their abilities, and their rights. As stigma is perhaps the greatest challenge facing people with disability (Cross et al. 2011a; Cross et al. 2011b), it is therefore something that should be given a high priority in the design and development of assistive technologies.

Figure 4.5 summarizes what we see as the potential for AT to challenge and counter stigma associated with disability and impairment.

In Figure 4.5 first consider attitudes towards disability. These are largely negative and stigmatizing; they are experienced within different domains mediated through cognition at the level of the individual (self), through social groups at the interpersonal level, and by social policy at the societal level. Stigma at the level of the self can impair the individual's motivation to interact with others, interpersonal experiences can result in exclusion, and societal barriers can prevent participation in social institutions. Coping, affect, evidence, and advocacy may mediate the extent to which stigma experienced within one domain is transferred to other domains.

Also, in Figure 4.5, attitudes towards AT can similarly be partitioned at the individual, interpersonal, and societal levels. These attitudes, while not unambiguously positive, are nonetheless relatively more positive than attitudes towards disability. If positive aspects of attitudes towards AT can become more closely associated with the users of the technology, then these attitudes may be transposed from the technology to the user, reducing stigma towards people with disability or impairment. Thus, we envision great psychological and social potential for AT in counteracting the widespread stigma toward people with impairment/disability, apparent in just about all cultures.

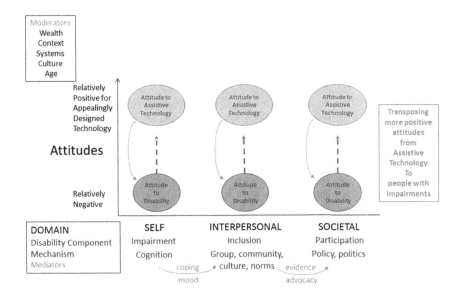

Figure 4.5 Schematic representation of how appealingly designed assistive technology can contribute to counteracting stigma and promoting social inclusion of people with physical or psychological impairments (Scherer & MacLachlan 2019).

Parette et al. (2004) noted that there had been little work on the relationship between stigma and the use of assistive technologies. Universal design has been suggested as one possibility for counteracting stigma associated with objects designed for people with disabilities. However, Bispo and Branco (2011) argue that for technology to overcome stigma it must directly challenge prejudiced assumptions concerning ability, perhaps promoting instead symbols of speed, sexiness, physical prowess, outdoor adventure, and so on.

A special open access issue of the journal *Disability & Rehabilitation: Assistive Technology* was dedicated to a series of position papers from the first GREAT Summit, held at WHO Headquarters in Geneva (Scherer, MacLachlan, and Khasnabis 2018). This produced a range of papers focusing on the primary beneficiaries of AT, that is, people or service users (Desmond et al. 2018), the main strategic drivers of AT, products (Smith et al. 2018), provision (de Witte et al. 2018), policy (MacLachlan, Banes, et al. 2018), and personnel or service providers (Smith et al. 2018), as well as a systems-thinking approach that incorporates the above five Ps and the additional five Ps that represent key contextual factors for AT – procurement, promotion, place, pace, and partnership (MacLachlan and Scherer 2018). Each of these ten Ps relates to different components of systems thinking and each of them may be influenced by psychosocial differences, such

Table 4.1 Assistive Technology Systems Components and Questions for Engineers

Component of System	Description and Psychosocial Questions for Engineers to Consider
Person (user)	Are you fitting the person to technology, or fitting technology to the needs of the person? How do you know you are doing the latter and not the former – what evidence do you have of your person-centered practice? To what extent have user values and needs been considered, perhaps through co-design?
Products	What types of assistive products are you focusing on – are they technologies that are commonly available (wheelchairs or hearing aids) or those less available (deafblind communication devices, or technologies for people with intellectual disability) – what are your reasons?
Policy	Is there an AT policy (or policies) in your country, who is responsible for providing AT, and which social groups or types of technology are prioritized in it?
Personnel	To what extent can/should engineers work directly with users and to what extent should other professionals be involved?
Provision	Is there the capacity within the existing system you work in to support the sort of technology you want to provide?
Procurement	Does the procurement of technology prioritize the needs of some groups over others? For instance, men over women, or technology for mobility over technology for intellectual disability?
Promotion	What ideas or images of technology use are promoted? Do they, for instance, reflect a charity model, a medical model, or a human rights model?
Place	What restrictions on AT use apply in your context – social attitudes (e.g., stigma), physical infrastructure (e.g., ramps), policy (e.g., lack of financial supports) – and how might this influence how you use the technology available to you?
Pace	If the technology you want to use or develop requires some sort of changes in the AT sector, how nimble is the sector, how quickly can change occur, and who needs to be involved to make this happen?
Partnership	Who else should be involved in bringing your engineered solution to fruition – the user, service providers, government, civil society, industry, others?

This table has two columns and ten rows describing components and questions for engineers about assistive technology. The first column lists the component of the system, and the second column lists psychosocial questions that the engineer should consider.

as culture, gender, or socioeconomic status. We therefore suggest that engineers consider the following ten questions when trying to think systemically about their work in the AT domain – see Table 4.1.

4.7 The inclusive engineer

The Royal Academy of Engineering (RAE) has turned the lens of inclusion upon itself, noting that "Engineering is unequal" (2018), that it is dominated by white males and that their outcomes from training are better than for those from other groups – women, ethnic minorities, people with disabilities. "Minority employees and students have lower satisfaction, experience exclusion and under achieve" (p. 11). The RAE therefore calls for a culture change in engineering. Some of the examples of engineering exclusion considered are of relevance here. For example, some washroom soap dispensers use invisible light from an infrared LED bulb, which is then reflected back to sensors to dispense soap. Darker skin colors absorb more light than lighter skin colors and therefore such dispensers may work less well, or not at all, for people with darker skins, giving rise to the discriminating effects of "racist" technology. Traffic crossings that assume everyone crosses the road at the same rate, may put those with mobility or visual impairments in greater danger; technology that evaluates the rate at which people approach crossings may be able to accommodate the length of time traffic is halted, to the needs of the pedestrian. Finally, seat belts are designed for "standard" people, being problematic for pregnant women – and a leading cause of fetal deaths in car accidents (Royal Academy of Engineering 2018), requiring better design solutions addressing the needs of, rather than marginalizing, this particular group of car users. While a description of the ethos of market shaping is beyond our scope here, the idea that markets can be shaped to address the needs of marginalized groups, is important for focusing more attention from engineers on perhaps lower volume, but equally valued markets (see MacLachlan, McVeigh, et al. 2018; MacLachlan 2019).

The RAE suggests that one route to a more inclusive approach in engineering is to take steps to increase engineers' self-knowledge (for instance understanding their own strengths and challenges through the use of psychometric testing), self-reflection (understanding how their own values and attitudes affect others they work with or clients they work for), and their ability to work in teams that are characterized by diversity, where different views can combine to create better solutions than are likely to arise from singular or narrow perspectives. Thus, the REA introduces the term, **the inclusive engineer**, by which they mean individuals who can "work effectively in a team, making adjustments and allowances for each individual's way of thinking and working, is able to consider a wide variety of users, and be creative and innovative in addressing users within designs and solutions" (Royal Academy of Engineering 2018, 45).

4.8 Conclusion

Good engineering design can actively question negative assumptions. For instance, the rough and tumble of Paralympic wheelchair rugby questions the fragility prejudice that is strongly associated with wheelchair use. This is only possible because Paralympic chairs have been designed with a different purpose in mind – wheelchair users are not "supposed" to play rugby! Such instances are imbued with contradictory symbolism, requiring the observers to reframe their conception, not just of the function of the technology, but also the "value" of the person using it. To overcome cognitive dissonance, the meaning ascribed to one or both has to change. The way that Bispo and Branco put it is that technology must produce an "argument" with automatic prejudicial assumptions about disability: "If a product creates an impression that it doesn't fit our expectations about how a disabled person should look, then it exposes our prejudice and gives us the chance to change our minds" (2011, 7)

Rehabilitation engineering has a crucial role, both in the functionality and design, of AT. This role is not an instrumental one only, it can also be a conduit for changing attitudes individuals have about themselves, as well as how others see them, and how society is structured to facilitate them. Rehabilitation engineering produces cultural artifacts – hardware and software – that symbolize something; they are never neutral; they can embody abstract ideas and attitudes that can either be enabling or disabling for people with impairments. Engineers themselves may also symbolize certain values and attitudes, even if they don't necessarily hold these views themselves. The inclusive engineer needs not only to understand and be open to others but also to understand how their own contribution can be strengthened by working with diverse teams, clients, and environments.

4.9 Future vision

User realization of benefits from the use of assistive solutions will depend largely on the service delivery process which begins with an initial and comprehensive assessment of the unique individual's needs and preferences. As we move increasingly towards person-centered approaches to healthcare, this will become all the more important. It additionally provides good baseline data for later addressing the outcomes achieved. The best technologies are those adapted to the user and those that do not require the user to adapt to them. Less complex designs, less consumer overload with choices and options, will also be trending. When engineers can lessen the "hassle index" for users, they will have achieved a milestone.

4.10 Discussion questions

1. How can the person – the user – be put at the center of assistive technology?
2. How is the ICF relevant to engineers?
3. How can technology be stigmatizing for its users?
4. In what ways might cultural differences be relevant to product design and use?

5. Should engineers partner with end users in the conceptualization and design of AT? Why, or why not?
6. Why are the unique, personal, characteristics of an individual important to understand?
7. What value does the MPT model have for the work of rehabilitation engineers?

Bibliography

American Medical Association. 1996. *Guidelines for the Use of Assistive Technology: Evaluation, Referral, Prescription: Primary Care for Persons with Disabilities: Access to Assistive Technology.* Washington, DC: American Medical Association.

Amin, M., M. MacLachlan, H. Mannan, S. El Tayeb, A. El Khatim, L. Swartz, A. Munthali, et al. 2011. "EquiFrame: A Framework for Analysis of the Inclusion of Human Rights and Vulnerable Groups in Health Policies." *Health and Human Rights* 13 (2): 1–20.

Baxter, Susan, Pam Enderby, Philippa Evans, and Simon Judge. 2012. "Barriers and Facilitators to the Use of High-Technology Augmentative and Alternative Communication Devices: A Systematic Review and Qualitative Synthesis." *International Journal of Language & Communication Disorders* 47 (2): 115–129.

Bispo, Renato and Vasco Branco. 2011. "Designing Out Stigma: A New Approach to Designing for Human Diversity." 9th International European Academy of Design Conference – The endless end. At: Faculade de Belas Artes da Universidade do Porto.

Cobigo, Virginie, H. Ouellette-Kuntz, Rosemary Lysaght, and Lynn Martin. 2012. "Shifting Our Conceptualization of Social Inclusion." *Stigma Research and Action* 2 (2): 75–84.

Craddock, Gerald and Lisa McCormack. 2002. "Delivering an AT Service: A Client-Focused, Social and Participatory Service Delivery Model in Assistive Technology in Ireland." *Disability and Rehabilitation* 24 (1–3): 160–170.

Cross, Hugh Alistair, Miriam Heijnders, Ajit Dalal, Silatham Sermrittirong, and Stephanie Mak. 2011a. "Interventions for Stigma Reduction–Part 1: Theoretical Considerations." *Disability, CBR & Inclusive Development* 22 (3): 62–70.

———. 2011b. "Interventions for Stigma Reduction–Part 2: Practical Applications." *Disability, CBR & Inclusive Development* 22 (3): 71–80.

de Witte, Luc, Emily Steel, Shivani Gupta, Vinicius Delgado Ramos, and Uta Roentgen. 2018. "Assistive Technology Provision: Towards an International Framework for Assuring Availability and Accessibility of Affordable High-Quality Assistive Technology." *Disability and Rehabilitation: Assistive Technology* 13 (5): 467–472.

Desmond, Deirdre, Natasha Layton, Jacob Bentley, Fleur Heleen Boot, Johan Borg, Bishnu Maya Dhungana, Pamela Gallagher, Lynn Gitlow, Rosemary Joan Gowran, and Nora Groce. 2018. "Assistive Technology and People: A Position Paper from the First Global Research, Innovation and Education on Assistive Technology (GREAT) Summit." *Disability and Rehabilitation: Assistive Technology* 13 (5): 437–444.

Dirks, S. and C. Bühler. 2018. "Assistive Technologies for People with Cognitive Impairments – Which Factors Influence Technology Acceptance?" In *Universal Access in Human-Computer Interaction. Methods, Technologies, and Users*, edited by M. Antona and C. Stephanidis. Cham: Springer. https://doi.org/10.1007/978-3-319-92049-8_36.

Federici, Stefano, Marcia Scherer, Andrea Micangeli, Caterina Lombardo, and M. O. Belardinelli. 2003. "A Cross-Cultural Analysis of Relationships between Disability Self-Evaluation and Individual Predisposition to use Assistive Technology." *Assistive Technology: Shaping the Future*: 941–946.

Filmer, Deon. 2008. "Disability, Poverty, and Schooling in Developing Countries: Results from 14 Household Surveys." *The World Bank Economic Review* 22 (1): 141–163.

Geyh, Szilvia, Claudio Peter, Rachel Müller, Jerome E. Bickenbach, Nenad Kostanjsek, Bedirhan T. Üstün, Gerold Stucki, and Alarcos Cieza. 2011. "The Personal Factors of the International Classification of Functioning, Disability and Health in the Literature–A Systematic Review and Content Analysis." *Disability and Rehabilitation* 33 (13–14): 1089–1102.

Goffman, E. 1963. *Stigma: Notes on the Management of Spoiled Identity.* Englewood Cliffs, NJ: Prentice-Hall.

Green, Sara E. 2003. ""What Do You Mean 'What's Wrong with Her?'": Stigma and the Lives of Families of Children with Disabilities." *Social Science & Medicine* 57 (8): 1361–1374.

Huss, Tessy and Malcolm MacLachlan. 2016. *The EquIPP Manual.* Global Health Press.

Kaye, H. S., P. Yeager, and M. Reed. 2008. "Disparities in Usage of Assistive Technology among People with Disabilities." *Assistive Technology* 20 (4): 194–203.

Lasker, J. P. and J. L. Bedrosian. 2001. "Promoting Acceptance of Augmentative and Alternative Communication by Adults with Acquired Communication Disorders." *AAC Augmentative and Alternative Communication* 17(3): 141–153.

Link, Bruce G. and Jo C. Phelan. 2001. "Conceptualizing Stigma." *Annual Review of Sociology* 27 (1): 363–385.

MacLachlan, Malcolm. 2004. *Embodiment: Clinical, Critical and Cultural Perspectives on Health and Illness: Clinical, Critical and Cultural Perspectives on Health and Illness.* London, UK: McGraw-Hill Education).

———. 2006. *Culture and Health.: A Critical Perspective Towards Global Health.* Hoboken, NJ: John Wiley & Sons.

———. 2019. "Access to Assistive Technology, Systems Thinking, and Market Shaping: A Response to Durocher Et al." *Ethics & Behavior* 29 (3): 196–200.

MacLachlan, Malcolm, David Banes, Diane Bell, Johan Borg, Brian Donnelly, Michael Fembek, Ritu Ghosh, Rosemary Joan Gowran, Emma Hannay, and Diana Hiscock. 2018. "Assistive Technology Policy: A Position Paper from the First Global Research, Innovation, and Education on Assistive Technology (GREAT) Summit." *Disability and Rehabilitation: Assistive Technology* 13 (5): 454–466.

MacLachlan, Malcolm, Hasheem Mannan, and Joanne McVeigh. 2016. "Disability and Inclusive Health." *Disability and Human Rights: Global Perspectives*: 150–172.

MacLachlan, Malcolm, Joanne McVeigh, Michael Cooke, Delia Ferri, Catherine Holloway, Victoria Austin, and Dena Javadi. 2018. "Intersections between Systems Thinking and Market Shaping for Assistive Technology: The SMART (Systems-Market for Assistive and Related Technologies) Thinking Matrix." *International Journal of Environmental Research and Public Health* 15 (12): 2627.

MacLachlan, Malcolm and Marcia J. Scherer. 2018. "Systems Thinking for Assistive Technology: A Commentary on the GREAT Summit." *Disability and Rehabilitation: Assistive Technology* 13 (5): 492–496.

MacLachlan, Malcolm, Grainne Ni Mháille, Pamela Gallagher, and Deirdre Desmond. 2012. "Embodiment and Appearance." In *Oxford Handbook of the Psychology of Appearance*, edited by N. Rumsey and D. Harcourt, 23. Oxford, UK: Oxford University Press.

Mann, William C., Kenneth J. Ottenbacher, Linda Fraas, Machiko Tomita, and Carl V. Granger. 1999. "Effectiveness of Assistive Technology and Environmental Interventions in Maintaining Independence and Reducing Home Care Costs for the Frail Elderly: A Randomized Controlled Trial." *Archives of Family Medicine* 8: 210–217.

National Academies of Sciences, Engineering, and Medicine. 2017. *The Promise of Assistive Technology to Enhance Activity and Work Participation.* Washington, DC: National Academies Press.

Nihei, M. S., I. Sugawara, N. Ehara, Y. Gondo, Y. Masui, H. Inagaki, T. Inoue, M. MacLachlan, and E. McAuliffe. 2019. "Assistive Products Use among Oldest-Old People in Japan: Differences in Personal Attributes and Living Situation." Retrieved from: https://extranet.who.int/kobe_centre/en/project-details/experiences-assistive-products-use-among-older-people-japan-2.

Orellano-Colón, Elsa M., Frances M. Morales, Zahira Sotelo, Nilkenid Picado, Edgardo J. Castro, Mayra Torres, Marta Rivero, Nelson Varas, and Jeffrey Jutai. 2017. "Development of an Assistive Technology Intervention for Community Older Adults." *Physical & Occupational Therapy in Geriatrics* 35 (2): 49–66.

Østlie, Kristin, Ingrid Marie Lesjø, Rosemary Joy Franklin, Beate Garfelt, Ola Hunsbeth Skjeldal, and Per Magnus. 2012. "Prosthesis Rejection in Acquired Major Upper-Limb Amputees: A Population-Based Survey." *Disability and Rehabilitation: Assistive Technology* 7 (4): 294–303.

Parette, Howard P., Mary Blake Huer, and Marcia Scherer. 2004. "Effects of Acculturation on Assistive Technology Service Delivery." *Journal of Special Education Technology* 19 (2): 31–41.

Pezzin, L. E., T. R. Dillingham, E. J. MacKenzie, P. Ephraim, and P. Rossbach. 2004. "Use and Satisfaction with Prosthetic Limb Devices and Related Services." *Archives of Physical Medicine and Rehabilitation* 85: 723–729.

Ripat, Jacquie and Roberta Woodgate. 2011. "The Intersection of Culture, Disability and Assistive Technology." *Disability and Rehabilitation: Assistive Technology* 6 (2): 87–96.

Royal Academy of Engineering. 2018. *Designing Inclusion into Engineering Education.* London: RAE.

Scherer, M. J. 1986. "Values in the Creation, Prescription, and Use of Technological Aids and Assistive Devices for People with Physical Disabilities." Doctoral Dissertation, University of Rochester. Graduate School of Education and Human Development.

———. 1993. "The Assistive Technology Device Predisposition Assessment: How Does it Measure Up as a Measure?" *Archives of Physical Medicine and Rehabilitation* 74 (6): 665.

Scherer, M. J., M. MacLachlan, and C. Khasnabis. 2018. "Introduction to the Special Issue on the First Global Research, Innovation, and Education on Assistive Technology (GREAT) Summit and Invitation to Contribute to and Continue the Discussions." *Disability and Rehabilitation: Assistive Technology* 13 (5): 435–436.

Scherer, M. J. and B. G. McKee. 1989. *But Will the Assistive Technology Device be Used.* Washington, DC: RESNA Press.

Smith, Emma M., Rosemary Joan Gowran, Hasheem Mannan, Brian Donnelly, Liliana Alvarez, Diane Bell, Silvana Contepomi, Liezel Ennion, Evert-Jan Hoogerwerf, and Tracey Howe. 2018. "Enabling Appropriate Personnel Skill-Mix for Progressive Realization of Equitable Access to Assistive Technology." *Disability and Rehabilitation: Assistive Technology* 13 (5): 445–453.

Smith, R. O., M. Scherer, R. Cooper, D. Bell, D. A. Hobbs, C. Pettersson, N. Seymour, et al. 2018. "Assistive Technology Products: A Position Paper from the First Global Research, Innovation, and Education on Assistive Technology (GREAT) Summit." *Disability and Rehabilitation: Assistive Technology* 13 (5): 473–485.

Tuazon, Joshua R., Alhadi Jahan, and Jeffrey W. Jutai. 2019. "Understanding Adherence to Assistive Devices among Older Adults: A Conceptual Review." *Disability and Rehabilitation: Assistive Technology* 14 (5): 424–433.

Wazakili, Margaret, Tsitsi Chataika, Gubela Mji, Kudakwashe Dube, and Malcolm MacLachlan. 2011. "Social Inclusion of People with Disabilities in Poverty Reduction Policies and Instruments: Initial Impressions from Malawi and Uganda." In *Disability and Poverty: A Global Challenge*, edited by A. H. Eide and B. Ingstad, 15–29. Bristol, UK: Polity Press.

Wessels, R., B. Dijcks, M. Soede, G. J. Gelderblom, and L. De Witte. 2003. "Non-Use of Provided Assistive Technology Devices, a Literature Overview." *Technology and Disability* 15 (4): 231–238.

Wielandt, Trish, Kryss McKenna, Leigh Tooth, and Jenny Strong. 2006. "Factors that Predict the Post-Discharge use of Recommended Assistive Technology (AT)." *Disability and Rehabilitation: Assistive Technology* 1 (1–2): 29–40.

World Health Organization. 2001. *International Classification of Functioning, Disability and Health: ICF.* Geneva: World Health Organization.

———. 2008. *Training Manual on Disability Statistics.* Geneva: United Nations Publications.

———. 2011. *World Report on Disability.* Geneva: World Health Organization.

Zapf, S. A. and R. B. Rough. 2002. "The Development of an Instrument to Match Individuals with Disabilities and Service Animals." *Disability and Rehabilitation* 24 (1–3): 47–58.

Zapf, Susan A., Marcia J. Scherer, Mary F. Baxter, and Diana Rintala H. 2016. "Validating a Measure to Assess Factors that Affect Assistive Technology Use by Students with Disabilities in Elementary and Secondary Education." *Disability and Rehabilitation: Assistive Technology* 11 (1): 38–49.

Chapter 5 Overview of disease, disability, and impairment

L.-J. Elsaesser

Contents

5.1 Chapter overview

Disease and impairment are recognized as primary indicators for disability lead-ing to poverty, inequality, and lack of fundamental human rights including health, social protection, education, and job opportunities that promote prosperity. This chapter presents global perspectives on socially responsible actions supporting the inclusion of persons with disabilities as full and equal members in society. Information on services, systems, and policies designed to reduce impairment and increase participation will focus on the value of rehabilitation and assistive technology interventions.

5.2 Background

The value of rehabilitation engineering and assistive technology for persons with disabilities is endorsed by international resolutions and initiatives with recom-mendations for effective actions.

DOI: 10.1201/b21964-6

The United Nations (UN) is an international organization whose mission is to maintain international peace and security, promote sustainable development, protect human rights, uphold international law, and deliver humanitarian aid. In January 2016, the UN 2030 Agenda for Sustainable Development Goals (SDGs) officially came into force. The SDGs build on the previous Millennium Development Goals of 2000, mobilizing efforts to end all forms of poverty, fight inequalities, and protect the environment while ensuring no one is left behind (Steele 2014).

The World Health Assembly in 2005, as the decision-making body for the World Health Organization (WHO), acknowledged that development goals contained in the United Nations Millennium Declaration of 2000, promoting international human rights and sustainable development, would not be achieved without addressing issues related to the health and rehabilitation of persons with disabilities (Leggett and Carter 2012). Health is viewed as both an outcome of and a precondition for economic, social, and environmentally sustainable development (Institute of Medicine 2014).

Globally sustainable actions assure that resources are and remain available. In 2010, the International Organization for Standardization (ISO) launched development of the future ISO 26000 standard on social responsibility to draw on and disseminate best practices for the good of the international community. ISO 26000:2010 provides guidance to businesses and organizations on translating sustainable principles into effective actions and best principles at a global level. The guideline principle on human rights states 'Every person, as a member of society, has economic, social and cultural rights necessary for his or her dignity and personal development' (ISO 2010). Socially responsible expectations and actions by organizations should be accessible, do not discriminate, and provide equal opportunities to all stakeholders including those with disability (ISO 2010). Figure 5.1 shows the 2010 schematic overview of ISO 26000.

The World Bank, whose motto is 'Working for a World Free of Poverty', is considered a leading institution for investments in health and development. Its overview on disability states that 'persons with disabilities, on average as a group, are more likely to experience adverse socioeconomic outcomes than persons without disabilities, such as less education, poorer health outcomes, lower levels of employment, and higher poverty levels'. 'One billion people, or 15% of the world's population, experience some form of disability, and disability prevalence is higher for developing countries' (The World Bank 2018).

As discussed in the earlier chapters in this section, the WHO is the body of the UN responsible for coordinating international public health and policy. The WHO

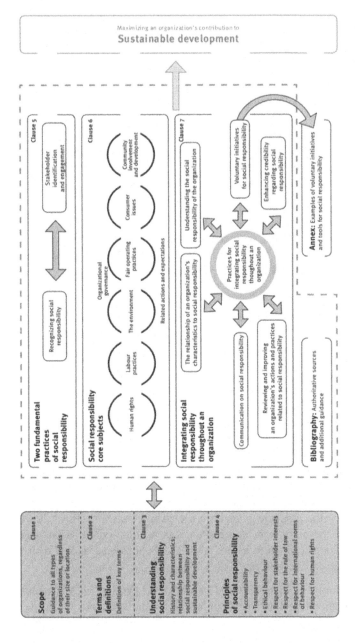

Figure 5.1 2010 schematic overview of ISO 26000 (https://www.iso.org/obp/graphics/pub/87f1a608-5bd8-4ea4-9e8d-749b2e00c79b_71a596ceb97e48c786ef205ab7456f3a.jpg).

and the World Bank jointly produced the first World Report on Disability in 2011. The World Report on

> Disability suggests steps for all stakeholders – including governments, civil society organizations and disabled people's organizations – to create enabling environments, develop rehabilitation and support services, ensure adequate social protection, create inclusive policies and programs, and enforce new and existing standards and legislation, to the benefit of people with disabilities and the wider community. People with disabilities should be central to these endeavors.
>
> **(World Health Organization 2011)**

The document includes a discussion on understanding the health of people with disabilities and the impact of rehabilitative medicine to improve functioning through treatment, therapy, and assistive technologies.

Rehab2030 is a call for action response to this report organized by the WHO in 2017. The meeting report states, 'With its objective of optimizing function, rehabilitation supports those with health conditions to remain as independent as possible, to participate in education, to be economically productive, and fulfil meaning life roles' (World Health Organization 2017).

5.2.1 Disease and health

Understanding the impact of disease and definitions of health as related to improving function is critical to provision of appropriate rehabilitation engineering services.

The WHO has chosen to define health as 'a state of complete physical, mental, and social well-being and not merely the absence of disease or infirmity' (World Health Organization 1948). General health care needs, to include health promotion and prevention activities, frequently are unmet for people with disabilities, resulting in greater vulnerability to secondary and age-related conditions (World Health Organization). Definitions of disease and health, however, have and continue to change due to increasing expectations for health, diagnostic ability, and social and economic factors. In addition, concepts such as disease and health in part 'embody value judgements and are rooted in metaphor' (Boyd 2000). The need to define these concepts and capture data using a common language and framework remains critical to assure ethical and appropriate global distribution of limited healthcare resources.

The WHO Family of International Classifications (WHO–FIC) is intended to support international and national health systems, statistics, and evidence (World Health Organization). To this end, and as previously described in previous chapters in this section, the WHO has developed reference classifications that can be used to describe the health state of a person at a point in time. Diseases are classified in the WHO International Classification of Diseases and Related Health Problems, now in its 10th revision (ICD–10). The ICD is used by healthcare providers, researchers, information and technology workers, policymakers, insurers, and patient organizations to classify and record diseases and other health problems such as symptoms and injury. These health records enable the storage and retrieval of diagnostic information for clinical, epidemiological, and quality purposes.

To contribute to shared global health objectives, the United States Centers for Disease Control and Prevention (CDC) works in close partnership with the WHO, UN agencies, the World Bank, and other federal agencies within the US Government, private foundations, and universities (Centers for Disease Control and Prevention 2017). The Centers for Medicare & Medicaid Services (CMS), an operating division along with the CDC in the US Department of Health & Human Services (HHS), requires reporting of medical events using ICD codes.

Functioning and disability are conceptualized in the context of health and classified separately in the WHO International Classification of Functioning, Disability and Health (World Health Organization 2013). A third reference classification, the International Classification of Health Interventions (ICHI), currently under development, will 'provide health care service providers and researchers with a common tool for reporting and analyzing health interventions between countries' (ICHI 2018).

While the ICD is used to 'monitor the incidence and prevalence of diseases and other health problems providing a picture of the general health situations of countries and populations' (ICD 2017), the WHO Global Burden of Disease (GBD) study measures what prevents the goal of achieving worldwide long life in full health. GBD measures burden of disease using the disability-adjusted life year (DALY). This time-based measure combines years of life lost due to premature mortality and years of life lost due to time lived in states of less than full health. Prevalence data, however, 'do not capture the burden of disease in terms of loss of functioning' (World Health Organization 2008b). People are living longer and the effects of illness due to chronic disease with loss of health may result in serious impairments and disability that affect a person's ability to participate in their life situations (World Health Organization 2017).

As early as 1983, H. Schipper raised the question 'Why measure quality of life?' as the final common pathway for healthcare delivery (Schipper 1983). Outcome measures for survival and disease-free lifetimes do not capture the relevance of care to patients in terms of physical, mental, emotional, and social functioning. Methodological development is still ongoing for participation measures which reflect individuals' assessment of the impact of their health on their social participation within their current environment. In 2015, Krahn et al. continued to support the need for research and policy directions to address health inequities for individuals with disabilities including 'improved access to health care and human services, increased data to support decision-making, strengthened health and human services workforce capacity, explicit inclusion of disability in public health programs, and increased emergency preparedness' (Krahn, Walker, and Correa-De-Araujo 2015).

Examples of this multidimensional concept of health-related quality of life and well-being can be found in the US Office of Disease Prevention and Health Promotion's Healthy People 2020 and the National Institute of Health Patient Reported Outcomes Measurement Information System (PROMIS) national initiatives. Healthy People 2020, based on priorities in the US National Health Security Strategy plan developed by the HHS, provided a national framework for people with disabilities to promote health, prevent secondary conditions, and work to eliminate disparities (Office of Disease Prevention and Health Promotion 2018) (see the overarching goals listed in Figure 5.2).

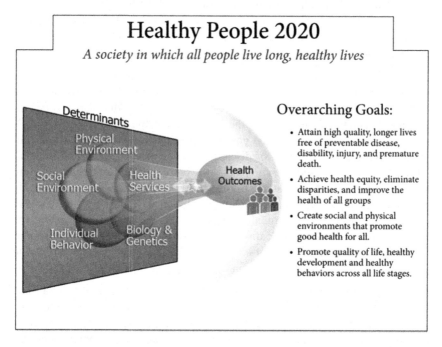

Figure 5.2 US National Health Security Strategy plan developed by the United States Department of Health and Human Services, Healthy People 2020 (https://www.healthypeople.gov/sites/default/files/HP2020Framework.pdf).

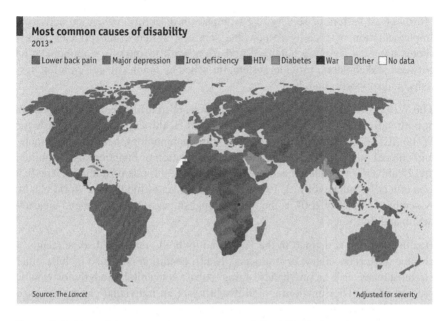

Most common causes of disability
2013*

Lower back pain   Major depression   Iron deficiency   HIV   Diabetes   War   Other   No data

Source: The *Lancet*   *Adjusted for severity

Figure 5.3 Map of the most common causes of disability internationally as reported in 2013 (http://www.thelancet.com/pdfs/journals/lancet/PIIS0140-6736(15)60692-4.pdf)(http://www.economist.com/news/science-and-technology/21654565-global-disability).

The health needs of people with disabilities vary with the type of limitation and by the health condition underlying the disability (Krahn, Walker, and Correa-De-Araujo 2015). While the types of illnesses and injuries causing death and disability are changing, findings are consistent in that disability is causing a greater and greater fraction of the burden of disease (Vos et al. 2015). Figure 5.3 illustrates the most common causes of disability internationally as reported in 2013 by *The Lancet*, a weekly peer-reviewed general medical journal.

5.3 Disability and functioning

Rehabilitation engineering professionals play a critical role in the application of science and technology to improve the quality of life of individuals with disabilities. They work as members of the transdisciplinary team in both indirect consumer service delivery and direct consumer service delivery.

(DiGiovine et al. 2018)

In 2005, World Health Assembly WHA58.23 resolution on 'Disability, including prevention, management and rehabilitation' urged member states to promote and strengthen national policies, strategies, and programs including coordinated efforts of all sectors of society to participate in disability prevention activities. Implementation of socially responsible services, systems, and policies necessitates use of a common language and framework to improve communication between stakeholders, provide systematic schemes for health information systems, and support research.

The WHO–FIC aims to provide such a framework to inform health management at both individual and population levels (World Health Organization). While the WHO–ICD is the standard diagnostic tool for epidemiology, health management, and clinical purposes, the International Classification of Functioning, Disability, and Health (ICF) is a classification of health and health-related domains. The ICF was officially endorsed by all 191 WHO member states in the 54th World Health Assembly on 22 May 2001 as the international standard to describe and measure health and disability.

Health condition is defined in the ICF as an umbrella term for disease (acute or chronic), disorder, injury, or trauma. A health condition may also include other circumstances such as pregnancy, aging, stress, congenital anomaly, or genetic predisposition. The functioning and disability of an individual can be assessed across different cultures and settings (World Health Organization).

The ICF organizes information in two parts. Part 1 deals with functioning and disability (body functions and body structures) while part 2 covers contextual factors. Disability is defined in the ICF as 'an umbrella term for impairments, activity limitations and participation restrictions. It denotes the negative aspects of the interaction between an individual (with a health condition) and that individual's contextual factors (environmental and personal factors)' (World Health Organization 2001). The term, functioning, denotes the positive aspects of these interactions. While functioning is conceptualized in the context of health, it does not associate specific health problems or diseases to disability and independently assesses the individual's activities and participation domains. The 'ICF places all health conditions on an equal footing, allowing them to be compared in terms of their related functioning, via a common framework' (World Health Organization 2013).

The WHO North American Collaborating Center is located at the National Center for Health Statistics (NCHS) within the CDC. The NCHS webpage describes the language of the ICF as 'neutral as to etiology, placing the emphasis on function rather than condition or disease' (Centers for Disease Control and Prevention 2018).

Rehabilitation engineering professionals are vital members of the assistive technology team working with persons with disabilities to optimize their function, whether in rehabilitation, home, community, educational, or vocational settings (RESNA 2018b).

The common language and framework of the ICF facilitate communication for the multidisciplinary collaboration seen as best practice to assure satisfactory outcomes in all settings. Without effective communication between all stakeholders to include consumers, providers, and researchers, there is the potential for a mismatch between the person and technology. As discussed previously in Chapter 3, such mismatches are known to result in sub-optimal outcomes and abandonment of technology at a cost to both persons with disabilities and society at large.

5.4 Impairment and participation

'It is the focus on, and collaboration with, individuals with disabilities that make rehabilitation engineering professionals unique in the engineering professions, and one of the most gratifying professions in engineering' (RESNA 2018b).

'People with disabilities are a diverse group who share the experience of living with significant limitations in functioning and, as a result, often experience exclusion from full participation in their communities', including access to healthcare (Krahn, Walker, and Correa-De-Araujo 2015). The WHO factsheet on disability and health, reviewed in November 2016, identifies barriers to healthcare to include prohibitive cost, limited availability of services, physical barriers, and inadequate skills and knowledge of health workers (World Health Organization). 'The way the health system contributes to social participation and the empowerment of the people, is defined as one of the main axes for the development of the Primary Health Care strategy' in the 2008 World Health Report (World Health Organization 2008a). Access to primary healthcare is viewed as the foundation of every healthcare system and essential to achieve the UN SDGs. The goal of universal health coverage is to ensure all people obtain the health services they need without incurring financial hardship and is 'a power mechanism for achieving better health and well-being, and for promoting human development' (World Health Organization 2013).

The United Nations Convention on the Rights of Persons with Disabilities (CRPD) of 2008 marked 'a shift in thinking about disability from a social welfare concern, to a human rights issue, which acknowledges that societal barriers and prejudices are themselves disabling' (United Nations 2008). The CRPD adopted a social model to define disability as including 'those who have long-term physical, mental, intellectual or sensory impairments which in interaction with various barriers may hinder their full and effective participation in society on an equal basis with others' to include education and employment (United Nations 2008).

The WHO–ICF offers an international, scientific tool to support this paradigm shift from 'the purely medical model to an integrated biopsychosocial model of human functioning and disability' (World Health Organization 2002). The

ICF clarifies that participation in everyday life cannot be inferred from medical diagnosis alone (Centers for Disease Control and Prevention 2018). Participation represents the societal perspective of functioning which, for a person with a disability, can be related to any one of a number of different health conditions. Given the rise of chronic disease, it has been proposed that the WHO definition of health as complete well-being be changed to emphasize the ability of humans to adapt and self-manage in the face of social, physical, and emotional challenges (Huber et al. 2011).

5.5 Barriers and facilitators

'Disability is not an unavoidable consequence of injury and chronic disease but is substantially affected by the actions that society takes' (Forum on Aging, Disability, and Independence et al. 2013). International and national initiatives for persons with disabilities have identified a need for greater awareness and advocacy, increased investment into rehabilitation workforce and infrastructure, and improved leadership and governance structures (World Health Organization 2017).

The preamble to the CRPD from 2008 includes the statement that despite 'various instruments and undertakings, persons with disabilities continue to face barriers in their participation as equal members of society and violations of their human rights in all parts of the world' (United Nations 2008). The CDC quotes the WHO definition of barriers to participation to include access to the physical environment, lack of relevant assistive technology, negative attitudes of people toward disability, and services, systems, and policies that are either nonexistent or hinder the involvement of all people with a health condition in all areas of life (Centers for Disease Control and Prevention 2018).

The WHO recognizes that 'Health or state of health can only be defined in terms of an individual and that person's goals and expectations' (World Health Organization 2001). Establishing a taxonomy of barriers and facilitators enables identification of unmet needs and tangible indicators for systems change. The WHO–ICF identifies two factors, personal and environmental, that may act as barriers or facilitators to individuals with health conditions. Personal factors are not classified in the ICF but are defined as the particular background of a person that are not part of a health condition but may play a role in disability and contribute to the outcome of various interventions. These personal factors may include gender, age, culture, life experiences, and psychological characteristics. Environmental factors represent the physical, social, and attitudinal environments in which people live their lives. Facilitating factors in a person's environment improve functioning and reduce disability (World Health Organization 2001). These factors include aspects such as a physical environment that is accessible, the availability of relevant assistive technology, and positive attitudes of people towards disability as well as services, systems and policies that aim to increase the involvement of all people with a health condition in all areas of life.

(Centers for Disease Control and Prevention 2018)

Qualifiers for environmental factors may be described from the perspective of the person's own situation or as a result of global factors such as poverty.

The WORLD Policy Analysis Center has collected and analyzed information on rights, laws, and policies in all 193 UN member states 'in a range of critical areas including education, health, adult labor and working conditions, child labor, poverty, constitutional rights, discrimination, childhood, gender, marriage, families, aging, and disability' (Global Partnership for Sustainable Development Data 2018). The map in Figure 5.4 identifies which nations include measures to promote equity for persons with disabilities in their constitutions (World Policy Analysis Center 2018).

A significant barrier to measuring progress in equity is that disability is defined differently across international legislation, classifications, and frameworks. In the US for example, the Americans with Disabilities Act defines disability to prohibit discrimination and the Social Security Act uses different definitions to determine eligibility for services and supports. The US Department of Labor states that definitions of disability vary depending on the purpose for which it is being used by federal and state agencies (US Department of Labor 2018). Lack of comparability

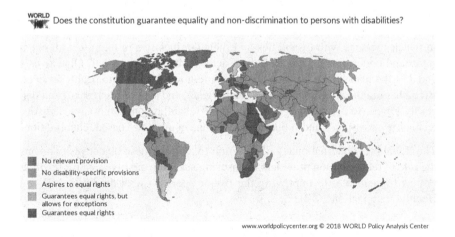

WORLD Does the constitution guarantee equality and non-discrimination to persons with disabilities?

No relevant provision
No disability-specific provisions
Aspires to equal rights
Guarantees equal rights, but allows for exceptions
Guarantees equal rights

www.worldpolicycenter.org © 2018 WORLD Policy Analysis Center

Figure 5.4 Map identifying which nations include constitutional measures promoting equity for persons with disabilities (https://www.worldpolicycenter.org/media/no-cdn-images/maps/161.png).

has been a major obstacle to developing a solid body of evidence on health and health disparities for disabled populations to guide development of effective services, systems, and policies (Krahn, Walker, and Correa-De-Araujo 2015).

The WHO Disability Assessment Schedule (WHODAS 2.0) operationalizes the concepts of the ICF and seeks to address this need for evidence through use of a single tool that can assess health and disability across different cultures and settings (World Health Organization). Additional guidance on use of the ICF as a tool for research, education, clinical, and policy development can be found in the Practical Manual. The 2013 WHO–ICF Practical Manual has not been finalized and published but describes its most important role as a planning and policy tool for decision-makers. The manual defines how standardized data collection, monitoring and evaluation of outcomes enables

> inferences to be drawn about the success of social measures such as anti-discrimination laws and policies, or service and rehabilitation programs designed to improve and equalize the participation of individuals with disabilities in all aspects of life. The Practical Manual provides real-life examples on how to apply the ICF concepts and framework in practice to include coding and statistical use, clinical documentation, education, social policy and programs, advocacy and empowerment.
>
> **(World Health Organization 2013)**

A high-level meeting of the United Nations General Assembly in September 2013 reaffirmed the need to realize internationally agreed upon development goals for persons with disabilities, 'acknowledging the value of their contribution to the general well-being, progress and diversity of society' (UN G. Assembly 2013). The succeeding WHO Global Disability Action Plan 2014–2021 envisions a world in which 'persons with disabilities and their families live in dignity, with equal rights and opportunities, and are able to achieve their full potential'. Objectives 1 and 3 of the plan's three objectives focus on removing barriers to health services, strengthening the collection of good quality data, and supporting research on disability. Objective 2 is to strengthen and extend rehabilitation, habilitation, assistive technology, assistance and support services, and community-based rehabilitation.

The Rehab2030 international call to action to address these objectives confirms the role of rehabilitation providers in ensuring access to quality assistive technology as fundamental to improving the lives of persons with disabilities (World Health Organization 2017).

5.6 Disability, rehabilitation, and assistive technology

As the fields of rehabilitation and assistive technology have advanced, 'so has the field of rehabilitation engineering in providing more educational, social, and vocational opportunities for individuals with disabilities' (RESNA 2018b). Recent public engagement activities, such as the Google Impact Challenge: Disabilities, support the role of rehabilitation engineers using 'big ideas' with technology at the core to expand opportunity and independence. The organization seeks to see how the lives of people with disabilities will be when successful innovative solutions and approaches are welcomed (Google Impact Challenge Disabilities 2018).

The 2005 World Health Assembly (WHA58) report, 'Disability, Including Prevention, Management and Rehabilitation', recognized that 'people with disabilities are important contributors to society and that allocating resources to their rehabilitation is an investment' (World Health Organization 2005). Rehabilitation is described as a set of interventions, along a continuum of care, designed to optimize functioning and reduce disability in individuals with health conditions in their environments. Access to rehabilitation can decrease the consequences of disease or injury, improve health and quality of life, and reduce the use of health services (World Health Organization 2011). Unfortunately, critical gaps remain in the evidence base for rehabilitation to include cost benefits, facilitators and barriers to access, and a standardized measure of rehabilitation impact (World Health Organization 2017). The international 'Rehabilitation 2030: A Call for Action' meeting 6–7 February 2017 at the WHO headquarters in Geneva, Switzerland, brought stakeholders together to discuss 'the strategic direction for coordinated action and establishing joint commitments to raise the profile of rehabilitation as a health strategy relevant to the whole population, across the lifespan and across the continuum of care' (World Health Organization 2017). The WHO supports rehabilitation as a process aimed at enabling people to reach and maintain their optimal physical, sensory, intellectual, psychological, and social functional levels. Rehabilitation provides disabled people with the tools they need to attain independence and self-determination through restoration of abilities. Habilitation has been defined as building abilities for the first time. Habilitation and rehabilitation interventions to optimize functioning and reduce disability for persons with disabilities include assistive technology (World Health Organization).

Assistive technology (AT), defined as including devices or products and services, can have 'a profound impact on safety, level of functioning and independence' (World Health Organization 2017). Access to AT, however, remains a barrier due to high costs, a lack of awareness, availability, trained personnel, policy, and financing with only one in ten people in need receiving the assistive products and services necessary to maintain or improve their functioning and independence (World Health Organization). The insertion of AT definitions into US legislation including the Rehabilitation Act of 1973, Assistive Technology Act 1998 as amended in 2004, and during reauthorization of acts supporting education, work, and independent living confirmed the value of AT to 'increase, maintain or improve functional capabilities of individuals with disabilities' (GovTrack.us 2020).

Recognizing the potential benefits of collaboration with international organizations that promote the field of rehabilitation and AT, the following associations in 2000 signed the Tokushima agreement to promote communication and information exchange: Rehabilitation Engineering Society of Japan (RESJA), Association for the Advancement of Assistive Technology in Europe (AAATE), Rehabilitation Engineering and Assistive Technology Society of North America (RESNA), and Australian Rehabilitation Assistive Technology Association (ARATA). The agreement was supplanted in 2016 by the Alliance of Assistive Technology Professional Organizations to also included the Rehabilitation Engineering Society of Korea (RESKO) and Taiwan Rehabilitation Engineering and Assistive Technology Society (TREATS). This formal agreement 'reflects a joint commitment to improving access to assistive technology through research, policy advocacy training, information sharing, and knowledge translation' (RESNA 2018a).

Recent international efforts to extend and expand rehabilitation strategies, including assistive technologies, are seen in the WHO Global Cooperation on Assistive Technology (GATE) initiative. GATE was established in 2014 with the single goal of improving access to high-quality affordable assistive products by persons with disabilities through capacity building (World Health Organization). AT, information and communication technology (ICT), accessible technology, universal design, and accessible or enabling environment are described as interlinked and preconditions for mainstreaming disability in development priorities. Investment in technology, to make it available and affordable, is identified as a practical step to establish the 'Promise of Technology to Achieve Sustainable Development for All' (World Health Organization). Stakeholders represent member states, international organizations, donor agencies, professional organizations, academia, industry, and consumer groups. The vision of the GATE initiative is 'A world where everyone in need has high-quality, affordable assistive products to lead a healthy, productive and dignified life' and will focus on four interlinked activities to include policy, products, personnel, and provision (World Health Organization). To further the aims of GATE, the 2017 Global Research, Innovation, and Education in Assistive Technology (GREAT) Summit brought together nearly 200 stakeholders to stimulate transformational change in assistive technology research, innovation, and education (Scherer, MacLachlan, and Khasnabis 2018). Position papers were developed to outline current thinking and possibilities regarding strategic drivers previously identified by GATE to include people (or users) personnel, policy, provision, and products (Scherer, MacLachlan, and Khasnabis 2018). Ninety-two (92) snapshots were gathered from global researchers, innovators, users, and educators of AT as a way to showcase AT innovation and foster global collaboration (Layton, Murphy, and Bell 2018).

Rehabilitation engineers and AT professionals are described as 'dedicated to increasing the personal independence and functional capability of individuals who are disabled' (US Department of Education 2017). This chapter offers a macro view of the overarching principles linking socially responsible actions to initiatives recognizing rehabilitation as critical to achieving healthy lives and well-being for all. Awareness of continually evolving global objectives with a clear understanding of system-level information, as well as the functioning of persons with disabilities, is essential for rehabilitation engineer professionals to continue to fulfill this critical role and remain at the forefront of transformative solutions creating a just and equal world.

5.7 Future vision

Strengthening interventions to optimize functioning and reduce disability in individuals with health conditions will begin with the inclusion of accurate data on rehabilitation across all health systems (World Health Organization 2017). Emerging health information systems will 'underpin decision-making in health policy, management and clinical care through the collection, standardization, coding and management of information' (World Health Organization 2017). Building capacity in the health and rehabilitation workforce will require disruptive innovation to create a new value network with fundamental changes in educational programming, practice, research, and policy. The following supplemental readings explore strategies to improve access to rehabilitation and AT by strengthening cooperative action between and within stakeholder groups.

5.8 Discussion questions

1. Why are socially responsible actions important?
2. In what way(s) does disease result in disability?
3. What does 'having a disability' mean?
4. When does impairment effect function?
5. Where are barriers to participation found by persons with disabilities and what types of facilitators should be considered?
6. How does rehabilitation and assistive technology impact individuals with disabilities?
7. Who must ensure that efforts to improving access to rehabilitation and assistive technology occur?

Bibliography

Boyd, K. M. 2000. "Disease, Illness, Sickness, Health, Healing and Wholeness: Exploring Some Elusive Concepts." *Medical Humanities* 26 (1): 9–17.
Centers for Disease Control and Prevention. 2017. "CDC's Global Health Partnerships." Accessed 08, 2018.

————. "The ICF: An Overview." 2017. Accessed 2018.

DiGiovine, Carmen P., Meghan Donahue, Patricia Bahr, Mark Bresler, Joseph Klaesner, Raj Pagadala, Brian Burkhardt, and Ray Grott. 2018. "Rehabilitation Engineers, Technologists, and Technicians: Vital Members of the Assistive Technology Team." *Assistive Technology* 28: 1–12.

Forum on Aging, Disability, and Independence, Sciences Policy Board on Health, Division of Behavioral and Social Sciences, and Education of Medicine Institute, and Research Council National. 2013.

Global Partnership for Sustainable Development Data. "World Policy Analysis Center." Accessed 08, 2018.

Google Impact Challenge Disabilities. "Meet the Innovators Working Toward a More Accessible Future." Accessed 08, 2018.

GovTrack.us. 2004. "H.R. 4278–108th Congress: Assistive Technology Act of 2004."

Huber, M., J. A. Knottnerus, L. Green, H. van der Horst, A. R. Jadad, D. Kromhout, B. Leonard, et al. 2011. "How Should We Define Health?" *BMJ (Clinical Research Ed.)* 343: d4163.

ICD, WHO. 2017. *Version: 2016*. Geneva: World Health Organization.

ICHI. 2020. "Classifications of Interventions."

Institute of Medicine. 2014. *Global Development Goals and Linkages to Health and Sustainability: Workshop Summary*, edited by Erin Rusch. Washington, DC: The National Academies Press.

ISO, ISO26000. 2010. "Guidance on Social Responsibility." Geneva: The International Organization for Standardization.

Krahn, Gloria L., Deborah Klein Walker, and Rosaly Correa-De-Araujo. 2015. "Persons with Disabilities as an Unrecognized Health Disparity Population." *American Journal of Public Health* 105 Supplement 2: S198–S206.

Layton, Natasha, Caitlin Murphy, and Diane Bell. 2018. "From Individual Innovation to Global Impact: The Global Cooperation on Assistive Technology (GATE) Innovation Snapshot as a Method for Sharing and Scaling." *Disability and Rehabilitation: Assistive Technology* 13 (5): 486–491.

Leggett, Jane A. and Nicole T. Carter. 2012. "Rio 20: The United Nations Conference on Sustainable Development, June 2012." Washington, DC: Library of Congress, Congressional Research Service.

Office of Disease Prevention and Health Promotion. 2020. "Health-Related Quality of Life and Well-Being."

RESNA. "International Efforts." Accessed 08, 2018.

————. "Rehabilitation Engineering Profession White Paper." Accessed 08, 2018.

Scherer, M. J., M. MacLachlan, and C. Khasnabis. 2018. "Introduction to the Special Issue on the First Global Research, Innovation, and Education on Assistive Technology (GREAT) Summit and Invitation to Contribute to and Continue the Discussions." *Disability and Rehabilitation.Assistive Technology* 13 (5): 435–436.

Schipper, H. 1983. "Why Measure Quality of Life?" *Canadian Medical Association Journal* 128 (12): 1367–1370.

Steele, K. 2014. *An Introduction for Mechanical Engineers*. Pennsylvania, PA: Springer.

The World Bank. "Understanding Poverty." Accessed 08, 2018.

UN G. Assembly. 2013. "Outcome Document of the High-Level Meeting of the General Assembly on the Realization of the Millennium Development Goals and Other Internationally Agreed Development Goals for Persons with Disabilities: The Way Forward, a Disability-Inclusive Development Agenda towards 2015 and Beyond." *Sixty-Eight Session*. New York.

United Nations. 2018. "Convention on the Rights of Persons with Disabilities and Optional Protocol, the United Nations." Accessed 08, 2018.

———. "Millennium Development Goals 2000." Accessed 08, 2018.

US Department of Education. "Careers in Rehabilitation: Rehabilitation Engineering." Accessed 08, 2018.

US Department of Labor. "Frequently Asked Questions." Accessed 08, 2018.

Vos, Theo, Ryan M. Barber, Brad Bell, Amelia Bertozzi-Villa, Stan Biryukov, Ian Bolliger, Fiona Charlson, Adrian Davis, Louisa Degenhardt, and Daniel Dicker. 2015. "Global, Regional, and National Incidence, Prevalence, and Years Lived with Disability for 301 Acute and Chronic Diseases and Injuries in 188 Countries, 1990–2013: A Systematic Analysis for the Global Burden of Disease Study 2013." *The Lancet* 386 (9995): 743–800.

World Health Organization. 2008a. *The Global Burden of Disease: 2004 Update*. Geneva: World Health Organization.

———. "Assistive Technology." Accessed 08, 2018.

———. "Classifications." Accessed 08, 2018.

———. "Disability and Health." Accessed 08, 2018.

———. 2005. *Disability, Including Prevention, Management and Rehabilitation*. Geneva, Switzerland: Author.

———. 2008b. "The Global Burden of Disease: 2004 Update." Geneva: World Health Organization.

———. "Global Cooperation on Assistive Technology (GATE)." WHO, last modified 2018, https://www.who.int/disabilities/technology/gate/en/.

———. 2013. "How to Use the ICF: A Practical Manual for Using the International Classification of Functioning, Disability and Health (ICF)." *Exposure Draft for Comment*. Geneva: WHO 26.

———. 2001. *International Classification of Functioning, Disability and Health: ICF*. Geneva: World Health Organization.

———. "The Need to Scale Up Rehabilitation." Accessed 08, 2018.

———. 1948. "Preamble to the Constitution."

———. 2017. "Rehabilitation 2030: A Call for Action."

———. "Rehabilitation: Key for Health in the 21st Century." Accessed 08, 2018.

———. "Social Determinants of Health." Accessed 08, 2018.

———. 2002. "Towards a Common Language for Functioning, Disability, and Health: ICF." *The International Classification of Functioning, Disability and Health*.

———. 2011. *World Report on Disability 2011*. Geneva: World Health Organization.

World Policy Analysis Center. 2017. "Does the Constitution Guarantee Equality and Non-Discrimination to Persons with Disabilities?". Accessed 08, 2018.

Chapter 6 Rehabilitation engineering across the lifespan

R. H. Wang and L. K. Kenyon

Contents

DOI: 10.1201/b21964-7

6.1 Chapter overview

The Oxford Dictionaries define lifespan as "the length of time for which a person or animal lives or a thing functions" (Dictionaries 2017). Practically speaking, in the field of rehabilitation engineering, the term lifespan refers to working with clients from the time of birth until the time of death. The time from birth to death encompasses a broad range of complex biological, psychological, and social developmental factors that must be acknowledged. While clinical practice, service settings, and funding programs are often defined by age cohorts (e.g., pediatrics or geriatrics) or the type of health issue being addressed (e.g., physical or mental health), in this chapter, emphasis is placed on the continuous nature of the lifespan and the holistic development of each individual client.

Whether working with a client during infancy or in old age, lifespan concepts directly influence how clients are viewed and understood, how interactions with clients are carried out, what expectations are placed on them, and what services are available to them. The chapter thus begins by introducing developmental stage theories, lifespan developmental theories, life course theories, and developmental systems theories as foundational considerations when working with clients in rehabilitation engineering practice. Normative development is reviewed along with differences in developmental trajectories and life course in the presence of health-related conditions that impact body functions and structures, activity, and participation. Client- and family-centered care approaches are briefly discussed to highlight the need to consider who clients are when working with clients across their lifespan. Finally, before presenting two cases that illustrate application of the theories, concepts, and principles outlined in this chapter, common misconceptions relevant to working with clients across their lifespan are discussed.

6.2 Theories relevant to examining lifespan

Human development is the process of continual change that occurs over the lifespan. Numerous theories have been proposed to describe the individual and interacting biological, psychological, and environmental factors that influence development. Selected prominent theories are presented to provide context related to the complexity of the developmental process.

6.2.1 Stage theories of human development

Stage theories suggest that development occurs in sequential, expectable, and universal stages. According to stage theories, an individual's abilities are determined by the chronological age or life stage of each individual. Often in stage theories, in order for an individual to progress to a subsequent stage, predefined challenges need to be overcome. An example of a stage theory is Erik Erikson's psychosocial

130

theory of development from infancy to late adulthood. According to Erikson, development is influenced by elements of the environment and comprises eight normative stages (Thies and Travers 2001). Each stage involves "developmental crises" which may have positive and negative results, and evolves from infancy (e.g., "trust vs mistrust") to senescence in older adulthood (e.g., "ego integrity vs disgust or despair"). Another stage theory is Piaget's constructivist theory of cognitive development which follows four stages of development from newborn to two years old ("sensorimotor"), two to seven years old (preoperational), seven to 11 years old (concrete operational), and 11 to 16 years old (formal operational) (Thies and Travers 2001). Piaget's theory also includes the environment as an influence in change. During development, operations (defined as more complex schemata arising from cognitive structures) evolve through the four stages (Thies and Travers 2001).

6.2.2 Lifespan developmental theories

Though still focusing on the individual, lifespan developmental theories present a continuous, rather than staged, view of human development (Baltes, Lindenberger, and Staudinger 2007). Lifespan development can be considered as a set of theories whereby development is an ongoing and adaptive process from the start of life (conception) until the end of life. Baltes (1987) outlined several "theoretical propositions" that depict the nature of lifespan development and stress the individual variation that can be expected from development. Beyond being a life-long process, lifespan development theories depict development as a multidirectional, plastic process that involves both gains and losses, and occurs within a complex context (Baltes, Lindenberger, and Staudinger 2007; Baltes 1987, 611). With respect to concepts of multi-directionality and the co-occurrence of gains and losses, development in the multiple dimensions of behavior may be reversed and may not always occur towards higher levels of function. Plasticity refers to variability that develops within an individual owing to individual experiences and the environment in which the individual resides. Relatedly, development is said to occur within complex contexts involving biological and environmental interactions with age-associated, history-associated, and non-normative factors.

6.2.3 Life course theory

In life course theory, developmental changes are viewed as occurring less within the individual, and more within the context of an individual's environment. Life course development stresses the dynamic interactions between a person's biological and psychological factors, as well as the forces imposed by the social environment. In life course theory, meaning in peoples' lives is socially constructed. Life course theory developed as more and more longitudinal studies were being conducted with children and people aging into their later years, in addition to the growing concerns over population aging (Elder Jr and Shanahan 2007). According to Elder Jr and Shanahan "life course is conceived as an age-graded sequence of socially defined roles and events that are enacted and even recast over time" (Elder Jr and Shanahan 2007, 706). Further, they describe lives as having a multitude of trajectories and transition states. Several principles are articulated within life course theory: "life span development", which is a life-long process; "human agency", where individuals' life courses are created via choices and actions made within the confines of their sociohistorical contexts; "timing", whereby timing influences the precursors and outcomes of life transitions, events, and behavior patterns; "linked lives", where interdependent individuals are related to each other through their socio-historical contexts; and "historical time and place", where individuals live within and are impacted by historical periods and locations.

6.2.4 Developmental systems theory

Developmental systems theory is an approach that integrates heredity (genetics and epigenetics), human development, and evolution. The approach goes beyond traditional perspectives of development in biology and psychology with their attribution of behaviors as arising from either primarily genetic or primarily environmental and experiential factors (Johnston 2010, 12–29). Several perspectives on developmental systems theory are actively being explored and debated, though some overarching tenets to describe the approach can be summarized (Oyama, Griffiths, and Gray 2001, 1–11; Johnston 2010, 12–29). In developmental systems theory, development involves multiple, interacting inputs that together determine behavior or behavioral patterns. Another important contributor to behaviors is the context in which development is occurring, which takes into account the current status of the system and all possible interacting inputs at the time. The notion of "extended inheritance" is also described, whereby a variety of transmittable resources beyond genes are available to support the development of behaviors. The mutual interactions between individuals and environments are developing and are additional inputs to development.

6.3 Development across the lifespan

When working with clients, it is important to keep in mind normative developmental factors in order to best serve clients at any age. This section examines what may be considered normative development and the associated biological, psychological, and social changes. Early development from birth to adolescence is when abilities, skills, and knowledge are intensely acquired and accumulated and hence involves rapid development. In adulthood and older adulthood, the individual is said to be undergoing an "aging" process that involves less intense development. While aging is not a disease process in itself, the aging process often reflects a decline within body structures and functions that results from interactions between personal characteristics, life habits, and choices (e.g., in diet or activity levels), environmental stressors, and the occurrence of disease conditions. Although normative development is outlined in this section, it should be noted that development is highly variable over the lifespan, and that an individual's capabilities, goals, expectations, and values are highly influenced by the social and cultural environment in which the individual lives.

6.3.1 Early development

Developmental milestones are age-specific behaviors or skills observed in infants and children within a particular age range. Sitting, walking, talking, and getting dressed are examples of developmental milestones. As children develop and achieve more developmental milestones, they progressively become more capable and independent. Typically, developing children acquire increasingly complex skills in all areas of development: gross motor, fine motor, speech and language, cognitive, and socioemotional. Gross motor skills are those skills that involve large muscle groups, such as standing and walking. Fine motor skills involve use of the hands to perform such tasks as coloring and writing. Speech and language skills involve receptive abilities (understanding what someone has said) as well as expressive abilities (communicating to others). Cognitive skills involve thought processes and include activities such as learning, problem-solving, and remembering. Socioemotional skills include interacting with others and developing relationships with other people.

Table 6.1 provides an overview of select developmental milestones at specific timeframes during infancy while Table 6.2 lists developmental milestones from 18 months to five years of age (Centers for Disease Control and Prevention 2016). Although each developmental milestone in the table is associated with a specific age, the actual age at which a typically developing child reaches a particular milestone is quite variable. Many factors contribute to a child's development including, but not limited to, the child's environment, the child's personality, and the cultural child-rearing practices of the child's family. For example, a child who does not have an opportunity to climb stairs very often may achieve stair climbing skills more slowly. A child who enjoys moving and movement may develop mobility skills sooner than a child who is content to sit and watch others move. Infants who are raised within cultures where babies are not placed on the floor or on the ground may not learn to crawl.

By the time children reach six to eight years of age, they are already able to perform many skills and activities. They can dress themselves, tie their shoes,

Table 6.1 Selected Developmental Milestones Observed at Specific Timeframes during Infancy

Developmental Skill Area	Two Months	Four Months	Six Months	Nine Months	Twelve Months
Social/emotional skills	• May smile at people • Tries to look at familiar people	• Spontaneously smiles at people • Likes to play and interact with people	• Starts to know if someone is a stranger • Likes to play and interact with people, especially caregivers • Responds to the emotions of other people • Looks at self in a mirror	• May be afraid of strangers and cling with familiar adults • Has preferred toys	• Maybe shy or anxious with strangers • Cries when a caregiver leaves • Repeats actions and sounds to get attention • Plays "peak-a-boo"
Motor skills	• Holds up head when lying on tummy	• Holds up head • May be able to roll over from stomach to back • Can hold and shake a toy • Brings hands to mouth • Pushes up to elbows when lying on belly	• Rolls over from front to back and from back to front • When held in supported standing, supports weight on legs	• Stands, holding onto furniture or other objects • Sits independently • Pulls to stand • Crawls	• Transitions into sitting • Pulls up to stand • Walks sideways holding on to furniture ("cruises") • May take a step and stands alone
Language/ communication skills	• Turns head toward sounds • Coos and makes gurgling sounds	• Babbles • Has different cries to show hunger, pain, or tiredness	• Takes turns with adults while making sounds • Responds to name • Makes noises to show joy and displeasure • Begins to babble using consonant sounds	• Understands the concept of "no" • Makes a variety of different sounds • Copies sounds and gesture of others	• Uses simple gestures such as waving "bye-bye" • Says "mama" and "dada"

(Continued)

Table 6.1 (Continued) Selected Developmental Milestones Observed at Specific Timeframes during Infancy

Developmental Skill Area	Two Months	Four Months	Six Months	Nine Months	Twelve Months
Cognitive skills	• Attends to people's faces	• Responds to attention • Reaches for toys with one hand • Uses hands and eyes together • Follows objects side to side with eyes • Recognizes familiar people and objects	• Visually explores things nearby • Brings objects to mouth • Shows curiosity about objects and tries to obtain objects out of reach	• Watches the path of a falling object • Picks up small objects using thumb and index finger	• Explores objects by shaking, banging, throwing • Easily finds hidden objects • Starts to use common objects correctly • Bangs two objects together • Puts objects in and out of a container

Source: Adapted from Centers for Disease Control and Prevention (2016).

Table 6.2 Selected Developmental Milestones Observed at Specific Timeframes during Childhood*

Developmental Skill Area	18 months	2 years	3 years	4 years	5 years
Social/emotional skills	• Gives objects to others as a form of play • May have tantrums • May be afraid of strangers • Demonstrates simple pretend play skills • Explores the environment with parent or caregiver near by	• Imitates others, especially adults and older children • Shows excitement when around other children • Demonstrates increasing independence • Demonstrates defiance (doing something that they were told not to do) • Plays alongside other children, but may start to include other children in simple games	• Beginning to demonstrate turn-taking skills • Shows concern for a friend who is crying • Demonstrates a wide variety of emotions • Separates easily from caregivers • May get upset when there are changes in routine • Begins to dress and undress self	• Is increasingly creative in pretend play • Prefers to play with other children than in solo situations • Cooperates with other children • Often has difficulty differentiating between what is real and what is pretend	• Wants to please and be liked by friends • More likely to comply with rules • Can differentiate between what is real and what is pretend • Shows increased independence • Sometimes is demanding and sometimes is cooperative
Motor skills	• Walks independently • May ascend steps • Helps to get self undressed • Drinks from a cup • Eats with a spoon	• Stands on tiptoes • Kicks a ball • Runs	• Climbs and runs well • Rides a tricycle • Walks up and down stairs	• Hops on one foot • Maintains a unilateral stance position for up to 2 seconds • Catches a bounced ball	• Maintains a unilateral stance position for 10+ seconds • Performs a somersault • Uses a fork and spoon well and sometimes a table knife

(Continued)

Table 6.2 (Continued) Selected Developmental Milestones Observed at Specific Timeframes during Childhood*

Developmental Skill Area	18 months	2 years	3 years	4 years	5 years
Language/ communication skills	• Says several words • Says and shakes head "no" • Using pointing and gestures to indicate wants	• Points to named objects or pictures • Knows names of familiar people and of body parts • Says two to four word sentences • Follows simple commands • Repeats words overheard in conversation	• Follows 2 or 3 step commands • Names most familiar things • Understands prepositions such as "in", "on", and "under" • Says name, age, and gender • Uses pronouns and some plural word forms • Can be understood by strangers most of the time	• Sings a song or says a poem from memory • Tells short stories • Can say first and last name	• Speaks very clearly • Uses future verb tense • Says name and address
Cognitive skills	• Knows that the use of ordinary objects • Points to get the attention of others • Correctly points to one body part • Scribbles • Follows one-step commands	• Begins to sort objects by shape or color • Builds towers of 4+ blocks • Follows two-step commands	• Does a 3–4-piece puzzle • Understand the concept of "two" • Copies a circle • Builds towers of 6+ blocks	• Names some colors and some numbers • Understands the concept of counting • Begins to understand the concept of time • Remembers parts of a story • Understands the concept of "same" and "different" • Can draw a person with two to four body parts • Starts to copy letters • Plays board or card games	• Counts ten or more objects • Draws a person with at least six body parts • Can print some letters or numbers • Copies geometric shapes

*Adapted from Centers for Disease Control and Prevention (2016).

may start to ride a bicycle, and often have started or will soon start to go to school. During this phase, children's social roles begin to change as they begin to seek independence from their parents and family and want to be liked and accepted by friends. Children of nine to 11 years of age often desire independence from their family as their interest in friendships with peers continue to strengthen and grow. In the young teen stage (ages 12–14 years), children begin experiencing many physical, cognitive, psychological, and social changes as puberty starts to unfold.

6.3.2 Adolescent development

Adolescence, or the period of time following the onset of puberty into early adulthood, marks the transition from childhood into adulthood (Dictionaries 2017). During this transitional period, social roles and responsibilities may fluctuate as many adolescents struggle with issues of independence and identity in the process of discovering themselves apart from their families. Peer pressures often magnify during this period in life and many adolescents find themselves struggling with choices and decisions related to a vast array of critical life issues such as the use of drugs and alcohol, sexuality and sexual orientation, and education and future career choices. Physical changes abound during this transitional period and by 15–17 years of age, most girls will have reached physical maturity while boys still may be physically developing throughout this stage. Responsibilities may increase as teens take on greater demands through school as well as paid and volunteer employment. Milestones such as obtaining a driver's license and graduating high school are also typically achieved during this stage. The end of adolescence and the beginning of adulthood are often a fluctuating line and are heavily influenced by a variety of cultural and societal factors. In the United States, 18-year-olds enjoy the autonomy and responsibility of being able to vote and serve in the military, but many adolescents at this age may live at home or rely on parental support while they attend college or attempt to establish a career.

6.3.3 Adult development

6.3.3.1 Early adulthood A variety of physical changes are associated with early adulthood. In the period between 20 and 30 years of age, physical abilities and performance reach their greatest extent (Thies and Travers 2001). Between the ages of 18 and 25, the epiphyses of the long bones have fused. An individual's peak bone mass (total bone growth in length and thickness) is achieved sometime between the late 20s and early 30s (Ondrak and Morgan 2007, 587–600; Kemper 2000, 198–216). After this period of maximum physical performance, muscle strength begins to decline, and reaction time stabilizes (Thies and Travers

2001). Further, skeletal system changes are notable as water proportions decrease in joints resulting in a concomitant increase in risk for knee, shoulder, and other joint injuries. Cardiovascular and pulmonary functions are also in their best performance states in the 20s (Thies and Travers 2001).

Knowledge of cognitive abilities over the lifespan is evolving as new research becomes available. Cross-sectional studies have shown that specific cognitive abilities that reflect processing efficiency or effectiveness such as reasoning, spatial visualization, memory, and speed peak and decline nearly linearly from early adulthood (Salthouse 2010, 754–760; Salthouse 2012, 201–226). Cognitive abilities for previously acquired information such as knowledge and vocabulary appear to increase until at least about 60 years of age, after which decline is noted (Salthouse 2012, 201–226; Salthouse 2010, 754–760). While these lab-based assessments showing cognitive changes may suggest that increased age is related to lower functional levels in real life, this is not the case. Possible reasons for this observation are the greater dependence on knowledge and experience in carrying out daily activities and the unnecessary need to perform at maximum efficiency in everyday situations. The cognitive control of behaviors, or executive functions, integrates several components which reach maturity at different periods during the lifespan (De Luca and Leventer 2010, 57–90). During early adulthood and continuing through middle adulthood, components such as cognitive flexibility, inhibitory control, working memory, and goal setting/problem solving are said to be at maturity (De Luca and Leventer 2010, 57–90).

Early adulthood is also the period of substantial change in psychosocial aspects of life. Major life events and transitions may occur in this period. This is a period of developing independent living and self-management skills in new facets of life (Quinn 1998). These may involve transitioning from school to work, career development, moving away from the family and living independently, seeking and developing intimate relationships, and purchasing property or other assets. This time period may also be marked by long-term relationships or marriage, pregnancy, or divorce (Quinn 1998; Thies and Travers 2001). With these life events, many individuals adopt and adjust to the roles of worker, romantic partner, parent, and the expectations and responsibilities of these roles.

6.3.3.2 Middle adulthood During middle adulthood, some bodily changes are notable with resultant declines in some physical abilities and comparatively stable cognitive abilities. In the musculoskeletal structures, bone and muscle mass decline, while the proportion of fat in the body increases (Thies and Travers 2001). Bone mass begins to decrease in the fifth decade for women and in the sixth decade for men and continues to steadily decrease as the individual ages (Ondrak and Morgan 2007, 587–600). As bone mass decreases, bone becomes more fragile and less able to withstand mechanical forces such as compression.

Water content decreases in supportive tissues such as cartilage, which can result in stiffness in joints (Thies and Travers 2001). Metabolism also decreases. Changes also occur in all of the sensory systems, with some marked decreases in vision (presbyopia, or decreased ability to focus on close objects) and hearing (presbycusis, or cumulative hearing changes from aging structures and environmental noise exposure) (National Institute on Deafness and Other Communication Disorders 2017; National Eye Institute 2010). The muscles in the cardiovascular and pulmonary systems do not change substantially, though the elasticity can change, and more fat develops in the muscles. There is also an increased risk for diseases such as cardiovascular disease. In women, middle adulthood is also the period in which menopause occurs (Thies and Travers 2001).

Middle adulthood is a time in the lifespan where personality development is relatively stable although several transitions and role changes may present. It is a time that may be marked by peaks in productivity and career. Roles in family life and the community may be more stable. This is also a time for contemplating plans for retirement. For some people in middle adulthood, it may begin a time when caregiving for both children living at home and aging parents become priority needs, as with the "sandwich generation" (Riley and Bowen 2005, 52–58). Conversely, middle adulthood may also be a time when children move out of the family home leaving parents with an "empty nest". Such transitions in middle adulthood may be viewed both positively and negatively depending on an individual's perspective and therefore may or may not contribute to what has been termed "midlife crisis" in some individuals.

6.3.3.3 Later adulthood   While many individuals are healthy and active in later adulthood, bodily changes are even more marked, and physical changes are also more apparent. Bone mass, lean body mass, and water content continue to decline (Thies and Travers 2001). Bones become progressively thinner, more porous and density is lost, resulting in a greater risk for fractures. There is a tendency toward increased muscle weakness. Deterioration of spinal discs occurs, partially as a result of changes in water content of supportive tissues. Skin changes include a loss of elasticity, subcutaneous fat, and collagen (Thies and Travers 2001). Skin changes result in thinned skin and a greater risk for damage. There is overall deterioration in sensory abilities for vision, hearing, olfaction, taste, and touch. Reaction time deteriorates for adjusting to varying light conditions in order to focus on objects. Cataracts may also develop as a result of oxidative damage. Hearing changes result in decreased ability to detect high frequencies during middle adulthood and lower frequencies in later adulthood. It may be more difficult to hear loud sounds and detect the location of objects through hearing (Thies and Travers 2001). There are also changes to the cardiovascular and pulmonary systems. The heart muscle becomes less elastic, and heart valves thicken and become more rigid.

Areas of cognitive change initiated during early adulthood continue and shift during later adulthood. As processing efficiency and effectiveness decline, there is now also a decline in abilities related to accumulated knowledge. Components of executive functions such as working memory and goal setting/problem solving will have started to decline while cognitive flexibility is observed to decline in later adulthood (De Luca and Leventer 2010, 57–90). It is also important to recognize what is part of development or aging compared to pathological conditions, such as with Alzheimer's disease or related dementias.

Significant psychosocial changes may occur during this stage involving multiple role changes. This stage is often characterized by retirement from paid work and new roles may be adopted in the community or in the family such as becoming a grandparent. There may be an expansion of the caregiving role with older parents or with a spouse. Key events may include the death of a spouse, parents, or friends. Multiple losses in social supports, social isolation, and loneliness are significant concerns beyond personal health changes (Gardiner, Geldenhuys, and Gott 2018, 147–157). Older adults often have a strong preference for aging at home, though some older adults may need to move elsewhere (e.g., to be closer to adult children or to a residential care home) because of changing health and care needs.

6.4 Variations in development with health-related conditions and disability

As previously described in this section, the International Classification of Functioning, Disability, and Health (ICF) (World Health Organization 2002) provides a structure for exploring the impact of a health condition on a specific individual. Consisting of broad dimensions related to body functions and structures, activities, participation, and contextual factors related to an individual and the environment in which that individual lives, the ICF provides a dynamic, multifactorial way to view the functional impact of a health condition. Various health conditions such as infectious disease and non-communicable disease, or life events such as injuries can occur over the lifespan that have a direct impact on body function and structures, activities that individuals are able to engage in, and their participation in community life. These conditions or events, interacting with personal and environmental factors, can result in disability. Approximately 15% of people worldwide have some type of disability (World Health Organization 2016). Factors such as when a condition or injury arises, and the nature of the condition, can influence how life circumstances and disability may be experienced differently by individuals.

Distinctions can be made between individuals aging with a disability and those aging into disability (Monahan and Wolf 2014, S1–3). When disability occurs early in life (for example, being born with a health condition such as spina bifida or having cerebral palsy), the health condition is assimilated in early developmental processes. If disability occurs later in life after an individual has experienced multiple facets of development, the individual is said to be aging into disability. Several differences such as in employment attainment, household income, and health and functional status, have been reported to indicate that the experiences and life course of these two groups are markedly different (Clarke and Latham 2014, S15–S23). If a life-changing health event occurs during the lifespan when certain normative activities are expected to be achieved, then the effects of the event may drastically alter future life trajectories. Experiences may also be influenced by a condition's nature such as whether it is temporary or chronic, whether the condition arises suddenly or progressively, and if progression of the condition is rapid, slow, or interrupted by periods of fluctuating symptom severity. In the following sections variations in development are discussed in the context of common health conditions and disabilities that may arise over the lifespan.

6.4.1 Early development

It is estimated that the number of children (0–14 years of age) living with disabilities ranges between 93 and 150 million (United Nations Children's Fund 2005; United Nations Department of Economic and Social Affairs Population Division 2009; World Health Organization 2008). Children may be born with a health condition such as spina bifida or a congenital limb difference that impacts their development. Some genetically based health conditions such as Down syndrome are apparent at or shortly after birth and immediately impact a child's development trajectory, whereas other genetic conditions such as Duchenne muscular dystrophy may not have an impact until later in childhood. Some genetic conditions may not even be evident or impact a person until adulthood. Acquired health conditions such as cerebral palsy (the most commonly occurring motor disability in childhood) occur as a result of events before, during, or shortly after birth and have an immediate and long-lasting impact on a child's developmental course. Other health conditions acquired during childhood such as severe brain injuries or traumatic limb loss immediately impact development across the lifespan. While infectious childhood diseases such as polio, measles, encephalitis, and meningitis are not commonly associated with disability in resourced areas of the world, such conditions may impact children in less-resourced areas of the world. For example, the number of polio cases worldwide fell from an epidemic state in 125 countries with an estimated 350,000 cases in 1988 to an estimated 1604 cases in 2009 (World Health Organization 2011).

Historically, many of the world's children with disabilities have been excluded from educational opportunities. Not only are such exclusions problematic from a learning perspective, but a lack of education is often associated with decreased opportunities for participating in work and other productive activities throughout the lifespan (World Health Organization 2011). In many resourced countries, legislation now requires including children with disabilities in educational systems. The United Nations Convention on the Rights of Persons with Disabilities (CRPD) (United Nations 2006) now asserts that all children with disabilities, no matter what country they live in, should be included in the general education programs available to children without disabilities. The CRPD further advocates that children with disabilities should receive whatever individual supports are needed to allow them to participate fully in education.

Regardless of the underlying cause of their disability, it is important to remember that some children may experience developmental delays that are directly related to their health condition whilst other children may experience delays related to factors associated with their health condition (such as prolonged hospitalization). Some children may experience delays across all areas of development while others may experience delays only in one developmental skill area (such as in gross motor skills). Some children with delays in development may eventually achieve all of their developmental milestones. However, some children may never achieve developmental milestones and may require long-term assistance and use of technology to help them to participate in daily activities and in the community.

6.4.2 Adult and older adult development

There are numerous health conditions and injuries that may result in disability during adulthood. Non-communicable diseases are now the most common health conditions worldwide (World Health Organization 2015). The leading causes of disability are hearing or vision loss, back and neck pain, osteoarthritis, chronic obstructive pulmonary disease, depression, falls, diabetes, and dementia. Depression is now considered a leading cause of disability worldwide (United Nations 2006). There is a growing trend of individuals having strokes at a younger age. Injuries resulting from sports, motor vehicle accidents, or work such as spinal cord injury or acquired brain injury are possible over the lifespan. As previously mentioned, aging itself is not a disease, but with aging comes a greater risk for disability. Increases in chronic health conditions and the increase in proportion of older people worldwide are resulting in higher disability rates (World Health Organization 2016). Health outcomes in older adults is the result of genetics as well as the amassing of stressors from the physical and social environment and the interactions of these stressors with an individual's health habits, and the opportunities they have had since a young age (World Health Organization 2015). For those who are aging with a health condition or disability, aging can be accelerated. Dementia prevalence increases with age. In people 85 years old or older, about 25–30% have some form of dementia (World Health Organization 2011). Older adults may have multiple concurrent health conditions resulting in an increased complexity of care. Conditions that arose during early development, though potentially stable or progressive in nature, continue to have an impact. Individuals aging with a disability will also be susceptible to cumulative physical injuries, for example, as a result of lifelong mobility disability and wear and tear on the physical body from using mobility aids such as wheelchairs (Quinn 1998).

In high-income countries, young adults with a disability often maintain the goals of developing autonomy and independence. Leaving the school system and transitioning to different services for health and social care are important life changes, as are leaving the family home to live more independently, developing social support systems and recreational lifestyles, and training for work opportunities. Finances and family planning for sustainable living for the future are big concerns. The World Report on Disability (World Health Organization 2011) indicates that people worldwide with disabilities are not as likely to be employed, earn less money, and incur additional monetary costs for medical care, assistive devices, and personal care services. Further, people with disabilities and their families often live with social and economic difficulties.

6.5 Care approaches across the lifespan: who is the client?

Whether it be developing a new assistive technology, assessing clients to determine the necessary intervention, or fitting clients for an existing technology, engaging clients in a meaningful way is critical to ensuring that the clients' goals are achieved, that they are satisfied with their experience, and that resources are used appropriately. Client-centered care (also known as, patient-, person-, and family-centered care), is now the preferred approach in many health settings (Grenness et al. 2014, S60–S67). Client-centered care emphasizes incorporating the client's subjective experience, goals, values, preferences, abilities, limitations, and interactions with the environment into a collaborative care process that supports an individual's choices and active participation in care. Literature suggests that client-centered care may improve client service satisfaction, adherence to recommendations and participation in health management activities, and health-related outcomes (Grenness et al. 2014, S60–S67). In care for individuals who have dementia, the use of person-centered care decreased neuropsychiatric symptoms and depression, and increased quality of life (Kim and Park 2017, 381–397).

When family members are involved, identifying who the actual client is may not be so straightforward. The primary client is often the person with the health condition. However, in many cases, in a family-centered approach, the client includes family members and others working in partnership (Bamm and Rosenbaum 2008, 1618–1624). For example, family members are often involved when individuals have difficulties making their own informed care decisions because they are not of legal age (such as in the case of a child), or if they have cognitive limitations as a result of their health condition. In some cases, the individual may require substantial care which is chiefly provided by a family member. As such, care decisions and intervention planning require the caregiver to ensure the person's as well as the caregiver's needs are met. Because of great demands associated with providing care for a family member with a disability, there is a potential for caregiver stress and burnout which can also be detrimental to the care recipient (Beach and Schulz 2017, 560–566). When multiple parties are involved, it may become unclear who the client is, and for practical purposes, whose goals and needs are being prioritized in care services. Often in the case of children or other clients who may require assistance in making informed care decisions, it is critical to involve these clients in the process as early as possible and on a continuous basis, rather than having the family members always make decisions by default.

6.6 Misconceptions related to working with clients across the lifespan

In our society, there are many misconceptions about individuals across the lifespan. It is important to recognize and be critical of conscious and unconscious biases that are often deeply ingrained in our society and culture, and to reflect on one's own biases when working with diverse client groups and individual clients so that we can best serve them. Intentional or unintentional discrimination on a societal or individual level, can result in unequal opportunities and the marginalization of clients and their families. Our interactions with, and services provided to, clients and their families may reflect our unconscious biases and may result in discriminatory language and behaviors. A focus on person-centered care as, described above, can help to address many of the following concerns.

6.6.1 Age discrimination

Age discrimination refers to unjust attitudes or actions towards people based on their age (Kydd and Fleming 2015, 432–438). Younger people, for example, may experience discrimination when they are not actively involved in decision-making processes related to their own care because they are considered "too young" to make informed decisions and parents are asked too often to speak on behalf of their children. Ageism refers to discrimination against people of older age (Kydd and Fleming 2015, 432–438). Older people are often described as frail or elderly, giving rise to images of physical or mental weakness. Older people may have ageist attitudes about older people, including themselves. For example, an older person may believe that they are too old to learn how to use technology (Wandke,

Sengpiel, and Sonksen 2012, 564–570) or perceive stigma related to older people who use canes or other mobility devices and thus decide not to use them. While younger people tend to use technology more than older people (Magsamen-Conrad et al. 2015, 186–196), it cannot be generalized that older clients will not want technology, as age is only one factor in the complex set of many reasons why people accept and adopt technology in their daily lives (Wandke, Sengpiel, and Sonksen 2012, 564–570). Older people can have positive attitudes toward technology and may wish to use technology, but several factors, including the usability of available technology or availability of training, can limit use.

6.6.2 Ableism

Ableism refers to the discrimination of individuals who have a disability of any type and placing a higher value on individuals who are able-bodied. Ableism stems from the notion that individuals who have a disability have something "wrong" with them and that they somehow need to be fixed in order to fully participate in society (Linton 1998). Ableism is deeply ingrained in our society. Examples include the lack of consistent accessibility features in the environment to accommodate people with mobility, cognitive, or sensory limitations, which result in a disparity of access to public spaces.

6.6.3 Assuming incompetence

Individuals who have disabilities cannot be automatically assumed to be less competent, and interactions with clients should not reflect this misconception. For example, individuals with severe physical disabilities or communication difficulties cannot be assumed to have cognitive disabilities as well since they may be fully cognitively intact. Children with a delay in one or more areas of development may be on target or even advanced in other areas of development. For example, a child who has significant motor delays and is unable to hold up his/her head, or sit, or walk may actually be at grade level academically and may in fact outpace his/her peers in reading or math or other areas. A child who is unable to communicate verbally may completely understand everything that is being said to him/her. Although well-intentioned, people sometimes mistakenly use a sing-song voice and interact with a child who has severe motor disabilities as if the child were an infant rather than a child who has thoughts and feelings. Interactions need to reflect the person's level of cognitive function and not use overly simplified language, or highly nurturing, or directive communication styles. Baby talk or elderspeak is characterized as communication that has slower speech, high volume and pitch, extreme intonations, and simplified vocabulary and grammar (Williams, Kemper, and Hummert 2016, 12–16). For an older person, communication needs to respect their abilities and life experiences. Baby talk and elderspeak are often viewed by older people as demeaning and can be detrimental to their health and well-being if they respond with social withdrawal, lowered self-esteem, or greater dependency (Williams, Kemper, and Hummert 2016, 12–16).

6.6.4 Therapeutic nihilism

Therapeutic nihilism refers to doubt in the benefit of a therapy and the subsequent withholding of therapy as a result of this doubt. The concept of therapeutic nihilism arises from the ethical principle of doing no harm, or non-maleficence, and balancing that with the principle of doing good, or beneficence (Gillon 1985, 130–131). For example, in older people who are at risk for health decline, it may be perceived that treatment is futile or that therapy may not be beneficial, and that resources may be better used for younger people who may have more years to live. Clients may be denied important opportunities if societal or individual biases related to disability, low expectations of what may be achieved, and the evaluation of benefits unduly restrict them from receiving therapy that may benefit them.

6.6.5 Expectations related to normative development

Individual biopsychosocial development can be highly variable. Looking at normative development is useful to offer a gauge for what may be expected in a general population at a certain part of the lifespan. Excessive focus on and expectations for the need to reach certain milestones or developmental tasks within normative time periods may be problematic. Development is embedded within a social context, and culture as part of the social environment has a strong influence on what is considered normative development. What is considered a developmental milestone in one culture, for example, may be unexpected in another culture, such as in the example of crawling before walking in early development. Also worth noting, is that for some individuals who have disabilities, it may not be possible to reach certain developmental milestones or achieve specific developmental tasks within the "typical" timeframe or even to achieve such milestones at all. As such, it is crucial to focus on working with individuals on goals that are relevant and realistic.

Case 1 – changing needs and priorities across the lifespan

Erica is a nine-month-old girl who has Down syndrome and a congenital heart defect (a ventricular septal defect). Her parents report that they are very concerned about her poor weight gain and the fact that she is well below the 10th percentile for both height and weight. Further conversation with her parents reveals that Erica is having a lot of trouble with feeding and that since she is not yet able to sit in a highchair, her parents are trying to hold her in their laps when feeding her. Both parents report that holding Erica and trying to feed her at the same time is very difficult. The team working with Erica suggests trying an adaptive insert for the highchair that might help to better position her for optimal feeding.

Erica is now an energetic 13-year-old who attends her local middle school. Although she receives special education services and speech-language therapy, Erica often becomes frustrated with her inability to be understood due to her severe disarticulation issues. The team working with Erica wonders if an augmentative communication device might be helpful. Erica is excited about this idea, but her parents are anxious and have many questions. Will using an augmentative communication device make it so that Erica is no longer motivated to work on improving her articulation? Erica is very active and involved in community activities. Will she be able to use an augmentative communication device "on the go" or will she always have to be sitting down at a desk to use it? How will using such a device impact how her peers see her? Her parents state that they are also afraid that she might misplace an augmentative communication device or that the device might be damaged during play activities. The team works with Erica and her parents to trial various augmentative communication devices and to provide education related to the nuances of integrating augmentative communication into daily activities.

Erica is now 44 years old. She had been living in an apartment with another adult who has Down syndrome and working at an area grocery store, but about a year ago, Erica's family noticed that her overall function was declining and that she was uncharacteristically irritable and seemed sad all the time. Testing revealed that Erica had developed Alzheimer-like dementia. Erica has started to have trouble living on her own and she and her family wonder if there is technology that might help Erica to be as independent as possible for as long as possible. A community-based care team experienced in home-based technologies works with Erica and her parents to learn about options available for home safety monitoring and assistance.

Case 2 - changing needs due to an unexpected health condition

Enrique is a 65-year-old man who had previously been in good health prior to a cerebral vascular accident (CVA) three months ago. Before his CVA, Enrique was the Chief Executive Officer for a large international company.

Although he worked long hours, he regularly made time for recreational activities such as racquetball, golf, and competitive ballroom dancing with his wife. He also spent time each week with his grandchildren and very proudly took the grandchildren on outings to the park, zoo, and community events. A voracious reader, he read multiple newspapers online each day and read several novels each month. Enrique's CVA changed all of this in an instant. Now, not only is he unable to walk even with assistance and unable to use his left arm at all, he has visual deficits including homonymous hemianopsia and a left-sided neglect. He still tries to read but between his visual deficits and constantly losing his place in the text, he is no longer able to enjoy reading. Despite these problems, he emphatically denies that he has any deficits. He requires constant supervision to ensure that he does not hurt himself by attempting to do things that he is no longer able to do such as stand up or go to the bathroom by himself. Enrique's wife has left her job and is intent on providing for his care needs, but she is beginning to appear worn out and discouraged by the changes in her husband's life and subsequently in her life. The team working with Enrique suggests exploring technological solutions and devices that might assist both Enrique and his wife in adjusting to life post-CVA. The team meets with Enrique and his wife to learn about the couple's rehabilitation goals together and evaluate the couple's priorities. Though Enrique denies that he has deficits, he sees that his wife is very concerned and worn out and he agrees to participate in the process. Together they identify that the greatest priorities for the couple are to explore options for Enrique to transfer from sitting to standing and to ambulate safely to where he needs to go, for example, to the bathroom. Also, because of his mobility concerns and risk of having falls, the team explores options in technologies, environmental modifications, and behavioral strategies to anticipate the potential for falls, prevent falls, and alert for help in case of a fall in the home. Another priority for Enrique is to be able to read again. Enrique and his wife are surprised at the wide range of technology available to help Enrique and his wife begins to realize that although things will always be different because of his CVA, both she and Enrique can enjoy life and participate in the community.

6.7 Future vision

Rehabilitation engineering is a diverse field and whether working in research and development or clinical practice, the clients that rehabilitation engineers encounter will span all age groups. Several trends related to working with clients across the lifespan are anticipated to impact rehabilitation engineering in the near future. The most notable trend pertains to population changes, with an increased proportion of older adults compared to a decreased proportion of younger adults who may be able to provide care. This trend is already significantly influencing how and how urgently technology is developed and applied to support clients and caregivers across the lifespan. With an increase in the number of older people, there is also an increase in the number of people with non-communicable diseases, or chronic health conditions that can result in long-term disability. Technology and services to support the management of or the prevention of chronic health conditions are also needed to support health, activity performance, community participation, and well-being.

6.8 Discussion questions

1. Compare and contrast the following theories of development: developmental stage theories, lifespan developmental theories, life course theories, and developmental systems theories.
2. Why is it important for rehabilitation engineers to have an understanding of normative development and developmental milestones across the lifespan?
3. Discuss some of the factors related to health conditions and disability that may impact an individual's life course and life trajectories during early and adult development.
4. Discuss the role of client-centered care and family-centered care in rehabilitation engineering practice.
5. A 12-year-old boy with Duchenne muscular dystrophy appears to have very different priorities and goals for his care than his parents. How can the professionals working with this young man and his family approach this situation to ensure the best possible outcomes? How might this approach be different if the client were a 65-year-old man with Alzheimer's disease whose priorities and goals were different than those of his grown children who care for him?
6. There are many misconceptions about individuals across the lifespan. Recognizing these misconceptions is important to ensure that we provide the best care and services possible to each of our clients. What are some misconceptions that you have observed? What can be done to overcome such misconceptions?

Bibliography

Baltes, Paul B. 1987. "Theoretical Propositions of Life-Span Developmental Psychology: On the Dynamics between Growth and Decline." *Developmental Psychology* 23 (5): 611.
Baltes, Paul B., Ulman Lindenberger, and Ursula M. Staudinger. 2007. "Life Span Theory in Developmental Psychology." *Handbook of Child Psychology* 1: 569–664.

Bamm, Elena L. and Peter Rosenbaum. 2008. "Family-Centered Theory: Origins, Development, Barriers, and Supports to Implementation in Rehabilitation Medicine." *Archives of Physical Medicine and Rehabilitation* 89 (8): 1618–1624.

Beach, Scott R. and Richard Schulz. 2017. "Family Caregiver Factors Associated with Unmet Needs for Care of Older Adults." *Journal of the American Geriatrics Society* 65 (3): 560–566.

Centers for Disease Control and Prevention. "Developmental Milestones." https://www.cdc.gov /ncbddd/actearly/milestones/index.html.

Clarke, Philippa and Kenzie Latham. 2014. "Life Course Health and Socioeconomic Profiles of Americans Aging with Disability." *Disability and Health Journal* 7 (1) Supplement: S15–S23.

De Luca, Cinzia R. and Richard J. Leventer. 2010. "Developmental Trajectories of Executive Functions Across the Lifespan." In *Executive Functions and the Frontal Lobes*, edited by V. Anderson, R. Jacobs and P. J. Anderson, 57–90. New York: Psychology Press.

Dictionaries, Oxford. 2017. "Apr. 2017." Web.

Elder Jr, Glen H. and Michael J. Shanahan. 2007. "The Life Course and Human Development." *Handbook of Child Psychology* 1: 665–715.

Gardiner, Clare, Gideon Geldenhuys, and Merryn Gott. 2018. "Interventions to Reduce Social Isolation and Loneliness among Older People: An Integrative Review." *Health & Social Care in the Community* 26 (2): 147–157.

Gillon, R. 1985. "'Primum Non Nocere' and the Principle of Non-Maleficence." *British Medical Journal (Clinical Research Ed.)* 291 (6488): 130–131.

Grenness, Caitlin, Louise Hickson, Ariane Laplante-Lévesque, and Bronwyn Davidson. 2014. "Patient-Centred Care: A Review for Rehabilitative Audiologists." *International Journal of Audiology* 53 (supl): S60–S67.

Johnston, Timothy D. 2010. "Developmental Systems Theory." In *Oxford Handbook of Developmental Behavioral Neuroscience*, edited by M. S. Blumberg, J. H. Freeman and S. R. Robinson, 12–29. Oxford, UK: Oxford University Press.

Kemper, Han C. G. 2000. "Skeletal Development during Childhood and Adolescence and the Effects of Physical Activity." *Pediatric Exercise Science* 12 (2): 198–216.

Kim, S. K. and M. Park. 2017. "Effectiveness of Person-Centered Care on People with Dementia: A Systematic Review and Meta-Analysis." *Clinical Interventions in Aging* 12: 381–397.

Kydd, Angela and Anne Fleming. 2015. "Ageism and Age Discrimination in Health Care: Fact Or Fiction? A Narrative Review of the Literature." *Maturitas* 81 (4): 432–438.

Linton, Simi. 1998. *Claiming Disability: Knowledge and Identity*. New York: NYU Press.

Magsamen-Conrad, Kate, Shrinkhala Upadhyaya, Claire Youngnyo Joa, and John Dowd. 2015. "Bridging the Divide: Using UTAUT to Predict Multigenerational Tablet Adoption Practices." *Computers in Human Behavior* 50: 186–196.

Monahan, D. J. and D. A. Wolf. 2014. "The Continuum of Disability Over the Lifespan: The Convergence of Aging with Disability and Aging into Disability." *Disability and Health Journal* 7 (1 Suppl): S1–3.

National Eye Institute. "Facts about Presbyopia." https://nei.nih.gov/health/errors/presbyopia.

National Institute on Deafness and Other Communication Disorders. "Age Related Hearing Loss." https://www.nidcd.nih.gov/health/age-related-hearing-loss.

Ondrak, Kristin S. and Don W. Morgan. 2007. "Physical Activity, Calcium Intake and Bone Health in Children and Adolescents." *Sports Medicine* 37 (7): 587–600.

Oyama, Susan, Paul E. Griffiths, and Russell D. Gray. 2001. "Introduction: What is Developmental Systems Theory." In *Cycles of Contingency: Developmental Systems and Evolution*, edited by R. D. Gray, P. E. Griffiths and S. Oyama, 1–11. Cambridge, MA: MIT Press.

Quinn, Peggy. 1998. *Understanding Disability: A Lifespan Approach.* Vol. 35. Newbury, CA: Sage Publications.

Riley, Lesley D. and Christopher "Pokey" Bowen. 2005. "The Sandwich Generation: Challenges and Coping Strategies of Multigenerational Families." *The Family Journal* 13 (1): 52–58.

Salthouse, Timothy. 2012. "Consequences of Age-Related Cognitive Declines." *Annual Review of Psychology* 63: 201–226.

Salthouse, Timothy A. 2010. "Selective Review of Cognitive Aging." *Journal of the International Neuropsychological Society* 16 (5): 754–760.

Thies, Kathleen M. and John F. Travers. 2001. *Quick Look Nursing: Growth and Development through the Lifespan.* Houston, TX: Jones & Bartlett Publishers.

United Nations. 2006. "Convention on the Rights of Persons with Disabilities." General Assembly United Nations, New York.

United Nations Children's Fund. 2006. "The State of the World's Children 2006: Excluded and Invisible." https://www.unicef.org/publications/files/SOWC_2006_English_Report_rev(1).pdf.

United Nations Department of Economic and Social Affairs Population Division. 2008. "World Population Prospects: The 2008 Revision Population Database: Highlights." http://www.un.org/esa/population/publications/wpp2008/wpp2008_highlights.pdf.

Wandke, H., M. Sengpiel, and M. Sonksen. 2012. "Myths about Older People's Use of Information and Communication Technology." *Gerontology* 58 (6): 564–570.

Williams, Kristine, Susan Kemper, and Mary Lee Hummert. 2016. "Enhancing Communication with Older Adults: Overcoming Elderspeak." *Journal of Psychosocial Nursing and Mental Health Services* 43 (5): 12–16.

World Health Organization. 2021. "Ageing and Health." http://www.who.int/mediacentre/factsheets/fs404/en/.

———. 2021. "Disability and Health." http://www.who.int/mediacentre/factsheets/fs352/en/.

———. 2008. "The Global Burden of Disease: 2004 Update."

———. 2011. "National Institute on Aging, National Institutes of Health, US Department of Health and Human Services." Global Health and Aging.

———. 2002. "Towards a Common Language for Functioning, Disability, and Health: ICF." In *The International Classification of Functioning, Disability and Health.* WHO, Geneva. http://www.who.int/classifications/icf/training/icfbeginnersguide.pdf

Section II
Key topics in rehabilitation engineering

Chapter 7 Policy and regulations in rehabilitation engineering

L. Walker and E. L. Friesen

Contents

DOI: 10.1201/b21964-9

7.1 Chapter overview

This chapter focuses on policies and regulations that affect the day-to-day work of a rehabilitation engineer. It begins by examining policies and regulations relating to initial training and certification (also known as preprofessional accreditation or attributes) that prepare an individual for entry into the engineering profession.

It then looks at the professional competencies and requirements associated with establishing oneself as a professional rehabilitation engineering practitioner, and requirements for ongoing professional development and training. Finally, the chapter looks at the policies, regulations, and standards that impact day-to-day work as a professional rehabilitation engineer.

7.2 Unique aspects of education and training in rehabilitation engineering

As described in more detail in Chapter 1, rehabilitation engineering can be broadly defined as the systematic application of engineering principles (including technical expertise and design methodologies) to the design, development, adaption, testing, evaluation, and application of technological solutions for individuals, that aid in the recovery of physical and cognitive functioning lost due to disease, injury, and human aging, in areas such as mobility, communications, hearing, vision, and cognition (adapted from the Rehabilitation Act of 1973, P.L. 93–112 (Rehabilitation Act of 1973, P.L. 93–112)) (National Institute of Biomedical Imaging and Bioengineering 2017; Cooper, Ohnabe, and Hobson 2006).

These technical solutions facilitate an individual's activities and participation across life domains such as daily living, employment, education, recreation, and community integration, and ultimately impact quality of life. As a result, rehabilitation engineers must not only demonstrate strong skills in technical thinking and design but must also understand the human component (including the consequences or impact of impairment and psychosocial factors), and the human–machine interface at which people directly interact with technology (Cooper, Ohnabe, and Hobson 2006; Szeto 2014, 277–331).

7.3 Formal education, training, and accreditation

Formal education, training, and accreditation for rehabilitation engineers often includes undergraduate training to attain an agreed set of graduate attributes, followed by workplace-based training to develop key competencies needed for independent practice. Alternatively, some rehabilitation engineers gain qualifications in other engineering, technical, or health disciplines, and then attain the agreed set of graduate attributes through postgraduate qualifications in rehabilitation engineering.

7.3.1 Graduate attributes in international accords

Many countries regulate professions and have developed processes to ensure consistent standards for engineering qualifications offered in that country. Typically, professional engineering education involves four years of advanced technical or university-level undergraduate study (including practical work). Across engineering disciplines there is no single, global standard for preprofessional accreditation, such as graduate attributes and program outcomes. However, there have been, and continue to be, international efforts to align on sets of key attributes for graduates of preaccreditation engineering qualifications.

In 1981, Australia, Canada, Ireland, New Zealand, the United Kingdom, and the United States observed substantial equivalence across the processes, policies, criteria, and requirements for granting accreditation to university-level programs. The Washington Accord was signed to facilitate recognition of engineering qualifications in these countries. Key graduate attributes of the Washington Accord are shown in Table 7.1. Other countries have since signed the Accord. In Europe, the European Network for Accreditation of Engineering Education (ENAEE) manages processes similar to those agreed in the Washington Accord, and there is mutual recognition of engineers trained in undergraduate programs in either system. Graduate attributes are broad, to ensure applicability to all disciplines of engineering.

7.3.2 Attributes for rehabilitation technologists, technicians, and associates

The International Engineering Alliance has two further accords that set international benchmarks for prequalification training of technologists and technicians (or associates) (International Engineering Alliance 2014).

- The Sydney Accord covers engineering technologists and incorporated engineers (UK), with most qualifications being degrees of three years duration post secondary school. The graduate attribute specification refers to broadly defined engineering problems.
- The Dublin Accord (2002) covers equivalence and international recognition of engineering technician qualifications. Most Dublin Accord qualifications are diplomas of two years duration post secondary school. The graduate attribute specification refers to well-defined engineering problems.

The engineering technologist is a relatively new level of competence. Generally, it gives a pathway for those trained in life or allied health sciences to bridge

Table 7.1 Graduate Attributes from the Washington Accord

Attribute	Description
Engineering knowledge	WA1: Apply knowledge of mathematics, natural science, engineering fundamentals, and an engineering specialization as specified in WK1 to WK4 respectively to the solution of complex engineering problems.
Problem analysis	WA2: Identify, formulate, research literature, and analyze complex engineering problems reaching substantiated conclusions using first principles of mathematics, natural sciences, and engineering sciences (WK1 to WK4).
Design/development of solutions	WA3: Design solutions for complex engineering problems and design systems, components, or processes that meet specified needs with appropriate consideration for public health, and safety, cultural, societal, and environmental considerations (WK5).
Investigation	WA4: Conduct investigations of complex problems using research-based knowledge (WK8) and research methods including design of experiments, analysis and interpretation of data, and synthesis of information to provide valid conclusions.
Modern tool usage	WA5: Create, select, and apply appropriate techniques, resources, and modern engineering and IT tools, including prediction and modeling, to complex engineering problems, with an understanding of the limitations (WK6).
The engineer and society	WA6: Apply reasoning informed by contextual knowledge to assess societal, health, safety, legal, and cultural issues, and the consequent responsibilities relevant to professional engineering practice and solutions to complex engineering problems (WK7).
Environment and sustainability	WA7: Understand and evaluate the sustainability and impact of professional engineering work in the solution of complex engineering problems in societal and environmental contexts (WK7).
Ethics	WA8: Apply ethical principles and commit to professional ethics and responsibilities and norms of engineering practice (WK7).
Individual and teamwork	WA9: Function effectively as an individual, and as a member or leader in diverse teams and in multidisciplinary settings.
Communication	WA10: Communicate effectively on complex engineering activities with the engineering community and society at large, such as being able to comprehend and write effective reports and design documentation, make effective presentations, and give and receive clear instructions.
Project management and finance	WA11: Demonstrate knowledge and understanding of engineering management principles and economic decision making and apply these to one's own work as a member and leader in a team, to manage projects and in multidisciplinary environments.
Life-long learning	WA12: Recognize the need for, and have the preparation and ability to engage in, independent and life-long learning in the broadest context of technological change.

Data from 25 years of the Washington Accord, p. 14–15, International Engineering Alliance, http://www.ieagreements.org/accords/washington/, June 2014 with a series of technical science subjects (certificate programs or credentialing) to achieve the Sydney Accord levels. Engineering technologists and technicians will usually train through certificate and diploma level programs with substantial on-the-job training and will combine technologies to meet an objective for someone with disability with significant supervision from a more senior engineer. The RESNA Professional Standards Group (PSG) paper "Rehabilitation Engineers, Technologists, and Technicians: Vital Members of the Assistive Technology Team" describes how this currently occurs in North America. (DiGiovine et al. 2018, 1–12)

7.3.3 Competencies for independent practice

After demonstrating the required attributes and therefore meeting the accreditation criteria for an engineering qualification (in a jurisdiction), graduates can seek employment as a graduate engineer and begin establishing themselves as a professional engineering practitioner. In addition to preaccreditation attributes demonstrated through undergraduate training, engineers must begin a process of demonstrating attributes associated with independent practice. As with graduate attributes, there is no single, global standard across engineering disciplines for this next stage of training. Further, minimum graduate qualifications specific to rehabilitation engineering vary across the world.

Rehabilitation engineering is currently not offered as a traditional undergraduate program in its own right. Engineers employed in rehabilitation settings may attain graduate attributes in related, broader disciplines such as biomedical, mechanical, electrical, electronic, or software engineering, as shown in Figure 7.1 (Cooper, Ohnabe, and Hobson 2006). In some cases, graduate engineers may have gained exposure to rehabilitation engineering through either elective design or research subjects within broader engineering programs, or in a specialization stream within the more general biomedical (or bioengineering) undergraduate

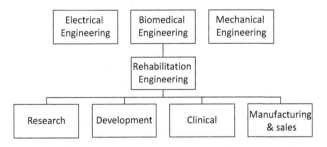

Figure 7.1 Example pathways (both undergraduate and graduate) to professional rehabilitation engineering and typical areas of employment. (Adapted from DeGiovine et al.; DiGiovine et al. 2018, 1–12; DeGiovine, Bresler, and Bahr 2014.)

program. Knowledge, experience, and skills specific to rehabilitation engineering are therefore largely attained in workplace settings, as part of initial workplace training and gaining of professional competence.

Internationally, various competency standards have been developed that define a minimum set of requirements to confirm that an engineer is capable of working either unsupervised, independently, or with minimal direction. Examples of these competencies include the UK Standard for Professional Engineering Competence (UKSPEC), the Chartered Professional Engineers Act 2002 (IPENZ), and Stage 2 Competencies produced by Engineers Australia. Professional bodies such as the Australian National Committee on Rehabilitation Engineering have then mapped rehabilitation engineering-specific examples of these competencies to each overarching competency element. An example of this is shown in Table 7.2.

7.3.4 Credentialing in rehabilitation engineering and assistive technology competencies

Credentialing and accreditation for professionals and services exist in many industries. In assistive technology (AT) provision, relatively few jurisdictions have developed and implemented credentialing and accreditation systems for engineers. The Rehabilitation Engineering and Assistive Technology Society of North America (RESNA) created the Rehabilitation Engineering Technology (RET) credential, in part to address this need. The RET is designed to build on knowledge, skills, and experience assessed for RESNA's Assistive Technology Provider (ATP) credential. In other jurisdictions, credentialing systems are either still in development, or are developed to establish minimum benchmarks for professionals assessing and/or prescribing assistive and rehabilitation technologies. Examples of such benchmarking systems can be found in many government-funded assistive AT funding schemes in Australia, Canada, and New Zealand. In these schemes, engineers and other professionals involved in AT provision apply for approval as assessors/prescribers, and supply evidence of knowledge, skills, and experience in AT as part of their application.

7.3.5 Ongoing and continuing professional development

Maintaining and enhancing the knowledge, skills, and experience related to professional practice is crucial for rehabilitation engineers throughout their careers. Ongoing and continuing professional development (CPD) is generally required as part of professional engineering registration to ensure current and up-to-date competence. Ideally, ongoing CPD should focus not only on technical requirements for professional practice, but also on non-technical and personal qualities required to carry out professional duties. Rehabilitation engineers should also

Table 7.2 Examples of Stage 2 Competencies for Rehabilitation Engineers, from Engineers Australia Biomedical College

Element of Competence and What It Means in Practice	Indicators of Attainment	Specific Examples for Rehabilitation Engineering
Identify, assess, and manage risks. Means that you develop and operate within a hazard and risk framework appropriate to engineering activities.	Identify, assess, and manage product, project, process, environmental, or system risks that could be caused by material, economic, social, or environmental factors. Establish and maintain a documented audit trail of technical and operational changes during system or product development, project implementation, or process operations. Follow a systematic documented method and work in consultation with stakeholders and other informed people to identify unpredictable events (threats, opportunities, and other sources of uncertainty or missing information) that could influence outcomes. Assess the likelihood of each event, and the consequences, including commercial, reputation, safety, health, environment, regulatory, legal, governance, and social consequences. Devise ways to influence the likelihood and consequences to minimize costs and undesirable consequences, and maximize benefits. Help in negotiating equitable ways to share any costs and benefits between stakeholders and the community.	Undertaken a risk analysis of an AT solution that aims to meet client need. The challenges of meeting competing (and changing) expectations that may conflict with clinical evidence. Examples of risk documentation appropriate for the therapeutic environment and/or the regulatory requirements (e.g., TGA). Experience in using guidelines, standards, and other protocols to mitigate risk. Recognition of the contribution to risk from changes post issue of AT.

(Continued)

Table 7.2 (Continued) Examples of Stage 2 Competencies for Rehabilitation Engineers, from Engineers Australia Biomedical College

Element of Competence and What It Means in Practice	Indicators of Attainment	Specific Examples for Rehabilitation Engineering
Meet legal and regulatory requirements. Means that you should be able to demonstrate an understanding of the laws, regulations, codes, and other instruments which you are legally bound to apply and apply these in your work.	Identify and comply with the codes, standards of compliance or legal instruments relevant to a particular product, project, process, or system. Draft commercial contracts that cover the procurement of services, equipment, materials, access rights, or access to information. Seek advice, rulings, or opinions from time to time to ensure that your understanding of legal and regulatory requirements is up to date. Practice within legal and regulatory requirements. Negotiate appropriate approvals from regulatory authorities for engineering activities Protect intellectual property.	Awareness and understanding of the Therapeutic Goods regulatory framework in Australia. Demonstrated experience in use of relevant standards and regulations in decision making. Use of standardized documentation and link to solution (including AT) specifications. Understanding of the roles and scope of self and others within clinical settings — including regulated professions.

Data from Engineers Australia Biomedical College and National Committee on Rehabilitation Engineering, Canberra, Australia, 2014.

document and retain an auditable record of CPD activities across their career, consistent with any requirements related to ongoing registration, accreditation, or credentialing.

7.4 Regulations affecting professional practice

Legislation, regulations, and policies relating to workplaces and employment impact the day-to-day work of rehabilitation engineers.

7.4.1 Workplace and industrial legislation and regulations

As an employee, rehabilitation engineers comply with employment protocols and norms of the workplace and industry. A formal role or job description outlines the legal scope of roles and responsibilities, expectations, and requirements for recruitment and performance management, and as the basis for compensation and remuneration. Role or job descriptions may also outline supervision requirements and line management for approved practice, as well as any supervisory responsibilities and delegations. Embedded in the role or job description may be other workplace requirements such as employment hours, internal policies and procedures, duties of care, responsibilities related to interests of the company or organization, and rights as an employee. The broader workplace may also be subject to industrial legislation, covering areas such as pay and working conditions, workplace/occupational health and safety, responsibilities for practitioner/professional registration and CPD, and standards of practice.

7.4.2 Industry – and service setting-specific legislation and regulations

Different industries and service delivery settings may have additional rules and regulations affecting the day-to-day work of rehabilitation engineers. In healthcare settings, rehabilitation engineers working as healthcare practitioners or professionals (HCPs) or in a clinical capacity have responsibilities relating to the collection, storing, and processing of health records and "sensitive personal information" about service users. This may be captured in legislation such as the Health Insurance Portability and Accountability Act of 1996 (HIPAA) in the USA, the General Data Protection Regulation (GDPR) in the European Union, other health- and privacy-related regulations applicable in the jurisdiction, and also in employer-specific policies and procedures. Similar requirements for storing, protecting, and sharing data exist in areas of practice such as education, human and social services, disability services, and non-government and non-profit sectors where rehabilitation engineers work directly with service users.

Rehabilitation engineers should also become familiar with the reimbursement, funding, and payment requirements for both professional engineering services and technologies. Historically, reimbursement for professional engineering services associated with AT service delivery has been challenging. Over several decades, rehabilitation engineers (and other AT practitioners) have worked to demonstrate the importance of professional skills, knowledge and practice in selection, delivery, and training in AT for individuals with disability to achieve optimal outcomes. Consequently, these elements of AT service delivery are being more adequately funded, with an emphasis on improved outcomes.

7.4.3 Statute, corporate, and case law

Engineers are subject to the laws of the location in which they provide their services. At their most basic, legislatures (e.g., parliaments, Congress, etc.) develop a new law (statute) that is then enforced by officials (police or regulatory authorities like the Environmental Protection Authority) and the judiciary. Governments have a hierarchy of powers, so a national government makes many of the laws regarding taxation, defense, or immigration, while state, regional, and local governments create laws for increasingly granular aspects of life such as workplace safety, traffic, and building codes. Each jurisdiction (level of government and court) is subject to working within its scope as granted by constitutions or treaties. This can even apply to national law which may be challenged through international law (such as the International Labor Organization) if the country is a signatory to relevant conventions, particularly in the European Union.

In addition to statute law, as courts deal with the cases that come before them, they build a body of reasoning that is known as case law. Law is often about interpretation, so judges are careful to read statute law and decide cases drawing on the knowledge and thinking of those who have gone before them. When a decision is made where one of the parties disagrees with the decision, that party usually appeals to a higher level of the judiciary for review of the decision. In some cases, a government may amend its statute law where a case (or cases) have not had an outcome that aligns with public expectation, such as a business successfully arguing that it was not responsible for an adverse outcome based on a particular interpretation (or loophole) of the current law.

There are two other key distinctions in law – criminal and civil law. Criminal law involves penalties brought by government authorities for breaching the "laws of the land" such as traffic infringements, deaths resulting from a person's action (or negligence), and so on. Civil law is between two parties, generally as the result of a breach of contract or obligation. If you damage your neighbor's garden, they may sue you to gain compensation for that damage.

Rehabilitation engineers will often work closely with legal professionals to ensure that their activity and the products that they supply are both compliant with the laws in the jurisdictions where they are provided, but also to avoid causing harm that may lead to a civil claim. In addition, as law is often subject to interpretation, independent professional engineers may be asked to provide their professional opinion to a court to assist in the understanding of technical matters (e.g., the causes of a product failure).

7.5 Technical policies and regulations relating to technologies

In addition to rules and regulations covering employment, rehabilitation engineers will find that their day-to-day work involves engineering and health standards, design guides, and regulatory codes. Some will apply across all stages of the technology life cycle: design, manufacture, implementation, maintenance and servicing, and end-of-life decommissioning and disposal. Others may only apply to an element (such as design standards).

7.5.1 Product and process standards

Standards are a common way for engineers to agree and share specifications for products, services, and systems, to ensure quality, safety, and efficiency. At an international level, groups like the International Organization for Standardization (ISO) and the International Electrical Commission (IEC) help coordinate and publish internationally agreed standards, ostensibly to establish global good practice and to facilitate compatibility and international trade. For example, structural strength tests for manual wheelchairs are covered in ISO 7176-8 and enable manufacturers in India to build and test their products to meet equivalent requirements in the USA. Similarly, the IEC 62280 series covers the technical specifications for universal serial bus (USB) interfaces to ensure the USB mouse made in China is compatible with the USB port on the electronic augmentative and alternative communication (AAC) device built in Germany. Some standards (such as ISO9001: Quality Assurance) outline the framework and elements of agreed processes and documentation to achieve a consistent outcome and facilitate auditing and compliance requirements. Most countries now adopt international standards into local or jurisdictional libraries. Local variations to address specific gaps or requirements can be added through the adoption processes. Some industries will also establish agreed standards that may eventually become national or international standards.

A key element of standards development is the contribution of expertise from multiple stakeholders such as technical experts, consumers, governments, regulators, manufacturers, and testers. Together stakeholders generate, debate, and refine standards documents for approval by member organizations. Standards can be understood as a consensus document, and always subject to regular review and updating. Some standards, particularly where they relate to safety, may be cited in jurisdictional law to make their requirements enforceable; others may be cited as part of a contract for product supply.

7.5.2 Medical device regulations

While more critical to biomedical engineers, medical device regulations also impact rehabilitation engineering technologies and assistive technologies. Such regulations are enforceable in the jurisdiction where they apply and set standards and processes that must be met in order to make available a medical device for human use. Most regulations apply even if the device is provided at no charge, and they are primarily aimed at providing a basic level of quality, effectiveness, and safety to users of those devices and the public. The frameworks for most medical device regulations have mostly been harmonized internationally (again to facilitate trade) around key elements:

- Global medical device nomenclature (GMDN) – a number and description of a type of medical device.
- Classes (e.g., low-risk Class 1 to high-risk Class III (or active implantable devices)).
- Conformity assessment (verification of the manufacturing efficacy, and similar to good manufacturing practice requirements for quality control).
- Vigilance (early identification of problems and taking corrective action).
- Surveillance (ensuring that manufacturers/providers meet their obligations).

Although the terminology and process to meet medical device regulations through design, development, and delivery of a device to a user may vary slightly between jurisdictions, the broad elements remain consistent and rehabilitation engineers will often be the key professional, in conjunction with an organization's legal counsel, who will have responsibility for ensuring the regulations are met – both initially and in an ongoing basis.

7.5.3 Protecting intellectual property

With the emergence of mass production, and particularly since the development of additive manufacture (for example, 3D printing), the value of a product depends less on the cost of fabricating it and more on the concepts and design that define it. Concepts, designs, prototyping outcomes, and manufacturing processes are all intellectual property (IP) and are a key contribution from rehabilitation engineers to both the final product and their engaging organization's profitability. Firms and individuals will protect their IP through copyright, patents, trademarks, and other legal tools. For some, their income is derived from the licensing (permission to use) or sale to manufacturers and others of their IP. Because of its value, employment or engagement contracts will often include detailed clauses about the confidentiality and ownership rights associated with IP generated in the course of work. Rehabilitation engineers should be particularly careful to understand their rights and obligations with regard to IP in two areas:

- Sharing IP (such as at a conference or meeting) without jeopardizing the ability to protect (and thus make money from) your IP, such as through patent protection and licensing.
- Ownership rights of IP generated during the course of employment (e.g., ideas, designs, or innovations).

7.6 Future vision

Across the world, markets for assistive, rehabilitative, and other health technologies are growing rapidly. Growth is being driven worldwide by many factors, including an aging population, and increased recognition of unmet needs for technologies in developed and developing countries. Demand for technologies that enable people with disabilities and/or disabling health conditions to remain active, healthy, and independent in their advancing years is increasing. This will also increase demand for competent rehabilitation engineering professionals. These changes present long-term regulatory challenges for the engineering profession in terms of workforce needs, and standards for technologies in the coming decades.

Increased demand will likely bring with it greater scrutiny of professional education, training, and accreditation of rehabilitation engineers, and the equivalence of this training across jurisdictions. This presents an imperative for accrediting organizations to further align on mutual recognition of qualifications across international borders, and for development of robust, transparent, and transferable credentialing systems. Harmonization of education, training, accreditation, and credentialing systems should therefore be a key priority for engineering regulators.

The regulatory environment for assistive and rehabilitation technologies will also change as demand grows. Convergence of technologies – either where assistive technologies become mainstream or mainstream technologies replace dedicated assistive technologies – means standards and product regulations must be adapted to reflect these new or broadening uses. Harmonization and alignment of standards will continue to facilitate international commerce, while local jurisdictions will continually adapt international standards to address unique factors in their environments. Rehabilitation engineers skilled in user-centered and participatory design methodologies will also be crucial to the design, adaptation, testing, approval, and implementation of these new technologies.

Another growing challenge is in the paradoxical demands for openness of scientific knowledge and information, and for the right to protect commercially or personally sensitive data. Advances in big data, artificial intelligence, and machine learning are creating new ways to link and analyze vast, disparate datasets. While there is great potential to gain new and broad insights into human health, behaviors, and interactions with technologies through these endeavors, it must be balanced with the rights of individuals to control and maintain privacy of their data, and to be recognized as a unique individual. From this perspective, rehabilitation engineers with a strong knowledge of data protection and privacy, and user-centered design philosophies that underpin AT systems, will bring distinctive perspectives to this work.

7.7 Discussion questions

1. What are some possible benefits of having different training and education pathways to achieving rehabilitation engineering competency?
2. How do harmonization and consistency of registration requirements for rehabilitation engineers enhance the global mobility of an engineering workforce?
3. Are there limitations to the creation of standards through stakeholder consensus?
4. What are some challenges, legal risks, or constraints on innovation in rehabilitation engineering?
5. What responsibility do professional rehabilitation engineers have for injury or damage caused by a product they design? How may professional rehabilitation engineers manage consumer responsibility for safe use of a complex product?
6. How could professional rehabilitation engineers share important scientific or technical developments in a professional context (e.g., a conference) without compromising potential or actual IP rights?
7. How would rehabilitation engineering input assist a provider of AT to avoid regulatory barriers to trade of their products?

Bibliography

Cooper, Rory A., Hisaichi Ohnabe, and Douglas A. Hobson. 2006. *An Introduction to Rehabilitation Engineering.* Boca Raton, FL: CRC Press.
DeGiovine, C., M. Bresler, and P. Bahr. 2014. "A Historical Overview of Rehabilitation Engineering." Indianapolis, IN: RESNA Annual Conference.

DiGiovine, Carmen P., Meghan Donahue, Patricia Bahr, Mark Bresler, Joseph Klaesner, Raj Pagadala, Brian Burkhardt, and Ray Grott. 2018. "Rehabilitation Engineers, Technologists, and Technicians: Vital Members of the Assistive Technology Team." *Assistive Technology* 28: 1–12.

International Engineering Alliance. 2014. "25 Years Washington Accord." Retrieved from: https://www.ieagreements.org/assets/Uploads/Documents/History/25YearsWashingtonAccord-A5booklet-FINAL.pdf.

National Institute of Biomedical Imaging and Bioengineering. 2017. "Rehabilitation Engineering." Accessed 06/01, 2017, https://www.nibib.nih.gov/science-education/science-topics/rehabilitation-engineering.

Szeto, A. Y. 2014. "Assistive Technology and Rehabilitation Engineering." In Assistive Technologies: Concepts, Methodologies, Tools, and Applications, edited by Information Resources Management Association, 277–331. Hershey, PA: IGI Global.

Chapter 8 Ethical issues in rehabilitation engineering

Mary Ellen Buning

Contents

DOI: 10.1201/b21964-10

8.1 Chapter overview—what is ethics?

Ethics is the branch of philosophy that seeks to guide and resolve issues of human morality. Ethics helps to define concepts such as good and evil, right and wrong, virtue and vice, justice and crime within a specific realm of human enterprise. Ideally, ethical behavior is guided by a person's internal compass in which moral values have been taught in the home and reinforced in educational and extracurricular settings like sports and community service. In this ideal progression, ethics subsequently serves as the foundation for personal and work-related relationships and commitments in all personal negotiations and obligations.

Professional organizations usually operationalize the concepts that guide practice with a document called a Code of Ethics. The wide scope of the work that engineers can engage in affects individuals at all levels of society and daily life, so professional engineering also has a code of ethics (National Society of Professional Engineers (NSPE) 2019). This engineering code of ethics has nine rules for practice and there is no question in the mind of NSPE that:

> engineers are expected to exhibit the highest standards of honesty and integrity. Engineering has a direct and vital impact on the quality of life for all people. Accordingly, the services provided by engineers require honesty, impartiality, fairness, and equity and must be dedicated to the protection of public health safety and welfare. Engineers must perform under a standard of professional behavior that requires adherence to the highest principles of ethical conduct.
>
> **(National Society of Professional Engineers (NSPE), 2007)**

As such, this code of ethics statement (National Society of Professional Engineers 2019) is a solid foundation for the further requirements of rehabilitation engineering, as a subset or specialization within engineering and which is the focus of this chapter.

8.2 What is "rehabilitation" engineering?

As described in Chapter 1, "rehabilitation engineering" is the name created by a small group of engineers from various engineering disciplines who gathered back in 1970 to discuss applying engineering principles to solving issues within rehabilitation systems. This same group of five engineers went on to found the Rehabilitation Engineering Society of North America (RESNA) in 1979 at their gathering in Chicago. As RESNA further developed to become a member organization, it also developed the RESNA Code of Ethics to guide practice within its new domain. Since RESNA's founders were professional engineers, there is an obvious overlap between RESNA's codes of ethics and that of the NSPE. This overlap will become more evident as we continue.

For most engineering students, practice with rehabilitation-related issues represents a significant broadening of the context for applying engineering principles, knowledge, and skills. Rehabilitation engineering requires considering the complexity of the human musculoskeletal (or biomechanical), cognitive, sensory, and psychosocial systems plus all the conditions that can cause impairment to typical human functioning. In addition, rehabilitation engineering requires the consideration of a range of qualitative factors such as social and cultural environments and human interactions. Those who will benefit from rehabilitation engineering, commonly called "clients," are typically vulnerable human beings who by their very nature have complex needs, lack the tools needed to create change for themselves, and yet have the desire for independence or improved ability to function effectively in everyday life. Once exposed to the possibilities offered by engineers with a rehabilitation focus, clients will likely continue to benefit from the knowledge, skills, and ethics of engineers and assistive technology (AT) professionals as they continue to fully live their lives.

We will explore rehabilitation engineering ethics more deeply as this chapter progresses but the most basic element of this code of ethics is to ensure that all behavior, actions, and interventions are carefully planned, communicated, and executed to "do no harm." This would include not only the client (i.e., the actual recipient of the engineer's services) with his or her performance limitations but also includes the manner in which these services are delivered. This service delivery aspect expands the "do no harm" mandate to include interpersonal, financial, legal, and social aspects of the service delivery processes in rehabilitation. This field has only existed for 40 years and even now, those who are currently rehabilitation engineers are working to better define themselves and their work. They are further defining their levels of engagement within a recently published "white paper." This document will be further discussed in Section 8.4 (DiGiovine et al. 2018, 1–12).

8.3 The AT evaluation process

As you have already learned in reading Section I, AT services (which include the contributions of the engineer) are typically delivered within a team setting with the client as the central focus of the process.

A successful outcome for the client will be the actual measure of a successful AT evaluation and treatment intervention. Sometimes a positive outcome is easy to achieve and measure; at other times, reaching a client's goal demands complex solutions and months or longer to achieve. It is also important to realize that an AT evaluation and intervention for a client is not a static process. Individuals grow and develop new skills both as they mature over time and through their successful use of an AT solution. A client's context can change as well. It is common to revisit AT options as students move from high school to university or when a

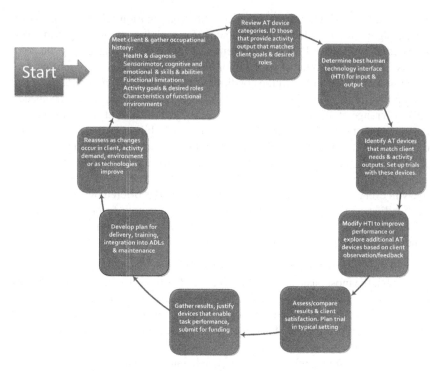

Figure 8.1 The assistive technology assessment process. All members of the AT Team participate in this process.

young adult moves from the suburbs to the city for a work opportunity. All of this variation and human difference requires an intervention process that starts with a client evaluation and moves systematically through a series of logical steps. The diagram in Figure 8.1 helps to show the steps in this process that lead from meeting the client and learning about their goals, to identifying categories of AT, to refining the human–technology interface, engaging in device trials and comparing outputs or results and client preferences, to determining the best AT option, and finally, making a plan for training and integrating the AT device(s) into daily tasks, routines, and environments.

8.3.1 Implementing the HAAT model

To help guide the problem-solving logic embedded within this multifaceted process a model is very helpful. As presented in Chapter 2, the human activity assistive technology (HAAT) model was introduced by Cook and Hussey in their initial text as a means to show the relationship of the client, with his or her desired activity output and the AT device or service that creates the bridge to function

(Cook and Hussey 2002; Cook and Polgar 2013). As seen below, "Context," the fourth component, (comprised of physical, social, cultural issues) is also a key factor in this system.

As in all models based on systems theory (Von Bertalanffy 1968), when change occurs within one factor, all other factors must be re-examined to restore balance to the system output, which in this case, is success for the client. The HAAT model (Figure 8.2) is one reason that a team approach is so important as it brings together varying skills, knowledge, and expertise. This diversity is needed to understand the client with his or her strengths and limitations, the desired activity output, and the contexts within which an activity will occur. Strong knowledge of AT device options and the range of user interfaces will also be needed to link the user to their desired activity output. The evaluation always starts with the client—not the AT device or the solution.

8.3.2 The value of the client-centered intervention

Because it's important to know where to begin in the AT assessment process, we start with the client in this key position. In some situations, due to impairment,

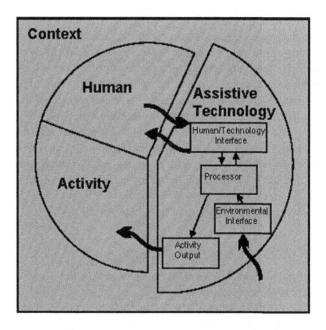

Figure 8.2 The human, activity, and assistive technology (HAAT) model. This model shows the interaction between the components of an assistive technology solution and the impact of the physical, social, and cultural context.

the client may not be able to speak for himself or herself and a family member or caregiver will need to serve as a proxy.

The power of a client's intrinsic motivation to accomplish something personally meaningful or of importance cannot be underestimated. It is the key to a successful AT outcome. Starting with this goal can also affect a client's willingness to trust the team and to consider additional, future AT solutions. For example, the power and feeling of accomplishment that comes from achieving the ability to move independently with a powered wheelchair is important in itself. However, it can naturally trigger interest and willingness to take on the work of learning to use a speech-generating or augmentative alternative communication (AAC) device. Independent communication is suddenly more relevant when one has the ability to move to a new location and interact with new people.

People with disabilities who are not yet empowered by use of AT may have difficulty expressing their goals or may feel that their goal is "too lofty" or unworthy of a team's time and efforts. An ethical approach will be sensitive to this issue and will work harder to allay fears, reinforce the path to success, and affirm their commitment to accomplish the goal.

8.3.3 Holistic intervention

In addition to placing a client at the center of the process it is important to use a *holistic* approach. This means considering the client's needs using a broad viewpoint that includes their strengths, limitations, supports, barriers, and their next steps in human development. For example, a young adult living in a group home in the community and working to acquire self-care and communication skills will have needs quite different from those of a young adult preparing to live independently on a college campus, participate in class discussions and, use a range of internet resources. Previous life experience and family attitudes toward disability and personal responsibility paired with encouragement to acquire new skills or take on age- and ability-appropriate levels of achievement will also factor into success with AT intervention. Here the ethical professional asks questions and expends the energy to fully understand their new client.

8.3.4 The other AT team members

It is important for the rehabilitation engineer to realize that they have the benefit of exposure to other types of knowledge and expertise within the AT team. As in many interdisciplinary teams, the client has the benefit of the knowledge brought by other disciplines to the process. An AT team creates a comprehensive set of evaluation and intervention skills. In addition to the rehabilitation engineer, this team may include: occupational therapist (OT), physical therapist

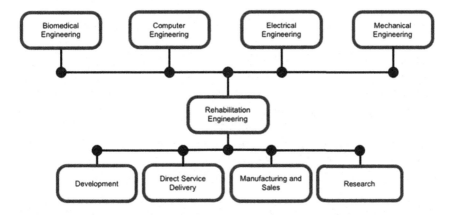

Figure 8.3 The focus of an engineer's work may be influenced by their engineering discipline and their clinical experience. This engineering discipline may also affect the focus area of rehabilitation engineering that they ultimately choose (DiGiovine et al. 2018).

(PT), speech-language pathologist (SLP), educator, vocational rehabilitation (VR) counselor, and rehabilitation technology supplier (RTS) (see Figure 8.3) (Casey 2011, 281–293).

OTs are knowledgeable about human "occupations" or the tasks and activities that people use to meet their daily living needs, define themselves as individuals, and express their interests and independence. The OT's knowledge of human functioning and development typically includes the motor, sensory, intellectual, and social-emotional aspects of human occupations as well as the limitations created by disease or disorder. All OTs are trained to consider modifying tasks, tools, and environments and to use adaptive equipment to enable human functioning (American Occupational Therapy Association 2014, S1–S48). Not all OTs know a lot about AT, so it is important for the one on the team to be open to the use of technology as a compensatory tool in today's world. AT can enable the client to move forward to participate in a valued role or life activity.

PTs are knowledgeable about human movement and its foundations in neuromuscular and biomechanical principles as well as consequences of developmental disability, disease, or injury processes. They are excellent diagnosticians and use their knowledge of physics, motor learning, and neuromuscular rehabilitation to build strength and restore the range of motion to build or restore function. PTs often specialize in types of dysfunction or clients of certain ages. Some PTs without exposure to AT can look at wheelchair use as a treatment failure or as a means of exercise and fail to see how a wheelchair increases mobility efficiency or allows greater participation in today's accessible environments.

177

SLPs are knowledgeable about both language and speech both from a developmental approach as well as from a pathological loss of language or speech. Language refers to the whole system of words and symbols—whether written, spoken, or gestures—that are used to communicate meaning. Speech refers to the system that produces the actual sounds of language, i.e., the lungs, lips, tongue, and teeth working together in a coordinated fashion to convey language. At times both speech and language are impaired. SLPs are the key team members when a client's impairment includes an inability to communicate. Not all SLPs have had strong exposure to AAC devices in their education and so can be reticent about seeing an AAC device as a means to acquire language or as a preparation for literacy.

Educators may be involved in early intervention (birth to three years), kindergarten to 12th grade (K–12) or in the post-secondary (college or technical) levels of education. Educators bring a clear vision of the tasks, social-emotional skills, and the demands of the family or classroom settings and so are helpful in guiding the selection or implementation of an AT solution that supports success in the academic tasks that lead to education and employment. Educators often work in school settings that are resource poor or that are unaware of the potential of AT to enable a student to acquire literacy or the skills to benefit from their education plan.

VR counselors help individuals prepare for the world of work or get the resources they need to return to work following injury. Counselors can help identify employment skills, provide support for education or job training and, in certain situations, fund the purchase of AT evaluation and training services, device purchase, and even fund home or adaptive vehicle modifications. VR counselors work with clients who have impairments that range from developmental to sensory to acquired physical limitations caused by accident or disease. Even though technology is a key to employment in many situations, some VR counselors have a limited exposure to how AT can accomplish this.

RTSs are the individuals who sell the device(s) recommended by an AT team. These individuals may represent one or more products which can range from AAC devices, manual or powered wheelchairs with specialized seating or alternative controls, and adaptive user interfaces for computers such as eye gaze devices or speech recognition. For clients with complex needs or overlapping impairments, the team may need to work with more than one supplier. In the absence of a rehabilitation engineer, the RTS may take the lead to integrate device controls or mount/position the devices needed. Technical skills and knowledge of the client's function and limitation are needed to ensure success for the client. The RTS becomes active on the AT team at a time that depends on the intervention setting or the needs of the client.

For each of the professions represented on an AT team, it is important to ensure that each has the continuing education, knowledge, experience, and even certification needed to function as an effective team member to support the client's goal(s). A professional lacking AT qualifications can become an ethical threat to the successful outcome of an AT assessment. They will not know what they do NOT know and cannot ensure that they "will do no harm." They also have codes of ethics specific to their professions, certification, and licensure and govern their ethics as they use their skills to evaluate client skills, the impact of impairments, and the nature of social supports, life roles, and performance contexts.

Ideally, you and each member contribute his or her expertise and blend their knowledge and skills to benefit the client. Team composition is often flexible and roles on the team can vary based on client needs. For example, a 16-year-old with motor impairment and the goal of attending college should have a team that includes a rehabilitation counselor, a seating and mobility specialist, and an adaptive computer access specialist. These skills and areas of expertise are not limited to a specific profession. OTs are often experts in seating and mobility and SLPs are frequently experts in computer adaptations for written communication and cognitive skills development. It would be an ethical problem if a team attempted to assess a client's needs in the absence of a member with a core expertise related to the client's goals or needs.

8.4 Your role on the AT team

A new rehabilitation engineer may find himself or herself focused on working to understand the needs of the client and integrating them with findings offered by other team members. This can lead to best use of technical skills to undertake device modification or change user interface preferences on a current or a future device. With input from other team members, the engineer might work independently on identifying device options while keeping tabs on client and team progress. Your specific contribution may vary based on your skillset, experience, or the needs of the client. Your role can range from device fabrication or modification to integrating the output or control of two or more AT devices. Your talents, and the experience you gain through being part of the rehabilitation process, will make you an even more important contributor to an AT team over time.

To illustrate, a client planning to return to paid employment following a cervical spinal cord injury may need not only a rehabilitation engineer with knowledge of workplace networks and software applications but also some awareness of strategies for alternate access to a computer keyboard. Over time and after learning more about the skills of a VR counselor you will recognize other issues and be ready to propose solutions to issues like workplace accessibility and/or vehicle modification. Learning more about adaptive driving technologies from a consulting OT specialist can help you broaden your skills and areas of expertise over time. Over time and in more technical situations, an experienced rehabilitation engineer might even serve as team lead to coordinate activities and guide the entire AT team.

Not all teams have the benefit of having a graduate engineer and may settle for a member with technical interests and/or skills that identify them as an engineering tech or technologist. To further document these ancillary roles, RESNA's engineers recently developed a white paper to help clarify the levels of expertise and responsibilities for an engineer (DiGiovine et al. 2018, 1–12). This paper was developed to help resolve ethical issues related to education, experience, and certification, guided by the mandate to "do no harm." This document (also posted on the RESNA website) provides multiple case studies and is meant to describe the typical rehabilitation engineering professions and roles, and reflects the majority perspective of current rehabilitation engineering professionals. It also provides a framework for future discussions on the advancement of rehabilitation engineering with the goal of improving the quality of life of individuals with disabilities through the application of science and technology (DiGiovine et al. 2018, 1–12) (see Figure 8.4).

Not all rehabilitation engineers work in clinical settings (although it is valuable baseline experience). With their measurement skills, engineers make great

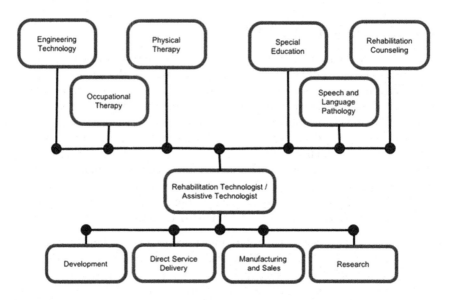

Figure 8.4 The professional disciplines included in the assistive technology team enrich the learning experience for the engineer and enable the best AT outcome for the client. There is a role for the engineer as a member of the clinical team or in product development, manufacturing and sales, or research roles (DiGiovine et al. 2018).

research partners with clinicians who want to engage in the type of research needed to prove the efficacy, benefits, and performance of all types of AT devices in applied settings. Other opportunities exist in product design with manufacturers, managing testing labs for device standards, and pursuing graduate work to the doctoral level.

8.5 The RESNA code of ethics for rehabilitation engineers

The RESNA Code of Ethics (CoE) was developed to cover all the issues that could arise in clinical practice and in all these other ways that an engineer might support the AT process and the development of AT devices and service delivery. These roles might include being an engineer on a research and development team, serving as a product developer and innovator, or as one who runs a product testing lab and develops standards. Engineers also lead and teach in academic programs that train therapists, technicians, and future rehabilitation engineers. They can staff federal agencies as program managers for Rehabilitation Engineering Research Centers (RERCs) or do quality control for manufacturers. Still others may work in public policy to establish safety guidelines for product compliance with standards. The RESNA CoE is intended to cover all aspects of these varied roles. RESNA has also developed a standards of practice document with statements that further elaborate on each item in the CoE (MindTools Content Team 2017).

In this section, each statement within the RESNA CoE will be discussed and how each applies to various engineering roles will be elaborated.

8.5.1 Hold paramount the welfare of persons served professionally

This first statement triggers the question, "What is professionalism?" The dictionary produces definitions that describe it as related to having specialized knowledge typically related to a level of education which supports competence and a commitment to excellence. In addition, professionalism also includes personal characteristics like honesty and integrity, accountability, self-regulation, politeness, and looking the part (MindTools Content Team 2017). The services of a professional are sought out by a client when there is a need for or an expectation of expertise with services delivered in an honest and ethical way. And so, around the world it is a fundamental precept in healthcare-related professions to "First, do no harm." Another way to state this is that, given an existing problem, it may be better **not** to do something, or even to do nothing than to risk causing more harm than good. Clearly, this restricts one to acting only within one's areas of knowledge and expertise. The inexperienced AT team member will do well to reflect on whether they would want someone with their current level of expertise to be providing service to one's own family member. Taking the ethical position on this means that once a client's goal or need is understood, the absence of appropriate knowledge would be explained and the client would be referred to someone with appropriate AT expertise, or credentials.

It is important to remember that not all clients will be agreeable and/or easy to work with. Some people with disabilities can be challenging and difficult. They will test interpersonal skills as well as professional knowledge. In this case, greater experience and coaching by mentors will assist with skill development and guide the young professional to modify approaches, set limits, and use distraction, negotiation, and humor to achieve success with interviewing or planning.

8.5.2 Practice only in their area(s) of expertise

When engaging in client interaction, it is important to be functioning solidly within one's area of expertise. Though there may be overlaps and common concepts, the implementation of an AT solution can be very different for a specific client even within the same type of disability. While one may know enough to help a visually impaired second-grader set up a text-to-speech application to begin keyboarding, the issues are much more complex for a blind English major who is formatting term papers and adding references from a bibliographic application while using JAWS™ to navigate the operating system and integrate the two applications. The complexity of today's AT solutions is now sufficient to require specialization to compare and make good product recommendations.

In other situations, client welfare and safety may demand more attention to the mandate to "do no harm." When a wheelchair user has left-sided neglect following a serious stroke, greater care needs to be taken when setting up user controls on a powered wheelchair. The typical stroke survivor may not be aware of this limitation and thus potentially risk serious injury on an urban sidewalk or unfamiliar doorway. This may not be part of the knowledge base for an engineer who typically does quality control for a wheelchair manufacturer, and who might otherwise be alerted to design a product safety warning feature as a wheelchair option.

There can also be situations in which the engineer who is clearly fascinated by technology and its potential for compensating for multiple limitations is unaware of the typical consumer's reluctance to surround themselves with "devices." Even children are aware of the social stigma of assistive devices and are known to refuse to use a speech recognition or an AAC device because they do not want to be perceived as "different" or "handicapped" by their peers.

Engineers newly engaged in the rehabilitation field need as much exposure as possible to clinical settings, the disciplines of other AT team members, and the range of conditions and functional limitations. This exposure helps one to understand the range of human differences. Even individuals with the same diagnosis and age can present very differently depending on culture, family expectations, and cognitive ability. The ability to develop appropriate self-assessment skills is a strong sign of an effective rehabilitation engineer. This knowledge is developed through supervised practice, mentoring by experienced team members, and a self-motivated request for review or input on next steps in an action plan.

8.5.3 Maintain the confidentiality of privileged information

Engineering students coming from a typical academic setting may be unaware of the demands of confidentiality. Though pre-professional education may have included issues like respecting a "non-compete" clause or protection of "intellectual property," personal privacy practices are essential in rehabilitation engineering. It is required in any situation related to disability, health condition, cognitive, or social-emotional factors. Very high value is placed on protecting the identity of clients or any details of their history or performance beyond their AT treatment team. Within the interactions of the AT team everyone is free to discuss, communicate, report, and document the AT services being offered. This information is also shared with the client and/or family. Patient confidentiality is also extended to those in related or business transactions such health insurance, ordering products, or making referrals, etc. De-identified information can be used when consulting on intervention planning, e.g., phoning a more experienced colleague or asking a question on a listserv.

Those working in non-clinical rehabilitation settings may need to focus on other elements of this ethical behavior. In product design, manufacturing, governmental agency, and standards development the engineer may need to be more focused on protecting intellectual property. Manufacturers invest huge sums in innovative design and product testing, and it becomes essential in maintaining their competitive edge. This factor plus loyalty to one's employer are important aspects of ethical behavior.

8.5.4 Engage in no conduct that constitutes a conflict of interest or that adversely reflects on the association, and more broadly, on professional practice

Self-interest is a very common source of motivation for violating this ethical practice. For instance, in a situation where one has been involved in developing an innovation that will change the market attractiveness of a device, it may feel great to reveal the identity of the developer of this feature in even though it is "privileged information." This action would clearly be a professional conflict of interest. One's own need for acclaim is being valued more than the manufacturer's intellectual property and product patent. An engineer knows that the corporation owns his or her design as part of their employment agreement.

This same ethical standard will apply to truthfulness in product testing and standards development. There is no room for carelessness, use of less rigorous methods, substitution of less reliable materials, or cutting corners on quality control. This has become very important as manufacturers have outsourced their processes to countries where lower quality is tolerated and/or may be overlooked. Federal agencies have been very alert to this potential and now demand the testing of imports to both International Standards Organization (ISO) and RESNA standards before allowing their sale in the United States (Hobson 2009, 79–125; Rehabilitation Engineering Research Center (RERC) on Technology Transfer 2009).

Engineers who take an academic path must remember that their professional integrity extends to conducting research. Healthcare professionals and sources of healthcare reimbursement are clearly seeking peer-reviewed evidence regarding the merits of one intervention approach over another (Minkel 1998; Sackett et al. 1996, 71–72; Sprigle and Sonenblum 2011, 203–213). The value of the entire academy of research enterprise is called into question when it is determined that, knowingly or not, data have been falsified or manipulated to show a desired outcome. Imagine the harm that would come from a team trusting inaccurate conclusions in a study on pressure distribution cushions or the efficacy of a new strategy in pelvic positioning.

Engineers can also find themselves in the role of serving as an expert witness in controversial cases regarding personal injury or product performance claims. These are often life-and-death deliberations with high dollar consequences. Consider an engineer called to testify about the correct use of wheelchair tie-down straps and occupant safety belts in a fatal public transit bus accident. Prior to accepting the invitation, the engineer's preparation included researching RESNA wheelchair transportation safety (WTS) standards, analyzing bus equipment for signs of failure, consulting with the engineer associated with several peer-reviewed articles on WTS, and reviewing the transit system's driver training manuals. The fatality was regrettable, but the case was settled through the engineer's meticulous preparation process and the uncovering of the fact *all* drivers were being taught to use an incorrect occupant restraint method. This action prevented future injuries and showed that compliance with the standards would reduce future deaths and injuries.

8.5.5 Seek deserved and reasonable remuneration for services

Engineers make a significant personal investment in pursuing their chosen field. To arrive where you are, you have competed for academic slots, and sacrificed time and effort in both academic classwork and summer internships. The intellectual and professional demands of this career plus the importance of their skills should result in good compensation. Along with this reality, is the expectation of fiscal honesty and clear communication with clients about the value/cost of services. Getting reimbursed for engineering services in a clinical rehabilitation setting is difficult as typical healthcare reimbursement does not include engineering. The only sources of reimbursement for engineering in clinical settings, at present, are State Offices of Vocational Rehabilitation—where rehabilitation engineering is in the language of the enabling legislation—the Veterans Administration Healthcare System, and in some academic settings.

Any variance in financial matters is a serious breach of ethics. This means that engineers must not permit use of their work by anyone engaged in fraud, nor can they issue public statements that are untruthful or incomplete or which do not fully disclose a conflict of interest to all relevant parties. The source of compensation for a project should always be clear and should never be received from more than one source unless fully disclosed.

There should always be an accurate and factual detailing of the merits of a recommendation to equate success with product features or the technical benefits of following a plan. By their very presence on an AT team the engineers contribute a level of confidence to a team's recommendation/plan and a likelihood of successful results

8.5.6 Inform and educate the public on rehabilitation engineering and assistive technology and its applications

The field of rehabilitation engineering is relatively new and, when mentioned, frequently evokes a quizzical expression from the listener. With even a brief explanation that it is a new field in which engineering knowledge, skills, and problem-solving approaches are used to reduce the consequences of impairment, heads begin to nod, and the relationship becomes obvious. Most people can relate this explanation to a story they have seen on the news about sensor-controlled wheelchairs that avoid obstacles and hazards or the use of the latest desktop speech recognition gizmo to dial the phone or check the accuracy of a fact for someone with multiple sclerosis or limited vision.

Engineers learn that it is part of their professional role to educate the public and explain, in non-technical language, the value of their work. The public likes rational explanations for the merits of a specific design with its flexible features or an accounting of the greater efficiency or value of proceeding on "Plan B" versus "Plan A." Rehabilitation engineers like the idea of turning kids on to careers in engineering with summer robotics camps. The added value is that robots allow customization of user interfaces so kids with disabilities can also compete and contribute to school robotic teams.

The cumulative effect of these efforts at increasing public awareness of rehabilitation engineering have the effect of influencing society's attitudes. It is these insights that lead to changes in public policy, to greater respect for the potential of individuals with impairment, and to leveling the playing field by adding a microprocessor to a toy or a better gearing system to increase mechanical advantage on a hand cycle.

Rehabilitation engineers, due to their experience with educating the public, can also relate well to the need for good training and user instruction to support the successful use of an AT device or system. Both consumers and their caregivers— whether home health aide, parent, or classroom teacher—will better support a new user in incorporating AT into daily routines and community participation if they have clear instructions, solid device mounting, and an appropriate user interface.

8.5.7 Comply with the laws and policies that guide professional practice

Engineers need to be familiar with the regulations that govern their type of rehabilitation work. This is a part of preparation for delivering services for any health-related profession. While this can seem like an onerous burden initially, it is necessary to learn about the specific demands of the Veterans Administration, Medicaid and Medicare, and private health insurance. Remember that laws and regulation apply to confidentiality, accuracy in charges and reimbursement, and licensure and certifications. OTs and PTs learn the rules of reimbursement and proper documentation to best serve their client's recovery and avoid even a suspicion of fraud and abuse. Such a tip-off can lead to a suspension of contractual agreements, generate unwelcome headlines, and lead to loss of reputation.

Some settings where rehabilitation engineers will practice are set by the ethics of academic honesty and respect for intellectual property. The foundations of research are deeply embedded in learning to use correct research designs, statistical methods, and data analysis to draw honest conclusions along with stated guidelines for their limitations. Credit should always be given to the source of or basis for ideas or innovation. For those practicing in commercial or manufacturing settings it should be clear that the employer sees an engineer as a trusted agent. The field of rehabilitation engineering is small and one's personal and professional ethics are soon noticed. In addition, this small field counts on the reliability of its research endeavors.

8.6 Conclusion

The process of developing a career marked by ethics and professional integrity is a commitment. It is shaped by making repeated decisions to do the right thing in your professional life and interaction with clients and professional colleagues. This may mean reordering priorities or putting personal convenience into a secondary position. The reward is both knowing that you are developing a reputation for integrity and that you have reached a point of personal and professional maturity.

Two case studies with extended or discussion points follow. They are intended to help you explore the course of action you would take or the advice you would offer to a novice colleague in a potential ethical challenge.

8.7 Case study #1

Ben has always had an interest in prosthetics. He grew up near a grandfather who had lost his dominant arm in combat. His grandpa adapted well to his limb loss and returned to work as a farmer which allowed him to support his family and earn the respect of other farmers in the community. His "Gramps" had rigged up adaptations with the help of an AgrAbility specialist that allowed him to continue to drive his tractor, hitch up the tiller, clear his land, and use a computer to communicate with his agricultural extension agent and get crop-related information from the internet.

Ben is in the last weeks of his internship experience and is intrigued with the issues of prosthetic design for a client, Jeff, who is just recovering from a traumatic forearm amputation of his dominant hand. Previously employed as a framing carpenter, Jeff has a wife and two kids under five years of age. He was referred to the AT team by an OT who referred him for training in speech recognition. This OT at the local community hospital has decided that Jeff should return to community college and get a degree in construction management. Ben, sensing a potential connection with Jeff, asks if he can follow Jeff more closely during his upcoming prosthetic evaluation and future visits with the AT team.

When going to the prosthetist with Jeff, Ben learns that Jeff won a generous financial settlement related to his amputation. It seems the prosthetist has already decided to fit Jeff with a top-of-the-line, myoelectric below-elbow prosthetic arm with interchangeable, computerized hands—the latest design to hit the marketplace. It appears that the prosthetist has not discussed the contraindications or "trade-offs" that will arise due to the features of this prosthesis. He has glossed over Jeff's past work as a framing carpenter relying on the OT's vision that Jeff should return to school and start preparation for computer use.

In addition, the prosthetist has glossed over Jeff's mention of jet skiing, his newly discovered interest in teaching his kids to fish, and his pre-amputation interest in rock climbing.

The prosthetist shows annoyance at Ben's questions, dismisses his technical knowledge, and criticizes his unexpected participation in this planning visit. To Ben, it seems that Jeff is still in a traumatized and discouraged state of mind and is mostly just focused on getting his "old lifestyle back." He is afraid of asking questions and is assuming that the prosthetist has his best interests at heart. Ben is really surprised by this situation. What actions should Ben take in this situation? After all, he is very new at this rehabilitation engineering "stuff" and things just don't seem right. What ethical violations is he having to deal with in this experience with his client?

8.7.1 Ethical response

Within your response to resolving these issues, describe the action you would take. Also, cite the number of the ethical standard(s) that is (are) being ignored or abused:

1. Issues with employment goal: First, firm up a client-centered goal. Introduce Jeff to another carpenter who uses an upper extremity prosthesis, so they discuss "real life" use of prosthesis in carpentry. There seems to be a failure in the OT's process of discussing future employment possibilities. She did not explore why Jeff had not pursued college in the first place (a learning disability? wanting to work outdoors?).
2. Issues with the recommended prosthetic device: Frequent repairs which are only done at a distant facility, fragility of the silicone gloves that cover and protect the finger articulation wiring, carpentry is a dirty environment, limitations of grip strength and grip angle, not waterproof, no discussion of other prosthetic options.
3. Issues with prosthetist's professional (ethical) behavior: Failure to consult with the hospital OT or the AT Team, failure to complete a full evaluation of Jeff's needs and justify the expense or functional value/versatility of the myoelectric computer-driven prosthetic limb, annoyance when Ben tried to ask questions on Jeff's behalf.
4. Issues with Jeff's inability to act on his own behalf: Discuss the situation with the larger AT team, alert the AT team's OT and his VR counselor to help clarify employment goals, provide education to Jeff about other prosthetic options, introduce Jeff to his farmer/grandfather to allow him to see someone functioning with a prosthesis.

8.7.2 Ethical principles being violated

1. Hold paramount the welfare of persons served professionally (lack of evidence of truthfulness and professional ethics in communication with the client).
2. Engage in no conduct that constitutes a conflict of interest or that adversely reflects on the association, and more broadly, on professional practice. (Prosthetist promoting a very expensive prosthesis which is inappropriate.)
3. Seek deserved and reasonable remuneration for services. (Prosthetist promoting a very expensive prosthesis which is also inappropriate.)
4. Inform and educate the public on rehabilitation/assistive technology and its application.
5. Comply with the laws and policies that guide professional practice.

The prosthetist's angry/annoyed expression when the engineer tries to ask questions on the client's behalf is out of line. Professionals should be open to well-intentioned questions that seek to serve the client. Professionals are committed to prevent fraud and abuse. Ben should feel free to consult with other AT team members to let them know about the broader issues related to the proposed prosthesis, need for support for emotional adjustment, and review of options for future employment.

8.8 Case study #2

Claire recently completed the graduate program at an accredited program in rehabilitation and AT education which was located at the same university as she completed her BS degree program in mechanical engineering. She got exposed to the idea of rehabilitation engineering (RE) as a career possibility during volunteer work that she did in the AT clinic back in her hometown. She loved the idea of transforming children's lives with AT devices that supported kids and enabled them to participate in their elementary education classrooms.

Claire responded eagerly to a job announcement seeking a rehabilitation engineer to lead an AT team in the Evans School District (ESD) just outside the city where she had completed her training. It meant that she would not have to relocate or move away and could stay in her same apartment. Feeling very knowledgeable and confident, having just recently finished her fieldwork experiences in RE and AT at the university, she "aced" the job interview. The administrator at ESD was pleased to find such an eager and promising employee. Parents had been increasing the pressure for competent AAC. None of the itinerant speech therapists assigned to ESD had training in AAC device evaluation or set up.

8.8.1 Additional questions for discussion for case study #2

1. How does a young professional balance the tension between needing to start paying for student loans versus and being offered a "convenient first job" in a very desirable setting. By asking about the skill level of ESD's SLPs, Claire has already indicated that she is concerned about her lack of knowledge about AAC devices. What advice would you give her?

2. Are there suitable options for supplementing her lack of knowledge about language acquisition and development? Do you think participating in manufacturer's device webinars and getting support from listservs can compensate for the absence of an SLP teammate? Are these sufficient to help her avoid "doing harm" to her young clients?

3. What are some important decision-making safeguards to remember and use when trying to decide among competing claims from AT product/device manufacturers? How do you know whether or not to believe manufacturers' claims?

4. How do rehabilitation engineers know or judge when they need to refer to a colleague with greater knowledge or experience (e.g., how do you know when you really do not have enough knowledge or experience and may inadvertently "do harm?").

5. What are some options for finding someone with more expertise who can assist? What are some options when travel distance is great, or resources are low?

Bibliography

American Occupational Therapy Association. 2014. "Occupational Therapy Practice Framework: Domain and Process (3rd ed.)." *American Journal of Occupational Therapy* 68 (Suppl 1): S1–S48. https://doi.org/10.5014/ajot.2014.682006.

Casey, Kelly Showalter. 2011. "Creating an Assistive Technology Clinic: The Experience of the Johns Hopkins AT Clinic for Patients with ALS." *NeuroRehabilitation* 28 (3): 281–293.

Cook, Albert M. and Janice Miller Polgar. 2013. *Cook and Hussey's Assistive Technologies-E-Book: Principles and Practice*. Amsterdam: Elsevier Health Sciences.

Cook, A. M. and S. Hussey. 2002. *Assistive Technologies: Principles and Practice*. St. Louis, MO: Mosby-Year Book.

DiGiovine, Carmen P., Meghan Donahue, Patricia Bahr, Mark Bresler, Joseph Klaesner, Raj Pagadala, Brian Burkhardt, and Ray Grott. 2018. "Rehabilitation Engineers, Technologists, and Technicians: Vital Members of the Assistive Technology Team." *Assistive Technology* 28: 1–12.

Hobson, D. A. 2009. "Voluntary Industry Standards for Wheelchair Technology: A Model for Successful Advancement of Assistive Technology." In *Industry Profile on Wheeled Mobility*, edited by S. M. Bauer and M. E. Buning, 79–125. Buffalo, NY: RERC on Technology Transfer, University at Buffalo.

MindTools Content Team. 2017. "Professionalism: Developing this Important Characteristic." https://www.mindtools.com/pages/article/professionalism.htm.

Minkel, J. L. 1998. "Evidence Based Practice: A Foundation." Paper presented at the Fourteenth International Seating Symposium, Vancouver, BC, Canada.

National Society of Professional Engineers. 2019. "Code of Ethics for Engineers. PUBLICATION #1102." https://www.nspe.org/sites/default/files/resources/pdfs/Ethics/CodeofEthics/NSPECodeofEthicsforEngineers.pdf.

Rehabilitation Engineering and Assistive Technology Society of North America. "Founders: The Founding of RESNA." http://www.resna.org/support-resna/founders/founders.

Rehabilitation Engineering and Assistive Technology Society of North America. "RESNA Code of Ethics." http://www.resna.org/sites/default/files/legacy/certification/RESNA_Code_of_Ethics.pdf.

Rehabilitation Engineering Research Center (RERC) on Technology Transfer. 2009. *Industry Profile on Wheeled Mobilty*, edited by S. M. Bauer, M. E. Buning. Washington, DC: NIDDR.

Sackett, D. L., W. M. Rosenberg, J. A. Gray, R. B. Haynes, and W. S. Richardson. 1996. "Evidence Based Medicine: What it is and What it isn't." *BMJ (Clinical Research Ed.)* 312 (7023): 71–72.

Sprigle, S. and S. Sonenblum. 2011. "Assessing Evidence Supporting Redistribution of Pressure for Pressure Ulcer Prevention: A Review." *Journal of Rehabilitation Research and Development* 48 (3): 203–213.

Von Bertalanffy, Ludwig. 1968. *General System Theory: Foundations, Development, Applications*. New York: George Braziller Publishers.

Chapter 9 Rehabilitation engineering in the assistive technology industry

Joseph P. Lane

Contents

DOI: 10.1201/b21964-11

9.1 Chapter overview

This chapter provides a framework for the assistive technology (AT) industry, as well as a context for the role of rehabilitation engineering (RE) within the AT industry. Both are equally challenging. The AT industry represents a combination of AT devices manufactured and distributed for sale by companies, along with a wide range of AT services delivered by professionals who may or may not be employed by the AT device companies. Further, both the AT devices and services lack any formal sanction or identification within standard industrial classification systems. Consequently, there is no established basis for formally recognizing or structuring the companies, products and services comprising this vital and expanding AT marketplace as a discrete and identifiable industry, or as a basis for analyzing a defined AT industry within the broader economic sector. Despite the lack of a formal industry classification there exists sufficient information available to provide an overall pastiche for the AT industry. That is a tenuous anchor for situating the role of RE, which ironically is quite appropriate. Rehabilitation engineers who plan to apply their professional skills within the AT industry must accept that role as more entrepreneurial and dynamic than the more structured roles in clinical, educational or government settings. Since there is no roadmap, the chapter serves as a guide to the essential information and resources necessary for rehabilitation engineers to orient themselves within this ill-defined domain.

9.2 The role of rehabilitation engineering in the AT industry

As described in Chapter 1, the practice of RE operates at the intersection of traditional engineering disciplines and the health professions. Furthermore, as presented in Chapter 8, RE practitioners typically maintain credentials and/or licensure within their traditional discipline while also passing one of two national standard exams offered by the Rehabilitation and Assistive Technology Society of North America (i.e., Assistive Technology Practitioner, ATP; Seating Mobility Specialist, SMS).

These RE professionals interact with the AT industry through their various professional roles. They may be university/college faculty and staff involved in sponsored research and development intending to increase the impact of AT products and services. They may be therapists or instructors delivering services through institutional or private practices, which creates a demand for AT products and services. They may even be career government staff administering related programs at local, regional or national levels, that in turn provide the resources to support all the stakeholders involved in AT product and service delivery.

An RE professional may be employed within the AT industry to support the supply side of the AT device and service marketplace. Some rehabilitation engineers own or work for established AT-oriented rehabilitation companies that are typically small to medium-sized enterprises (SMEs). These companies provide both AT commercial products (i.e., durable medical equipment; DME) and customized AT services (i.e., home medical equipment services). The rehabilitation engineers working for home medical equipment providers are responsible for a wide range of tasks involving the client, their environment and regulatory/reimbursement structures (Kuka 2016):

- Delivery of DME to the client
- Home assessment to verify DME safety and appropriateness
- DME set-up and testing
- Operation instructions to client, family, care providers
- Determine relevant insurance coverage (if it exists) and prepare supporting documentation
- Submit invoices to relevant insurance carriers and defend client's requirements when challenged
- Uninstall and retrieve DME if/when claim is denied on appeal
- Ensure technical support staff whenever needed around the clock

All of these tasks consume time and effort. The reimbursement process typically involves government agencies, such as the Centers for Medicare and Medicaid in the US, or the Ministry of Health in Canada and the European Union. Consumers and providers also look for reimbursement through supplemental private insurance carriers. These reimbursement agencies have codes for devices and services eligible for payment, with limits set on amounts paid for devices or for services rendered. The codes are fairly comprehensive and harmonized in the single-payer system of North America. In contrast, there remains substantial variability in the codes and payment structures across individual countries in the European Union. The challenge for home medical equipment providers operating under any of these systems is to provide the highest quality of devices and services, while securing sufficient payment to keep the company solvent. Getting the necessary devices qualified for payment and obtaining sufficient reimbursement for professional services define and constrain the entire AT industry operation.

Other rehabilitation engineers prefer the role of entrepreneurs who start new firms around a device innovation or a service region. These entrepreneurial firms may eventually be acquired by – or merge with – other firms, where the rehabilitation engineers may continue to be employed, or they may leave the field to satisfy the non-compete clauses of the merger/acquisition contract. Due to the fluid nature of RE qualifications and of the AT field itself, many individuals move across these various roles throughout their careers as circumstances and opportunities allow.

In order to describe the role of rehabilitation engineers within the AT industry, it is first necessary to define the AT industry. Unfortunately, the AT industry is more of a fuzzy concept than an established reality. The AT industry encompasses both AT products (devices) sold in the commercial marketplace, and AT services dispensed through clinics and community settings. Yet there is no standard industrial classification code for AT products or AT services, no formal structure for recognizing and classifying the for-profit and not-for-profit companies operating in the AT marketplace as a discrete and identifiable industry. More importantly for policy and practice, there is no basis for analyzing and supporting the role of a defined AT industry within the broader economic sector.

What we have instead is a variety of ad hoc efforts to gather and list information about AT companies and the products and services they offer in the marketplace. The balance of this chapter summarizes such information as it exists, explains why the information is not as comprehensive as found in other industries and provides some assessment of the AT industry's current status and future directions. That is the context in which to place the role of RE, a role all too familiar to practitioners in this amorphous field.

9.3 AT classification systems

An industry profile is a market tool typically compiled by a trade association or market research enterprise, then offered for sale to members of that industry as well as to other stakeholders interested in that industry segment's activity. Components of an industry profile include an overview, financial information, related industries, top companies, recent developments, future trends, etc. Detailed profiles exist for hundreds of industries. These are published in standard and comparative formats by commercial firms like IBIS*World*. These standardized industry profiles are assembled from data repositories based on government-level coding systems. Canada, Mexico and the United States established the North American Industrial Classification System (NAICS Association 2018) that assigns codes according to the underlying manufacturing processes involved in each company's products. These three countries are currently building a complementary North American Product Classification System that will eventually offer codes at the level of individual products or services as well as their prices. The North American Product Classification System (NAPCS) is currently in development phase (Beta 2017 1.0) undergoing testing for a subset of classification categories. The presence of official codes within a government-sanctioned classification system makes an industry visible to policymakers and for econometric analyses.

Unfortunately, the AT industry is one that very much needs – but does not have – official NAPCS and NAICS codes. As a result, it also lacks reliable industry profiles or valid marketing reports on which to base policies or practices. Instead of a dedicated code for the AT industry, some AT company listings under NAPCS/NAICS are scattered across various existing input/process categories. Most AT companies do not appear under any NAICS code whatsoever, and there is little expectation that they will be a category under wholesale or retail products and services without a concerted effort from within the AT industry.

There are some examples of industry-level profiles that address at least a significant portion of the AT marketplace. Grand View Research (Grand View Research 2017) has analyzed the rehabilitation device/equipment market according to product type, application, end use, region and market segment with forecasts from 2018 to 2025. These customized profiles are labor intensive and therefore command high prices; access to the electronic download is nearly US$6,000 for a single user. The company offers a free sample and the Table of Contents, offering a preview of the market segments addressed. As titled, this report focuses on devices used during medical rehabilitation (e.g., bathing, toileting, transfer, mobility and exercise).

The absence of a standard industrial classification for the AT industry means the key stakeholders responsible for supporting national economic activity have no basis for formally recognizing the companies and products that comprise this vital and expanding marketplace as an industry. Instead, publications such as this must piece together an incomplete industry profile from multiple and varied sources. This is challenging because products with functional benefits for persons with disabilities – and therefore the companies that manufacture, distribute and sell them – cross a range of markets. Figure 9.1 shows the range of the market sector containing products that fall within the definition of AT devices (Hersh 2010).

9.3.1 Formal classification systems

The United States government maintains a formal coding system for a subset of AT called durable medical equipment (DME). The DME designation is restricted to devices and services that are medically necessary. The US Centers for Medicare and Medicaid (CMS) maintain the Healthcare Common Procedure Coding System (HCPCS), a formal coding system for devices and services deemed medically necessary. The HCPCS Level I is comprised of numeric codes and descriptive terms of medical services and procedures performed by physicians and other healthcare professions. Level II provides codes to identify product, supply and service categories that are not covered under Level I, such as durable medical equipment, prosthetics, orthotics and supplies (DMEPOS). The HCPCS codes standardize information to help plan, implement and evaluate procedures, for billing and collections, and to conduct comparative efficacy studies. Given that the HCPCS codes drive the payment/reimbursement systems, companies within the

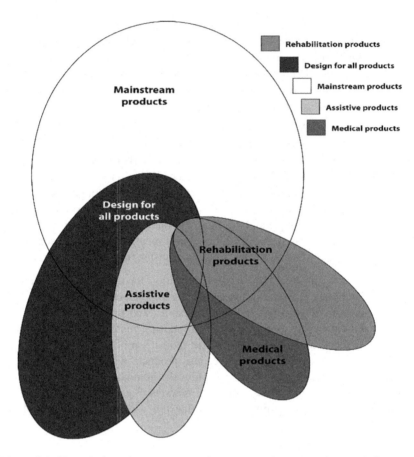

Figure 9.1 The relationships between mainstream, universal design, assistive, medical and rehabilitative products.

AT industry are eager to comply with all reporting requirements, thereby keeping the content comprehensive and accurate. Unfortunately, the criteria requiring medical necessity justification preclude the HCPCS system from coding and covering the wide range of AT products and services that are non-medical (e.g., vision, hearing, speech and haptic interfaces for information and communication technologies; environmental modifications).

The US Food and Drug Administration (FDA) maintains the Global Unique Device Identification Database (GUDID), to serve as a reference for every medical device tagged with a unique identifier, which is affixed by the manufacturer, or some other agent involved in preparing that device for interstate commerce within the United States. All device identification information is freely available to the public through the Access GUIDID portal (Food and Drug Administration 2018). Database query categories include device identifier, brand name, company name or key words describing the type of device, but no more detailed information is presented.

The GMDN Agency is a non-profit organization (registered charity) in the United Kingdom, maintaining a coding structure for all medical devices and their components called the Global Medical Device Nomenclature (GMDN Agency 2018). While similar to the GUDID, the GMDN contains a massive number of key words and phrases, each with a definition. GMDN access is through fee or permission, and then searchable by terms representing the device name, or by terms representing the device use. However, only the top-level terms have so far been assigned codes. There is a code for disability-assistive products (CT1000) with a master list of 1,571 terms as of this access date. The CT1000 code contains 12 subcategory codes, each containing anywhere from a dozen to several hundred terms. These terms must be mutually exclusive – with assignment to only one subcategory – because they collectively sum to the total number of terms under CT1000. The subcode CT103 (personal mobility assistive products) contains eight coded subcategories and 254 unique terms. While one can find 144 terms containing the term "wheelchair," a cursory inspection shows that codes are not yet assigned to them.

Both the GUDID and the GMDN should currently be treated as works in progress. The GUIDID does include a reference to GMDN terminology (see below) where one exists. There is a reciprocal effort underway to cross-reference the GMDN codes to the GUDID codes.

9.3.2 Informal classification systems

In the absence of a formal system encompassing all AT, two informal organizing structures are in use – one in the United States and another in the European Union. Both of these informal systems were created by government-sponsored stakeholders who sought to bring some structure and order to information about AT devices in the marketplace.

9.3.2.1 United States　All AT devices are intended to address functional limitations by providing interventions for the person, the task or the environment. Consequently, human functions are, so far, the most successful organizing constructs for AT products. The US web-based AT product information system AbleData (Abledata 2018) strives to capture the widest range of AT products by establishing broad categories of function under descriptive terms only. For example, Abledata lists 20 general product headings (e.g., computers, wheeled mobility), with about a dozen major categories under each one. However, the products are not divided by the major categories, but instead are only listed alphabetically under the product heading (e.g., Computers lists 6,207; Wheeled Mobility lists 4,102). AbleData offers a key word search function for more experienced users.

A parallel system established in 2001 is no longer supported, but the archived content still provides an example of an alternative approach. The Assistivetech (Assistivetech 2018) system was designed to facilitate searches by cross-classifying products by 11 functions and/or by 15 activities. Further, each of the 15 activities contained a list of numerous subactivities to help users narrow their search for a set of related products.

9.3.2.2 European Union The European Union applied the structure found within the International Standards Organization (ISO) to create the first alphanumeric classification system for AT devices consisting of a hierarchical structure of classes, subclasses and divisions (ISO – International Standards Organization 2018). The ISO 9999 system also contains codes, titles, notes and cross-references within each of these hierarchical levels. Table 9.1 contains an excerpt from the ISO 9999 showing these levels (Heerkens, Bougie and de Kleijn-de Vrankrijker 2010, 1–10) (reprinted here with permission).

The ISO 9999's numeric structure permits finer distinctions between groups of products for search, sort or analytic purposes, than does the US key word system. As a result, the ISO 9999 system includes components used for the installation of AT devices, combinations of multiple AT devices, devices used in healthcare and rehabilitation settings (e.g., external and implantable medical devices), non-technical solutions to functional limitations and information about financial support for device acquisition. Under the ISO 9999 system, AT products are organized by subclasses and divisions, leaving a specific category for each product application area (European Assistive Technology Information Network (EASTIN) 2018).

The ISO 9999's overarching alpha-numeric structure provides a level of adaptability and expansion conducive to inclusion of the wide variety of products and companies comprising the AT industry. Its structural malleability permits stakeholders to envision new applications. For example, a team of scholars and clinicians is calling for additional codes so that AT devices can be categorized according to the World Health Organization's International Classification of Function (ICF). Their idea is to require companies to identify the core functional capabilities of each AT device, and ensure every capability is linked to the code for every relevant ICF category (Bauer, Elsaesser and Arthanat 2011, 243–259). These linkages would further streamline the search, identification and matching process for all stakeholders.

At present, both the United States and European Union classification systems provide only the most basic information about AT product (specifications) and even

Table 9.1 The Classes of ISO 9999 and Some Examples of Subclasses and Divisions

Classes (One-Level Classification) of ISO 9999

04	Assistive products for personal medical treatment
05	Assistive products for training in skills
06	Orthoses and prostheses
09	Assistive products for personal care and protection
12	Assistive products for personal mobility
15	Assistive products for housekeeping
18	Furnishings and adaptations to homes and other premises
22	Assistive products for communication and information
24	Assistive products for handling objects and devices
27	Assistive products for environmental improvement, tools and machines
30	Assistive products for recreation

Subclasses (Two Level) of Class 12 Assistive Products for Personal Mobility

12 03	Assistive products for walking, manipulated by one arm
12 06	Assistive products for walking, manipulated by both arms
12 07	Accessories for assistive products for walking
12 10	Cars
12 12	Car adaptations
12 16	Mopeds and motorcycles
12 18	Cycles
12 22	Human driven wheelchairs
12 23	Powered wheelchairs
12 24	Wheelchair accessories
12 27	Vehicles
12 31	Assistive products for transfer and turning
12 36	Assistive products for lifting
12 39	Assistive products for orientation

Divisions (Three Level) of Subclass 12 31 Assistive Products for Transfer and Turning

12 31 03	Sliding boards and sliding mats and turning sheets
12 31 06	Turntables
12 31 09	Free-standing rails for self-lifting
12 31 12	Grip ladders
12 31 15	Lifting belts and harnesses
12 3118	Carrying chairs, harnesses and baskets
12 31 21	Transfer platforms

less information about AT companies (contacts) or the AT industry as a whole. Both systems lack the type and depth of information typically found in standard industry profiles, such as the distribution of customers across AT device market segments, or the distribution of sales among companies operating within each market segment.

9.4 Obstacles preventing a clear definition of the AT industry

9.4.1 Primary obstacle to AT industry definition

The AT industry arose from product/service offerings in multiple fields. The medical field drove much of the early industry from the Civil War era's demand for mechanical prosthetics and wheelchairs through subsequent applications of electronics and synthetic materials, to the present-day use of information technology in the form of software, sensors and actuators. In parallel, non-medical needs to support individuals in educational, vocational and recreational settings drove the introduction of vision, hearing, speech and even haptic products for the senses. Current advances in neuro-prosthetics (e.g., direct brain interfaces and functional electrical stimulation) offer even more possibilities to support or even supplant human functions.

This organic growth from within the field of AT led to a plethora of competing terms and territories. As a result, companies and products listed under the legally defined term "assistive technology" can also be found in different web-based catalogs and listings under a variety of other terms as shown in Table 9.2.

The lack of clear criteria for differentiating one term from another – at national or international levels – led to the present circumstance where redundancies across

Table 9.2 Many Terms Compete with the Term Assistive Technology

Term
Adaptive Technology
Assistive Health Technology (AHT)
Assistive Health Products (AHP)
Rehabilitation Technology
Accessible Technology
Independent Living Aids
Durable Medical Equipment (DME)
Durable Medical Equipment Prosthetic & Orthotic Services (DMEPOS)
Home Medical Equipment (HME)

categories coexist with gaps within categories. With no resolution in sight, the best rehabilitation engineers can do is to know the content and implications of each term and treat all as resources falling within the scope of their profession.

For example, within the home medical equipment (HME) industry, the critical distinction is between DME products and HME services. DME is what devices/equipment the professional uses, while HME services are what services the professional provides through application of the DME. In the US, the CMS has over 1,000 coded categories for products, components, systems and services, and any product or service must be officially classified under one of those codes to be eligible for reimbursement by CMS and typically by any other health insurance carrier.

A device is recognized as a DME eligible for reimbursement by public and private health insurance carriers, when a physician stipulates that the device is required to support a medical need on an ongoing basis – the device meets the criterion of medical necessity. This criterion of medical necessity is the single criterion creating a chasm between DME and AT devices. Many AT devices are necessary on an ongoing basis to support a person's need to complete ADL/IADL activities, participate in school or the workplace, to access transportation and recreation and generally to participate in all aspects of society. However, since none of these needs meet a medical need, the devices are not considered DME nor are they and associated services eligible for reimbursement. From the 1960s onward, persons with disabilities, family members and their advocates strove to separate themselves from the medical model, arguing that most of their device and service needs for living a full and independent life were not medically necessary. They were and are right to view their access to many enabling devices and services (e.g., information and communication interface devices, accessible materials and environments, assessment, referral and training) as a civil right rather than a medical necessity. The downside is the very same separation eliminated such non-medical devices and services from reimbursement through the healthcare system, which happens to drive most markets and industries.

The reimbursement situation for AT devices and services in the United States stands as follows: those deemed as medically necessary may be eligible for reimbursement through the healthcare system. For children up to age 18, a school district is required to pay for AT identified through an individualized assessment as necessary for a full and equal educational experience. Persons who need AT to secure employment may be eligible for assessment, training and equipment through state-level vocational programs. Similarly, people who qualify for homemaker status may also receive support through these same vocational programs. Of course, support for AT devices and services across other countries varies widely.

All companies operating within the HME industry use the Berenson-Eggers Types of Service (BETOS) codes: a classification system assigning unique codes to general categories of devices and procedures recognized as qualifying for reimbursement by the CMS system under the Health Care Financing Administration Common Procedure Code System (HCPCPS). There are six general BETOS codes. There is also a crosswalk between the six general BETOS codes and the more than 1,000 specific HCPCS codes on a fee-based site with a free example from 2016 (Find A Code LLC 2016).

The HME industry publishes a table showing all allowable charges under the six BETOS codes representing different general categories of DME devices and reports annual expenditures under each of the BETOS codes on a rolling seven-year basis as shown in Table 9.3 (HME News 2018).

9.4.2 Secondary obstacles to clearly define the AT industry

While the absence of clear boundary criteria is the major obstacle to characterizing the AT industry, here are five additional obstacles compounding the problem:

1) Ambiguity in legislative language – The United States passed the Technology Related Assistance for Individuals with Disabilities Act in 1988. This legislation established the term "assistive technology," and further defined two categories of AT as "devices" and "services" (US Congress 1988):

> AT devices: "Any item, piece of equipment, or product system, whether acquired commercially off the shelf, modified, or customized, that is used to increase, maintain, or improve functional capabilities of individuals with disabilities."

> AT services: "Any service that directly assists an individual with a disability in the selection, acquisition, or use of an assistive technology device."

The language demonstrated intent for the term "assistive technology" to be treated as an adjective describing two categories of nouns (devices and services). Despite this intent, the common vernacular adopted the term and the initials "AT" as a noun encompassing both devices and services. Nor did this 1988 legislation describe or list the specific devices and services to be considered AT. The level of ambiguity regarding AT was reinforced in subsequent US legislation (e.g., ADA, IDEA, Olmstead) and similar legislation in other nations, because the specific criteria for inclusion or exclusion were never articulated.

In the US, the broad definition of AT in 1988 and subsequent legislation left the field open to interpretation and to competing terminology. The legislative language added an additional level of jargon to the mix. As noted in the previous section, the gradual and organic growth of the

Table 9.3 BETOS Codes, DME Definitions and Annual Expenditures (2010–2016)

BETOS	Product	2009	2010	2011	2012	2013	2014	2015	2016
DIA	Med/Surg	202M	198M	198M	183M	153M	203M	231M	300M
DIB	Hospital beds	224M	255M	240M	230M	139M	120M	112M	86M
DIC	Oxygen and supplies	2.0B	2.2B	2.1 B	1.9B	1.3B	1.4B	1.5B	1B
DID	Wheelchairs	1.4B	1.4B	1.05B	1.1B	622M	615M	625M	588M
DIE	Other DME	3.4B	3.8B	3.6B	3.9B	2.5B	2.6B	3B	2.6B
DIG	Respiratory meds	588M	629M	637M	709M	605M	836M	890M	863M
	Total	**7.9B**	**8.5B**	**7.8B**	**8.1B**	**5.3B**	**5.8B**	**6.3B**	**5.5B**

What is a BETOS bucket?
BETOS stands for Berenson-Eggers type of service, and it's the name of a coding system developed to analyze the growth in Medicare expenditures. The coding system covers all HCPCS codes; assigns an HCPCS code to only one BETOS bucket; consists of readily understood clinical categories that permit objective assignment; is stable over time and is relatively immune to minor changes in technology or practice patterns.
Source: CMS

AT industry from both medical and non-medical arenas, predated this legislation and persists in complicating the articulation of a clear industry profile.

2) Non-commercial AT devices – Given the limited distribution of commercial AT devices and the lack of consumer information about them, the field contains many custom-made devices, one-off modifications and do-it-yourself kits. Rapid prototyping capabilities are increasing the presence of such offerings from the well intentioned to the uninformed. The commercial marketplace requires structure, regulation and financing under both for-profit and non-profit models, which are safeguards lacking in the maker movement. A legitimate and accurate industry profile focuses on commercial devices and the companies offering them for sale. However, most web-based compilations of AT devices typically include both commercial and non-commercial items.

3) Complexity of AT product mix – The AT industry presents a major challenge to structuring a definitive classification system because AT devices span a wide range of even the most general industrial categories. They include various product categories and applications: everything from aids to daily living, through sensory products (hearing, vision, speech, haptics) and out to environmental modifications. They represent a wide range of the materials, components and production systems that form the basis of most industrial classification systems (mechanical and electrical, hardware and software). A related and increasing trend is for AT components (e.g., software applications) to be added to or downloaded into mainstream products (e.g., cellphones), which increases the challenges of identifying and classifying AT devices at the category and subcategory levels.

4) Corporate diversity – There is no single financial, geographic or business criterion capable of capturing all AT companies. Some companies exclusively manufacture and sell AT devices, while other companies make and offer AT devices along with a range of mainstream products. Some mainstream companies intentionally design their products to include features and functions that make them easier to use by persons with disabilities.

   a) Large companies – There are three relatively large corporations within the AT industry. Two are public corporations (Invacare HCS LLC and Tobii Group Inc.), while the third (Ottobock) is a multi-generational private company. Invacare HCS LLC is the AT industry's single largest company with reported annual revenue of US$1.05 billion and about 5,000 employees in 2016 (Invacare 2017). Although Invacare is well known in AT circles for wheelchairs, cushions, transfer aids and related mobility products, its sales units include respiratory equipment, hospital beds and related furnishings not typically classified as AT products. As one of the few publicly traded companies, the detailed information available about Invacare is not common to most AT companies.

Tobii Group Inc. is another public company that falls within the AT industry. However, its annual sales of US$750 million and 600 employees account for both AT augmentative and alternative communication (AAC) applications within its Tobii Dynavox division, and mainstream applications of its eye-tracking technology in computer, gaming, virtual reality and automobile interfaces in its Tobii Technology division (Tobii Group 2018). Ottobock Group is another company that is difficult to classify. Its orthotic, prosthetic, powered prosthetic and wheelchair products straddle the medical and AT markets. Ottobock is privately owned, reporting 2014 revenue of US$1.05 billion and employs 7,300 people within its Ottobock Group division (Ottobock Group 2017).

Invacare HCS LLC, Tobii Group Inc. and Ottobock Group are the only three operating as multinational corporations within the AT industry. These three companies are exceptional due to their size and breadth of operations. At present there are very few medium-sized AT companies, with most having been acquired or merged over the past decade (e.g., Tobii & Dynavox). Therefore, the AT industry has a yawning gap between three large multinational corporations and the multitude of small companies.

b)   Small companies – Most AT companies meet the United States definition of a small business by employing fewer than 500 people in manufacturing enterprises or generating less than US$7.5 million in average annual receipts for non-manufacturing enterprises. Europe refers to small businesses as small and medium-sized enterprises (SMEs), defined as employing fewer than 250 people or with sales of less than EUR50 million. This is further divided into medium (> 250 employees, > EUR50 million sales), small (> 50 employees, > EUR10 million sales) and micro (> 10 employees, > EUR2 million sales) enterprises (OECD 2016).

These small AT companies typically operate within single nations or occupy regional market boundaries within a single country. The fragmented marketplace in which companies operate results in fragmented information available to customers about these companies and their products. Even web-based information systems have limited value because the small AT companies are usually privately owned, so there is little information in the public domain about them, and what information exists is difficult to identify through key word searches.

c) AT product distributors – Another business model is to distribute AT products manufactured by others, e.g., Performance Health LLC in the United States and the ERP Group in Canada. The European Union has a wide range of distributors operating in different countries, organized in the early 1990s as the European Medical Device Distributors Alliance (EIDDA). Distributors offer a wide range of products to capture revenue through resale, ranging from those serving non-medical ADL/IADL functions, through various classes of medical devices. They represent another path for rehabilitation engineers who are comfortable working with a wide range of products, suppliers, operating environments and customer bases.

One final example is AliMed Inc. a US-based privately held corporation, which combines all of the above business models. AliMed Inc. manufactures and sells direct a wide range of medical and non-medical products, distributes products manufactured by others, and operates a global network of distributors.

5) Heterogeneous consumer marketplace – People with disabilities are not readily classified or categorized because they represent a heterogeneous mix of factors. Users of particular AT devices may vary widely in age, ethnicity, education, vocation, geographic distribution and socioeconomic status. Although some people are born with a disability, the term "temporarily able-bodied" reminds us that anyone can become disabled at any time through accident, illness, longevity or other life circumstances.

This heterogeneity is a challenge to anyone attempting to collect marketing information on market size, trends, or other aspects of the consumer landscape. Some studies try to assess markets by applying statistics to the number of people within some diagnostic categories. These studies typically misrepresent the actual market because not everyone in the same diagnostic category has the same functional requirements (overreporting for that diagnostic category), while those who do use specific AT devices may only represent a subset of users for any given AT product (underreporting full range of users). Underreporting also occurs when people in certain age cohorts, or those with particular diagnoses or functional limitations, carry some stigma about their impairments, making them less likely to disclose pertinent information.

Broader population-based surveys are frequently used to collect marketing information for mainstream products, but the AT device marketplace adds serious barriers. Many countries have laws protecting the confidentiality of personal health, medical and welfare data, particularly for what are considered vulnerable populations, so either the target populations are excluded from the survey, or the results cannot be reported in meaningful ways. Further, most surveys about disability, impairment and functional limitations do not routinely gather information about the use of AT devices, either by type of device or frequency, breadth or duration of use. So even appropriately de-identified data from surveys does not contain information useful for market analysis or policy planning and decision making.

The six barriers outlined above are not reasons to discourage rehabilitation engineers from engaging with AT companies. In fact, the barriers should encourage rehabilitation engineers to support the creation of a standard industrial classification system for the AT industry. The AT industry's lack of cohesion as an identifiable industry segment limits its ability to organize, plan and fund the creation of a unique classification code. Lacking this code, AT companies cannot generate the information and data necessary to inform public policies, support future entrepreneurs and investors, or direct sales and marketing in an efficient and effective manner.

9.5 Provisional profile for the AT industry

There is very little public information available about the number, size and role of individual companies within the AT industry. Aggregated lists of AT companies on websites are incomplete, difficult to search and navigate and tend to offer little beyond the name, address and website link. Even individual company websites tend to provide few details on size, internal operations, sales and marketing or future plans. As noted, most are privately held, and small to medium-sized, so they have limited resources and likely are very protective of their internal information. This lack of information on individual corporations precludes the kind of macro-level analysis on impact and trends required to support public policy actions in support of the AT industry.

Our ability to properly describe the AT industry is further complicated by the array of business models operating in this field. Some companies manufacture products and offer them for direct sale as vendors. Other companies manufacture products but prefer to have them distributed in quantities by distributors who function as the vendors. Another type of vendor is called a "value-added retailer" because they staff bricks-and-mortar locations with staff who are qualified to offer advice and guidance which is a value beyond the point-of-sale transaction. Even beyond these business models, practicing clinicians may have arrangements with selected vendors to which they refer a majority of clients, adding a link of value-added brokers to the AT product supply chain.

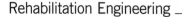

The following content summarizes what is known about the AT industry in general.

9.5.1 A sample of AT companies

There are two types of AT device companies. The first type is any company focusing on and limited to the production and sale of AT devices. The second type is any company that includes AT devices amongst a broader range of mainstream products, including those designing products with features and functions that make them more useful for persons with disabilities (i.e., accessible thermostat features). Some of the largest global medical device companies have product lines that fall within the definition of AT (MPO 2017).

There are hundreds of both types of AT companies in today's marketplace. These companies can be divided into groups based on the functional use of the products they create. Functional areas include prosthetics/orthotics, wheeled mobility/seating, hearing, vision, education, aids to daily living, software and AAC.

A sample of AT device companies in the market today is listed in the following web link:

http://sphhp.buffalo.edu/content/dam/sphhp/cat/kt4tt/pdf/assistive-technology-companies-leahy.pdf

9.5.2 AT industry factors and dynamics

Figure 9.2 identifies key forces shaping the AT industry's overall dynamics. These forces fall under the four industry-based headings of: (1) Economic Drivers, (2) Supply Industries, (3) Demand Industries, (4) Related Industries.

Given that the AT industry is highly fragmented, the influence of these forces is spurious and opportunistic, rather than deliberate and systemic. The economic forces have the broadest potential impact, but they are the most constrained by government and private insurance policies. As the aging demographic shifts more citizens into functional impairments, the market may appear to be growing, which may induce more small businesses to enter the AT marketplace. This will perpetuate or even expand the industry fragmentation while ensuring market concentration remains low. Low market concentration makes all AT product and service deployment efforts more expensive, while higher concentrations would yield economies of scale that increase both efficiency and effectiveness.

Social forces have a related impact on the AT industry. The continued integration of persons with disabilities into mainstream society led to additional challenges in ensuring that consumer products as well as features of the built environment

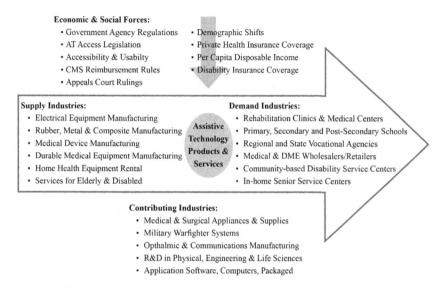

Economic & Social Forces:
- Government Agency Regulations
- AT Access Legislation
- Accessibility & Usabilty
- CMS Reimbursement Rules
- Appeals Court Rulings
- Demographic Shifts
- Private Health Insurance Coverage
- Per Capita Disposable Income
- Disability Insurance Coverage

Supply Industries:
- Electrical Equipment Manufacturing
- Rubber, Metal & Composite Manufacturing
- Medical Device Manufacturing
- Durable Medical Equipment Manufacturing
- Home Health Equipment Rental
- Services for Elderly & Disabled

Assistive Technology Products & Services

Demand Industries:
- Rehabilitation Clinics & Medical Centers
- Primary, Secondary and Post-Secondary Schools
- Regional and State Vocational Agencies
- Medical & DME Wholesalers/Retailers
- Community-based Disability Service Centers
- In-home Senior Service Centers

Contributing Industries:
- Medical & Surgical Appliances & Supplies
- Military Warfighter Systems
- Opthalmic & Communications Manufacturing
- R&D in Physical, Engineering & Life Sciences
- Application Software, Computers, Packaged

Figure 9.2 Key forces shaping the AT industry's dynamics.

are accessible as well as usable to persons with any type of functional impairment. Disability is no longer considered a condition of the person, but instead is a barrier in the design of products or environments that present a disabling situation to the person. Design concepts that reflect an effort to accommodate a wide range of functional abilities – physical, sensory and cognitive – can be found in terminology such as Universal Design, Inclusive Design, Design for All, Design for More and Accessible Design.

These trends seem to create a paradox for companies operating in niche markets such as AT. When the functional needs of customers can be met by mainstream products, the consumer benefits from lower prices (economies of scale) and easier access (broader distribution). However, reducing the demand for specialized AT products threatens the viability of the companies that make and supply them. The AAC field has experienced this paradox because functions once only available on dedicated speech output devices, are now widely available through inexpensive software applications that operate on laptops, pads and even smartphones. Some AT companies need revenue streams from products with broader markets in order to cover the losses accrued from the cost of sales in very small markets. Without those revenue streams the availability of truly customized products is imperiled. Despite the market broadening achieved through universal design practices, there will always remain a need for products and services tailored to an individual's unique and likely complex requirements. Rehabilitation engineers will always play an important role in AT product customization.

211

Understanding the requirements of human access in the context of product and environmental interfaces, presents a rich opportunity for rehabilitation engineers to participate in both the AT and mainstream marketplace, by constructively delivering products and services which are more accessible and usable. However, it is important to frame these principles within the competitive market context of the AT industry. While corporate managers may support the principles, they can only invest the additional resources necessary to make interfaces more accessible and usable if they can demonstrate a return on that investment. The critical argument is grounded in the concept of **market share** – the percentage of the total customers for a type of product or service who purchase your company's version. By increasing my company's share of the market, I'm diminishing the share held by my competitors – a zero-sum perspective given the finite number of actual customers. By making a product or service more accessible and more usable by a broader range of the population, the company can increase its share of the market for that type of product or service, and in two ways. First, it can become a preferred product or service for the current total number of active customers. Second, it can become the only option for additional people who could not access or use the existing market offerings. Expanding market share brings increased economies of scale and expanded profits, so the social principles of access and use relate directly to the economic considerations of scale and profit.

9.5.3 Barriers to entry

Barriers to entry into the AT device industry are low but barriers to sustaining a successful business enterprise are high. There are limited major players in the industry, indicating that no operator has monopolized any market segment, product, service or geographic region. The absence of territorial monopolies reduces barriers for new entrants. Many countries have government agencies offering grant/contract assistance to small business start-ups, and to entrepreneurs commercializing some new technology-based product, especially for industries such as AT which offer beneficial socioeconomic impacts. The continuing growth stage for the AT industry's life cycle allows for new entrants into the market. Because the market is yet to be concentrated or fully defined, customers welcome new brands and often consider them as equals to already existing brands. This can be good for the new company but potentially bad for the customer if the new option lacks proper field testing, clinical evaluation or features/functions rendering it less accessible or usable. Rehabilitation engineers have a role to play in helping people conduct a proper comparative analysis, choose the proper product or service and provide training and follow-through support.

There are few avenues for accessing start-up capital for a new AT business venture. The US Small Business Administration offers two highly competitive programs targeting new product research and development, with the field of application defined by the funding agency. Small Business Innovation Research (SBIR) grants are made to small businesses operated by individuals dedicating more than half of their time to the business venture. They receive funding in two increments from the sponsor agency, with the funding for scale-up, deployment and promotion left to the recipient or their commercialization partners. The Small Business Technology Transfer (STTR) program is similar, although the primary recipient may operate from a university or non-profit setting.

The US National Science Foundation's I-Corps Program provides resources to scientists and engineers determined to become entrepreneurs. Canada's version is the National Research Council's Industrial Research Assistance Program (IRAP–NRC). The European Union offers a wide range of support from investment funding, through coaching and incubation through the European Institute of Innovation and Technology. All of these government-sponsored options require lengthy commitments of time and effort, and usually a matching or majority investment from the outside sources.

9.5.4 Crucial information gaps in the AT industry

The absence of a standard industrial classification code for the AT industry, and the fragmented nature of the AT marketplace, both limit the amount and range of publicly available information about AT products, services and the companies providing them. Government policies and industry representation are both hampered by the absence of information on the AT industry as a whole. There are four specific categories where aggregated information is essential for performing analyses concerning the health, scope and direction of any industry. Information is currently unavailable in all of them for the AT industry:

1) Capital intensity – This metric compares the cost of goods sold (labor, materials) to sales revenue. Doing so requires data on a representative set of companies within the subject industry. The more comprehensive the set becomes, the more precise becomes the aggregation and stratification – and therefore the more accurate the numbers generated.

2) Competition level – This analysis determines the degree to which competition exists, which in turn helps stakeholders assess the barriers to entry, anticipate mergers and acquisitions and determine the potential risk/return on investment. The competition level can encourage or discourage future investment in the subject industry, even in the presence of positive projections for growth from demographics, legislation or technological advances.

3) Revenue volatility – Revenue volatility describes the increase and decrease in annualized revenue growth for an industry over any prior five-year timeframe. This statistic requires annual revenue reports from

a representative sample of companies within the same industry over a sustained period of time.

4) Key success factors – A profile for a subject industry draws from a list of several hundred known critical success factors, to create a subset of factors thought to be most relevant to that industry's context. Doing so requires having sufficient information about an industry to identify the most relevant factors, which requires input from the companies comprising that industry. Collecting this information requires identification, contact and agreement with subject companies, so the AT industry remains a long way away from compiling and applying such important information.

These gaps in information about the AT industry leave participants – including rehabilitation engineers – at a disadvantage when charting a career, launching a new business or planning for future growth and sustainability.

9.6 Future of the AT industry

9.6.1 AT industry performance as an indicator of future trends

The general US trend during the past five years has been positive for the AT device industry, with the aging baby boomer population cohort driving up demand for AT devices and services, as part of the mix of products and services for the growing population of persons who are elderly or aging into disabilities. Nations around the world are facing similar demographic and societal trends, so the following industry analysis of elderly and disabled services in the United States can be readily generalized:

> During the next several years, the number of people aged 65 and older and the number of people with disabilities are expected to increase. As the population ages, more individuals require [AT] industry products because aging adults are more susceptible to injuries and illnesses that prevent them from performing daily activities. Medical advancements and superior nutrition have helped people live longer, contributing to the size of the baby-boomer demographic. As a result, an aging population and increased life expectancies are fueling demand for [AT] industry devices. According to the US Census Bureau, about 56.7 million people living in the United States had some kind of disability in 2010 (latest available data). Almost half of all people with disabilities have a severe disability that affects their ability to see, hear, walk or perform other basic functions. US Census Bureau data show that about 12.0 million adults need assistance with one or more activities of daily living. Demand for [AT] industry services has been further underpinned by an increase in the number of individuals receiving disability payments. Disability payments have been on the rise because workers with modest health problems

are, like many in the labor force, unable to find jobs, leading to an increase in the number of applicants who are approved for disability payments.

Despite these growth projects, demand for AT will be inhibited by multiple factors. Limitations on meeting the growing demand will largely come from government restrictions on AT device eligibility for reimbursement, capitation on reimbursement levels for specific AT devices or components, limited private insurance coverage. At the same time, constraints on discretionary income among persons with disabilities will persist, because as a group they remain unemployed or underemployed at higher levels than other segments of society. There is no foreseeable improvement in these constraining factors.

9.6.2 AT industry life cycle path

The expansive demographic and social drivers will play out against the countervailing economic constraints. However, from a purely technological standpoint the AT device industry remains in an accelerating growth phase of its life cycle. One key characteristic of a growing industry is technological change. The introduction of integrated circuits and internet connectivity has certainly revolutionized the opportunities to deliver new or improved features and functions. Less than 30 years ago, the solitary software package capable of providing text entry via speech recognition was Dragon Dictate which required discrete speech – a pause between each word – and cost US$12,000 per unit. Some versions of Dragon Naturally Speaking – which now permits continuous speech – sell for less than US$50, while similar speech recognition capabilities come installed in desktop operating systems at no additional cost.

Accelerating advances in information, communication, nanoscale and biomedical technologies – along with their applications in materials, components and software systems – will continue to push the frontiers of AT device capabilities and AT service deliverables. Because innovation is constrained by the economics of purchasing power and reimbursement capitation, advances will first appear in those application areas with the most resources, such as military and private rehabilitation facilities. Companies operating across the broader public areas will continue to focus their discretionary resources on making their existing AT products less expensive to manufacture and support and increasing their efficiency in the delivery of AT services.

All of these points emphasize the need for rehabilitation engineers to accrue a breadth of skills through higher education degrees and through professional practice credentials. People who enter the field from technical engineering backgrounds may find it useful to become credentialed on an allied health or social service field. That combination allows them to apply their technical knowledge within settings that permit them to secure reimbursement for time spent in clinical service settings.

9.6.3 AT industry globalization efforts

The World Health Organization (WHO) recently redefined AT by inserting the world "health" into the term and introducing the following new terms (World Health Organization 2018):

Assistive Health Technology (AHT) – A subset of health technology, which encompasses a wide range of Assistive Health Products (AHP) and their service provisions. AHT is defined as the application of organized knowledge, skills, procedures and systems related to the provision of AHP. The need for AHT is rapidly increasing as people continue to live longer despite health conditions and functional status.

Assistive Health Products (AHP) – a subset of health products, which include any form of an external tool, whether specially designed and produced or generally available, whose primary purpose is to maintain or improve an individual's functioning and independence, facilitate participation, and enhance overall well-being.

Redefining the terms was the first step in the WHO's Global Cooperation on Assistive Health Technology (GATE) initiative, which intends to improve global access to high-quality and affordable AT products representing both high-tech and low-tech solutions. The four main goals of GATE are:

1) Remove physical barriers to health facilities, information and equipment
2) Make health care affordable
3) Train all health care workers in disability issues including rights
4) Invest in specific services such as rehabilitation

Given the WHO's mission it is not surprising that any topic targeted for intervention must carry a health-oriented brand. The challenge will be to consider the health implications of AT without forcing it back into the mindset and control of a medical model. This is a highly sensitive issue to persons with disabilities who spent more than 30 years arguing to move from a medical to a social model, and that independent living was a civil right not a medical outcome – the argument being that people living their daily lives with disabilities are not sick, nor should their lives be dominated by treatments imposed by others. Of course, the independent living movement has not reached many countries so there remains much work to enlighten people with disabilities, family members, service providers and government policy makers about these critical and hard-won distinctions.

Distancing disability, and functional impairment as a consequence, from the medical treatment of illness or trauma as a cause, remains a necessary component of individual choice, empowerment and self-determination. At the same time, this

216

important distinction should not ignore the point that the manufacture, delivery and support of AT is a matter of public health and welfare. Conversely, many public health technologies – water purification, mine detection, vaccinations – can be considered AT in that they prevent the occurrence of illness or trauma.

GATE's current challenges include limited funding, weak procurement systems, lack of clear understanding of AHT needs and benefits, lack of needs assessment and the absence of a properly trained workforce. The WHO is yet to take implement this initiative which has potential to invigorate the AT industry around the world. Rehabilitation engineers who engage with the GATE program should be mindful of the sustained efforts to clarify distinctions between the medical and social perspectives, and to help advocate for maximum independence and self-determination among persons with disabilities everywhere.

9.7 Discussion questions

1. How would you define the state of the AT industry and the rehabilitation engineer's role in it?
2. What kind of categorization schema do most industries have that the AT industry lacks, and what are the consequences of lacking it?
3. Why so many names for the same market, and what impact does that have on business?
4. What are some of the issues facing an AT company or an AT professional when trying to make a living through product or service delivery?
5. What should rehabilitation engineers know about the social movement surrounding AT devices and services and how does the medical/social dichotomy influence stakeholders?
6. Distinguish between the social principle and business practice of universal design as a construct, and explain how to best apply it within the context of the AT industry?
7. Talk about some of the roles a rehabilitation engineer can perform within the AT industry to improve its economic and social standing?
8. Given all of the social and demographic factors driving an expanding market for AT products and services, why is the future forecast constrained?

Bibliography

Abledata. "Abledata." Accessed 04/09, 2018, https://abledata.acl.gov/.

Assistivetech. "Assistive Tech." Accessed 04/09, 2018, http://assistivetech.net/.

Bauer, Stephen M., Linda-Jeanne Elsaesser, and Sajay Arthanat. 2011. "Assistive Technology Device Classification Based upon the World Health Organization's, International Classification of Functioning, Disability and Health (ICF)." *Disability and Rehabilitation: Assistive Technology* 6 (3): 243–259.

Centers for Medicare and Medicaid Services. "Berenson-Eggers Type of Service Codes." Accessed 04/09, 2018, https://www.cms.gov/Research-Statistics-Data-and-Systems/ Statistics-Trends-and-Reports/MedicareFeeforSvcPartsAB/downloads/betosdesccodes .pdf.

———. "HCPCS General Information." Accessed 04/08, 2018, https://www.cms.gov/medicare /coding/medhcpcsgeninfo/index.html.

———. "HCPCS Release and Code Sets." Accessed 04/08, 2018, https://www.cms.gov/Medicare/ Coding/HCPCSReleaseCodeSets/Alpha-Numeric-HCPCS-Items/2017-Alpha-Numeric-HCPCS-File.html.

European Assistive Technology Information Network (EASTIN). "Guided Search – Assistive Products." Accessed 04/10, 2018, http://www.eastin.eu/en/searches/products/index.

Find A Code LLC. "HCPCS-BETOS Code Matching Table." Accessed 04/09, 2018, https:// www.findacode.com/hcpcs/HCPCS-BETOS-2016.pdf.

Food & Drug Administration. "Access Guide for Global Unique Device Identification Database (GUDID)." Accessed 04/08, 2018, https://www.fda.gov/MedicalDevices/Dev iceRegulationandGuidance/UniqueDeviceIdentification/GlobalUDIDatabaseGUDID/ ucm444831.htm.

GMDN Agency. "Global Medical Device Nomenclature (GMDN)." Accessed 04/08, 2018, https://www.fda.gov/MedicalDevices/DeviceRegulationandGuidance/UniqueDeviceIde ntification/GlobalUDIDatabaseGUDID/default.htm.

Grand View Research. "Rehabilitation Devices/Equipment Market Analysis by Product Type and Segment Forecasts 2018–2025." Accessed 04/11, 2018, https://www .grandviewresearch.com/industry-analysis/rehabilitation-products-market/toc.

Heerkens, Y. F., T. Bougie, and M. W. de Kleijn-de Vrankrijker. 2010. "Classification and Terminology of Assistive Products." *International Encyclopedia of Rehabilitation*: 1–10.

Hersh, Marion A. 2010. *The Design and Evaluation of Assistive Technology Products and Devices Part 1: Design*. Edited by M. Blouin Cirrie. http://cirrie.buffalo.edu/ encyclopedia/en/article/309/.

HME News. "State of the Industry 2017 (Supplement – December 2016)." Accessed 04/09, 2018, http://www.hmenews.com/white-paper/state-industry-2017.

IBISWorld. "About IBISworld." Accessed 04/18, 2018, http://www.ibisworld.com/.

———. "Elderly and Disability Services in the U.S.: Market Research Report." Accessed 04/10, 2018, https://www.ibisworld.com/industry/default.aspx?indid=1607.

Invacare, HCS L. "2017 Annual Report." Accessed 04/10, 2018, http://www.invacare.com/HQ/ EDITORIAL/InvestorRelations/2017%20Annual%20Report%20and%20Form%2010-K .pdf.

ISO - International Standards Organization. "ISO 9999:2011 Assistive Products for Persons with Disabilities – Classifications and Terminology." Accessed 04/10, 2018, https://www. iso.org/obp/ui/#iso:std:iso:9999:ed-5:v1:en.

Kuka, G. "DME is What We Use, HME Services is What We Do." *HME News*. United Publications, http://www.hmenews.com/blog/dme-what-we-use-hme-services-what-we-do.

MPO. "Medical Product Outsourcing: Top 30 Global Medical Device Companies." Accessed 04/10, 2018, https://www.mpo-mag.com/issues/2015-07-01/view_features/top-30-global-medical-device-companies.

NAICS Association. "History of the NAICS Code." Accessed 04/10, 2018, http://www.naics. com/history-naics-code/.

OECD. "What is an SME?" Accessed 04/10, 2018, http://ec.europa.eu/growth/smes/business-friendly-environment/sme-definition/index_en.htm.

Ottobock Group. "Facts and Figures." Accessed 04/10, 2018, http://www.ottobock.com/en/company/facts-figures/.

Tobii Group. "Tobii Group Business Units." Accessed 04/10, 2018, http://www.tobii.com/group/about/.

U.S. Census Bureau. "Introduction to NAICS." Accessed 04/10, 2018, http://www.census.gov/eos/www/naics/.

———. "North American Product Classification System (NAPCS)." Accessed 04/10, 2018, http://www.census.gov/eos/www/napcs/index.html.

U.S. Congress. "Technology-Related Assistance for Individuals with Disabilities of 1988. Public Law 105–394 (as Amended)." Accessed 04/08, 2018, http://www.gpo.gov/fdsys/pkg/STATUTE-102/pdf/STATUTE-102-Pg1044.pdf.

World Health Organization. "GATE Project." Accessed 04/08, 2018, http://www.who.int/phi/implementation/assistive_technology/en/.

Chapter 10 Understanding the end user

Jennifer Boger, Tony Gentry,
Suzanne Martin, and
Johnny Kelley

Contents

10.1 Chapter overview

Think about the technologies you reach for every day. Why do you choose to use them? What makes them useful? A straightforward answer to these fundamental questions is that we engage with the technologies that enable access to meaningful tasks that would be difficult or impossible to accomplish without them. Regardless of a person's abilities, interventions of any kind must complement the needs, preferences, and abilities of the people they are intended for if they are to be usable and useful. While the terms "usable" and "useful" are not always teased apart, there is a distinct difference. A person may find it easy to use a technology but that does not mean it enables them to achieve a meaningful goal; it is usable but not useful. Conversely, a technology may be intended to support a desired

DOI: 10.1201/b21964-12

goal, but if it does not mesh with a person's abilities or context, the technology may not provide the necessary support and may be abandoned. How can rehabilitation engineers ensure technologies and systems fit the needs and contexts of the people using them? This chapter explores ways of connecting with, understanding, and incorporating the perspectives, abilities, and needs of the people the technology is intended to support – the end users – so that they may be embedded into the design of the technology itself, resulting in solutions that will improve the lives of the people who use them.

10.2 Introduction

An assistive technology (AT) "solution" that fails to meet the needs of the person it was intended for will be abandoned or not even adopted in the first place. Studies have shown AT abandonment rates ranging from 15–65% (Steel, Steel, and Gray 2009, 129–136), leading to investigations examining the causes of this problem. A study of AT users in Colorado, USA, by Riemer-Reiss and Wacker (2000) found that end user (consumer) involvement was the primary factor determining adoption or discontinuance of an AT solution. The authors concluded that "assessment practices for assistive technology should concentrate on involving the consumer as extensively as possible in all aspects of decision-making" (p. 49). In a study of patients discharged from hospital with AT recommendations, Wielandt et al. (2006, 29–40) similarly found that consideration of patient needs and patient involvement in selecting AT were primary factors in AT adoption at home. Martin et al. (2011, 225–242) surveyed AT consumers and found that being informed about options, feeling that personal needs were considered, and being included in the decision-making process led to increased end user satisfaction and AT adoption. AT provision frameworks such as the human activity assistive technology (HAAT) (discussed in Chapter 2) and matching person and technology models (discussed in Chapter 4) emphasize end user participation in all stages of the assessment and implementation process to assure successful outcomes.

As the evidence shows, including the user throughout the process is key to assuring applicability, usability, and technology adoption. Without this first-hand perspective, technology developers can fall into the trap of "thinking we know better" or of failing to anticipate the context of use, both of which result in technologies that reflect what we imagine people want or are able to do rather than what they actually want or can do. Moreover, while there may be a single "primary" end user of a device or system, almost always there are "secondary" users who may also interact with or support the use of the technology, such as carers and service providers. The consideration of user types becomes more complex with contemporary AT as separate devices are integrated onto single platforms to become integrated at a systems level and there may be multiple (sometimes simultaneous) users, systems, and services accessing the technology.

Whether considering technology design at a micro (i.e., individual) or macro (i.e., generalized population) level, the technology needs to fit into a person's specific context for it to be accessible and sustainable. This requires consideration of a multitude of contextual domains (e.g., lived environment, socioeconomic factors, culture, and related policies/services). It is crucial that the AT team complements the goals, scope, and stage of the development process to ensure a good fit with intended users. This team is usually from one or more disciplines and sectors that may include engineers, clinicians, occupational therapists, and service providers. This chapter argues that the end user and his or her needs must be the focal point of the entire design process; we need to engage in **user-centered design**. The key to this approach is to effectively engage the end user as a member of the design process for its entirety – from conceptualization to implementation. The rest of the chapter provides an overview of techniques that have been developed as well as examples of their use in real-world situations.

10.2.1 The evolution of user-centered models of technology design

Everett Rogers's *Diffusion of Innovations Theory* (Rogers 2003) articulates a stepwise process for adopting or rejecting new technologies that has been applied to assistive technology provision. The stages of the diffusion process include knowledge, persuasion, decision, implementation, and confirmation. In the initial **knowledge** phase, a person learns of an innovation and how it works. During the **persuasion** phase, that person explores the innovation and forms an appreciation of its benefits and drawbacks, deciding whether to adopt the innovation or reject it in the **decision** phase. The person puts the innovation to use in everyday life during the **implementation** phase and seeks agreement from others that this is a good solution to the identified functional problem during the final **confirmation** phase. At each step along the way, the person actively evaluates the usefulness of the innovation in everyday life. If the innovation successfully answers the questions inherent to each phase, then adoption is assured. The Diffusion of Innovations Theory implies that the end user is the final arbiter; all other members of an AT team serve only to support her/him in the stepwise process of adoption or rejection.

In line with this theory, the US Tech Act Amendments of 1994 articulate support for active end user and family participation in decisions about AT provision, including establishing goals and objectives, device assessment and selection, and preferences and evaluation in service delivery across all users of state-wide technology-related assistance programs. Over time, instructive frameworks have emerged to assure collaboration among all of the partners involved in AT provision, with the end user seen in all of these models as the central participant and final arbiter of an accommodation's success.

Over the past two decades, our understanding of disability has changed dramatically. We no longer think primarily of physical or other impairments, but rather of environmental factors and social situations that act as barriers to participation in everyday activities. The World Health Organization's Social Model of Disability (World Health Organization 2001) positions AT as a vast and evolving tool kit incorporating accessibility law, universal design, and the importance of personal agency in the use of devices and methods that promote function. At the same time, the worldwide Disability Rights Movement has sparked demands for end user-driven access, which puts the end user at the center of decisions about technology design and implementation.

In Europe, the Empowering End Users Through Assistive Technology (EUSTAT) project has developed guidelines for end user–designer interactions (Cook and Polgar 2014). In the US, the Technology-Related Assistance to Individuals with Disabilities (TRAID) project provides robust resources to support awareness and identification of appropriate AT solutions and a peer mentoring model for accessing and using such tools. The internet has become a "clearing house" of information about AT solutions, and social networking among consumers has opened a world of options to anyone with computer access.

Historically, the cost, tools, and expertise required to create and develop AT limited this role to a relatively small group of people and places. The rapid rise of the **maker movement** (i.e., the ability for people to create products from computer-based devices) is fundamentally changing how AT is created. Using machines such as 3D printers and Arduinos, people are able to self-create complex devices with relatively low cost and ease. Often, people are able to forgo collaborations with experts and create the solutions they want for themselves. Not only can this be an empowering experience, but it provides a valuable opportunity for AT developers to gain knowledge regarding desired features and functionality directly from people with disabilities themselves. With this democratization of AT design and access, the field is progressively shifting toward more end user-driven solutions; the practitioner is increasingly becoming a facilitator and vendor rather than a "gatekeeper". Moreover, with the increasing connectivity and complexity of technology, we must recognize how the technologies we create can enable access to social, medical, and other systems. With this in mind, it is increasingly important that people in the field of rehabilitation engineering take the time and care to thoroughly understand the people they are working with and for – the end users of AT.

10.3 Methods for understanding the user

Including end users as partners in the design and development of technology enables them to guide the process and discourages the obsolete notion of designing for a "condition that needs to be fixed". Shifting epistemological views are increasingly challenging technology developers to delve deeper into how technology can be made to inherently support more complex ideas of selfhood. For example, Lazar, Edasis, and Piper (2017, 2175–2188) leverage the concept of **critical dementia** (i.e., the legitimacy of context, embodiment, sensorial experiences, and emotion as perceived by a person living with dementia) to explore how the creators of human–computer interfaces can complement four related concepts: meaning-making as contextualized (i.e., embracing existing abilities and interactions rather than externally-imposed ones), physical and embodied interaction as valued forms of knowing, the importance of multisensory experiences, and embracing emotion without rationalization. By doing so, Lazar et al. point out that "we no longer focus on what an individual can or cannot do; the focus shifts to what an individual actually **does**" (Lazar, Edasis, and Piper 2017, 2175–2188). Technology design powerfully influences perceptions; the technologies used by a person can profoundly impact his or her sense of self as well as how others perceive him or her. As such, technology developers are responsible for going beyond basic functionality and should consider how a technology can be made to positively support aspects that are crucial to a person's sense of self but can be difficult to characterize, such as citizenship, culture, and creativity.

User-centered design is often used to include the targeted end users in the development process. Based on ISO 9241-210, user-centered design is the inclusion of the person the technology is intended to support (or representatives of the target population) at every stage of the design and development process; this begins with user-identified problems through the creation and evaluation process to a finished product (International Standards Organization 2010). User-centered design advocates that all identified end users should be included at some level in the development team, thereby inherently guiding the process and driving design choices toward a useful and usable product. This is (ideally) an ongoing process to reflect any changes in the needs, abilities, and/or context of the AT end users; it is an iterative rather than a one-time effort, where the team members and the technology itself evolve over time.

Early end user-focused strategies looked only at the implementation and confirmation phases of the Diffusion of Innovations Theory, seeking to assess satisfaction with AT. Studies based on the Quebec User Evaluation of Satisfaction with Assistive Technology (QUEST) assessment (Demers, Weiss-Lambrou, and Ska 2002, 101–105) demonstrated the importance of items such as comfort, simplicity of use, safety, and availability of repair services for end users of AT such as wheelchairs (Vachon et al. 1999, 25–29) and smart homes (Andrich et al. 2006, 492–499).

More recent models have engaged the end user as a proactive participant in exploration and decision phases.

As described in Chapter 2, the HAAT model, for instance, is a widely used framework focused on supporting the activities a person seeks to perform within the everyday contexts where those tasks occur (Cook and Polgar 2014). To remind the reader, the HAAT model has four elements: (1) **activity**, which describes what the person is trying to achieve, such as a self-care, employment, or a leisure task, (2) **the person**, including descriptors regarding physical, cognitive, emotional, and sensory performance, as well level of expertise, roles, and meaning, (3) **context**, which encompasses location, social, cultural, financial/reimbursement resources, living arrangements, and so on, and (4) **technology**, which describes the AT itself, including how it interfaces with the person and his or her environment, the technology type, and its output. The model intentionally focuses on the activity first, then the person and their context, and lastly on the technology itself. Putting technology last underscores the importance of AT complementing the user and his or her needs rather than the other way around. The purpose of the HAAT model is to capture information that is required to execute effective product development, service delivery, and outcome evaluations. In practice, the model requires collaborative assessment and problem-solving among all partners, and ongoing follow-along to support everyday function as a person's needs and goals and the technologies available to support them evolve. Two key elements of the HAAT model – usability and usefulness – are easily confused. Under this model, it is not enough for an end user to demonstrate **usability** or the ability to operate an assistive technology; the end user must also find the device **useful** in performing everyday tasks in a manner that fits how (s)he prefers to engage in those tasks.

The comprehensive assistive technology (CAT) model (Hersh and Johnson 2008, 193–215) follows HAAT in appreciating the importance of end user-centered design focused on everyday tasks in real-world environments. CAT was developed by electrical engineers and differed from HAAT in a closer attention to each element of AT iteration with less emphasis on collaborative interaction among all partners. While models and frameworks such as those discussed above can be useful tools, they are just one aspect of the process; they should be augmented with other approaches to fit the particular person and context, with all their related (macro and micro) circumstances. What is most important is that the users of the technology or intervention are involved in its conception, development, testing, and implementation as they are the true experts of their own situation.

10.4 Connecting with the user

Whether working with individuals in a rehabilitation program or developing cutting-edge technologies as part of a research program or engaging in product

development in industry, rehabilitation engineers have a primary goal in mind –
to facilitate improved function for people with disabilities. The place to start in
this process is with the person. Key questions to ask include:

1) What is their medical condition, prognosis, physical, emotional, and
   cognitive state?
2) What are their needs, skills, and functional challenges in performing
   everyday tasks?
3) In what contexts and environments are these activities performed?
4) What do they want to do that they cannot do now?
5) What do people do for them that they would like to do on their own?
6) What tools have they tried previously to help and how have they failed
   them?
7) What are their own ideas about what constitutes a solution?
8) What financial resources do they have to fund an AT solution?

The answers to questions such as these will determine the focus of a rehabilitation engineer's work, allowing a truly client-centered and client-driven solution.
It is important to meet with the client herself and (if applicable) with her carers
to learn firsthand what she wants to do and what obstacles may lie in the way of
doing those things. If possible, observe not just what people say but what they
do. Getting people to demonstrate how they perform everyday activities with the
tools at their disposal can provide a deeper understanding of the problem space
and allow the rehabilitation engineer to draw out information about the situation
that may otherwise have been missed. Often a rehabilitation therapy team can
assist with this assessment, since occupational therapists, physical therapists, and
others may be keenly aware of the functional challenges their clients face.

With this information in hand, discussion can progress to explorations of current
and emerging technologies that the client may not know about, a comparison of
various technologies and adaptive strategies to support function, and a trial of a
chosen tool with close attention to the features of usability, usefulness, ease of use
and likeability. Often an off-the-shelf device, judged by these rules, will require
some customization for an individual (for instance, see the work done to perfect
a steering post to help Johnny Kelley drive his car, as discussed in Section 10.5.1:
Case Study 1). As the end user tries out the chosen tool in the context of her
everyday life, it is important to follow along, noticing any difficulty that may lead
the end user to reject the solution and making adjustments as needed, to ensure
adoption. At each stage, an attentive, collaborative, problem-solving approach is
essential, since the final proof of any AT intervention is whether the end user continues to use the tool to support improved everyday function or whether it ends up
gathering dust in a corner. This process may take lots of tweaking – patience and
good communication are central to success, as is demonstrated in the following
case studies.

10.5 Case studies

10.5.1 Case study 1: user-directed implementation of adapted controls for driving (written by Johnny Kelley)

I am a 38-year-old man with severe spastic cerebral palsy (CP). I use a motorized wheelchair that I have customized to fit my unique way of life. I also use augmentative communication software to convey my thoughts. As a proactive user of AT, over the years I have collaborated with occupational therapists (OT), speech therapists, DME vendors, rehabilitation engineers, and others to adapt the AT to my own needs. I have fashioned many of these devices myself (see my "AT in Action" Youtube Playlist: https://youtu.be/P55lYEPF474).

Two years ago, I set out on a mission that many thoughts were impossible for someone with my physical disability, learning to drive. Fortunately, the Virginia Department of Aging and Rehabilitation Services (DARS) sponsored my driving evaluation at Wilson Workforce Rehabilitation Center (WWRC). I was also fortunate to work with Mary, a resourceful OT with over 20 years of adaptive driving experience who recognized my intelligence, skill, and experience, and recognized that I should take the lead in designing my driving adaptations. Since Mary and her colleagues had never seen someone with my level of CP successfully drive, doubts were made known. I told her at the onset, "I've been the first to do many things. Help me be the first once again". In the end, her entire staff contributed to my success.

Mary evaluated my vision, reaction time, strength, and core stability before getting in a vehicle. We both recognized that my startle reflex might be a danger, as my arm might jerk the wheel, which could cause an accident. We worked together to figure out how to manage problems like that as we drove together on the grounds of WWRC. Like an athlete learning a new skill, I insisted on recording every driving session. To improve my performance, I analyzed the footage to improve my positioning, body mechanics, and coordination. I asked Mary to randomly scream as loud as she could to provoke my startle reflex. Over time, I learned how to maintain full control of the vehicle even when startled. Car horns, sirens, and other loud noises still affect me, but I maintain control.

As you may know, vendors can modify minivans with kits that include lowered floors, automated ramps, and wheelchair lockdown features that allow a motorized wheelchair to take the place of a driver's seat. The electronics package installed in most adapted vans allows a key fob to remotely operate the wheelchair ramp. But once at the driver's console, there were individualized challenges to surmount. For instance, because of limited mobility, I had to drive with one hand while operating a hand brake and accelerator with my other hand, so we needed to modify the steering wheel for one-handed operation. We installed a steering post that eliminates the need to grab and release the wheel while turning. That helped, but I wanted to further customize the post, replacing its foam padding with a spray-on truck bed liner that made it easier to let go when I needed to shift gears. Hours were spent sanding and polishing the adapted post to perfectly fit my needs. The liner material sparkles, so now the post looks cool, too! By far, that has to be my favorite piece of AT in my van.

Most hand controls are mechanically connected to the accelerator and brake pedals leading up to a lever that is positioned beside the steering wheel. Pulling and pushing that lever applies the accelerator and brake. However, I wanted more fine control over my brake. So I designed a little pulley between the brake pedal and the lever to increase the mechanical advantage and the gradient of braking I can apply. A mechanic at the adapted vehicle dealership did a wonderful job of implementing my design, allowing me to apply the brake more easily and smoothly.

With those adaptations in place, I could safely drive the van, but I couldn't safely release the hand controls to activate my lights, turn signals and wipers. I wondered if there might be a way to operate those secondary controls with a head switch. Working in AT in the school system had taught me about different types of button switches and mounts. Mary introduced me to button switch arrays that can control everything from the wipers to the radio. I knew that I wanted to keep this array as simple as possible to avoid distractions while driving, so I decided on three head-controlled tap switches, two to activate my turn signals and the other to activate my wipers. Mary and her team had not seen such an array before, but they mocked it up and it worked!

While I was at WWRC, I calculated that I practiced driving with Mary for around 80 hours in total. I was fortunate to find a wonderful pre-owned van with low mileage and some of the equipment I needed already installed. Technicians at the Mobility Supercenter completed customization. Within two months of practicing in my new van, to the amazement of my assessor, I aced my driver's license test. All of the equipment and all of my strategies worked perfectly. I've driven, as of this date, over 20,000 miles in 20 months. Many of those miles have been as an **Uber** driver. But I'm not done yet. It's not enough for me to simply prove driving is possible with my disability. My goal is to take driving to its ultimate expression – racing.

AT, when designed and implemented correctly, will always be unique to its user. For that to be possible, the user must participate in its implementation. However, in the ideal situation the user directs the creation of that AT, thereby ensuring a perfect fit that can provide liberating, life-changing opportunities.

10.5.2 Case study 2: involving end users in research to design and develop novel assistive technologies for home use

The case scenario above is from the very personal perspective of an individual with motivation and desire to gain a new skill. This case study focuses on a novel AT design for a vulnerable population – those with acquired brain injury (ABI) – to support everyday function at home. The goal of the Adaptive Multimodal Interfaces to Assist Disabled People in Daily Activities (AIDE) project* has been to work with individuals who have a neurological condition, and are currently stable, able to communicate, and live in the community following rehabilitation.

The AIDE consortium seeks to explore two questions: 1) how might we use everyday household smart technologies to support physical function and mobility, and 2) what tools might we integrate into a final comprehensive AIDE digital platform, as shown in Figure 10.1, that may compensate for physical impairment.

The opportunity in the marketplace was to develop a home-based platform that a mobility-impaired person can access (operate) using a range of technologies, for example a brain-computer interface (using electroencephalogram (EEG) signals), eye tracking, or electromyography (EMG). Based on personalized requirements

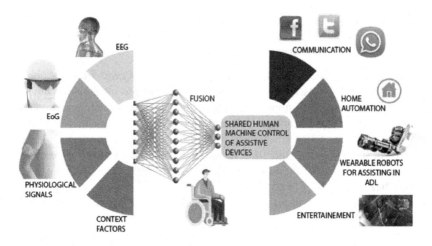

Figure 10.1 System design for the AIDE platform (European Union's Horizon 2020 Research and Innovation Programme, 2015).

* Funded by the European Union's Horizon 2020 Research and Innovation Programme under Grant Agreement No. 645322

the person was encouraged to use any one of these technologies or a combination. Within the platform, a range of software enables the person to engage with an environmental control system that enables access to social media applications, such as **Facebook** and **Twitter**, along with the ability to control smart home lights and appliances or even a robotic arm or exoskeleton.

In designing this platform, we first sought to identify and describe end users who might be interested in using it. As the AIDE project targets people with ABI, who may have both physical and cognitive challenges, there were trade-offs to be made regarding ethical governance, merit of the engagement, and timelines for the research, all of which influenced the reflections and refinement of the end users who engaged directly in the project. In addition, there was an awareness of the need to engage with informal and formal carers, therapists, and non-government organizations representing the views of those with ABI.

Following the user-centered design process discussed earlier in this chapter, we set out first to gather end user requirements. This conversation needed a structure and focus to be meaningful for the researcher and the individual(s) giving their precious time. Preliminary work involves developing use case scenarios to help explain the utility of the AIDE platform alongside videos and mock-ups to visually describe the technological ambition. The methodological tools to help gather information for AIDE are focus groups (8–10 people), face-to-face interviews, telephone interviews, surveys (online, hard copy, or telephone), storyboarding, and brainstorming sessions. By analyzing this rich body of data, the technology development team was able to focus on design requirements driven by the needs and wants of potential end users. A range of principles and characteristics provided our designers with the tools to approach design and development in a human-centered way. These include ISO 9241-210 (International Standards Organization 2010), Nielsen's usability heuristics (Nielsen 1994), and Principles of Human Computer Interaction (Shneiderman and others 2016). In technology development it is often necessary to embark on an iterative approach, with two or three prototype presentations and "check ins" with target end users. This is outlined in Figure 10.2.

Moving towards system integration and end user validation, it is prudent to have a series of lab-based tests with non-target users mapped against a clearly defined experimental protocol. This provides the opportunity to explore the system's reliability and robustness, confirming the time expectations for testing and teasing out any emerging issues that have not previously been foreseen.

An iterative approach therefore emerges at this second point of system integration and validation testing, with a focus on the three constructs of effectiveness, efficiency, and satisfaction, in line with ISO 9241-210. Experience has shown that working closely with end users supports truly user-centered design, however this is not by any means a simple or trivial undertaking. The challenges can be

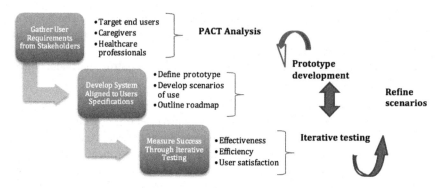

Figure 10.2 Systematic user-centered design approach.

the logistics of finding a convenient time for the end user and arranging suitable transport and practical assistance. While the challenges may be significant, particularly with large and complex projects, the payoff is a collaborative exchange of knowledge and skill between the engineer, researcher, occupational therapist, and end user, with all benefiting from the connection and engagement.

10.6 Ethical considerations

In Chapter 8 an in-depth exploration of ethical considerations in relation to AT is provided. It would be remiss of us, however, not to highlight the necessity for an ethical approach to meaningful engagement with end users. Within developed countries ethical governance is fairly well established and aligned to traditional empirical research. The type of work outlined in this chapter explores the engagement of end users well in advance of intervention-based studies. An ethical framework with associated protocols to support engagement with the end-user should be a routine gold standard approach as the people who need AT the most are often the most vulnerable in society. A clear and sensible approach within an ethical framework minimizes the risk of harm to the people you intend to support and indeed supports the researcher or provider as well.

10.7 Conclusions

Rehabilitation engineers are important struts for a team-based bridge that connects people to AT. As such, rehabilitation engineers recognize that a working knowledge of the field is not enough. One of the most powerful and useful skills of a proficient rehabilitation engineer is being able to engage with end users to understand their abilities, identify where support is missing, establish what goals they want to reach, and use this information to provide AT that is both usable and useful. This is not a cookie-cutter approach, as every person is different. How this process is executed will change on a case-by-case basis.

Understanding the end user can be a complex and challenging undertaking. The approaches presented in this chapter are by no means exhaustive. Rather, the chapter is intended as a starting point that orients the reader to the concepts of user-centered design and development and seeks to convey the importance of end user participation in design decisions. We should never forget that the end user is the ultimate expert when it comes to his or her own experience. When your work is done, the ultimate test of your collaborative effort will be whether that end user adopts or abandons the solution you agreed on. Including them at every step of the process goes a long way toward assuring adoption.

10.8 Future vision

It is an exciting time to be in the field of rehabilitation engineering! The increasingly rapid progress of technology, as well as social inclusivity, has, over the past few decades, profoundly and positively altered the work we do. It is likely that rehabilitation engineering will continue to become more user-centric and transdisciplinary, as well as more complex. With the rise of global networks, artificial intelligence, and the internet of things, intangible "digital" solutions will become increasingly ubiquitous, connected, and autonomous. Collaborative teaming, which includes end users, as well as the providers and systems that will support ongoing use, will be increasingly emphasized in the growing age of customized technology. At the same time, technology is enabling increasing end user engagement not only in the process, but as the expert who is driving the process. In a growing age of do-it-yourself AT creation, the users themselves are creating their own solutions. With users playing a more active role in creating solutions for their challenges, rehabilitation engineers may often become creation partners or "guides", rather than providers, helping the end user understand and connect with requisite best practices and resources. It is the responsibility of rehabilitation engineers and their partners in the rehabilitation therapy field to ensure that the future of AT is shaped in partnership with the people it is intended to support – the users themselves.

10.9 Discussion questions

1. Where do I start my discussion with a client about possible solutions I may be able to offer?
2. How does end-user participation in AT decision making support adoption and use?

3. What AT provision models support collaborative AT assessment and implementation? How do I choose which ones should be used?
4. What is the role of an occupational therapist and other professionals in rehabilitation engineering design?
5. How do you determine who should be involved in identifying, creating, and evaluating each AT solution?
6. How can I facilitate the sort of collaborative problem solving among clients and practitioners recommended in this chapter?

Bibliography

Andrich, Renzo, Valerio Gower, Antonio Caracciolo, Giovanni Del Zanna, and Marco Di Rienzo. 2006. *The Dat Project: A Smart Home Environment for People with Disabilities.* New York: Springer.

Cook, Albert M. and Janice Miller Polgar. 2014. *Assistive Technologies-E-Book: Principles and Practice.* Amsterdam: Elsevier Health Sciences.

Demers, Louise, Rhoda Weiss-Lambrou, and Bernadette Ska. 2002. "The Quebec User Evaluation of Satisfaction with Assistive Technology (QUEST 2.0): An Overview and Recent Progress." *Technology and Disability* 14 (3): 101–105.

Hersh, Marion A. and Michael A. Johnson. 2008. "On Modelling Assistive Technology Systems–Part I: Modelling Framework." *Technology and Disability* 20 (3): 193–215.

International Standards Organization. 2010. "Ergonomics of Human-System Interaction—Part 210: Human Centred Design for Interactive Systems, ISO 9241-210." Geneva: International Standards Organization.

Lazar, Amanda, Caroline Edasis, and Anne Marie Piper. 2017. "A Critical Lens on Dementia and Design in HCI." *Proceedings of the 2017 CHI Conference on Human Factors in Computing Systems.* May 2017, 2175–2188.

Martin, Jay K., Liam G. Martin, Norma J. Stumbo, and Joshua H. Morrill. 2011. "The Impact of Consumer Involvement on Satisfaction with and Use of Assistive Technology." *Disability and Rehabilitation: Assistive Technology* 6 (3): 225–242.

Nielsen, Jakob. 1994. *Usability Engineering.* New York: Elsevier.

Riemer-Reiss, Marti L. and Robbyn R. Wacker. 2000. "Factors Associated with Assistive Technology Discontinuance among Individuals with Disabilities." *Journal of Rehabilitation* 66 (3): 44–51.

Rogers, Everett M. 2003. *Diffusion of Innovations/Everett M. Rogers.* New York: Simon and Schuster, 576.

Shneiderman, Ben, Catherine Plaisant, Maxine Cohen, Steven Jacobs, Niklas Elmqvist, and Nicholas Diakopoulos. 2016. *Designing the User Interface: Strategies for Effective Human-Computer Interaction.* London: Pearson.

Steel, Dianne M., Dianne M. Steel, and Marion A. Gray. 2009. "Baby Boomers' Use and Perception of Recommended Assistive Technology: A Systematic Review." *Disability and Rehabilitation: Assistive Technology* 4 (3): 129–136.

Vachon, Brigitte, Rhoda Weiss-Lambrou, Michele Lacoste, and Jean Dansereau. 1999. "Elderly Nursing Home Residents' Satisfaction with Manual and Powered Wheelchairs."

Wielandt, Trish, Kryss McKenna, Leigh Tooth, and Jenny Strong. 2006. "Factors that Predict the Post-Discharge Use of Recommended Assistive Technology (AT)." *Disability and Rehabilitation: Assistive Technology* 1 (1–2): 29–40.

World Health Organization. 2001. *International Classification of Functioning, Disability and Health: ICF.* Geneva: World Health Organization.

Chapter 11 Rehabilitation engineering in less resourced settings

Jamie H. Noon,
Stefan Constantinescu,
Matthew McCambridge,
and Jon Pearlman

Contents

DOI: 10.1201/b21964-13

11.1 Chapter overview

An estimated 15–20% of the world's population – more than one billion people – live with some form of disability according to the World Report on Disability, published by the World Health Organization (WHO) in 2011 (WHO 2012). People with disabilities constitute the world's largest minority. It is also estimated that 80% of persons with disabilities live in less resourced settings (LRS) (United Nations 2006).

The WHO estimates that more than 70 million people need a wheelchair and only 5–15% have access to one (WHO 2010). The importance of mobility is reflected in the United Nations Convention on the Rights of Persons with Disabilities (CRPD) (United Nations 2006), which states that "effective measures to ensure personal mobility with the greatest possible independence for persons with disabilities".

This chapter will explore some of the ways in which rehabilitation engineering (RE) has been applied to address the needs of persons with disabilities (PWD) in LRS as well as the challenges and opportunities seen in these environments. Examples will be given with lessons learned from the perspective of organizations and individuals that have been engaged in provision of assistive technology (AT) for PWD living in LRS. In addition, this chapter will focus on how RE in LRS differs from RE in more resourced settings (MRS).

Mobility aids (i.e., prosthetics and wheelchairs) have comprised a major portion of efforts toward development and provision of AT in LRS. The many examples and lessons that focus on wheelchairs will be applicable toward other AT.

11.2 History

Since the mid-1900s AT has grown with major contributions from a relatively small group of international non-governmental organizations (INGOs) working toward provision of wheelchairs and prosthetics and orthotics (P&O). Contributing professionals included prosthetists and orthotists, P&O technicians, orthopedic surgeons, rehabilitation doctors, physiotherapists, occupational therapists, orthopedic shoemakers, nurses and biomechanical/rehabilitation engineers, and product designers. PWD have always played an integral part in program design as well as product design, testing, production, and provision of assistive devices. In 2008 WHO released *Guidelines on the Provision of Manual Wheelchairs in Less Resourced Settings* (WHO 2008). In the decade following release of the wheelchair guidelines, WHO wheelchair service training packages (WSTP) were developed and have seen worldwide use (WHO 2012). Parts of these training packages have been adopted in academic settings in North America and Europe.

The International Society of Wheelchair Professionals (ISWP) was launched in February 2015 in order to serve as a global resource for wheelchair service standards and provision through advocacy, education, standards, evidence-based practice, innovation, and a platform for information exchange. Based on global data, the ISWP estimates that 23 million wheelchairs (both manual and powered) are needed annually. Currently, about three million wheelchairs are produced each year, resulting in a 20 million per year deficit. The ISWP helps to professionalize wheelchair services and improve wheelchair quality around the world.

11.3 Context

While RE activities in LRS have obvious limitations compared to working with more resources, it is often the limitations and constraints that lead to the most innovative solutions. Many of these solutions, easily transfer to MRS.

> Working in a developing country is often more like working as a gourmet chef than a fast food cook. You may need to be involved in every preparatory step until the final product is ready to meet the individual needs, preferences and expectations of your customer.

(Borg 2018)

> Being a wheelchair user and also a wheelchair Technologist and Provider I've learned to understand better the importance of involving users in the process of providing rehabilitation services, especially in less resourced settings. Sometimes it is very challenging working in this context due to limitations in materials, tools, and technology. However, you will always have an opportunity to get new ideas from the users or family members because of the deep experience that they have. You cannot separate the user involvement in the rehabilitation engineering process. It is essential to clearly identify the needs and opinions of the user, in their own words, in order to have the best results.

(Munish 2018)

As discussed in previous chapters, disability is an interaction between a person's physical impairment and the physical and social environment in which that person lives. While humans globally are much more similar than we are different, there remain differences both in the physical impairments (prevalence of different types of diagnoses such as polio), anthropometric measurements of the population, and, most significantly, the physical and social environments. Therefore, development of AT should draw on successful AT experience in MRS but cannot assume that a technology successful in MRS will be successful in LRS, or that some other solution, not typically used in MRS, may be appropriate. For example, hand cycles that are used typically as recreational products in MRS may be more appropriate than wheelchairs as a primary mobility device in LRS where individual car use is less common and sitting on the floor in the home is more culturally appropriate (hand cycles are generally not used indoors). Knowledge of the specific local culture (not LRS in general) is essential. At an absolute bare minimum, people with disabilities from LRS should be involved in the design process. However, due to challenges in communication within cross-cultural teams, mere "involvement" (interviews, meeting attendance, etc.) may not guarantee that the team fully heeds local user expertise. Thus, ideally people with disabilities from LRS should occupy positions of real authority within governments and nongovernment organizations (NGOs) and should have the opportunity to exercise leadership or at least formal sign-off/veto power during the process of creating AT for LRS.

When working in LRS that do not have established healthcare systems we are in a position to help initiate efficient practices from the beginning. In some situations, the outcomes can be more effective because of the lack of existing systems. Starting from scratch can sometimes be easier than adapting or eliminating systems that are inefficient. Similarly, the development and uptake of new technologies can take place with more speed and wide support where existing technologies are not established.

This practice of giving "hand-me-down" technology has proven to have damaging effects on existing local efforts as well as preventing development of more appropriate sustainable solutions. Whether it's handing down used devices or transplanting technology and services that have evolved for use in MRS the results are often that of the ubiquitous pile of rusting wheelchairs seen behind hospitals, schools, and rehab centers in LRS.

11.4 Availability of materials in LRS

A common challenge when developing AT in LRS is availability and suitability of materials and technologies which will vary enormously throughout the world and among different regions within a country. Local investigation into available tools and materials can be facilitated by partnership with local counterparts with skills and experience in building. We will explore in depth a few of the more commonly used materials for designing and producing AT in LRS and some challenges encountered.

11.4.1 Wood

Plywood is often available but can be poor quality and cost prohibitive for local production of AT. The dimensional stability of plywood and ease of working may be useful when making custom solutions and simple jigs and tools for consistent production. Figure 11.1 shows an example of an adjustable foam cutting jig used for small scale but consistent production of pressure relief wheelchair cushions.

"The AT's suitability to a given context depends on the culture, traditional craftsmanship and availability of raw materials which are all interwoven. The wooden, Motivation developed Mekong wheelchair in Cambodia is a prime example for this" (Pakirisamy 2018).

The "Mekong" wheelchair shown in Figure 11.2 below was developed and produced in the 1990s in Cambodia by Motivation Charitable Trust. The frame was made primarily of mahogany to avoid dependence on an expensive and inconsistent supply of steel tubing and is still produced and distributed in Cambodia as of 2018.

11.4.2 Metals

Different metals (e.g., steel, stainless steel, aluminum) offer different advantages in terms of performance, local manufacturability, and field repairability. Steel bars and shapes, as well as tubing made of thin steel formed into round or square profiles in a variety of sizes, are a common building material globally, used for doorways, window frames, roof trusses, etc. Thus, the materials, tools, and skills to form and weld steel are very common throughout the world, and the additional capacity to weld thin steel tubing is available through the most skilled subset of local builders. Materials and equipment suitable for fabricating devices from steel tubing such as wheelchairs and hand cycles can be sourced in most small cities, and devices made of steel tubing can potentially be repaired even in very small towns. That said, experience suggests that the quality of repair may vary considerably as the repair requires not just welding skill but creativity, experience, and judgment regarding reinforcement of the failed structure. Making

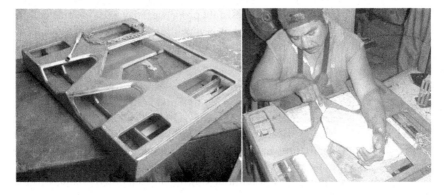

Figure 11.1 Adjustable foam cutting jig (courtesy of Jon Pearlman, 2018).

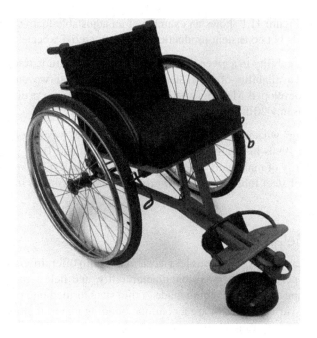

Figure 11.2 Mekong wheelchair (courtesy of Jon Pearlman, 2018).

devices from thin steel tubing that are used in the presence of moisture (rain, bathing water) and specifically salt water (ocean spray, sweat, urine) demands meticulous attention to painting by the manufacturer and maintenance by the user. Thin steel that has been structurally damaged by rust can be very challenging to repair.

Stainless steel and aluminum greatly reduce but do not entirely eliminate the corrosion challenges associated with steel. Capacity to weld stainless steel while preserving its structural and corrosion-resistant properties may exist in some coastal areas with a strong marine industry but is much less common than capacity to work with mild steel. Capacity to weld aluminum appears to be extremely scarce in LRS.

The "Roughrider" wheelchair shown in Figure 11.3 was developed and produced, beginning in the early 2000s, in small workshops throughout Southeast Asia, Central America, and Southern Africa with assistance from Whirlwind Wheelchair. The frame is made of low-cost mild steel tubing formed by hand over simple bending fixtures and welded using simple jigs to maintain alignment. It is still produced, as of 2018, in larger factories using more sophisticated production equipment but without significant functional changes to the design.

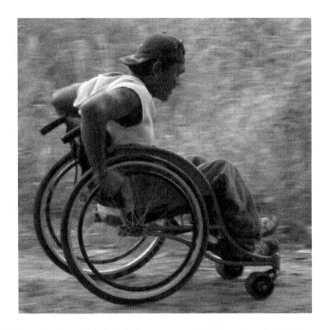

Figure 11.3 Roughrider wheelchair (courtesy of Jon Pearlman, 2018).

11.4.3 Rubber

Heat-vulcanized rubber and production equipment is common in many cities in LRS. Components such as specialized caster wheels, as seen in Figures 11.2 and 11.3, and crutch tips have been designed, tooling ordered, and production initiated at local, small- to medium-scale rubber parts factories without great investment cost. Quality control and spot check monitoring of rubber parts quality is important as the mix of rubber versus filler can be easily changed after the initial sample part is approved.

11.4.4 Foams and fabrics

Foams and fabrics are used in the manufacture of furniture, transportation seating, bedding, clothing, shoes, packaging, sports equipment, and luggage and thus many types may be available via supply chains established by local industry. Common examples of foams include polyurethane (PU) foams, latex rubber foams, expanded polyethylene (EPE), and vinyl foams (PVA/EVA). Foams vary in terms of their stiffness, durability, ability to return to their original shape once compressed over time, breathability, resistance to damage from temperature and moisture, resistance to contamination by microorganisms, weight, and cost. For good quality foam for cushions, it is best to get the heaviest foam you can find.

The more it weighs, the better it will perform and the longer it will last. Available fabrics may include woven or knitted synthetic and natural fibers as well as leathers and plastic sheets. Fabrics vary by their strength, flexibility, breathability, resistance to damage from temperature, moisture, and abrasion, resistance to contamination by microorganisms, weight, and cost. Designers using these foams and fabrics must note that the demands of the wheelchair application of these materials may not be identical to the demands of the industry application for which they were manufactured. For example, tolerance for sweat and urine, or performance over long-duration use, may be especially important in a wheelchair application. Furthermore, the designer must identify whether the material is in a safety critical role. Sometimes foam and fabric are used to increase comfort, and other times to preserve life, for example as part of a strategy to prevent pressure sores. The rigor with which these materials are selected and tested must match the consequences for poor product performance.

11.4.5 Plastics

In developing countries, polypropylene thermoplastics are commonly used in prosthetic and orthotic applications; they offer great advantages over other materials because they are cheaper, lighter, and easier to transport and store. Prosthetic sockets are fabricated by vacuum forming a heated thermoplastic sheet over the positive model of the residual limb.

Because they are recyclable and durable, thermoplastics were recommended by ISPO as the material of choice for prostheses in low-income countries (Pearlman et al. 2008, 12–22). Consequently, the International Committee of the Red Cross (ICRC) uses injection-molded polypropylene (a process of injecting molten plastic into a cavity mold) for almost all of its prosthetic component production.

Plastic parts offer potential advantages for wheelchair part fabrication due to their light weight (when used in low-load applications), low cost when manufactured in high quantity, and unmatched resistance to moisture. The strength of plastic parts varies widely and may not be intuitively obvious. Subtle variations in the ingredients used to form the plastic have enormous effects on durability, which may vary with temperature and exposure to sunlight in ways that are unexpected by craftsmen used to working with wood and metal. Different types of plastics fail in different ways, some (such as LDPE) bending or stretching rather than breaking into pieces, others (such as PVC pipe) shattering and leaving sharp edges. Designers are responsible for selecting plastics with qualities appropriate for their individual application and verifying that those qualities are consistently maintained.

The ability to locally repair plastic parts varies widely. In Vietnam, where motorcycles with plastic fenders are ubiquitous and suffer frequent minor damage, skillful repair of damaged fenders and thus other plastic parts are readily available. Similarly, in the Philippines, where plastic tanks are used in agriculture, rapid watertight repair is similarly available. In other places broken plastic objects are discarded.

11.5 Availability of tools in LRS

11.5.1 Hand tools

The availability of hand tools for fabrication and maintenance and the skills to use them varies widely across the globe, and locally with respect to local industries and proximity to cities. In some circumstances local craftspeople can achieve astonishing results with simple tools, creating custom-fabricated solutions much more quickly and cheaply than would be possible in a commercial context in a wealthy community. The availability of tools to turn fasteners (bolts and nuts) will depend on the ubiquity of cars, trucks, motorcycles, bicycles, and agricultural equipment. Anecdotally, bolts in imperial sizes (i.e., measured in inches) and Allen bolts (bolts with hexagonal holes into which Allen keys, also known as hex keys, are inserted) present a challenge to mechanics in LRS who are most accustomed to hex-head fasteners (fasteners with a hexagonal head which can be gripped on its outer surface by a wrench) and specifically hex-head fasteners in metric sizes.

11.5.2 Power tools

Manufacturing machinery in LRS varies enormously in the availability and sophistication of manufacturing machinery and the associated skilled labor to operate it. As the manufacturing of products for wealthy markets may occur in LRS, the local availability of manufacturing capacity may be extremely high, and vendors may offer advanced services at very low cost, especially if orders can be consolidated into high-volume purchase. In other LRS, where there is little local industry and most products are imported, it may be challenging to find anything other than hand tools or basic power tools.

11.6 Product development for LRS

New technologies, products, or processes in or for LRS often come to life very quickly. For this reason, it is incumbent upon the developer to employ a responsible pacing and design cycle which includes stakeholder involvement throughout, prioritizing user-identified needs, as well as careful trials, testing, and improvement before production and final market.

Design of AT should always consider the systems within which it will be provided, used and sustained. The best designed device could become redundant due to complex training on its use, lack of spare parts or skills to repair, or ineffectual systems to ensure provision, adjustment and maintenance. Be as creative with design of systems and training as with the actual technology. Keep it simple and intuitive – complex items will often be discarded, feared or even simplified on the ground.

(Seymour 2018)

Based on decades of experience developing and producing new AT in LRS, the list below shows a recommended sequence of activities for effective local product development:

1. Identify a local partner
2. Location research or questionnaire to the local partner to identify:
   - Availability, method of purchase, pricing, and user preferences regarding existing products
   - Availability of parts, materials, and manufacturing processes, including prices
   - Level of clinical services currently offered along with existing products and training needs
   - Obtain anthropometric data from local population (combine with existing larger databases if large local sample is not possible)
3. Analyze collected data and start design concept development, involving end users
4. Evaluate design concept and adapt it according to the reality on the ground to allow for use of local materials, local reparability, use of locally available spare parts
5. Additional cycles of evaluation and concept development as needed
6. Develop first working prototype (may not use only locally available materials/methods)
7. Iterative cycles of prototype development as needed within local context including:
   - Use of local materials and production methods
   - User feedback, with repeated quick trial for each set of changes
   - Involvement of distribution networks in trials and feedback
   - Small production for multiple extended user trials
   - Evaluate product (redesign, prototype, and trial if needed)
   - Design finalization
8. Medium production for final extended user trial (replace prototypes from first trial)
9. Finalize distribution methods and networks including availability of spare parts

When we serve in contexts where the available products could not meet the needs of the user population, we might intend to convince ourselves and the clients

(clients-service providers and the service users combined) that the products are supposed to meet the spectrum of 'usual' population. Such false justification gainsays our own philosophy of adapting the products according to the user needs. One fine example of such scenario is the wheelchair users in South Sudan where the users could be falling totally out of the size range that the existing products could cover (In SSUD, the civilian, as well as the armed personnel, mark one of the tallest league of world population. The statistics of wheelchair service provision shows that most of the products are customized to accommodate length related issues).

(Pakirisamy 2018)

Product durability warrants special consideration in LRS due to challenges posed by terrain and usage, the unpredictable nature of distribution (for example sporadic donation by INGOs), and challenges associated with maintenance. In the case of mobility devices, users may be traveling over rougher terrain and covering more distance (in the absence of motorized transport). Products may be essential to perform physical labor such as farming or manual construction, subjecting the devices to more-than-average outdoor environmental conditions (moisture and dust). Meanwhile, there may not be a set interval at which the device will be replaced. For example, in the case of international donations, it may be impossible to predict the content and timing of the next donation. Maintenance is a particularly important aspect of AT provision, prolonging the life of the product by preventively or reactively fixing individual parts rather than replacing the whole device. Furthermore, if the product has unique parts, a supply chain must be established and maintained that reaches each and every end user. If the product is meant to be maintained using commonly available local parts and locally common technical skills (e.g., needle and thread, bicycle tires, motorcycle bearings), then the fact that the product can be maintained and how to do it must be communicated clearly to users and providers. Finally, the economic condition of the expected users must be understood to predict what maintenance activities are possible and reasonable even if parts are in fact locally available. The provision of spares and/or repair service is a particularly important but often overlooked aspect of AT product development.

In past years the goal of AT programs in LRS was to design and build AT that could be entirely built and repaired locally. Trends have shifted toward designing for central/mass production with local reparability in mind. There is no one design that fits all environments, target user group, service provider level of skill, target price, and method of service provision. In small local production it is easier to adapt the design in order to use locally available materials and parts as much as possible. However, in mass production in a central location it is very difficult to design products that are locally repairable in all locations worldwide. The design must be more universal in order to be able to cover as many potential beneficiaries as possible. Also, a range of products and sizes rather than one product design will allow buyers and users to have access to a product that meets most of their needs and the freedom to mix and match.

It is often far too easy to overlook the issue of spare parts until after the development cycle is almost complete. Suppliers must make sure that spare parts are made available to local buyers through the distribution channels. Local service providers must make sure that trained technicians are available to attend to maintenance and repair work. Local service providers must train users and their families in product maintenance, prolonging the useful life of the product.

11.7 Product testing in LRS

Evaluating the performance of AT through standardized testing methods is important during the design process, as well as once a device is in production. During the design process, iterative testing is essential to determine whether the device meets the design specifications, is appropriate for the intended environment(s), and performs desirably for the user and other stakeholders involved in the production, supply, and delivery of the device. Once a device is in production, standardized testing is important to ensure the device is compliant with national regulations, and to determine whether manufacturing quality has changed over time.

In the section below we provide an overview of the types of testing available and best practices on how to apply them. We describe them in two subcategories:

Qualifying tests are commonly used to qualify a product for sale in a certain country. Qualifying tests are often prescribed by national or international bodies as a prerequisite before the product can be provided. Examples include the Food and Drug Administration (FDA) which requires qualifying tests in the United States of America. In the context of LRS, the WHO *Guidelines on the Provision of Manual Wheelchairs in Less Resourced Settings* indicates that ISO 7176 should be considered a minimum standard for wheelchairs being provided, and national standards should be applied if they exist.

Research and development (R&D) tests are used to elicit failures and performance issues in prototype designs so that the design can be improved prior to production. The goal of these tests is to try to subject a prototype to worst-case scenarios to highlight weak links within the design. These tests include user evaluation and will solicit feedback from users about the design, and support verification and modification of the design prior to production.

11.7.1 Testing principles

There are several testing principles that are important to keep in mind when designing and performing testing. These best practices are to help ensure the test results accurately reflect the performance of the wheelchair, and that they are defensible. These principles apply in cases for LRS and MRS. The differences between these settings have to do with contextual factors, such as what would be defined as worst-case scenarios and differences in environmental factors.

Worst-case scenarios: It is important to know the conditions that are related to the worst-case scenario when designing and carrying out tests. For instance, for the safety of the users, tests are often performed to determine whether a wheelchair will fail catastrophically when it is in use. Performing tests under conditions that are average (e.g., average user weight) would only predict whether the wheelchair will be safe for approximately half of the population of users; any user who weighs above average could be at risk. Instead, testing conditions should be set to reflect the worst-case scenario. Using the same example as above, the user weight condition should be selected to be the maximum weight of a user who may use a wheelchair. In conditions where the parameter is normally distributed, a maximum value is typically considered two standard deviations above the mean (mean + 2*SD).

Repeated trials: There is variability in all tests that are performed which leads to a variation in the testing results. The variability could be from many sources, some known and some unknown. For instance, the welds on a wheelchair frame may not be consistent which could lead to failures during load testing of one frame but not another. Testing methods are also sometimes difficult to reproduce, which can lead to different test results even with all other variables being fixed. To address this variability, it is important to perform multiple trials and investigate the average and standard deviation of the test result (or other applicable statistical test). A rule of thumb is that as the variability increases, so does the required number of repeated trials. Validation testing (e.g., ISO 7176) of wheelchairs is a common test and has limited variability due to the standardized test methods. It is critical to document all testing methods and results. This helps ensure that the test is defensible when questioned, and that it can be repeated by others if necessary. A general rule of thumb is that all tests must be documented with enough detail that the test can be replicated by someone else. In many cases, documentation such as test reports is required to satisfy regulatory requirements.

11.7.2 Qualifying tests

The goal of qualifying tests is to demonstrate performance of a device according to set standards. Table 11.1 provides some examples.

11.7.2.1 R&D tests Introduction: When a new wheelchair is designed, an existing design is modified, or new components are designed or modified it is important to perform tests prior to launching the product. Testing will help ensure the product is safe and durable for the user. Testing can also provide valuable

Table 11.1 Examples of Qualifying Standards for Wheelchairs Are Listed with a Description of How They Are Applicable

Name	Scope
ISO 7176	Covers testing for manual and powered wheelchairs and is used as reference for most national standards
Whirlwind ISO+	Low-cost approach to ISO 7176, with additional tests focused on conditions in LRE
ISO 16840	Tests for Wheelchair seating systems
WC 19	Wheelchair crash testing
ISWP Wheelchair Standards	Caster, rolling resistance, corrosion, and whole-wheelchair testing

feedback about design changes that may improve performance. There are several testing approaches, and we present them in the order in which we recommend they be performed.

All testing performed should be in compliance with local regulations and good practices. In many cases, this may require an ethics board review and approval prior to human subject testing. Specifically, hazards related to the testing of a particular technology are the responsibility of the testing agency to identify and communicate. Examples include the risk of pressure sores from sitting in any unfamiliar seat or posture support system, or the risks of falling while maneuvering any unfamiliar device. See Section 11.13 "Ethics" below.

Any safety concerns that are found at each of the stages of testing described below should be addressed, and then testing should be repeated at that stage to check if the design changes addressed the safety concerns.

In-lab qualifying test: A first step when evaluating a new design is to perform qualifying tests that are relevant to the strength and durability of the product. This is done prior to any user testing to ensure that there are no obvious failure modes or safety concerns with the product. The appropriate subset of qualifying tests listed above should be applied. For instance, a newly designed wheelchair would likely need to be tested to ISO 7176 Section 8 (static strength, impact, and fatigue) prior to user testing. If a new foot support has been designed, then only the subset of testing relevant to the foot support (e.g., static strength and impact) would need to be tested.

Controlled environment user testing: Once the new design has passed the relevant qualifying test, a user test can be performed in a controlled environment, such as indoors in a laboratory or office space, and outdoors in a specified space. A single-user test is often performed first, and if the product is safe and reliable, then multiple individuals may be invited to test the product to gather feedback from a range of potential users. These types of tests often require a test subject to perform a series of mobility tasks, while a data collector records real-time feedback while the test subjects are performing the tasks, and then a discussion occurs after the testing to gather more broad feedback.

11.8 Extended user trials

User trials take place when the design team believes the device is ready to use in the real world. After controlled-environment testing is complete and relevant modifications have been made to the design based on the feedback, it is recommended that a single user is provided with the device to perform community-based testing. Ideally a "lead user", who will benefit from new technology and places extreme demands on the device is the best individual to recruit for this stage of testing. This user would need to understand the risks of using a prototype product and would need to be open to providing detailed feedback on how to improve the product.

Multi-user community test: Once the design revisions have been made from the single-user test, a multi-user test is valuable to gather feedback from a diverse range of potential users. These trials can produce conflicting feedback, some of which the design team may act on. One of the key values of this trial, if performed correctly, is that it reflects the experience of the intended to be users.

After multi-user testing is completed and the feedback is positive about the product, it is typically ready to launch into the market. Best practice is to provide a channel for continuous feedback about the product from the clinical service providers and wheelchair users, so that quality and safety issues are identified immediately and can be addressed through design revisions.

It is useful to perform three repeated trials of each wheelchair to determine the test results. As variability increases, the number of repeated trials should increase. In-home trials with users is an example where there may be wide variability, and thus at least ten repeated trials may be necessary.

> When designing AT for low and middle income contexts thorough research and trials in the intended context is essential. There is a substantial amount of learning already out there and highly likely that the problem you wish to solve is not unusual and similar solutions have been tried before. This does not mean there is no scope for new innovations but does mean more time should be spent on researching and planning prior to the fun part of design to avoid falling into already known pitfalls. Extensive and thorough trial in the context and really being responsive to the user's voice is key. The impact and interaction of environmental and contextual factors cannot always be anticipated. If at all possible observe and gather feedback your self – receiving from others who have different experience, language, culture can affect results.

(Seymour, personal communication, 2018)

11.9 The user experience

I found Peer Training to be very useful to both new and experienced wheelchair users. This training provides knowledge and skills in life changing ways. Those who have been trained describe themselves as having higher self-esteem, confidence and independence. In this training they have opportunities to learn different subjects including; what it is to live with a disability; what is an appropriate wheelchair; bladder and bowel management; sports and wheelchair skills. If you look at all these subjects, you will agree that, in order for a user to be more active and participate in any community activity, they need to have the kind of confidence and self-esteem that can only be found in Peer Training.

(Munish, personal communication, 2018)

The wheelchair user and his or her caregivers should be assessed with respect to their abilities to use the wheelchair in their everyday lives. If they do not have the capacity and confidence they need to perform these skills, they should be provided training. The Wheelchair Skills Program is a free, evidence-based, safe and effective set of protocols for the assessment and training of wheelchair skills (Kirby et al. 2019). Because the Wheelchair Skills Program is low-tech and high-impact, it is suitable for use in less- and more-resourced settings. To date, the Wheelchair Skills Program website (www .wheelchairskillsprogram.ca) has been used by over 75,000 users from 178 countries.

(Kirby 2018)

In the provision of assistive technology, the user should have choices to determine what is right and suitable for his or her needs. A professional should respect and consider the opinions of the user when developing or selecting technology. This good relationship will be essential in other stages of the process such as user training and follow up.

(Munish, personal communication, 2018)

11.10 Organizations engaged in LRS

NGOs bring many skills and resources to LRS, often with financial support from large donors. Contributions range from education and training, clinical services, product sales, local product development, to research. Table 11.2 lists organizations currently active in the area of AT provision in LRS and indicates the AT areas in which they have been primarily engaged.

11.11 Sustainability

When endeavoring to introduce improved O&P services anywhere, I'm in favor of first exploring and learning about existing in-country O&P service programs and providers whether private enterprises, NGOs or, especially, any government funded entities. If you just come in and start something new, local entities may be undercut and destroyed. It is far better to find what, if any, service providers are worthy of support and go from there.

(Carlson, personal communication, 2018)

Table 11.2 Organizations Currently Active in the Area of AT Provision

Organization	Link	Prosthetics & Orthotics	Wheelchairs	Seating & Positioning	Design & Production	AT Provision Training	Rehabilitation Training	Guidelines & Certification	Publication	Donor	NGO	Enterprise
CE Mobility	http://www.cemobility.co.za		X		X							X
DDO	http://diversable.org		X	X	X						X	
FWM	https://www.freewheelchairmission.org		X		X						X	
GTZ (now GIZ)	http://www.giz.de	X								X		
Hesperian Foundation	http://hesperian.org	X	X			X			X			
HI	https://hi.org/en/index	X	X	X	X	X	X		X			
Hope Haven	https://www.hopehaven.org		X	X	X	X					X	
ICRC	https://www.icrc.org	X	X	X		X	X				X	
ISPO	http://www.ispoint.org	X	X	X		X		X	X		X	
ISWP	http://www.wheelchairnet.org		X	X		X		X	X		X	
LDSC	https://www.ldscharities.org		X	X	X	X				X	X	
MCT	https://www.motivation.org.uk	X	X	X	X	X	X				X	
Ottobock	https://www.ottobock.com/en	X		X	X							X
ROC Wheels	http://www.rocwheels.org		X								X	

(Continued)

251

Table 11.2 (Continued) Organizations Currently Active in the Area of AT Provision

Organization	Link	Prosthetics & Orthotics	Wheelchairs	Seating & Positioning	Design & Production	AT Provision Training	Rehabilitation Training	Guidelines & Certification	Publication	Donor	NGO	Enterprise
Shonaquip	https://shonaquip.co.za		×	×	×	×						×
UCP/WFH	http://ucpwheels.org		×	×	×	×					×	
USAID	https://www.usaid.gov							×		×		
WFK	https://wheelchairsforkids.org		×	×	×						×	
WF	https://www.wheelchairfoundation.org		×		×			×			×	
WHO GATE	http://www.who.int/phi/implementation/assistive_technology/phi_gate/en	×	×	×		×	×	×	×		×	
WWI	https://whirlwindwheelchair.org		×		×						×	

Respect and support for existing local products and service is key when offering input. Donor funding constraints and international NGO models of operation can make it difficult to take advantage of local strengths. It is common for well-meaning programs to replace or eclipse smaller local efforts. Local NGOs often find themselves either competing with visiting NGOs or flexing their core principles in order to collaborate and benefit from the larger budget for the project period. Chasing the changing objectives of visiting organizations can leave local NGOs struggling to stay true to their mission and vision.

Developing a national tender (or procurement policy) is a very delicate undertaking that requires constant updating. A good national tender is one that does not stop at procuring products that users are historically familiar with but requires improvements to existing products based on feedback from users and providers. A fair and informed tender committee can establish pricing that is realistic and does not drive manufacturers to cut features and quality.

> Working in a developing country is basically like working anywhere else: Use resources that are sustainably available. If they are not, do not use them or else make them sustainably available.
>
> **(Borg, personal communication, 2018)**

11.12 Working in LRS

Humility, mutual respect, and cultural understanding are easy concepts to understand when preparing to contribute in LRS. However, these are also the easiest principles to forget once the work begins. For input to be effective it is critical to bake these principles into a plan in concrete ways.

> Be humble and rid yourself of preconceptions. The way assistive products are designed, manufactured, prescribed and funded in your native context is likely not the only possible way, and not necessarily the best way. Do not let what you take for granted in one context limit the opportunities of what is possible in another context.
>
> **(Borg, personal communication, 2018)**

> It is ultimately pretty hard to show any true respect for the people if you don't spend some time learning about them, their practices and constraints. We need to learn from them as we teach so that there is a genuine mutual component to the process.
>
> **(Carlson, personal communication, 2018)**

> Understand the culture and how people works, understand things and how they interpret things to their existing environment. But the most important is listen, listen and be able to learn from different cultural context which will enable to grow

as an individual but also as professional as you will have wider ability to compare things/ products and how they work from one context to another.

(Munish, personal communication, 2018)

11.13 Ethics

Because there is a greater unmet need in LRS, the potential to help is greater. However, for the same reasons, potential to harm is also greater. The perception that there is "nothing" in place to serve the needs of people in LRS can tempt practitioners to set a very low bar for quality of the service delivered. If the notion that "better than nothing" drives the level of diligence in LRS, then the outcome can never reach its potential. A better notion might be, "how would I serve my family if they were in the situation of my clients?". The decision regarding how to allocate scarce resources should be made in close collaboration with local stakeholders who know the situation intimately and are accountable to the people who are impacted. When developing new AT products, keep in mind that product development does not typically require institutional review board approval, as with human subjects' research. At the same time, responsible innovators must follow safe and equitable practices when developing products with the help of AT users. It is recommended to implement many of the practices one uses when conducting human subjects research. General guidelines for the ethics of conducting research in the developing world can be found at https://d-lab.mit.edu/lean-research, while product improvement efforts typically do not fall under the formal definition of research, the ethical issues raised are worth considering in cooperation with local partner organizations.

In many LRS a flexible labor force exists which is often exploited for low-cost production. In MRS, laws are in place to protect the natural environment and the labor force from exploitation. These upstream issues should be considered as early as concept ideation. A good idea that endangers the environment and the people involved in its realization is actually a bad idea.

The "market" for AT products in LRS is approaching a time when investor capital may begin to replace donor funding when it comes to AT innovation and provision systems. Emerging economies will ideally follow most developed nations in the prioritization of AT in such a way that the commercial sale of products does not dictate service models and practices.

Often the service users are expect to pay for rehab services when the projects come to a point of stoppage of external funding. We all know poverty and disability contribute to each other in a vicious cycle. Rehab services should be made as a basic right just like access to primary healthcare or education. A person cannot be expected to pay for the products or services for the very reason that anyone can become disabled at any time in life.

(Pakirisamy 2018)

11.14 The future of RE and provision of AT in LRS

Development opportunities have often been based on donor funding and therefore limited by the ability of large donors to envision and lead the industry through a better future. NGOs tend to fit their goals to match those of specific large donor grants. At times, this makes it difficult to develop and follow a long-term organizational strategy. This is especially true for smaller, local NGOs that survive or perish based on successfully winning the next grant, regardless of what activities the grant requires. Global tools such as the WHO Community Based Rehabilitation Guidelines, WHO Wheelchair Guidelines, and related training packages are being used in many countries as a foundation for building their own system of services and product development. These new systems can take advantage of the donor funding that now exists. As higher-quality products become more available in larger quantities for LRS, designs and provision systems should strive for a blend of local and global solutions. This "two-way" approach is much harder to achieve but at the same time much more important to strive for. As always, the best results can be realized when more AT users are engaged at all levels and all stages of planning and implementation of AT programs and product development.

In a positive future, commercial AT product developers working in MRS will dedicate a portion of efforts toward a new kind of universal design (UD) which considers the needs of persons with and without disabilities but also the needs of those living in both MRS and LRS. With globalization we use more products, resources and services that originate in LRS. In this environment the only true UD is global universal design (GUD). With global solutions entering all socioeconomic levels, a clear and constant awareness of the need and available resources is essential for effectively meeting the needs. The ISWP is leading an effort to develop and a global common data set for this purpose. The dataset may include details such as the need for wheelchairs, location of qualified service providers, and list of appropriate products.

It is likely that in MRS the future will include more development of robotics and artificial intelligence. A lack of funding will no longer be an adequate reason to withhold these developments from LRS. User-centered innovations from LRS may soon find their way to the products and models of provision in MRS.

I met a young American named Rob Singer, who spent some significant amount of time working in the Jaipur program in India, learning their prosthetic technology.

255

He then spent extended periods establishing prosthetic services for a program in Sri Lanka. He took a very caring and mature approach to the task. He did not come in and do some isolated lectures and then disappear. He spent month after month after month on several visits to firmly gain the respect of the local technicians and administration, and to teach practical things. He also learned practical things and really help to establish a large facility doing a very practical job.

(Carlson, personal communication, 2018)

Since Rob Singer's time in Sri Lanka, there have been great developments in the field and a surge in number of users served worldwide. Yet there is a clear sense of something lost in the process. Balance can be restored with more two-way sharing of knowledge and skills.

11.15 Discussion questions

1. Discuss examples of AT in LRSs that students and instructors are already familiar with
2. Some of the best practices described in this chapter appear to make the job of AT development and implementation more complicated and difficult. How do these practices actually save time and cost and, in the end, produce better results?
3. How can AT be developed in/for LRS in a way that is inclusive of AT users in that setting?
4. What is an existing example of a GUD?
5. Describe and discuss elements of an ideal AT product development cycle considering the ethics concerns of working in or for LRS
6. In the early 2000s the trend in AT programs for LRS has been from local to global product solutions, allowing for far greater numbers of AT users served but fewer users and local providers engaged in the design process. To win large grant funding, NGOs are under pressure to shift their approach from building local capacity and local solutions to selling their products to an increasingly global market. An NGO would see a "profit" on the global sale of proprietary products. This "profit", in turn, is meant to subsidize internal programs and services according to the NGO's long-term strategy. This would be fine except that the market for the products is also funded by large donors and their global strategies. The result of this trend is a smaller number of higher-quality designs available worldwide in larger numbers. These products then fit into a system of distribution determined by an increasingly smaller group of professionals who, for the most part are not users of AT and do not live in LRS. Discuss possible product and system solutions to navigate through this future dilemma

Bibliography

Borg, Johan. 2018. Personal Interview.

Carlson, J. M. 2018. Personal Communication.

Kirby, R. L. 2018. Personal Communication.

Kirby, R. L., P. W. Rushton, C. Smith, F. Routhier, K. L. Best, J. Boyce, R. Cowan, E. Giesbrecht, L. K. Kenyon, and A. Koontz. 2019. "Wheelchair Skills Program Manual Version 5.0." Wheelchair Skills Program Manual Version 5.0. Published Electronically at Dalhousie University, Halifax, NS, Canada.

Munish, Abdullah. 2018. Personal Communication.

Pakirisamy, Venkatakannan. 2018. Personal Communication.

Pearlman, Jon, Rory A. Cooper, Marc Krizack, Alida Lindsley, Yeongchi Wu, Kim D. Reisinger, William Armstrong, Hector Casanova, Harvinder Singh Chhabra, and Jamie Noon. 2008. "Lower-Limb Prostheses and Wheelchairs in Low-Income Countries [An Overview]." *IEEE Engineering in Medicine and Biology Magazine* 27 (2): 12–22.

Seymour, Nicky. 2018. Personal Communication.

United Nations. "Convention on the Rights of Persons with Disabilities: Some Facts about Disability." *New York United Nations*, https://www.un.org/development/desa/disabilities/convention-on-the-rights-of-persons-with-disabilities.html.

WHO. *Assistive Devices/Technologies: What WHO is Doing.* Geneva: WHO. Accessed 18/06/2010, www.who.int/disabilities/technology/activities/en/.

———. 2008. "Guidelines on the Provision of Manual Wheelchairs in Less Resourced Settings."

———. "Wheelchair ServiceTraining Package." http://www.who.int/disabilities/technology/wheelchairpackage/en/.

Section III

Rehabilitation engineering and areas of application

Chapter 12 Rehabilitation engineering seating and mobility

Saleh A. Alqahtani,
Cheng-shui Chung,
Theresa M. Crytzer,
Carmen P. DiGiovine,
Eliana C. Ferretti,
Sara Múnera Orozco,
S. Andrea Sundaram,
Brandon Daveler,
María L. Toro-Hernández,
Amy Lane, Tamra Pelleschi,
Rosemarie Cooper, and
Rory A. Cooper

Contents

DOI: 10.1201/b21964-15

12.1 Chapter overview

In this chapter, the reader will be able to learn about rehabilitation engineering, seating, and mobility. After providing a brief introduction, the chapter describes the model for assistive technology service delivery, transportation options for wheelchair users, and principles of basic seating. The text then explains the different options of advanced robotic wheelchairs, followed by the principles of basic wheelchair design. In addition, the chapter will highlight the guidelines that wheelchair users can follow to maintain their wheelchairs at home. The chapter then proceeds to discuss rehabilitation engineers' role in the customization and integration of assistive technology solutions for clients.

12.2 Introduction

The World Health Organization (WHO) estimates that 1% of the world's population, approximately 75 million people, needs or could benefit from using a wheelchair as their primary means of mobility (World Health Organization 2008). This need will be more pressing in future years due to the global increase of chronic health conditions as well as the aging of the world's population (World Health Organization 2015). In the United States, for instance, 3.6 million people are wheelchair users (US Census Bureau 2015). However, it is more common not to have accurate measures of the need as in low- and middle-income countries. For example, in Colombia, the Registry for Localization and Characterization of the population with disabilities measures limitations in activities, but it is unspecific to the need or use of assistive technology, especially wheelchairs (Health Ministry and Social Protection 2016). Unfortunately, the WHO estimates that only between 5% and 15% of people who need a wheelchair have access to an appropriate one (World Health Organization 2008).

Due to the immense need, it is still common to see massive deliveries of donated products, especially in developing countries without the appropriate associated services (Jefferds et al. 2010, 221–242; Pearlman et al. 2008, 12–22; Visagie et al. 2015, 201). The United Nations Convention on the Rights of Persons with

Disabilities mandates ratifying member states to guarantee that persons with disabilities exercise all human rights, including the right to personal mobility (United Nations 2006). Discrimination against people with disabilities, lack of access to appropriate technology, lack of funding, and a lack of trained personnel on how to deliver wheelchairs are significant barriers to the human right of personal mobility (Jefferds et al. 2010, 221-242). Wheelchairs and their services are a necessary step to access the right of individual mobility (World Health Organization 2011).

The term community participation is used to refer to returning to the mainstream of family and community life, engaging in roles and responsibilities, and actively contributing to one's social groups and society. The ability of people who require a wheelchair to successfully participate in their community and regain independence depends on access to appropriate and adequate wheelchairs. An appropriate wheelchair is one that meets the user's needs, provides fit and postural support, meets the needs of the environment, and is maintainable and repairable (World Health Organization 2008). Greater satisfaction with a wheelchair should result in enhanced use of that technology and contribute to a better subjective quality of life (J. Scherer, Laura A. Cushman, Marcia 2001, 387–393). Additionally, when a wheelchair is not appropriate, it is likely to cause secondary complications such as pressure sores or repetitive strain injury, a decrease in independence and self-esteem, and a decrease in the chances to access education and employment that can lead to abandonment and wasting resources (Visagie et al. 2015, 201; Phillips and Zhao 1993, 36–45).

In 2008, the WHO published Guidelines for the Provision of Manual Wheelchairs in Less Resourced Settings (World Health Organization 2008). The guidelines aimed to encourage personal mobility and enhance the quality of life of wheelchair users by helping countries to develop a system of wheelchair provision. The guidelines served as the foundation for the development of the Wheelchair Service Training Packages (WHO WSTP), which described the eight steps needed for appropriate wheelchair provision: referral, assessment, prescription, funding and ordering, product preparation, fitting and adjusting, user training, and follow-up and maintenance and repairs. The WHO WSTP aims to expand wheelchair service provision, focusing on developing countries where the need is the greatest, to support the minimum skills and knowledge required by the personnel involved in wheelchair service delivery, including managers, stakeholders, rehabilitation professionals, and technicians.

In 2015, the International Society of Wheelchair Professionals (ISWP) was founded with the goal to professionalize the wheelchair sector. There are vast disparities in the world and even between urban and rural settings in the same countries. Wheelchairs can be covered through a healthcare plan, through programs in ministries or departments of social welfare, out-of-pocket purchases, and donations, among others. Even though there are different organizations conducting training in wheelchair provision globally, each organization uses different curricula and methodologies. Moreover, there is not an internationally accepted way to measure competency in providing wheelchair services. As previously mentioned, one of the barriers to access to appropriate services is the lack of competent personnel. The ISWP is working to increase awareness about wheelchairs and related services as well as coordinate education and training initiatives.

In conclusion, even though significant efforts have been made over the last decade in helping countries in developing and improving a system of wheelchair provision, there is still a lot to do, especially in developing countries. The amount of information on the effectiveness of these technologies in improving function and, in particular, increasing independence and community participation is relatively sparse. Professionals involved in the provision of wheelchairs globally should apply outcome measures to raise the standard of practice, support evidence-based practice, and improve the level of accountability. This would allow us to understand wheelchair service provision in each country better and contribute to professionals increasing their knowledge related to wheelchair services and ultimately inspire individual mobility and enhance participation as well as contributing to a better quality of life for wheelchair users.

12.3 Assistive technology service delivery

Assistive technology (AT) includes the environment and physical structures within it, assistive devices for mobility (Arledge et al. 2011) and communication (American Speech-Language-Hearing Association 2004; Government of New South Wales, Australia 2019), and the interaction of a person with the environment and devices (Cook and Hussey 2001; Gitlin 2002). A stepwise process may be used to obtain AT devices that include, when appropriate, assessments by a physician and a therapist (i.e., physical therapist, occupational therapist, or speech and language pathologist) and input from an assistive technology supplier (Arledge et al. 2011). The person with a disability is at the center of the process and has the final decision-making authority. Obtaining reimbursement for assistive devices from insurance companies in resourced countries, including the United States, requires specific documentation procedures that include gathering objective outcome measures (Fuhrer et al. 2003, 1243–1251) and following a timeline for completion of required paperwork (Arledge et al. 2011; Cook and Hussey 2001). In less-resourced settings, the process may follow similar methods but adapted to the local culture and the resources available; however, an eight-step process for service provision has been created and tested by the WHO (Toro et al. 2016, 1753–1760). Regardless of the setting or location, a successful AT service delivery model includes the multidisciplinary collaboration of the person with a disability and the specialists who have knowledge and expertise in the design and application of AT (Cook and Hussey 2001). Following the ethical and legal parameters is expected of all professionals involved in the service delivery process. With strong collaboration between the person with the disability and the healthcare professionals, and adherence to the documentation and ethical and legal processes, the AT service delivery process can positively impact the integration of people with disabilities into the community and improve quality of life.

A model AT assessment team consists of the client, a physiatrist, physical therapist or occupational therapist, speech and language pathologist, rehabilitation engineer, and an equipment supplier who has training and certification in AT. Depending on the needs and goals of the client, additional professionals who are engaged with the client and may be consulted to contribute to the AT assessment and delivery process include family members, rehabilitation counselors, nurses, personal care assistants, and teachers.

The AT service delivery process begins with the client making an appointment with either a multidisciplinary AT clinic or with a physiatrist for a mobility evaluation. After seeing the physiatrist, the client schedules an evaluation with a physical or occupational therapist, ideally one who has an ATP, and a wheelchair supplier with an ATP. RESNA provides a searchable list of ATP providers (e.g., therapists and suppliers) across the United States. If the client attends a multidisciplinary AT clinic, the visit starts out with the introduction of the client to the AT Assessment team. Regardless of the setting in which the AT service process takes place, clients must be empowered to be active decision-making members of that team.

A proper AT assessment begins with an initial interview that involves listening and paying attention to the client's needs, concerns, and goals for a device. It is important to understand the medical variables that were assessed by the physiatrist and shared with the team how underlying medical conditions may impact the recommendation of an AT device. It is also important to understand the medical, social, physical, behavioral, and functional variables assessed by the therapist and how physical capacity and limitations affect mobility and the conduct of activities of daily living (ADL). Therapists and physiatrists often use the International Classification for Functioning and Disability as a model or guideline when completing AT evaluations. In collaboration with the physiatrist, a plan for the use of AT to compensate for limitations and augment task performance is developed. Allowing the user to try the equipment and compare devices informs the AT team and the client's decision on the device that meets the majority of their needs. Understanding environmental barriers that clients face (e.g., access to home and community environments and transportation) is also an important consideration, especially when transporting the wheelchair is required to complete the activities of daily living.

265

Following the assessment, the AT team members will explain to the client the findings of the assessment, the interpretation of the outcome measures, and the reasoning upon which the team based their final recommendation(s) to the client. The final decision on the mobility device lies with the client, the family, and/or the caregivers, although some constraints within the insurance industry should be included in the discussions with the client and caregivers that may be limiting factors in obtaining the needed equipment. Additional discussion may include secondary or tertiary funding that covers the cost of AT.

Delivery of the new device to the client is one of the final steps in the AT service delivery process. Ideally, the therapist and supplier should both be present during the delivery of the device to whatever location is chosen (e.g., clinic, school, home, or another community environment). Only when the therapist is present at the final fitting can he or she assess the fit and function of the device, and if needed, make further recommendations for any modifications or additional components. When the therapist attends the final fitting, he or she is in a position to advocate for his or her client if the device does not fit or work well for the client. Once the AT device is fitted properly, education and training have been provided, and the client demonstrates that they can operate the device, the client signs forms provided by the wheelchair supplier to indicate that he or she received the device. The therapist documents the final fitting process (i.e., fit, demonstration, education, practice). Follow-up by the AT team is also recommended and clients should be provided with contact information for the AT team should their condition change, or he or she requires maintenance on the device in the future. The AT service delivery process may be a lifelong experience for some clients and strong collaboration and continued communication by the AT team with the client can help make this process smoother for the client.

12.4 Transportation for wheelchair users

Transportation options, including driving, allow individuals greater opportunities to engage in their community. Driving is essential for many adults to participate in meaningful activities, carry out valued roles, and be mobile outside their home environments. For many individuals with a disability, the automobile is not only a preferred method of transportation, it is often the only means of transportation available in suburban and rural areas (Field, Jette, and Institute of Medicine (US) Committee on Disability in America 2007).

Driver rehabilitation programs across North America and worldwide provide a range of services for individuals whose critical driving skills are significantly affected by medical or age-related changes. Typically, these programs offer clinical and driving skills assessment, education, and training in the use of adaptive driving equipment, and experience in using modified vehicles (Lane et al. 2014, 177–187).

Certified driver rehabilitation specialists (CDRS) are trained professionals who aid in determining the type of adaptive driving technology best suited to a client's goals and ability. Consideration of the client's wheelchair, transfer skills, functional abilities and limitations, ability to maintain an appropriate position as a driver or passenger, and vehicle type are included in the assessment process. Many persons who use wheelchairs can continue or return to driving given appropriate education and training on adaptive equipment and modifications.

Vehicle structural modifications are indicated when barriers impede vehicle ingress/egress, affect safe wheelchair transport and securement, or limit access to the driver or passenger position. Examples of significant structural modifications include lowered floor mini-vans with side or rear entry ramps, gull-wing style door designs, and side entry hydraulic platform lifts installed on sport utility vehicles or trucks. Less invasive modifications for ingress/egress and wheelchair transport include wheelchair hoists or loading devices. Modifications that address access to the driver or passenger position include transfer seat bases or retractable transfer boards that bridge the gap between the wheelchair and the car seat.

Accessibility features are often added to vehicles that have undergone significant structural changes. These may include powered door openers and automatic ramp deployment. Kneeling systems lower the vehicle floor closer to ground height and decrease the angle of a ramp entry system.

Adaptive driving equipment used when operating the vehicle's primary or secondary controls can be categorized as high tech or low tech. High-tech devices are those that can control the vehicle functions or driving controls and operate with a designed logic system or interface/integrate with an electronic system of the vehicle. Examples include powered gas or brake systems, reduced effort steering systems, or remote panels that interface with the installation of the original equipment manufacturer (OEM) electronics. Low-tech modifications are all other devices that do not meet the criteria for high tech, including manual gas and brake hand controls, a remote horn, extensions for OEM devices such as turn signals, parking brake extensions, and transmission shifter levers.

Items such as seat cushions and lumbar or lateral supports can be used for comfort and positioning while riding in a vehicle. Upper torso positioning belts can be used when the client is unable to sit unsupported or requires external support to maintain an upright position while in a moving vehicle. It is important to note that these items do not replace the use of an OEM shoulder and lap belt system.

When traveling in a vehicle, it is generally safest for wheelchair users to transfer to a vehicle seat and use the OEM seatbelt system. The wheelchair should be stored and secured in the vehicle. If transferring is not feasible, the wheelchair should be forward facing, secured to the vehicle, and the rider should use a crash-tested lap and shoulder belt. A WC-19 compliant wheelchair is optimal due to its design and testing for use as a seat in a vehicle (University of Michigan Transportation Research Institute n.d.).

Wheelchair securement using four-point tiedown systems is typically designed for someone other than the wheelchair rider to apply. Wheelchairs can also be secured using a docking tiedown device in the vehicle. Although this allows for greater independence, the wheelchair user should be aware that additional hardware is attached to the wheelchair.

To prevent injury to the client, wheelchair, equipment, or vehicle, it is important to adhere to the highest level of industry standards and practices. In the United States and Canada, vehicle modifiers who are members of the National Mobility Equipment Dealers Association comply with Federal or Canada Motor Vehicle Safety Standards and Society of Automotive Engineers' recommended practices when modifying vehicles for people with disabilities (National Mobility Equipment Dealers Association 2017).

Drivers who use adaptive driving equipment and/or vehicle modifications must adhere to the regulatory structure and requirements of the driver licensing authority. Driver rehabilitation specialists ensure client compliance with these standards and can assist in navigating the licensing system.

Due to the cost of modifying a vehicle, the client should be assessed in an evaluation vehicle with equipment that is functionally equivalent to what will be prescribed, assuring that it meets the client's needs. Additional training in the client's vehicle ensures optimal functioning of the devices, that it was installed as prescribed, and most importantly, the client has demonstrated proficiency with the technology (Association for Driver Rehabilitation Specialists 2016).

12.5 Basic seating principles

Understanding the physical presentation and its progression will allow the clinician to determine the selection of the wheelchair base and frame on the seating system and where they will be mounted, either to a "static" frame, meaning all seat angles of the system are fixed, or a "dynamic" seat frame, with adjustable seating features such as tilt, backrest recline, and elevating leg rests. The dynamic seat features can be manually or power-adjusted and will be addressed later within this section. For the person to be considered a "dynamic" sitter, he/she must be able to conduct independent, functional, and safe transfers and independent and effective weight shifts for positioning, pressure relief, and comfort.

For a "dynamic" person, a "static" seat frame like a manual wheelchair, a push-rim-activated power-assist wheelchair, or a power base with a captain-style seat would be appropriate. For a person to be considered a "static" sitter, he or she is no longer able to conduct independent transfers and independent weight shifts. Losing the ability to conduct independent weight shifts compromises and limits effective pressure relief and exposes the person to an increased risk of pressure sores and skin breakdown. For a "static" sitter, a "dynamic" seat frame, for example, a power wheelchair base with a power seating system to include power tilt, recline, seat elevator, and leg rests, would be indicated, given the person is cognitively able to independently operate and safely control a power wheelchair; if not, then the alternative would be a manual tilt-in-space with manual recline and elevated leg rest.

12.5.1 Manual wheelchairs

Manual wheelchairs are typically classified into three categories: standard/depot/transport wheelchairs that weigh more than 36 lbs., are non-adjustable and low cost, and are intended for indoor use, that is, hospital or nursing facility for multiple user transports; lightweight wheelchairs that weigh 34–36 lbs., are minimally adjustable, and are intended for short-term use by users who are not able to self-propel a standard wheelchair; and ultra-lightweight wheelchairs generally weigh less than 25 lbs. Since manual wheelchair propulsion is like "walking on your hands" and therefore not a natural phenomenon, people who propel manual wheelchairs are known to have very high incidences of upper extremity repetitive strain injuries (RSI) that significantly impair function. Reducing the weight of the wheelchair as well as a proper fit and alignment of the rear axle position can significantly reduce the potential for these injuries. Only ultra-light manual wheelchairs have an adjustable axle position, camber, and seat angle needed to fit the user, as well as a positive impact on propulsion mechanics to preserve the upper extremities and reduce the risk of RSI associated with wheelchair propulsion. They come in different frame styles: rigid, folding, and with suspension. Rigid wheelchairs tend to be lighter than folding chairs, which, in turn, have the advantage of allowing easier stowage; whereas suspension chairs absorb surface irregularities for people that have to travel over uneven terrain or have to hop down curbs. The "right" ultra-lite wheelchair depends on the user's height and weight, environment, lifestyle, and personal preference.

Pushrim-activated power-assist wheelchairs (PAPAW) require users to stroke the hand rims to activate small, lightweight motors, which then drive the wheels for a brief period of time (seconds; Figure 12.1). To keep a PAPAW moving, users must continue to stroke the hand rims as they would if they were propelling manual wheelchairs. The combination of an ultra-lightweight manual wheelchair and the pushrim-activated power assist wheels provides the end user with an ideal set-up

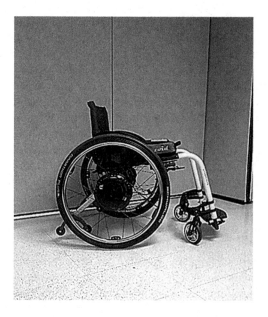

Figure 12.1 PAPAW wheelchair.

that will allow for continuation with active self-propulsion of a manual wheelchair and allow for loading the wheelchair into other vehicles, as it incorporates the benefits of a lighter wheelchair frame equipped with quick-release wheels for ease of stowage. Research studies have found that the power assist wheels have the potential to reduce stress on upper extremities during wheelchair propulsion, reduce metabolic energy expenditure, reduce the cardiovascular demand over manual wheelchair propulsion, improve function during daily activities, and improve mobility and participation within the user's community.

The "SmartDrive" is a power assist system that is designed to provide auxiliary power to manual wheelchairs to reduce the pushing power and push frequency (Figure 12.2). The system is lightweight and attaches to the back of a manual wheelchair, including folding, tilt-in-space, one-arm drive, and standing. The system assists the user to go up the steepest ramps, sidewalks, thickly padded carpets, and so on. The smart drive has an anti-rollback feature that allows the user to stop on a hill and then easily get going again. SmartDrive power assist can be individualized as it is equipped with different selectable modes, where the user can easily pick the one that is best for a desired activity level and needs.

An attendant-propelled manual wheelchair frame usually comes equipped with a tilt/recline combination seating system (Figure 12.3) for gravity-assisted postural support, which is recommended for a person who is not able to operate a power wheelchair with power seat functions and is considered a "static" sitter having

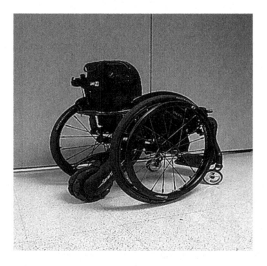

Figure 12.2 SmartDrive system.

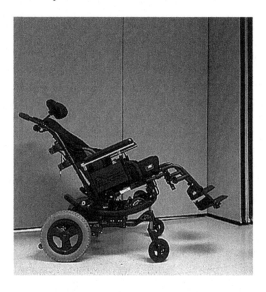

Figure 12.3 Wheelchair with tilt/recline seating system.

lost the physical ability to conduct independent weight shifts required for effective pressure relief and is at increased risk for pressure sores and skin breakdown.

12.5.2 Powered wheelchairs

Power wheelchairs are motorized devices driven by a joystick or alternative input device (Figure 12.4). The location of the drive wheels determines how the chair

271

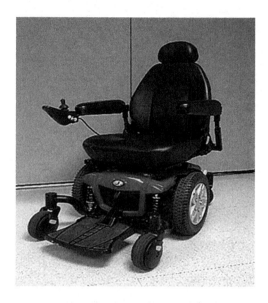

Figure 12.4 A standard power wheelchair.

will steer and handle various terrain. A rear-wheel drive power chair provides good directional stability while driving forward. Rear-wheel drive chairs handle uneven terrain well. Front-wheel drive chairs are good at climbing obstacles as the drive wheels, which tend to be larger, face the front and help to power over objects; yet they are harder to drive straight and are prone to "fish-tail" while going up and down ramps. Mid-wheel and center-wheel drive chairs are easily recognizable by having six wheels, two casters in the rear, two casters or anti-tip wheels in the front, and the drive wheels in between. This type of power base is most intuitive for maneuvering in tight areas due to the small turning radius. The selection of the appropriate powerbase is based on the frequency of usage, outside terrain, and home environment.

Power seat features that can be accommodated on a power wheelchair base include tilt-in-space, recline, elevating leg rests, and seat elevation (Figure 12.5). With the activation of power tilt, the backrest angle remains unchanged while both the backrest and seat will change orientation. Power tilt-space will promote postural stability, pressure redistribution, increase comfort by providing gravity-assisted redistribution, and prevent sliding out of the seat; 45 degrees of tilt is recommended for effective pressure relief.

Power recline, when used in combination with tilt, will safely accommodate limited hip flexion, provide pressure relief (120 degrees), and increase comfort. Power elevating leg rests, when used in combination with tilt and recline, assist with the management of lower extremity edema and allow for adjustment to fluctuation in

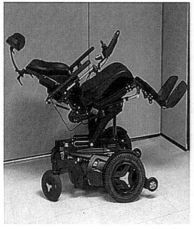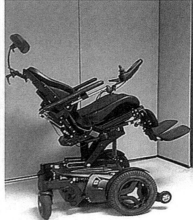

Figure 12.5 Seating system functions.

tone; they also assist with curb and obstacle clearance when operating the chair in outdoor terrain. The seat elevator allows the user to adjust the seat height to accommodate the limited range of both upper extremities as well as promote safe functional transfers (Figure 12.6). Also, the user can elevate the seat height to eye level for natural and healthy social interactions.

12.5.3 Control system

The most common control system for power wheelchairs is a joystick that is typically mounted at the end of either the right or left armrest, depending on the user's preference. Other types of joysticks, mini or micro, can be mounted in locations such as on the footplate. For users who are unable to use a joystick due to limited extremity strength or movement, alternative controls such as sip and puff, head control, and chin control are additional options. Many power wheelchairs are also capable of adding expandable controllers to control devices such as an augmentative speech device or computer, an attendant control joystick, or an enhanced display.

12.6 Robotic and connected wheelchairs and seating

12.6.1 Robotic-powered wheelchairs

In the United States, about 15% of wheelchair users use electric-powered wheelchairs (Cooper et al. 2008, 1387–1398)—and even smaller percentages in some other parts of the world; significant efforts have gone into

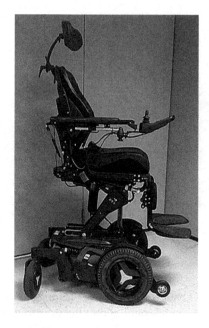

Figure 12.6 Power elevating seating system.

advancing the state-of-the-art for this category of mobility aid. While electric power wheelchairs (EPWs) provide community integration, independence, and increased quality of life for persons with disabilities (Edwards and McCluskey 2010, 411–419), current commercial wheelchairs are still unable to surmount many architectural barriers—including curbs, steps, and significant slopes—presenting obstacles that limit where wheelchair users may freely go (Ding and Cooper 2005, 22–34; Wretstrand, Petzäll, and Ståhl 2004, 3–11). Additionally, based on a survey sent to 200 clinicians, Fehr, Langbein, and Skaar (2000, 353–360) found that anywhere from 9% to 50% of EPW users had difficulty steering/maneuvering their wheelchairs, depending on what criteria were used. For EPWs to provide greater independence and ease of use, research has focused on ways to incorporate the ability to sense and avoid or overcome architectural barriers, as well as providing autonomous, or semiautonomous, navigation.

Advanced powered wheelchairs can be divided into two basic categories. The first category consists of devices with some ability to sense and respond to their environments—these are sometimes referred to as "smart wheelchairs." The second category consists of devices with mechanical and electronic configurations that allow them to perform tasks that are difficult or impossible to complete using standard powered wheelchairs, for example, climbing stairs. Several devices bridge both categories—combining sensors and algorithms with sophisticated mechanical systems.

In his 2005 review of the topic, Simpson noted that smart wheelchairs have been a topic of research since the 1980s. His survey of the literature found that most examples have been built by attaching seats to robots or modifying existing EPWs. Technologies that have been used for navigation and obstacle avoidance include machine vision, sonar, infrared and laser rangefinders, and tape tracking (Simpson 2005, 423). By far, the most common feature of smart wheelchairs is obstacle detection.

In a particularly advanced implementation of a smart wheelchair, a Toyota MOBIRO personal mobility robot was fitted with a laser rangefinder (LRF) that swept along the ground to detect and map stationary obstacles, another stationary LRF to detect moving objects, and a camera to recognize features in the environment. By using the device to gather information about features in its surroundings, adding data about traffic patterns collected by other means, and analyzing the data in an off-board computer system, the researchers were able to create a sufficiently detailed map for their smart wheelchair to navigate autonomously (Hatao et al. 2014, 281–296).

Despite the number of research projects on smart wheelchairs, in 2005, only two were available for purchase in the United States, and those only for research purposes (Simpson 2005, 423). Smile Rehab Ltd. (Berkshire, United Kingdom) continues to sell the "Smart Wheelchair," which includes contact sensors, tape tracking, and an optional ultrasonic sensor, but it is intended for use as a training tool, rather than as a product for daily use (Simpson 2005, 423). A search conducted at the time of writing did not uncover any other commercially available obstacle detecting or path following wheelchairs. As recently as 2014, interviews with wheelchair users, caregivers, and clinicians continued to show a high level of interest in such products, with all three groups feeling that intelligent wheelchairs would improve social interaction by increasing safety and reducing anxiety (Kairy et al. 2014, 2244–2261).

Obstacle negotiating wheelchairs have been designed with a number of different mechanisms. The simplest implementations involve exceptionally large wheels and all-wheel-drive or tank-like treads. Such designs can handle rough terrain and some types of architectural barriers but have difficulty navigating indoors and often damage the surfaces they traverse.

Other companies and researchers have tried more complex systems with greater flexibility to work in built environments. In 2017, a literature review on step-climbing wheelchairs found 13 devices that were, or had been, in active development since 2005 (Sundaram et al. 2017, 98–109). These 13 devices were divided into four basic types. Leg-wheel hybrids consist of wheels mounted at the end

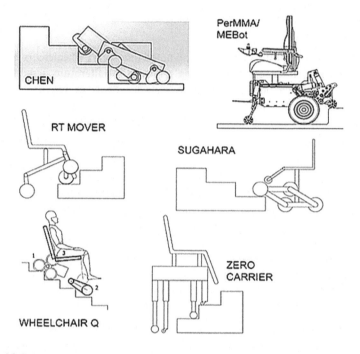

Figure 12.7 Leg-wheel hybrid wheelchairs.

of structures that use sliding and/or swinging motions to position the wheels on surfaces at different levels (Figure 12.7). Another approach separates the leg and wheel mechanisms. Spider wheels comprise small wheels mounted radially around a central hub (Figure 12.8). The small wheels drive and support the chair on level surfaces. When the device encounters an obstacle, the central hub turns to put a new set of wheels in contact with the higher or lower surface. The last category uses tank-like treads, but also incorporates other features (e.g., the ability to switch between tread in wheeled operation or the ability to change track shape to better conform to stair geometry).

The most famous stairclimbing wheelchair was the Independence Technology iBOT 3000—the balancing technology that led to the Segway. The iBOT employed four wheels in two rotatable clusters enabling four driving modes: standard two-wheel-drive, four-wheel-drive for rough terrains or small obstacles, a balancing mode in which the iBOT rotated one-wheel cluster above the other to lift the user to typical standing eye level, and a stairclimbing mode that used the movement of the wheel clusters to step up and down the stairs (Figure 12.9). Although the iBOT did eventually obtain FDA approval and was enthusiastically received by a significant number of wheelchair users, limitations of its seating

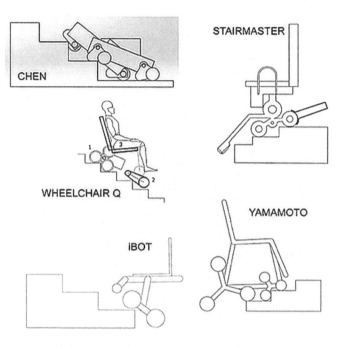

Figure 12.8 Examples of spider wheel designs.

system combined with a high price prevented it from being adopted by enough users to make it a viable product, and it was discontinued in 2009. In 2016, however, DEKA Research and Development—creators of the iBOT—and Toyota USA announced a partnership to further work on the iBOT and bring it back to the market.

12.6.2 Assistive robotic manipulators

In the United States, about 19.9 million people aged 15 years and older have difficulties with physical tasks related to upper extremity functioning, including lifting, grasping, pushing/pulling, reaching, dressing, and eating (Brault 2012). Assistive robotic manipulators (ARMs) have been developed and provide enhanced assistance to people with impairments in completing ADL while a care attendant is not on site (Prior and Warner 1993, 1194–1200). An ARM can be mounted either on a powered wheelchair or a mobile base. ARMs have also demonstrated enhanced independence in ADL tasks at home and work (Bach, Zeelenberg, and Winter 1990, 55–59; Hammel et al. 1989, 1–16).

The research and development of ARMs, including wheelchair- and desktop-mounted robotic manipulators, can be traced back to the 1960s. Over the past

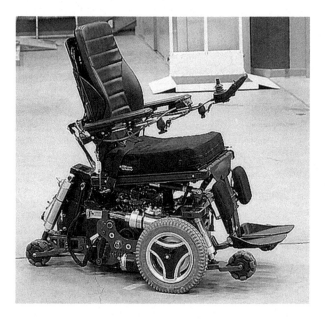

Figure 12.9 Mobility enhanced robotic wheelchair.

50 years, nearly a dozen ARMs have been developed and evaluated for their performance in usability and functionality. Different user interfaces have been designed for each of these assistive robotic manipulators to improve the performance of accomplishing functional ADLs. The involvement of user experiences and feedback from the target population has kept the design and development progressing. In addition, with the benefit of increasing computational power, more research groups have developed automation and artificial intelligence for object recognition and path planning so that people with disabilities may perform ADLs and vocational tasks more independently and efficiently. However, despite these attempts, there are only a few commercialized assistive robotic manipulators currently available on the market.

Literature reviews summarized the results of nine surveys that identify the task priorities of the robotic devices (Stanger et al. 1994, 256–265) and new commercial ARMs (Yanco and Haigh 2002, 39–53). A literature review article compared 19 commercial and developing ARM with five criteria: interaction safety, shock robustness, adaptability, energy, and position control (Groothuis, Stramigioli, and Carloni 2013, 20–29). These robotic manipulators were compared through their functionalities and specifications. A recent literature review discussed the clinical effectiveness of the most recent commercialized ARMs (Chung, Cheng-Shiu, Wang, and Cooper 2013b, 273–289).

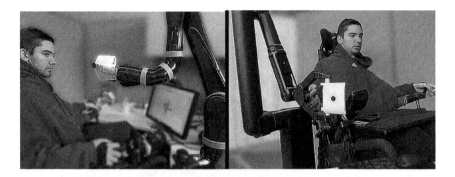

Figure 12.10 Two commercialized wheelchair-mounted robotic manipulators: JACO manipulator (left) and Manus ARM (right).

Currently, two commercialized ARMs (iARM and JACO manipulator, shown in Figure 12.10, with six degrees of freedom and minimized fold-in position). The iARM has a two-finger gripper manufactured by Exact Dynamics. It can be controlled by keypad, joystick, or single-button switches (Driessen, Evers, and van Woerden 2001, 285–290; Driessen et al. 2005, 165–173). Alternatively, the JACO manipulator has a three-fingered hand manufactured by Kinova Technology. The hand can grasp objects using either two or three fingers. It can be controlled by its own three degrees of freedom joystick, single switches, or wheelchair joystick (Chung, Cheng-Shiu and Cooper 2012; Maheu et al. 2011, 1–5). Their performance in ADL and users' perceived loading were evaluated in a study (Chung, Cheng-Shiu et al. 2016; Chung, Cheng-Shiu et al. 2017a, 395–407).

The Personal Mobility and Manipulation Appliance (PerMMA) is the first wheelchair to integrate bimanual manipulation for enhancing the quality of life for people with severe physical impairments (Figure 12.11). PerMMA integrates both a smart powered wheelchair and two dexterous robotic arms to assist its users in completing essential mobility and manipulation tasks during basic and instrumental activities of daily living (Cooper et al. 2012, 2505–2511).

PerMMA aims to improve functional performance and independence with three integrated user interfaces: a local control interface, a remote-control interface, and an assistive interface. In the local control interface, the local user has full control of PerMMA. The user can operate them with a smartphone. In the remote-control interface, a remote operator can operate both robotic manipulators using either the haptic joysticks, touchscreen, or keyboard. In the assistive interface, the local user or a remote operator work together in conjunction with autonomous functions to complete mobility and manipulation tasks. PerMMA was evaluated with end users in completing ADL tasks and showed improved independence

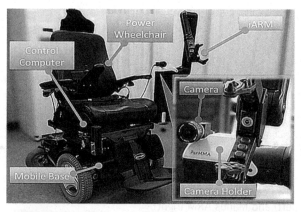

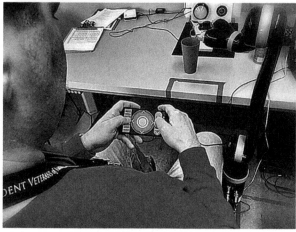

Figure 12.11 Personal mobility and manipulation appliance (PerMMA).

and ADL performance (Chung, Cheng-Shiu 2015; Chung, CS et al. 2014; Chung, Cheng-Shiu, Wang, and Cooper 2013a, 1–6; Chung, Cheng-Shiu, Wang, and Cooper 2013b, 273–289; Chung, Cheng-Shiu and Cooper 2012; Chung, Cheng-Shiu et al. 2017a, 395–407; Chung, Cheng-Shiu et al. 2017b, 16–27; Wang et al. 2013, 1613–1619; Wang et al. 2012, 3324–3327).

12.7 Basic wheelchair design principles

12.7.1 User needs and characteristics

The most important principle when designing a wheelchair is having a thorough understanding of the characteristics and needs of the user. These may include the user's demographics (age, weight, location of residence, residence type, work status, lifestyle, etc.), health information (diagnosis, physical limitations, mental limitations, etc.), and preferences (drive controls, folding/rigid, manual/power, front-/mid-/rear-wheel drive, etc.). This information is helpful when creating a list of design criteria for the device (length/width, maximum user weight, turning radius, manual/powered, control method, etc.). Other factors to consider are the environment (dry/humid, cold/hot) and drive surface (smooth/rough, hard/soft) that the user travels in and over, respectively.

12.7.2 Manual wheelchairs

Manual wheelchairs should be designed to allow the user to carry out the tasks that they need to do, which include transferring, propelling, and transporting the wheelchair for daily activities. They are designed to either be folding or rigid (Figure 12.12). Rigid frame designs are customized to perfectly fit the body of the user whereas the design of a folding frame is primarily designed to fold. A rigid frame's design is optimized for performance. Its design allows for more weight to be put on the rear wheels because of the short distance between the front casters and footrests. This allows less weight to be placed on the front casters, resulting in easier turning for the user. The casters for folding wheelchair designs must be positioned behind the footrests for the chair to fold properly, which places more weight on the front casters. The customized design of a rigid frame places the user in an optimal position for propulsion unlike the universal design of a folding frame wheelchair.

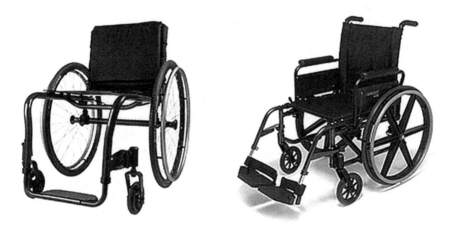

Figure 12.12 Rigid frame (left); folding frame (right) (www.sunrisemedical.com, 2018).

Folding frame wheelchairs have an X-style frame that allows them to fold when a locking mechanism is released and they usually have removable footrests and armrests. The frames are most commonly made from titanium or aluminum and are heavier compared with a rigid frame design. Folding wheelchairs are not as durable and require more maintenance than rigid frame designs due to the additional movable parts of the folding mechanism. The folding capability allows them to be placed in the rear of a vehicle without needing to remove the wheels. Typical users are those with minimal or no upper body strength who are unable to be independent and are either very young or elderly. These types of wheelchairs are most commonly used in long-term and acute care settings.

The design of a rigid frame wheelchair is most commonly made from aluminum or titanium and sometimes even carbon fiber. The lightweight advantage allows them to be easily transported with the addition of quick-release wheels that let the user remove the wheels with the push of a button located on the axle. A rigid frame without wheels could weigh as little as 5 kg. Their light weight allows them to be easier to propel and places less stress on the shoulder joints, which reduces the likelihood of repetitive strain injuries.

The customized design of a rigid frame takes into consideration the user's body size to determine the chair's length and width of the seat, height and width of the footrests, height and width of the backrest, and angle of the seat also known as the dump. The shape of the frame should conform to the user's body, making it appear as though the wheelchair and the user are one. Other customizable components include types of cushions, push rims, tire compounds and tread patterns, armrests, and colors. The fewer number of moving parts of a rigid frame typically last longer and are stronger than that of a folding frame wheelchair. In general, rigid wheelchairs are used by independent, active individuals with good upper body strength.

12.7.3 Powered wheelchairs

The design and components of a power wheelchair can be separated between its base and seating system. The base includes the batteries, electric motors, wheels, and a suspension system. When designing the base of a power wheelchair, the base's length and width determine the stability and maneuverability of the device. Larger bases are better suited for outdoor use due to their increased stability, while small bases allow for better maneuverability indoors. The seating system can either be an automotive—"captain" style—seat with a manually reclining backrest or a complex—"rehab" style—seat with power seating functions.

12.7.4 Drive wheel configurations

The configuration or location of the drive wheels for a power wheelchair determines its maneuverability, stability, and obstacle climbing capability. These characteristics are the main differentiators between the three configurations (Figure 12.13); rear-wheel drive (RWD), front-wheel drive (FWD), and mid-wheel drive (MWD). RWD and FWD wheelchairs are designed to have four main wheels (two drive wheels and two caster wheels) in addition to two wheels used as anti-tippers for safety when going up or down slopes. For RWD wheelchairs, the drive wheels are located toward the rear of the frame behind the wheelchair's center of gravity (CoG) while FWD wheelchairs have the drive wheels located toward the front of the frame and in front of the CoG. RWD wheelchairs are the most stable at higher speeds but lack the maneuverability of FWD and MWD. FWD wheelchairs perform better when going over rough terrain or climbing obstacles due to the larger diameter driving wheels being the first contact of the obstacle. MWD wheelchairs have a six-wheel design (two drive wheels and four caster wheels). The location of the driving wheels on MWD wheelchairs are directly in the center of the frame, thus close to the wheelchair's CoG. Maneuverability is highest with an MWD wheelchair because the chair is able to turn 360 degrees within its own wheelbase.

12.7.5 Seating system

The seating systems for power wheelchairs are either a captain style or a rehab style (Figure 12.14) and are determined based on the physical characteristics of

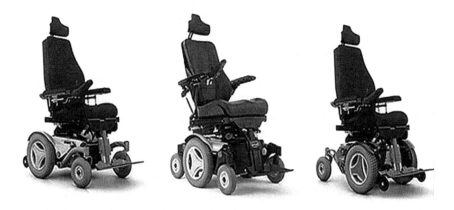

Figure 12.13 Rear-wheel drive (left); mid-wheel drive (center); front-wheel drive (right) (www.sunrisemedical.com, 2018).

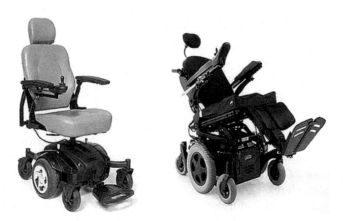

Figure 12.14 Captain style seat (left); rehab style seat (right) (www.sunrisemedical
.com, 2018).

the user. Captain style seating provides limited postural support for the user, thus
requiring them to be able to maintain their stability when using the device. Users
of this type of seating are typically also capable of performing pressure relief
independently. However, rehab-style seats are for users that are unable to independently perform pressure reliefs and may require additional postural support.
They are also capable of being configured with power seating functions such as
tilt, recline, elevating leg rests, and seat elevators. These functions allow the user
to reposition themselves for comfort and perform pressure reliefs. Rehab seating
systems are customized to the user using different types of seat cushions (gel, air,
foam, or a combination), backrests, head rests, armrests, and footrests.

12.8 Wheelchair maintenance

The World Health Organization in its guidelines for appropriate wheelchair
provision recommends that wheelchair users have to receive training on how to
maintain their wheelchairs at home (step 7) and there needs to be readily available wheelchair maintenance and repairs services for the user (World Health
Organization 2008). The main reason for this is that an appropriate wheelchair
can be a mechanism to ensure social participation; nonetheless, if the wheelchair
is in a disrepair state, it can be a barrier to this participation. Additionally, a
wheelchair in a disrepair state can cause secondary health-related problems such
as abrasions or lacerations (reported by Chen et al.), sprain or contusions, head
injuries, fractures, and organ injuries (Chen et al. 2011, 892–898).

Research has shown that up to 99% of the inspected wheelchairs needed maintenance to perform correctly (Hansen, Tresse, and Gunnarsson 2004, 631–639;

Young et al. 1985, 1388–1389). Moreover, there has been an increase in wheelchair failure rates; users have reported the need for wheelchair repairs increasingly in the last couple of years, from 44.8% in 2009 to more than 63.8% in 2016 (Calder and Kirby 1990, 184–190; Toro et al. 2016, 1753–1760; Worobey et al. 2012, 463–469; Worobey et al. 2014, 597–603). Additionally, wheelchair users have reported experiencing an increase in consequences due to a failure, from 22% in 2006 to 30% in 2011 (Worobey et al. 2012, 463–469).

More than half (63.8%) of the individuals surveyed in a study (n=591) reported needing at least one repair in a six-month period, and 27.6% reported at least one adverse consequence because of the breakdown (Toro et al. 2016, 1753–1760). Common adverse consequences reported were being injured or stranded, having less mobility, and decreased quality of life (Toro et al. 2016, 1753–1760). This same study reported that 6.9% of those needing a repair did not complete it. The number of repairs completed at home by wheelchair users was 40% for manual wheelchairs and 14% for power wheelchairs, showing a willingness of users to complete repairs independently. In contrast, 50% of repairs were completed by a vendor, suggesting that users may not know how to perform maintenance on their wheelchairs (Toro et al. 2016, 1753–1760).

A study by Chen et al. reported three significant findings: properly maintained wheelchairs could reduce the risks of wheelchair accidents; wheelchair users perceive that wheelchair-related problems (component failures or technical issues) are one of the main causes of accidents; and some of these component failures can be easily solved if performing regular maintenance (Chen et al. 2011, 892–898). When maintenance is performed, wheelchairs are in better working condition (Arledge et al. 2011) and accidents and injuries for users are significantly less likely to occur (Chen et al. 2011, 892–898; Hansen, Tresse, and Gunnarsson 2004, 631–639). It is important to train wheelchair users on how and when to perform maintenance on their wheelchairs to reduce adverse consequences related to wheelchair malfunction.

12.9 Key concepts

Wheelchairs are one of the most common mobility tools that can be provided to people with mobility impairments. A wheelchair can be a reflection of a person and help them to achieve their goals if properly matched to the user and their goals. If done poorly, a wheelchair can be a trap that limits a person's mobility and can cause harm. Engineers need to learn basic medical principles to understand biomechanics and ergonomics, collaborate with healthcare professionals, and engage with end users to design and assist in the selection and fitting of the most appropriate wheelchair for each individual. Wheelchairs are used for a variety of activities and may be highly specialized for a specific purpose. For example, the design of a racing wheelchair is entirely different from the design of a powered off-road wheelchair, although some basic design principles may apply to both. Some basic principles hold for most sports wheelchairs.

1. *Weight.* In most wheelchairs, especially those where speed or agility are required, the lowest possible weight is often a design goal. Lower weight tends to reduce the force required to propel, power, and maneuver the wheelchair, making it faster, more agile, and easier to transport.

2. *Stiffness and strength.* Ideally, wheelchair frames would be very light, extremely strong, and highly stiff. This would allow the energy transferred from the user or by the motors to the chair to be applied to the desired motion without dissipation However, design trade-offs need to be made to optimize stiffness, strength, and weight.

3. *Resistance.* Mobility is critical to wheelchairs, the goal of designing the wheelchair is to minimize resistance. The most common type of resistance that designers of wheelchairs attempt to control are the following: rolling resistance, and internal friction. Rolling resistance is commonly minimized by choice of wheels, tires, and bearings, and by careful alignment of the wheels. Internal friction is commonly referred to as "flex" or "movement" resulting from the person moving within the seat, the seat moving with respect to the frame, and bending and warping of the frame that causes wheel misalignment or user energy to be dissipated by the frame.

4. *Ergonomics.* The biomechanical and ergonomics goal of wheelchair design is for the device to become one with the user at a subconscious level. At the same time, the fitting and positioning of the user should maximize the control and motion of the wheelchair in response to the volitional movement of the user, with minimal physiological effort. The user interface and interaction are often the most complex design challenges.

These four factors must be weighed against the abilities (physical, physiological, skill) of the user, the safety of the user and other participants, and the goals of the user. The materials, manufacturing, and fitting techniques are determined by these factors, as well as the sport-specific needs and the abilities of the user or users. The design and provision of wheelchairs are complex and require training and experience to become proficient. This chapter only provides some of the basic concepts.

12.10 Custom wheelchair accessories through digital fabrication

The United States Department of Veterans Affairs (VA) is a federal government agency that operates 150 hospitals around the country for veterans of the US military. The VA employs several clinical rehabilitation engineers and during the past five years, they have introduced the use of digital design and fabrication to several rehabilitation clinics. The rehabilitation engineers work side by side with therapists to provide customization and integration of assistive technology solutions for veterans. When assessing a client for mobility, occasionally the assistive technology solution that would best meet the client's needs is not commercially available and so the rehabilitation engineer will use digital design software and additive manufacturing (i.e., 3D printing) to create a custom solution for that client. The most easily implemented additive manufacturing method in clinical settings is FDM followed by the more expensive stereolithography (SLA), selective laser sintering (SLS), and materials jetting methods. Each additive manufacturing technology offers different material selections suited for different applications. FDM lends itself to the clinical rehabilitation setting as printers can be small, easily operated, and produce functional parts for client usage.

Anecdotally, clinical rehabilitation engineers have seen that when clients are given the chance to co-create a custom assistive technology device tailored to their exact needs, they have a much greater sense of ownership in the device and it is less likely to be abandoned.

The following examples illustrate the application of additive manufacturing for commercial product customization and how the implementation of additive manufacturing can enhance current fabrication practices available to rehabilitation clinicians. Specifically, the usage of additive manufacturing can produce more refined end products than traditional clinical fabrication and customization methods. Additionally, 3D-printed solutions can be easily reproduced for the same or additional clients without any substantial fabrication time investment from the clinician.

Example 1: Refining clinician-based customizations

A client with quadriplegia was having difficulty reliably actuating the small power/mode and speed toggle switches on his powered wheelchair (Figure 12.15). Due to no commercial solutions being available, the client's occupational therapist created a press-on adapter from low-temperature moldable thermoplastic that fitted over the toggle switches to enlarge them. This solution was successful, however, the adapters would easily become dislodged and fall to the floor. The clinical rehabilitation engineer noticed this problem and designed a similar adapter with precise dimensions, which, when 3D printed, provided a much tighter fit along with a more ergonomic design. The client reported that he now actuates the switches completely reliably and does not need to even look at his hand anymore.

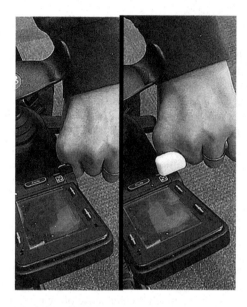

Figure 12.15 Wheelchair joystick toggle switch adapter.

Example 2: Customizing commercially available products based on client needs

An occupational therapist recommended a flexible mount arm containing an air tube and water tube that allowed a client with quadriplegia to drive his powered wheelchair with breath control and independently stay hydrated. However, the two tubes were not supported well enough where they exited the mount arm so the client could not reliably reach them with his mouth due to the extremely limited range of motion of his head. The therapist then requested help from the rehabilitation engineer to develop a solution for the client. Initially, an industrial strength twist tie was used to hold the tubes in a semi-functional location. With feedback from the client, the rehabilitation engineer designed and 3D printed a tray that was attached to the end of the flexible mount arm and held the air tube and water tube at the exact position and angle needed (Figure 12.16). The tray contained a magnetically attached lid to allow for the saliva trap in the air tube to be changed. An embossed message on the tray lid cautioned caregivers to move the arm by handling the flexible portion and not the 3D printed tray. The client chose the color red for the final design as this was his favorite color.

Example 3: Modifying commercial products for alternative usage

A client using a powered wheelchair with a mounted augmentative communication device needed a smartphone mounted next to it. The brand of

288

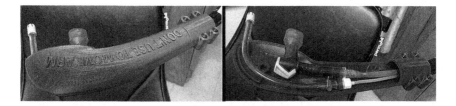

Figure 12.16 Tray for air and water tubes that allow the user to drive a powered wheelchair with breath control independently and stay hydrated.

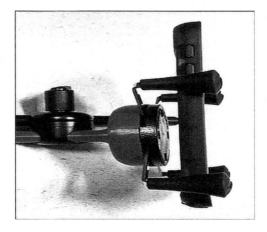

Figure 12.17 Mixing mounting products via adapter provided a universally designed solution.

mount used for the communication device only offered an iPhone-compatible mount cradle. The rehabilitation engineer recommended the client use a universal phone mount from a different brand. To make the two products compatible, a custom adapter was designed and 3D printed (Figure 12.17). This allowed the client to leverage the mount product already on the wheelchair, while at the same time providing a universal smartphone mount compatible with any smartphone the client might use. This adapter was also 3D printed several more times for other clients, thereby distributing the design time cost over several clients.

12.11 Discussion questions

1. List the steps involved in assistive technology service delivery, which of these steps is the most important and why?
2. Describe the optimal methods to keep a wheelchair user secured when traveling in a vehicle.

3. Describe two different types of wheelchairs and their advantages in addressing the seating issues.
4. What are the two basic categories of advanced powered wheelchairs? Give an example for each category.
5. What is the most important principle when designing a wheelchair?
6. Describe the role of rehabilitation engineers in customizing and integrating assistive technology solutions for wheelchair users.
7. What gaps do you wish the authors had filled in? Were there points where you thought they shared too much?

Bibliography

American Speech-Language-Hearing Association. 2004. "Roles and Responsibilities of Speech-Language Pathologists with Respect to Augmentative and Alternative Communication: Technical Report." Rockville, MD: American Speech-Language-Hearing Association.

Arledge, Stan, William Armstrong, Mike Babinec, Brad E. Dicianno, Carmen Digiovine, Trevor Dyson-Hudson, Jessica Pederson, Julie Piriano, Teresa Plummer, and Lauren Rosen. 2011. "RESNA Wheelchair Service Provision Guide." *Resna (Nj1).*

Association for Driver Rehabilitation Specialists. 2016. "Best Practice Guidelines for the Delivery of Driver Rehabilitation Services." http://c.ymcdn.com/sites/www.aded.net/resource/resmgr/docs/ADED_BestPracticeGuidelines_pdf.

Bach, J. R., A. P. Zeelenberg, and C. Winter. 1990. "Wheelchair-Mounted Robot Manipulators. Long Term Use by Patients with Duchenne Muscular Dystrophy." *American Journal of Physical Medicine & Rehabilitation* 69 (2): 55–59.

Brault, Matthew W. 2012. *Americans with Disabilities: 2010.* US Department of Commerce, Economics and Statistics Administration.

Calder, C. J. and R. L. Kirby. 1990. "Fatal Wheelchair-Related Accidents in the United States." *American Journal of Physical Medicine & Rehabilitation* 69 (4): 184–190.

Chen, Wan-Yin, Yuh Jang, Jung-Der Wang, Wen-Ni Huang, Chan-Chia Chang, Hui-Fen Mao, and Yen-Ho Wang. 2011. "Wheelchair-Related Accidents: Relationship with Wheelchair-Using Behavior in Active Community Wheelchair Users." *Archives of Physical Medicine and Rehabilitation* 92 (6): 892–898.

Chung, Cheng-Shiu. 2015. *Development and Assessment of Advanced Assistive Robotic Manipulators User Interfaces.* http://d-scholarship.pitt.edu/25771/1/JoshuaChung_ETD 2015.pdf.

Chung, Cheng-Shiu and R. A. Cooper. 2012. "Literature Review of Wheelchair-Mounted Robotic Manipulation: User Interface and End-User Evaluation." RESNA Annual Conference.

Chung, Cheng-Shiu, Hongwu Wang, and Rory A. Cooper. 2013a. "Autonomous Function of Wheelchair-Mounted Robotic Manipulators to Perform Daily Activities." IEEE.

———. 2013b. "Functional Assessment and Performance Evaluation for Assistive Robotic Manipulators: Literature Review." *The Journal of Spinal Cord Medicine* 36 (4): 273–289.

Chung, Cheng-Shiu, Hongwu Wang, Dan Ding, and Rory A. Cooper. 2016. "Feasibility Analysis of Daily Activities Using Assistive Robotic Manipulators." RESNA Annual Conference.

Chung, Cheng-Shiu, Hongwu Wang, Matthew J. Hannan, Dan Ding, Annmarie R. Kelleher, and Rory A. Cooper. 2017a. "Task-Oriented Performance Evaluation for Assistive Robotic Manipulators: A Pilot Study." *American Journal of Physical Medicine & Rehabilitation* 96 (6): 395–407.

Chung, Cheng-Shiu, Hongwu Wang, Matthew J. Hannan, Annmarie R. Kelleher, and Rory A. Cooper. 2017b. "Daily Task-Oriented Performance Evaluation for Commercially Available Assistive Robotic Manipulators." *International Journal of Robotics and Automation* 3 (1): 16–27.

Chung, C. S., M. J. Hannan, H. Wang, A. R. Kelleher, and R. A. Cooper. 2014. "Adapted Wolf Motor Function Test for Assistive Robotic Manipulators User Interfaces: A Pilot Study." RESNA Annual Conference.

Cook, AM and SM Hussey. 2001. *Assistive Technologies: Principles and Practice*, Volume 2nd ed. Mosby-Year Book.

Cooper, Rory A., Brad E. Dicianno, Bambi Brewer, Edmund LoPresti, Dan Ding, Richard Simpson, Garrett Grindle, and Hongwu Wang. 2008. "A Perspective on Intelligent Devices and Environments in Medical Rehabilitation." *Medical Engineering & Physics* 30 (10): 1387–1398.

Cooper, Rory A., Garrett G. Grindle, JJ Vazquez, Jijie Xu, Hongwu Wang, Jorge Candiotti, C. Chung, Ben Salatin, Elaine Houston, and Annmarie Kelleher. 2012. "Personal Mobility and Manipulation Appliance—Design, Development, and Initial Testing." *Proceedings of the IEEE* 100 (8): 2505–2511.

Ding, Dan and Rory A. Cooper. 2005. "Electric Powered Wheelchairs." *IEEE Control Systems Magazine* 25 (2): 22–34.

Driessen, B. J. F., H. G. Evers, and J. A. van Woerden. 2001. "MANUS—A Wheelchair-Mounted Rehabilitation Robot." *Proceedings of the Institution of Mechanical Engineers, Part H: Journal of Engineering in Medicine* 215 (3): 285–290.

Driessen, B. J. F., T. K. Ten Kate, F. Liefhebber, A. H. G. Versluis, and J. A. Van Woerden. 2005. "Collaborative Control of the Manus Manipulator." *Universal Access in the Information Society* 4 (2): 165–173.

Edwards, Kara and Annie McCluskey. 2010. "A Survey of Adult Power Wheelchair and Scooter Users." *Disability and Rehabilitation: Assistive Technology* 5 (6): 411–419.

Fehr, Linda, W. Edwin Langbein, and Steven B. Skaar. 2000. "Adequacy of Power Wheelchair Control Interfaces for Persons with Severe Disabilities: A Clinical Survey." *Journal of Rehabilitation Research and Development* 37 (3): 353–360.

Field, Marilyn J., Alan M. Jette, and Institute of Medicine (US) Committee on Disability in America. 2007. "Transportation Patterns and Problems of People with Disabilities." In *The Future of Disability in America*. National Academies Press.

Fuhrer, Marcus J., Jeffrey W. Jutai, Marcia J. Scherer, and Frank DeRuyter. 2003. "A Framework for the Conceptual Modelling of Assistive Technology Device Outcomes." *Disability and Rehabilitation* 25 (22): 1243–1251.

Gitlin, Laura N. 2002. "Assistive Technology in the Home and Community for Older People: Psychological and Social Considerations." In *Assistive Technology: Matching Device and Consumer for Successful Rehabilitation*, edited by M. J. Scherer, 109–122. Washington, DC: American Psychological Association.

Government of New South Wales, Australia. 2016. "Augmentative and Alternative Communication (AAC) Guidelines for Speech Pathologists Who Support People with Disability." http://www.adhc.nsw.gov.au/__data/assets/file/0011/302402/Augmentative _and_Alternative_Communication_Practice_Guide.pdf.

Groothuis, Stefan S., Stefano Stramigioli, and Raffaella Carloni. 2013. "Lending a Helping Hand: Toward Novel Assistive Robotic Arms." *IEEE Robotics & Automation Magazine* 20 (1): 20–29.

Hammel, Joy, Karyl Hall, David Lees, Larry Leifer, Machiel Van der Loos, Inder Perkash, and Robert Crigler. 1989. "Clinical Evaluation of a Desktop Robotic Assistant." *Journal of Rehabilitation Research and Development* 26 (3): 1–16.

Hansen, Rich, S. Tresse, and R. K. Gunnarsson. 2004. "Fewer Accidents and Better Maintenance with Active Wheelchair Check-Ups: A Randomized Controlled Clinical Trial." *Clinical Rehabilitation* 18 (6): 631–639.

Hatao, Naotaka, Satoshi Kagami, Ryo Hanai, Kimitoshi Yamazaki, and Masayuki Inaba. 2014. *Construction of Semantic Maps for Personal Mobility Robots in Dynamic Outdoor Environments.* Springer.

Health Ministry and Social Protection. "Registry for the Localization and Characterization for People with Disabilities." https://www.minsalud.gov.co/proteccionsocial/Paginas/DisCapacidad_RLCPD.aspx.

Jefferds, A. N., N. M. Beyene, N. Upadhyay, P. Shoker, J. L. Pearlman, R. A. Cooper, and J. Wee. 2010. "Current State of Mobility Technology Provision in Less-Resourced Countries." *Physical Medicine and Rehabilitation Clinics of North America* 21 (1): 221–242.

Kairy, Dahlia, Paula Rushton, Philippe Archambault, Evelina Pituch, Caryne Torkia, Anas El Fathi, Paula Stone, François Routhier, Robert Forget, and Louise Demers. 2014. "Exploring Powered Wheelchair Users and Their Caregivers' Perspectives on Potential Intelligent Power Wheelchair Use: A Qualitative Study." *International Journal of Environmental Research and Public Health* 11 (2): 2244–2261.

Lane, Amy, Elizabeth Green, Anne E. Dickerson, Elin Schold Davis, Beth Rolland, and Janet T. Stohler. 2014. "Driver Rehabilitation Programs: Defining Program Models, Services, and Expertise." *Occupational Therapy in Health Care* 28 (2): 177–187.

Maheu, Veronique, Philippe S. Archambault, Julie Frappier, and François Routhier. 2011. "Evaluation of the JACO Robotic Arm: Clinico-Economic Study for Powered Wheelchair Users with Upper-Extremity Disabilities." IEEE.

National Mobility Equipment Dealers Association. "Guidelines 2017 Edition." http://www.nmeda.com/wp-content/uploads/2017/01/QAP-103-2017-Guidelines.pdf.

Pearlman, Jon, Rory A. Cooper, Marc Krizack, Alida Lindsley, Yeongchi Wu, Kim D. Reisinger, William Armstrong, Hector Casanova, Harvinder Singh Chhabra, and Jamie Noon. 2008. "Lower-Limb Prostheses and Wheelchairs in Low-Income Countries [An Overview]." *IEEE Engineering in Medicine and Biology Magazine* 27 (2): 12–22.

Phillips, Betsy and Hongxin Zhao. 1993. "Predictors of Assistive Technology Abandonment." *Assistive Technology* 5 (1): 36–45.

Prior, Stephen D. and Peter R. Warner. 1993. "Wheelchair-Mounted Robots for the Home Environment." IEEE.

RESNA. "Find a Certified AT Professional." http://www.resna.org/member-directory/individual.

Scherer, Marcia J. and Laura A. Cushman. 2001. "Measuring Subjective Quality of Life Following Spinal Cord Injury: A Validation Study of the Assistive Technology Device Predisposition Assessment." *Disability and Rehabilitation* 23 (9): 387–393.

Simpson, Richard C. 2005. "Smart Wheelchairs: A Literature Review." *Journal of Rehabilitation Research and Development* 42 (4): 423.

Stanger, Carol A., Carolyn Anglin, William S. Harwin, and Douglas P. Romilly. 1994. "Devices for Assisting Manipulation: A Summary of User Task Priorities." *IEEE Transactions on Rehabilitation Engineering* 2 (4): 256–265.

Sundaram, S. Andrea, Hongwu Wang, Dan Ding, and Rory A. Cooper. 2017. "Step-Climbing Power Wheelchairs: A Literature Review." *Topics in Spinal Cord Injury Rehabilitation* 23 (2): 98–109.

Toro, Maria Luisa, Lynn Worobey, Michael L. Boninger, Rory A. Cooper, and Jonathan Pearlman. 2016. "Type and Frequency of Reported Wheelchair Repairs and Related Adverse Consequences among People with Spinal Cord Injury." *Archives of Physical Medicine and Rehabilitation* 97 (10): 1753–1760.

United Nations. 2006. *Convention on the Rights of Persons with Disabilities and Optional Protocol*. United Nations.

University of Michigan Transportation Research Institute. "Wheelchair Transportation Safety." http://wc-transportation-safety.umtri.umich.edu/.

US Census Bureau. "FFF: 25th Anniversary of Americans with Disabilities Act: July 2016." https://www.census.gov/newsroom/facts-for-features/2015/cb15-ff10.html.

Visagie, S., T. Mlambo, J. van der Veen, C. Nhunzvi, D. Tigere, and E. Scheffler. 2015. "Is any Wheelchair Better than no Wheelchair? A Zimbabwean Perspective." *African Journal of Disability* 4 (1): 201.

Wang, Hongwu, Garrett G. Grindle, Jorge Candiotti, Chengshiu Chung, Motoki Shino, Elaine Houston, and Rory A. Cooper. 2012. "The Personal Mobility and Manipulation Appliance (PerMMA): A Robotic Wheelchair with Advanced Mobility and Manipulation." IEEE.

Wang, Hongwu, Jijie Xu, Garrett Grindle, Juan Vazquez, Ben Salatin, Annmarie Kelleher, Dan Ding, Diane M. Collins, and Rory A. Cooper. 2013. "Performance Evaluation of the Personal Mobility and Manipulation Appliance (PerMMA)." *Medical Engineering & Physics* 35 (11): 1613–1619.

World Health Organization. 2008. *Guidelines on the Provision of Manual Wheelchairs in Less Resourced Settings*. World Health Organization.

———. 2011. "United States Agency for International Development." *Joint Position Paper on the Provision of Mobility Devices in Less Resourced Settings*.

———. "Wheelchair Service Training Package - Basic Level." http://www.who.int/disabilities/technology/wheelchairpackage/en/.

———. "Wheelchair Service Training Package - Intermediate Level." http://www.who.int/disabilities/technology/wheelchairpackage/wstpintermediate/en/.

———. "Wheelchair Service Training Package for Managers." http://www.who.int/phi/implementation/assistive_technology/wheelchair_train-pack_managers/en/.

———. "Wheelchair Service Training Package for Stakeholders." http://apps.who.int/iris/bitstream/10665/246227/5/9789241549080-stakeholders-eng.pdf.

———. 2015. *World Report on Ageing and Health*. World Health Organization.

Worobey, Lynn, Michelle Oyster, Jonathan Pearlman, Benjamin Gebrosky, and Michael L. Boninger. 2014. "Differences between Manufacturers in Reported Power Wheelchair Repairs and Adverse Consequences among People with Spinal Cord Injury." *Archives of Physical Medicine and Rehabilitation* 95 (4): 597–603.

Worobey, L., M. Oyster, G. Nemunaitis, R. Cooper, and M. L. Boninger. 2012. "Increases in Wheelchair Breakdowns, Repairs, and Adverse Consequences for People with Traumatic Spinal Cord Injury." *American Journal of Physical Medicine & Rehabilitation* 91 (6): 463–469.

Wretstrand, Anders, Jan Petzäll, and Agneta Ståhl. 2004. "Safety as Perceived by Wheelchair-Seated Passengers in Special Transportation Services." *Accident Analysis & Prevention* 36 (1): 3–11.

Yanco, Holly A. and Karen Zita Haigh. 2002. "Automation as Caregiver: A Survey of Issues and Technologies." *American Association for Artificial Intelligence* 2: 39–53.

Young, J. B., P. W. Belfield, B. H. Mascie-Taylor, and G. P. Mulley. 1985. "The Neglected Hospital Wheelchair." *British Medical Journal (Clinical Research Ed.)* 291 (6506): 1388–1389.

Chapter 13 Universal design and the built environment

J. Maisel and E. Steinfeld

Contents

13.1 Chapter overview

Universal design (UD) has been adopted enthusiastically by many members of both the rehabilitation technology and environmental design communities. It offers these two disciplines a great opportunity to influence society at large by taking a leadership role in re-shaping the physical world using human-centered design. Moreover, it provides a vehicle through which the two disciplines can forge a partnership and demonstrate how creative ideas can be developed and implemented to serve people who have disabilities, and the broader population as well. This chapter describes the need for universal design, its evolution, and its application across various domains of the built environment. It concludes with speculation on the future role that universal design will play in advancing rehabilitation goals and transferring knowledge from rehabilitation to general environmental design practices.

DOI: 10.1201/b21964-16

13.2 The need for universal design

Disability is part of the human condition. It results from a mismatch between the goals and abilities of an individual and the demands of both the social and physical environment. Almost everyone will be temporarily or permanently impaired at some point in life, and those who survive to old age will experience increasing difficulties in body function. The importance of disablement as a cultural condition will grow as life expectancies continue to increase because the prevalence of disability increases with age. People with disabilities experience greater barriers to participation in the environment (Nary, Froehlich, and White 2000, 87–98) and these barriers impede their full involvement in community life (Clarke et al. 2011, 1674–1684). Physical access to the built environment plays an important role in creating an inclusive society because it supports participation in workplaces, educational programs, healthcare, the community, transportation, and social and recreational activities.

Rehabilitation practice focuses primarily on helping individuals with disabilities to overcome their daily barriers to independence and participation. Environmental design can reduce those barriers and make the rehabilitation practitioner's job easier, reduce the cost of rehabilitation technology, and increase freedom of action for people with disabilities. Prior to the development of the UD concept, designers sought to remove barriers for people with disabilities alone. However, experience with "barrier-free design" quickly demonstrated that the broader population could benefit as well. Good examples are lever-handled doors and curb ramps. Universal design, therefore, seeks to bring the benefits of more usable, healthier, and friendlier settings to the entire population, recognizing that everyone encounters disablement at some time. It is aligned with other progressive environmental design practices like design for inclusion of minority groups, design for active living, and design for health, all of which position human needs and aspirations as the central focus of design practice. As the population ages, traditional rehabilitation practices will not be able to address all of the needs of people with disabilities; community-wide solutions that do not require one-on-one rehabilitation care will be necessary.

13.3 Evolution of universal design

Most highly developed countries and many other countries have laws that have some level of physical access to the built environment for people with disabilities. For example, in the United States, the Americans with Disabilities Act (1990; 2008) requires accessibility to all types of buildings with the exception of privately financed housing, and the Fair Housing Act and its Amendments (1968; 1988) require accessibility to multifamily housing. The Australian Disability Discrimination Act (1992), the Canadian Constitution—Charter of Rights and

Freedoms (1982), the UK Disability Rights Act (1999), and the Irish Disability Act (2005) are other examples. Some countries have specific minimum standards included or referenced by their anti-discrimination laws, while others have minimum accessibility requirements included in their building regulations rather than regulations for anti-discrimination laws, and others have both. The Disability Education Defense Foundation has developed a list of anti-discrimination laws, although it may not be completely up to date.*

"Accessibility," or removing barriers to access and use of resources in buildings, was the initial paradigm of physical access for people with disabilities (Thapar et al. 2004, 280–289). Accessibility regulations include both rules about construction, incorporated in design standards and guidelines referenced by the regulations, and policies and practices for managing the environment (e.g., facilities management). The rehabilitation community has contributed greatly to the development of these policies, regulations, and practices, but, because they are implemented by government, they are limited in both scope and effectiveness to minimal conditions of access, safety, and usability. Instead, they need to be implemented throughout the entire construction sector and across all economic levels. For example, accessibility regulations focus on giving people access to buildings and facilities, but not on other issues that support social integration, remove stigma, promote health, or increase employment opportunities. Rehabilitation and environmental design professions have extensive knowledge that can be brought to bear not only for improving regulations, but also for advancing voluntary efforts that have larger goals to improve usability, wellness, and social participation.

In response to the limitations of current regulations, the concept of universal design emerged in the mid-1980s as a new paradigm for physical access. UD does not eliminate the need for standards that define the legal baseline for minimum accessibility. Instead, UD seeks to provide more aspirational goals than minimum regulatory requirements. UD initially sought to raise the bar on accessibility, address issues not yet covered by regulations, and make access an integral part of good design. UD was initially defined as "the design of products and environments to be usable by all people, to the greatest extent possible, without the need for adaptation or specialized design" (Mace 1985, 147–152). In keeping with the evolving conception of disablement, as embodied by the revisions to the WHO's International Classification of Diseases, UD has evolved from initially focusing on supporting independent function to addressing additional goals (Hammel et al. 2008, 143–149; Steinfeld and Maisel 2012; Watchorn et al. 2014, 65–88). Furthermore, the application of UD has expanded beyond building and product design and is now reflected in policies and practices in urban design,

---

* See https://dredf.org/legal-advocacy/international-disability-rights/international-laws/ for a list of laws by country.

town planning, transportation, and even education (World Health Organization 2007; Bringa 2007; Steinfeld 2001; Meyer, Rose, and Gordon 2014).

In order to encompass these new ideas, Steinfeld and Maisel (2012) offered a new definition: "Universal design is a process that enables and empowers a diverse population by improving human performance, health and wellness, and social participation." In short, UD benefits everyone. Moreover, it is a process that should be based on a commitment to continual improvement even, in the case of built environments, after a building or facility is constructed.

Steinfeld and Maisel (2012) developed eight Goals of Universal Design to clarify the outcomes of UD practice:

- Body fit: accommodating a wide range of body sizes and abilities
- Comfort: keeping demands within desirable limits of body function and perception
- Awareness: ensuring that critical information for use is easily perceived
- Understanding: making methods of operation and use intuitive, clear, and unambiguous
- Wellness: contributing to health promotion, avoidance of disease, and hazard protection
- Social integration: treating all groups with dignity and respect
- Personalization: incorporating opportunities for choice and individual preferences
- Cultural appropriateness: respecting and reinforcing positive cultural values and the social and environmental context of any design project.

Complementing the earlier Principles of UD (Mace et al. 1997), the Goals define the outcomes of UD practice in ways that can be measured and applied to all design domains within the constraints of existing resources. In addition, they encompass functional, social, and emotional dimensions. Moreover, each Goal is supported by an interdisciplinary knowledge base (e.g., anthropometrics, bio-mechanics, perception, cognition, safety and health promotion, social interaction, and cultural values and practices). Thus, the Goals can be used effectively as a framework for both knowledge discovery and knowledge translation to practice. Moreover, the Goals help to tie policy embodied in disability rights laws to UD and provide a basis for improving regulatory activities by adopting an outcomes-based approach.

13.4 Who benefits from universal design?

The two largest target stakeholder groups that benefit from UD are people with disabilities and older adults. About 15% of the world's population lives with some form of disability, of whom 2–4% experience significant difficulties in functioning (Officer and Posarac 2011). In the United States, almost 19% of the US adult population reports some form of disability, and close to 13% report a severe disability (Brault 2012). In addition, 8.5% of people worldwide (617 million) are aged 65 and over. This percentage is projected to jump to nearly 17% of the world's population by 2050 (1.6 billion; He, Goodkind, and Kowal 2016). Due to aging populations, the higher risk of disability in older people, as well as the global increase in chronic health conditions such as diabetes, cardiovascular disease, cancer, and mental health disorders, the prevalence of disability will continue to rise.

Demographic factors interact in complex ways. For example, those experiencing disability are much more likely to be unemployed and in poverty (Brault 2012). Gerontologists also point out that older African American women are subject to a "triple threat" in quality of life. Each demographic category—gender, minority status, and age—increases the likelihood that a person will have lower disposable income, worse health, and other low quality of life outcomes (Bowen, Tomoyasu, and Cauce 1992, 123–143). Although accessibility laws focus primarily on design for mobility, and to a more limited extent, vision and hearing, UD addresses a full spectrum of disability concerns and recognizes the interrelationship of other demographic factors such as income, age, race, and ethnicity. It is critically important to remember that all people, at one time or another, are "disabled" by the demands of the environment or when they are sick, injured, tired, in an unfamiliar place, carrying a heavy burden, dealing with adverse conditions, homeless, or victims of disasters. Reducing the stress of everyday life, promoting health, and supporting social participation are valued by everyone.

Since UD is not mandated by laws, it needs to appeal to building owners and design professionals in order to be widely adopted. Thus, understanding and communicating the benefits of more usable, healthier, and socially sustainable environments, and establishing a business case for its adoption, that is, proving that the cost of UD is minimal or that any additional cost incurred is worth the investment, is paramount.

13.5 Universal design and housing

Most countries that have signed on to the UN Convention on the Rights of People with Disabilities have legal mandates to provide accessible housing. These mandates require various degrees of accessibility and cover different types of housing. Some countries only require the provision of accessibility in publicly funded housing, and sometimes only for a few units. Others require accessibility in every unit. There are only a few countries that require accessibility to owner-occupied single-family homes.

Researchers and policymakers expect the need for accessible housing in the United States, and other developed countries, to increase substantially in the next few decades as the population ages. Approximately 70% of Americans, for example, live in single-family homes (US Census Bureau, Housing and Household Economic Statistics Division 2011), and the overwhelming majority of these housing units have barriers that make it difficult or impossible for someone with physical disabilities to enter/exit or live independently. Many houses have steps at all entrances and hallways and doorways too narrow for users of wheelchairs or walkers to pass through easily, if at all. Furthermore, architectural barriers make it difficult for other households to accommodate visits from friends and relatives who need basic accessibility.

These barriers often result in significant consequences. In addition to social isolation and dependence, many people with severe mobility impairments may be unable to exit their homes independently in an emergency and risk injury from falling. Barriers within a home can also increase the work and stress of the caretakers who assist older adults and people with disabilities. Many family caregivers report that they suffer physical injuries as a result of lifting and handling their relatives, as well as psychological health problems such as fatigue, anxiety, and depression (Brown and Mulley 1997, 21–23). Young people with disabilities who live in inaccessible housing have little chance of leading independent lives or seeking employment.

Barriers can make it difficult for older people to remain in their homes as they encounter age-related physical limitations. According to a survey conducted for AARP, a nonprofit, nonpartisan membership organization that seeks to address the needs and interests of the 50+ population in the United States, 87% of adults age 65+ want to stay in their current residence for as long as possible (AARP PPI 2014). Aging in place offers numerous social and financial benefits. Research shows that independent living promotes life satisfaction, health, and self-esteem, three keys to successful aging. Furthermore, older adults get a sense of familiarity, comfort, and meaning from their own home (Herzog and House 1991).

Changes in public policy and new design practices emerged in response to the need for more accessible homes. Visitability represents a highly focused strategy in the continuing evolution of accessible housing policy and practice. Visitability is an affordable, sustainable, and inclusive design approach for integrating basic accessibility features as a routine construction practice in all newly built homes. Although visitability does not provide the same level of usability as older forms of accessible housing, it is a UD strategy because it provides a foundation for improving the home with additional UD features, thereby lowering the cost of housing adaptations. Visitability includes a few basic accessibility features. In the United States, they are as follows: one zero-step entrance at the front, side, or rear of the home; 32-inch wide clearances at doorways and hallways with at least 36 inches of clear width; and at least a half bath on the main floor (Maisel, Smith, and Steinfeld 2008, 1–34). Figure 13.1 shows visitable homes in Oak Hill, PA, which confirms that visitability can be introduced in cold weather regions that have homes with basements. Visitability provides benefits to a wide range of users, including those with disabilities, their nuclear family, friends, and other relatives who may, from time to time, need to use wheelchairs or other adaptive equipment.

A more extensive array of features can improve usability, safety, and health for people with disabilities, and also support aging in place. In many countries, new housing designs are being produced in order to reduce the need for relocation and supportive services over time. This type of housing, sometimes called "lifespan housing" (Steinfeld et al. 2010, 51–67) has many universal design features and represents a noteworthy development in the field of housing. Figure 13.2 shows the interior of the LIFEHouse, a UD concept house built in the award-winning planned community of Newport Cove, IL. The home demonstrates that UD can easily be incorporated into track housing without sacrificing aesthetics or marketability.

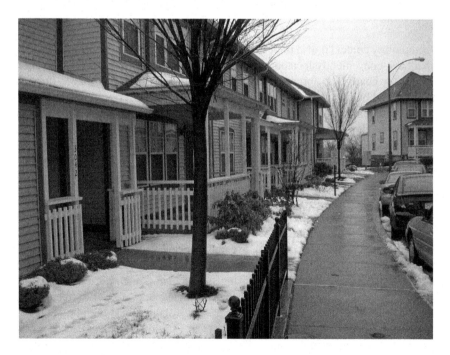

Figure 13.1 Visitable homes in Oak Hill, PA (courtesy of Jordana Maisel, 2017).

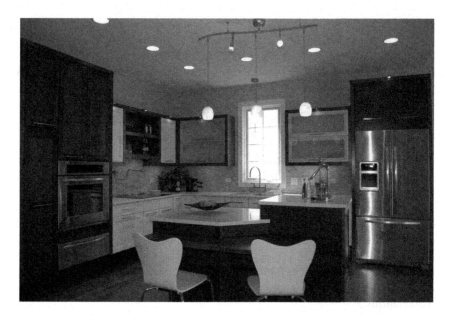

Figure 13.2 LIFEHouse interior in Newport Cove, IL (courtesy of Jordana Maisel, 2017).

Community context is also important for aging in place. It requires neighborhoods that have conveniently located community services, opportunities for recreation and work nearby, a vibrant street life, and informal gathering places through which neighbors can more easily get to know each other. Traditional neighborhood development, or TND, is an example (Smith 2015, 15–32). But traditional neighborhoods have a high degree of inaccessible buildings and streetscapes. Applying UD to TND-type planning ensures that redeveloping both newer and older neighborhoods will have the benefits of traditional walkable and balanced neighborhoods, while not perpetuating the barriers of the past.

Existing neighborhoods can initiate developing small housing for older adults, including assistive living options, so that residents can maintain existing social networks when they cannot live alone anymore. But building new units alone will not address the total demand. So, another key component of UD in neighborhood planning includes affordable housing residential repair and renovation services that can adapt existing housing for occupants with disabilities. At the neighborhood scale, initiatives to improve neglected sidewalks and streetscapes, and key neighborhood resources like places of worship, must accompany housing improvements. Figure 13.3 shows streetscape improvements in Park Heights, an older Baltimore neighborhood. These improvements were initiated by a local nonprofit neighborhood development organization that also initiated several programs to support older residents in their homes, including home adaptation

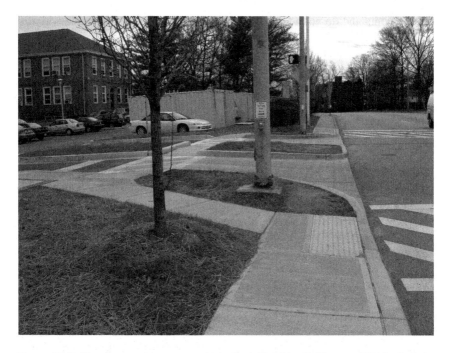

Figure 13.3 Streetscape improvements in Park Heights, Baltimore, MD, included marked street crossings, pedestrian signals with countdown signs, increased crossing time, benches at bus stops, improved street lighting, and curb ramps (courtesy of Jordana Maisel, 2017).

services, outreach and supportive services, and community management of existing apartment buildings with large numbers of older people.

There is a tendency to view design for aging in place as something desirable only by people over the age of 50. However, the same features that assist older residents to age gracefully in their homes and neighborhoods are also desirable for other age groups. Stress on families due to an increase in single-headed households, a need for both parents to work, time demands of competitive work environments, concerns for the safety and security of children, rising rates of asthma, and the health effects of inactive lifestyles all contribute to the desirability of safe, convenient, and healthy housing and neighborhoods.

13.6 Universal design and public accommodations

Most developed and developing countries have regulations that require accessibility to public accommodations, although enforcement of these regulations varies significantly from country to country. These regulations, however, are minimum requirements and do not address the full spectrum of needs of people with disabilities or older adults. The rehabilitation community has participated in the development of standards and regulations (see, for example, Steinfeld et al. 2010, 51–67). But there is a lot more knowledge within the community that could be translated to improve their effectiveness. In some cases, rehabilitation research actually contradicts standard requirements. For example, research on the design of grab bars suggests that older people in assistive living facilities need different types of grab bars than those provided in public buildings (Sanford, Echt, and Malassigné 2000, 39–58).

In 2004, an expert panel was convened in the United States to set an agenda for UD. To advance UD adoption, they recommended developing "tools suitable for use in a variety of practical applications" in forms that "communicate effectively to all of the diverse stakeholders of universal design" (National Endowment for the Arts (NEA) 2004a; NEA 2004c). They noted that UD "is still marginalized and not integral to mainstream design education and practice" (NEA 2004b). Barriers to UD adoption include the following: confusion about how it differs from conventional accessible design (ArchVoices 2002; NEA 1999); lack of flexibility in codes (NEA 1999); and a perception that UD will cost more and not be worth it. The panel concluded that such tools can demonstrate how UD differs from conventional accessible design, supports improvements in standards and codes, and illustrates cost-effective solutions that will help to overcome these barriers.

Mandatory standards and regulations are a vehicle for evidence-based building design. Experts usually develop them to translate research and practical knowledge into guidelines for practice. Architects, product designers, and other design professionals rely on these guidelines rather than directly consulting the research literature (Vaughan and Turner 2013). Mandatory regulations and standards, however, are time consuming to develop, cannot be changed easily, and are politically contentious. Thus, the knowledge embodied in typical regulations and standards often lags behind the growth of scientific evidence and practical experience, especially in the early stages of a field of knowledge. UD can be implemented much faster by using expert opinion to identify guidelines, updating them regularly, and creating incentives for adopting solutions, that is, the carrot instead of the stick. To this end, the Center for Inclusive Design and Environmental Access developed innovative solutions for universal design, or isUD (www.thisisud.com) with funding support from the National Institute on Disability, Independent Living, and Rehabilitation Research (NIDILRR). isUD has higher and more inclusive goals than accessibility standards and regulations, and addresses usability, safety, wellness, and social participation. The isUD business model is based on the success of the US Green Building Council and the Green Building Initiative, both developed standards (i.e., LEED and Green Globes, respectively), and provides services like

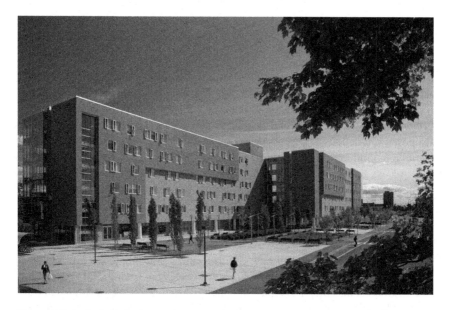

Figure 13.4 Greiner Hall at the University at Buffalo (courtesy of Jordana Maisel, 2017).

certifying buildings that recognize competency in sustainable design practices. isUD is designed to offer similar resources and services to support and recognize UD adopters. Figure 13.4 shows Greiner Hall, a relatively new residential facility at the University at Buffalo that was designed using an early version of isUD.

IsUD certification will provide several benefits to UD adopters: (1) a means to implement UD solutions; (2) a branding opportunity for engaging in socially responsible activities; (3) reduced liability in the operation of buildings by increasing accessibility and safety, and creating healthier environments; and (4) increased employee and visitor satisfaction that leads to increased productivity, repeat visits, and other benefits. Proponents of UD could also use the program as a focus of public education programs to increase demand for UD among consumers. The isUD system also provides a framework for developing a "community of practice," through which many participants with key knowledge, including the rehabilitation community, can contribute relevant evidence to support UD solutions.

13.7 Universal design and streetscapes

Public rights-of-way (ROW) include roads, bicycle paths, and sidewalks that support multiple transportation modes (e.g., motor vehicles, bicycles, and pedestrians).

Over the last decade, new ROW design principles increased the priority given to non-automotive, or "active transportation" modes, and to the needs of diverse user groups.

There are few guidelines or resources for designing accessible public ROWs. The ADA Accessibility Guidelines (ADAAG) and the ABA Accessibility Guidelines for Buildings and Facilities address features such as curb ramps, sidewalk routes, ground and floor surfaces, and bus stops and shelters. The US Access Board's Proposed Guidelines for Accessible Rights-of-Way provide guidance for space limitations and conditions unique to public ROW and people with disabilities (US Access Board 2011). The Federal Highway Administration produced similar design guidelines for sidewalks and trails (Federal Highway Administration 1999; Federal Highway Administration 2001).

From a UD perspective, there are important design challenges associated with public ROWs, including excessive cross-slopes, rough and slippery surface materials, irregular pavement, and lack of curb ramps. Many injuries are related to outdoor ramps used by wheeled mobility users (Xiang, Chany, and Smith 2006, 8–11; Edlich et al. 2010, 150–154). In a national poll of people over 50 years old, 47% said it was unsafe to cross the street near their home. Almost 40% said their neighborhood lacks adequate sidewalks (Lynott et al. 2009), creating a disincentive to walking. The oldest pedestrians (75+ years) incur fatality rates nearly twice the national average for those under 65 years of age (Ernst and Shoup 2009). Since residents with disabilities drive less frequently and already feel more isolated from their communities (BTS 2003), any barrier to outdoor mobility further impedes their ability to function independently and participate in the community (Clarke, Ailshire, and Lantz 2009, 964–970; Glass and Balfour 2003, 303–334).

The growing number of federal initiatives (e.g., the Partnership for Sustainable Communities by HUD, EPA, and DOT, and the US National Physical Activity Plan), and local policies that stress the importance of safe and accessible pedestrian environments, reinforce the need to address ROW design challenges. Nearly 1000 municipalities have adopted "Complete Streets" (CS) policies to date. The CS approach encourages ROWS to be "designed for the safety and comfort of all road users, regardless of age and ability" (Lynott et al. 2009) and introduces public health and economic vitality as critical transportation goals.

CS encourages changes to planning efforts that balance the needs of pedestrians, bicyclists, public transportation users, and motorists, regardless of age, ability, income, ethnicity, or mode of travel (National Complete Streets Coalition 2010). The community benefits of the CS approach include urban revitalization, traffic calming, improved pedestrian safety, reduced vehicle usage and the concomitant fuel consumption and greenhouse gas emissions, improved population health due to increases in walking and bicycling, and improved access to daily services for older adults and people with disabilities (Boarnet et al. 2005, 301–317; McCann

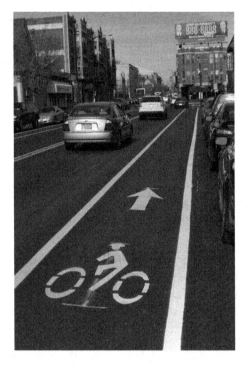

Figure 13.5 A Complete Street with a bike lane in Buffalo, NY (courtesy of Jordana Maisel, Information Classification: General 2017).

and Rynne 2010). Figure 13.5 shows an example of a Complete Street with bike lanes in Buffalo, NY.

Limited research has explored the implementation and evaluation of CS projects on a national scale, thus the effectiveness of existing guidelines is still unclear. Two recent field studies conducted by the IDeA Center, and funded by NIDILRR, found that municipalities around the United States are generally not capturing data regarding the impact of their Complete Streets projects (Lenker et al. 2016). In fact, many municipalities are not even maintaining systematic quantitative descriptions of their Complete Streets project outputs. A recently completed study, however, funded by the New York State Energy Research and Development Authority, found that when pre- and post-implementation data points are available, CS corridors absorb higher volumes of vehicles, pedestrians, and cyclists, and become safer in terms of total crashes and injuries. Additionally, survey responses from 2200 residents, merchants, and streetscape users indicated a positive and substantial increase in walking and biking behaviors, suggesting that Complete Streets corridors support and elicit healthy behaviors.

13.8 Universal design and public transportation

Transportation is critical for ensuring community engagement, productivity, and social participation for individuals with disabilities (Sundar et al. 2016, 682–691). The accessibility of a transportation system has to be understood from the perspective of the entire **travel chain** (Iwarsson, Jensen, and Ståhl 2000, 3–12). The links in the travel chain include trip planning, traveling to the station, using the station/stop, boarding vehicles, using vehicles, leaving vehicles, using the stop or transferring, and traveling to the destination after leaving the station or stop. If one link is not accessible, then access to a subsequent link is unattainable and the trip cannot be completed. Thus, the travel chain defines the scope of potential research and development in accessible public transportation. The "last mile" problem is a persistent issue in the creation of an accessible travel chain; the inability to get to and from stops/stations results in a lack of mobility or a dependency on costly paratransit.

In the United States, more than half a million people with disabilities cannot leave their homes because of transportation difficulties (BTS 2003). Without access to transportation, older adults and people with disabilities are more likely to be excluded from services, social contact, and become stuck in a disability-poverty cycle (Roberts and Babinard 2004; Venter et al. 2004, 23–26), which, in turn, can lead to social isolation, depression, and health deterioration (Sundar et al. 2016, 682–691; Steptoe et al. 2013, 5797–5801). Since the loss of driving ability often triggers individuals to relocate to long-term care settings, public transit availability and use can lead to large healthcare-related savings.

In many countries, citizens depend on private transportation more than transit. But this is rapidly changing due to increased traffic congestion, an aging population, the fluctuation in gasoline prices, and changes in lifestyle. The Transportation Cooperative Research Program (TCRP) reported that nationally there has been an increase in individuals with disabilities using public transit, including large accessible transit vehicles (LATVs) and paratransit services (Thatcher et al. 2013). Barriers to public transportation particularly affect older adults with lower incomes because they rely on transit more regularly (Houser 2005). In the United States, one of the most auto-dependent countries in the world, one in seven nondrivers over 75 use public transit as their primary mode of transportation (Ritter, Straight, and Evans 2002). Transit use by people over 65, as a share of all the trips they take, increased by a remarkable 40% between 2001 and 2009 in the United States (Lynott and Figueiredo 2011).

In most communities, public transit cannot be affordable without subsidies from local governments. When subsidies are not sufficient, cuts in services lower ridership, even though demand may be increasing, leading to a vicious downward cycle in transportation availability. There is a pressing need for new knowledge and technology to produce more cost-effective solutions.

Current LATVs do not adequately address the accessibility needs of all riders and lead to challenges and frustrations for riders with disabilities, bus operators, and transit agencies. Although LATVs are generally thought to be a safe means of transportation (Shaw and Gillispie 2003, 309–320; Shaw 2000, 89–100), research demonstrates that public transit may present unique safety challenges for wheeled mobility device users (Shaw and Gillispie 2003, 309–320; Songer, Fitzgerald, and Rotko 2004, 115–129). Individuals who use wheeled mobility devices specifically cite securement while riding LATVs as an important concern relating to safety, independence, and dignity (Frost, Bertocci, and Salipur 2013, 16–23). Innovations in securement technology could reduce the challenges related to effective securement, including the need for assistance, receiving unwanted attention, lengthy securement times, and improper and unsafe securement.

Conventional public transportation practices are currently being challenged by the disruptive technologies of ride hailing, ride sharing, and crowdsourcing used by companies like Uber and Lyft. Although these services initially competed only with taxis, they are rapidly entering the public transit arena by contracting with public transit agencies to provide services, particularly where agencies have limited resources. Ride sharing with small buses and vans could replace many fixed route LATV services. Services based on small buses have a good future in accessible transportation. In particular, as the population ages, it will be necessary to increase service to low-density neighborhoods like those in suburbs, and, in older cities, deep into neighborhoods with narrow streets. Further, where demand is low, small buses are much less expensive to purchase and operate. Figure 13.6 shows a low-floor shuttle bus with a deployed ramp. The low-floor models, with kneeling features and ramps, provide more inclusive access than buses with lifts.

There are major controversies about whether these new forms of public transportation are covered by existing accessibility regulations. Are they a public service, which clearly is regulated by laws such as the Americans with Disabilities Act, or are they a private transaction between two individuals not covered by the laws? While litigation and consumer advocacy are addressing this question, Uber and Lyft report that they have internal policies in place to support riders with disabilities which, in some cases, are influenced by negotiated agreements with states and local municipalities (e.g., Portland, California). Even though these companies may take the position that they are not covered by the ADA, in negotiating with local municipalities, they agree to offer services to riders with disabilities to gain access to a market and promote goodwill in the community. Both companies also explicitly prohibit discrimination against people with disabilities.

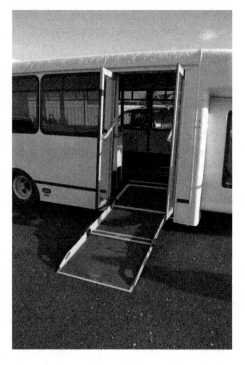

Figure 13.6 A low-floor shuttle bus with a deployed ramp (courtesy of Jordana Maisel).

13.9 Universal design and products

Innovative products conceived for special populations often evolve into mainstream consumer products. When innovations are first designed and developed, they are typically crude and/or expensive. Once perfected through limited use by special populations, the broader benefits are often recognized. The products or technologies are then transformed into mass-manufactured products for the general market. Thus, the special markets can be viewed as proving grounds in which unique needs justify the higher cost of innovative products.

Assistive technology (AT) has the most relevance to UD because of its emphasis on supporting everyday life. AT is now a well-established field for the development of products that compensate for lost function. The Technology Assistance for Individuals Act of 1988 (TECH Act of 1988) defined AT as "any item, piece of equipment or product system, whether acquired commercially off the shelf, modified or customized, that is used to increase, maintain or improve the functional capabilities of individuals with disabilities" (Morrissey and Silverstein 1989); however, the creation of new markets influenced by changing demographics and technological innovations is slowly erasing the line between what is assistive and what is mainstream (Morris, Mueller, and Jones 2010, 131–146).

Despite this blurring of the lines, AT has yet to find a solid place in the larger context of consumer products. The industry needs to explore new directions that will provide it with the resources to realize its full potential. Practicing UD is emerging as an opportunity. AT companies have the knowledge to address usability needs for a wide range of individuals, knowledge that can be applied in UD. However, to be effective, the overall quality of product design must improve. Creating mediocre products would only "result in people being further stigmatized by the very products that are intended to remove barriers for them" (Pullin 2009). It would also continue to lead to high rates of abandonment. Without improving design quality, costs will remain high and may become unaffordable for those who really need AT. Designers need to tackle these challenges and look for ways in which their designs can appeal to larger markets and be more sustainable.

Universally designed products are marketable because they appeal to a diverse group of people. They would not be as successful if only people with disabilities used them, but to be successful in the broader marketplace they must appeal to a broader population. For example, consider the built-up handles commonly used by occupational therapists to adapt silverware and utensils for people who have gripping limitations. It was not until OXO International applied this concept to a mass-marketed product so well that other companies in the utensil industry began to include built-up handles on their products too. The availability of inexpensive utensils with large, easy-to-grip handles in the local discount store and supermarket radically increased the availability and lowered the cost of this feature for everyone. The OXO Good Grips products eventually eliminated the stigma associated with built-up handles and made them an element of style on their own. This is an example of UD as assistive technology for the masses. Moreover, the widespread emergence of smart products is providing additional opportunities to develop new generations of UD products.

Ultimately, the AT community has an excellent opportunity to bring its knowledge about design for diversity and customization to bear in the mainstream market. In addition, the AT community can also benefit from studying how mainstream companies are successfully applying UD ideas to address the increasing diversity of the population.

13.10 The future

UD can increase function and social integration through improved design of physical, virtual, and social environments. Supporters contend that UD helps all people become more self-reliant and reduces the economic burden of special programs and services designed to serve designated groups of people. Making products, services, and environments more accessible to everyone reduces stigma and allows people with disabilities, individuals with low socio-economic status, members of minority groups, and others to more fully engage in the community, which benefits society as a whole (Danford and Maurer 2005, 123-128). In many respects, UD expands the application of knowledge from rehabilitation science and assistive technology to broader domains of practice.

Rehabilitation science has made contributions to improving accessibility to the built environment. However, it could be more effective by using organizations like RESNA, which has member status on consensus standards committees like ANSI A117 and ICC/ANSI A117, to advocate for improved knowledge translation to design guidelines. The rehabilitation community could also be more active in the development of building codes through the consensus process used by the International Code Council to promulgate the International Building Code, a model code used in North America. Alliances with other organizations like the Human Factors and Ergonomics Society, the American Public Health Association, the Congress of New Urbanism, and the Environmental Design Research Association could further advance standards development based on scientific evidence. Certification programs, like isUD, can incorporate guidelines that are not widely accepted in reference standards and mandatory regulations, and their benefits can be proven.

UD advancement could benefit from a re-positioning to align it with other progressive design goals, including design for social justice, health, and sustainability (Steinfeld et al. 2010, 51–67; Steinfeld and Maisel 2012). This includes design for active living to prevent future disability, planning to provide access to healthy food, and interventions to address environmental justice. The intersections between UD and these movements are becoming more evident. Research repeatedly demonstrates that efforts that support environmental design support human health and wellness (Gossett et al. 2009, 439–450; Mikiten 2013). There is also growing awareness among practitioners that true sustainability encompasses not only ecological concerns, but also economic, social, and human health considerations (Vavik and Keitsch 2010, 295–305). By bringing attention to these intersections and finding common ground, UD advocates can gain support from a larger constituency in the design community, learn from the experience and successes of other evidence-based design movements, and demonstrate how the adoption of UD can help reach broader design goals.

Universal design is a new paradigm that replaces the older accessibility paradigm. In the new way of thinking, accessibility regulations are only the first step on a ladder toward improving usability, health and wellness, and social participation for all. There are several major challenges and opportunities in the road ahead. Clarifying the concept of UD is critical at this point in time. In housing, there is a need to promote visitability in all new housing and support and develop innovative ways to deliver renovation and repair services to residents of existing dwellings, especially older people aging in place. Neighborhood improvement strategies focused on safety, comfort, and security must accompany housing improvements to ensure that people with disabilities are able to fully engage in community life and access transportation. In public accommodations, coordinating the many threads of rehabilitation knowledge to improve the development of evidence-based standards would increase the effectiveness of regulations. The isUD program could be a focus for such efforts and a conduit for bringing rehabilitation science and practical knowledge to the design disciplines and business community. In transportation, there is still a lot of work needed to make conventional public transportation safe for riders with disabilities. But there is also a need to identify strategies to ensure that disruptive new technologies do not reduce access to public transportation. Finally, building bridges with other related design movements and organizations (e.g., RESNA) is another important priority to identify common ground and joint advocacy opportunities.

13.11 Discussion questions

1. What are the origins of universal design? Explain how universal design differs from accessible design.
2. What other contemporary design issues have a relationship to universal design? Explain the relationships using examples.
3. Name at least three target populations of universal design. Describe how each can benefit from universal design.
4. Explain how human performance knowledge and other bodies of research specifically relate to universal design and the Goals of Universal Design.
5. Explain the concept of visitability and describe how it is an example of universal design.
6. Explain the role of neighborhoods in supporting aging in place.
7. Describe isUD and discuss how it can serve as a tool for UD implementation in public accommodations.
8. What are Complete Streets and how do they support UD?
9. Describe at least two barriers to public transportation for people with disabilities.
10. Discuss at least two ways rehabilitation science can contribute even more to the built environment.

Bibliography

AARP PPI. "What is Livable? Community Preferences of Older Adults." http://www.aarp.org/livable-communities/info-2014/livable-communities-facts-and-figures.html.

ArchVoices. "Universal Design." http://www.archvoices.org/index.cfm?pg =Resources&s=Is sueArchive&d=newsD&NID=241&MaxResults=30&StartRow=1&searchwords=U niversal%20Design&lineNbr=1.

Boarnet, Marlon G., Kristen Day, Craig Anderson, Tracy McMillan, and Mariela Alfonzo. 2005. "California's Safe Routes to School Program: Impacts on Walking, Bicycling, and Pedestrian Safety." *Journal of the American Planning Association* 71 (3): 301–317.

Bowen, Deborah J., Naomi Tomoyasu, and Ana Mari Cauce. 1992. "The Triple Threat: A Discussion of Gender, Class, and Race Differences in Weight." *Women & Health* 17 (4): 123–143.

Brault, Matthew W. 2012. *Americans with Disabilities: 2010.* US Department of Commerce, Economics and Statistics Administration.

Bringa, Olav Rand. 2007. "Making Universal Design Work in Zoning and Regional Planning: A Scandinavian Approach." In *Universal Design and Visitability: From Accessibility to Zoning.* Boston, MA: Disability Rights Fund.

Brown, Alex R. and Graham P. Mulley. 1997. "Injuries Sustained by Caregivers of Disabled Elderly People." *Age and Ageing* 26 (1): 21–23.

BTS. 2003. "Transportation Difficulties Keep Over Half a Million Disabled at Home." https:// www.bts.gov/archive/publications/special_reports_and_issue_briefs/issue_briefs/num-ber_03/entire.

Clarke, Philippa J., Jennifer A. Ailshire, Els R. Nieuwenhuijsen, and de Kleijn–de Vrankrijker, Marijke W. 2011. "Participation among Adults with Disability: The Role of the Urban Environment." *Social Science & Medicine* 72 (10): 1674–1684.

Clarke, Philippa, Jennifer A. Ailshire, and Paula Lantz. 2009. "Urban Built Environments and Trajectories of Mobility Disability: Findings from a National Sample of Community-Dwelling American Adults (1986–2001)." *Social Science & Medicine* 69 (6): 964–970.

Danford, Gary Scott and James Maurer. 2005. "Empirical Tests of the Claimed Benefits of Universal Design."

Edlich, Richard F., Angela R. Kelley, Karrie Morton, Richard E. Gellman, Richard Berkey, Jill Amanda Greene, Larry Hill, Roy Mears, and William B. Long III. 2010. "A Case Report of a Severe Musculoskeletal Injury in a Wheelchair User Caused by an Incorrect Wheelchair Ramp Design." *The Journal of Emergency Medicine* 38 (2): 150–154.

Ernst, Michelle and Lilly Shoup. 2009. "Dangerous by Design: Solving the Epidemic of Preventable Pedestrian Deaths (and Making Great Neighborhoods)." https://www .inist.org/library/2009-11-09.Ernst%20Shoup.Dangerous%20by%20design.Surface %20Transportation%20Policy.pdf.

Federal Highway Administration. 1999. *Designing Sidewalks and Trails for Access - Review of Existing Guidelines and Practices.* US Department of Transportation, Federal Highway Administration.

———. 2001. "Designing Sidewalks and Trails for Access Part II of II: Best Practices Design Guide." *Designing Sidewalks and Trails for Access, Part 2, Best Practices Design Guide.* Federal Highway Administration.

Frost, Karen L., Gina Bertocci, and Zdravko Salipur. 2013. "Wheelchair Securement and Occupant Restraint System (WTORS) Practices in Public Transit Buses." *Assistive Technology* 25 (1): 16–23.

Glass, Thomas A. and Jennifer L. Balfour. 2003. "Neighborhoods, Aging, and Functional Limitations." *Neighborhoods and Health* 1: 303–334.

Gossett, Andrea, Andrea Gossett, Mansha Mirza, Ann Kathleen Barnds, and Daisy Feidt. 2009. "Beyond Access: A Case Study on the Intersection between Accessibility, Sustainability, and Universal Design." *Disability and Rehabilitation: Assistive Technology* 4 (6): 439–450.

Hammel, Joy, Robin Jones, Janet Smith, Jon Sanford, Cathy Bodine, and Mark Johnson. 2008. "Environmental Barriers and Supports to the Health, Function, and Participation of People with Developmental and Intellectual Disabilities: Report from the State of the Science in Aging with Developmental Disabilities Conference." *Disability and Health Journal* 1 (3): 143–149.

He, Wan, Daniel Goodkind, and Paul R. Kowal. 2016. "An Aging World: 2015." https://www.census.gov/content/dam/Census/library/publications/2016/demo/p95-16-1.pdf.

Herzog, A. and James S. House. 1991. "Productive Activities and Aging Well." *Generations: Journal of the American Society on Aging* 15 (1): 49–54.

Houser, Ari N. 2005. *Community Mobility Options: The Older Person's Interest.* AARP Public Policy Institute.

Iwarsson, Susanne, Gunilla Jensen, and Agneta Ståhl. 2000. "Travel Chain Enabler: Development of a Pilot Instrument for Assessment of Urban Public Bus Transport Accessibility." *Technology and Disability* 12 (1): 3–12.

Lenker, James A., Jordana L. Maisel, and Molly E. Ranahan. 2016. *Measuring the Impact of Complete Streets Projects: Preliminary Field Testing.* The New York State Department of Transportation.

Lynott, Jana and Carlos Figueiredo. 2011. *How the Travel Patterns of Older Adults are Changing: Highlights from the 2009 National Household Travel Survey.* The New York State Department of Transportation.

Lynott, Jana, Jessica Haase, Kristin Nelson, Amanda Taylor, Hannah Twaddell, Jared Ulmer, Barbara McCann, and Edward R. Stollof. 2009. *Planning Complete Streets for an Aging America.* The New York State Department of Transportation.

Mace, Ronald. 1985. "Universal Design: Barrier Free Environments for Everyone." *Designers West* 33 (1): 147–152.

Mace, Ronald L., B. Connell, Mike Jones, Jim Mueller, Abir Mullick, Elaine Ostroff, Jon Sanford, Ed Steinfeld, Molly Story, and Gregg Vanderheiden. 1997. "Principles of Universal Design." Last Accessed March 24.

Maisel, Jordana, Eleanor Smith, and Edward Steinfeld. 2008. "Increasing Home Access: Designing for Visitability." *AARP Public Policy Institute* 14: 1–34.

McCann, Barbara and Suzanne Rynne. 2010. *Complete Streets: Best Policy and Implementation Practices.* American Planning Association.

Meyer, Anne, David Howard Rose, and David T. Gordon. 2014. *Universal Design for Learning: Theory and Practice.* CAST Professional Publishing.

Mikiten, E. 2013. "Redefining Sustainable Design." *Universal Design Newsletter.*

Morris, John, James Mueller, and Michael Jones. 2010. "Tomorrow's Elders with Disabilities: What the Wireless Industry Needs to Know." *Journal of Engineering Design* 21 (2–3): 131–146.

Morrissey, P. A. and Silverstein, R. "The Technology-Related Assistance for Individuals with Disabilities Act of 1988." http://findarticles.com/p/articles/mi_m0842/is_n2_v15/ai_820 0899/.

Nary, Dorothy, A. Katherine Froehlich, and Glen White. 2000. "Accessibility of Fitness Facilities for Persons with Physical Disabilities Using Wheelchairs." *Topics in Spinal Cord Injury Rehabilitation* 6 (1): 87–98.

National Complete Streets Coalition. 2010. *Complete Streets Policy Inventory and Evaluation.* National Complete Streets Coalition.

National Endowment for the Arts (NEA). "Executive Summary. Envisioning Universal Design: Creating an Inclusive Society – October 2–3, 2004." http://www.arts.gov/resources/resources/Accessibility/ud/execsum.html.

———. "Introduction and Meeting Overview. Envisioning Universal Design: Creating an Inclusive Society – October 2–3, 2004." http://www.arts.gov/resources/Accessibility/ud/intro.html.

———. "Issues and Perspectives: Accomplishments, Challenges and Recommendations. Meeting on Universal design—June 7–8, 1999." http://www.nea.gov/explore/ud/issues.html.

———. "Issues and Perspectives. Envisioning Universal design: Creating an Inclusive Society – October 2–3, 2004." http://www.arts.gov/resources/Accessibility/ud/issues_b.html.

Officer, Alana and Aleksandra Posarac. 2011. *World Report on Disability.* World Health Organization.

Pullin, Graham. 2009. *Design Meets Disability.* MIT Press.

Ritter, Anita Stowell, Audrey Straight, and Edward L. Evans. 2002. *Understanding Senior Transportation: Report and Analysis of a Survey of Consumers Age 50.* AARP, Public Policy Institute.

Roberts, Peter and Julie Babinard. 2004. "Transport Strategy to Improve Accessibility in Developing Countries." Washington, DC: World Bank.

Sanford, Jon A., Katharina Echt, and Pascal Malassigné. 2000. "An E for ADAAG: The Case for ADA Accessibility Guidelines for the Elderly Based on Three Studies of Toilet Transfer." *Physical & Occupational Therapy in Geriatrics* 16 (3–4): 39–58.

Shaw, Greg. 2000. "Wheelchair Rider Risk in Motor Vehicles: A Technical Note." *Journal of Rehabilitation Research and Development* 37 (1): 89–100.

Shaw, Greg and Timothy Gillispie. 2003. "Appropriate Protection for Wheelchair Riders on Public Transit Buses." *Journal of Rehabilitation Research and Development* 40 (4): 309–320.

Smith, Russell M. 2015. "Planning for Urban Sustainability: The Geography of LEED®–Neighborhood Development™(LEED®–ND™) Projects in the United States." *International Journal of Urban Sustainable Development* 7 (1): 15–32.

Songer, T. J., S. G. Fitzgerald, and K. A. Rotko. 2004. "The Injury Risk to Wheelchair Occupants Using Motor Vehicle Transportation." *Annual Proceedings. Association for the Advancement of Automotive Medicine* 48: 115–129.

Steinfeld, Edward. 2001. "Universal Design in Mass Transportation." *Universal Design Handbook.* McGraw Hill.

Steinfeld, Edward and Jordana Maisel. 2012. *Universal Design: Creating Inclusive Environments.* John Wiley & Sons.

Steinfeld, Edward, Jordana Maisel, David Feathers, and Clive D'Souza. 2010. "Anthropometry and Standards for Wheeled Mobility: An International Comparison." *Assistive Technology* 22 (1): 51–67.

Steptoe, A., A. Shankar, P. Demakakos, and J. Wardle. 2013. "Social Isolation, Loneliness, and All-Cause Mortality in Older Men and Women." *Proceedings of the National Academy of Sciences of the United States of America* 110 (15): 5797–5801.

Sundar, Vidya, Debra L. Brucker, Megan A. Pollack, and Hong Chang. 2016. "Community and Social Participation among Adults with Mobility Impairments: A Mixed Methods Study." *Disability and Health Journal* 9 (4): 682–691.

Thapar, Neela, Grace Warner, Mari-Lynn Drainoni, Steve R. Williams, Holly Ditchfield, Jane Wierbicky, and Shanker Nesathurai. 2004. "A Pilot Study of Functional Access to Public Buildings and Facilities for Persons with Impairments." *Disability and Rehabilitation* 26 (5): 280–289.

Thatcher, Russell, Caroline Ferris, David Chia, Jim Purdy, Buffy Ellis, Beth Hamby, Jason Quan, and Marilyn Golden. 2013. *Strategy Guide to Enable and Promote the Use of Fixed-Route Transit by People with Disabilities.* Transportation Research Board.

US Access Board. 2011. *Proposed Guidelines for Pedestrian Facilities in the Public Right-of-Way.* U.S. Access Board.

US Census Bureau, Housing and Household Economic Statistics Division. "Historical Census of Housing Tables." https://www.census.gov/hhes/www/housing/census/historic/units.html.

Vaughan, Ellen and Jim Turner. 2013. "The Value and Impact of Building Codes." *Environmental and Energy Study Institute White Paper.* Transportation Research Board.

Vavik, Tom and Martina Maria Keitsch. 2010. "Exploring Relationships between Universal Design and Social Sustainable Development: Some Methodological Aspects to the Debate on the Sciences of Sustainability." *Sustainable Development* 18 (5): 295–305.

Venter, Christo, Mac Mashiri, Tom Rickert, David Maunder, Joanne Sentinella, Khaimane de Deus, Anand Venkatesh, Alister Munthali, and Hendrietta Bogopane. 2004. *Towards the Development of Comprehensive Guidelines for Practitioners in Developing Countries.* Citeseer.

Watchorn, Valerie, Helen Larkin, Danielle Hitch, and Susan Ang. 2014. "Promoting Participation through the Universal Design of Built Environments: Making it Happen." *Journal of Social Inclusion* 5 (2): 65–88.

World Health Organization. 2007. *Global Age-Friendly Cities: A Guide.* World Health Organization.

Xiang, H., A. M. Chany, and G. A. Smith. 2006. "Wheelchair Related Injuries Treated in US Emergency Departments." *Injury Prevention: Journal of the International Society for Child and Adolescent Injury Prevention* 12 (1): 8–11.

Chapter 14 Wireless technologies

John Morris and Mike Jones

Contents

14.1 Chapter overview

Wireless information and communication technology (ICT) includes cellphones, tablets, wearable devices, home automation and control functions, and other ICT that connects wirelessly. Accessibility, usability, and utility of wireless ICT are as important to people with disabilities as to their non-disabled peers. In part, its importance derives from the central place wireless ICT has come to occupy in all our lives – for school, work, communicating, getting information, and navigating physical and social environments. Additionally, as these technologies have become more powerful, they have more features and capabilities that can serve assistive technology functions, including functions that were previously available only through specialized assistive technology.

This chapter describes how mobile wireless ICT has profoundly affected the independence of people with disabilities. First, this chapter will review the relatively short but fast-paced history of wireless ICT, beginning with the two-way pager

DOI: 10.1201/b21964-17

and cellular phones, how this technology has affected people with disabilities, and how these users helped to shape the technology. The chapter will then discuss technological, social, and policy trends related to the adoption of wireless ICT and its expanding capabilities and potential uses. This discussion includes a review of survey research on the use and attitudes toward wireless ICT. Central to this discussion is the smartphone, which has emerged as the ICT platform of choice for most people. The smartphone continues to be the essential ICT device for most users even with the advent of the so-called Internet of Things technologies (activity trackers, environmental sensors and controls, and home automation).

14.2 Evolution of mobile phone use by people with disabilities: 1990s–present

Since 1990, mobile wireless technology has evolved from relatively simple phones for voice communication to robust ICT systems. For increasing numbers of wireless users, mobile devices have replaced not only their landline phones but also desktop and laptop computers. Several important developments have been instrumental in accommodating the needs of mobile phone users with disabilities. At the beginning of the 1990s, speech recognition could be used in desktop computers, but the training of the devices was tedious and the error rate (5–10%) was unacceptably high. Today, effective voice recognition is a common feature among smartphones. Mobile telephone short message service (SMS) became popular, leveling the field for deaf and hard-of-hearing wireless customers. While hearing aid compatibility has improved, it remains an issue for some users, requiring a trial period with a new device to assure compatibility. Integration of global positioning system (GPS) functionality into mobile phones offered advantages in navigation to users with and without disabilities (e.g., fast and efficient access to emergency services). Software such as BlissCat and WordCat was created to assist people with cognitive difficulties to communicate independently.

When mobile phones were simply instruments for voice communications, they often served as a backup phone at home during power interruptions, or as a security device for people with disabilities and elders venturing out into the community (Mann and others 2004). While the adoption of mobile phones into daily life rapidly gathered momentum among young people, elders found themselves challenged to understand and use this technology effectively. Simple "feature phones," including the GreatCall Jitterbug, Pantech Breeze (Figure 14.1), and the Raku-Raku series from Fujitsu (Furuki and Kikuchi 2013) and NTT Docomo, emerged to offer this large and growing market an entry-level option. As competition for this market segment increased, mainstream devices began to incorporate many of the usability features first found in specialized feature phones. However,

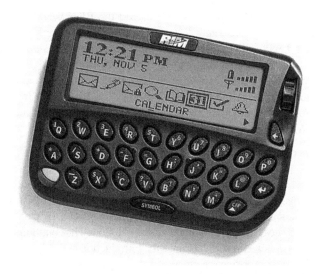

Figure 14.1 "A Prehistoric Blackberry." Retro Thing: Vintage Gadgets and Technology (courtesy of James Grahame, www.retrothing.com/2011/06/a-prehistoric-blackberry.html).

many customers with specialized needs tend to retain their devices to avoid the challenging learning curve associated with a new device.

Fast forward to 2007, the introduction of the Apple iPhone was a game-changer in mobile wireless ICT like nothing that had come before. The iPhone's icon-based touchscreen interface and rapidly growing ecosystem of mobile wireless applications (apps), single-handedly revolutionized mobile ICT usage, redefining the smartphone concept and capabilities. Although revolutionary, the iPhone was met with almost universal concern by the disability community because of its touchscreen interface that was inaccessible for blind users. By 2014, the combination of technological advances in mobile devices and services, intense market competition among manufacturers of wireless devices and service providers, growth of the population of people with disabilities, and a more demanding regulatory environment related to technology access have transformed mobile phone use by people with disabilities.

14.2.1 Deaf consumers

Deaf individuals were enthusiastic early adopters of mainstream mobile phones. Prior to 1999, deaf users had access to two-way communications only via the teletype (TTY) device, also known as a telecommunications device for the deaf (TDD). These devices were about the size of a small electric typewriter or laptop computer with a QWERTY keyboard and a small screen to display typed text.

In 1999, Research in Motion (RIM) introduced the Blackberry, an evolution of the company's Inter@ctive Pager 900 and 950 two-way pagers with full physical QWERTY keyboards, which also offered email functionality (Figure 14.2). Blackberry also introduced technology to "push" new emails and calendar updates to user devices, making the exchange of information automatic and immediate, a useful feature for deaf individuals who relied on text-based information for mobile communication. Other two-way pager competitors included Motorola T-900, PageWriter, and TimePort.

Deaf consumers embraced the T-Mobile Sidekick (also sold at the Danger Hiptop) when it came to market in the fall of 2002. This device offered a full physical QWERTY keyboard and mobile email and came loaded from the factory with AOL Instant Messenger (AIM; TDI, n.d.; Wikipedia, n.d.). In March 2003, the Sidekick (Figure 14.3) became the first mobile phone to offer unassisted TTY and relay operator calls, with devices from other manufacturers to follow. The continuing evolution of touchscreen smartphones and tablets since the introduction of the iPhone in 2007, and the rollout of mobile broadband networks in recent years, opened new opportunities for deaf users to use video calling for simultaneous, two-way mobile communication.

14.2.2 Hearing aid users

Hard-of-hearing users generally do not rely solely on text-based communications. However, those who use hearing aids often have experienced their own

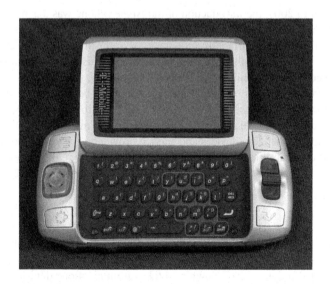

Figure 14.2 T-Mobile SideKick II (source: https://commons.wikimedia.org/wiki/File:SidekickII.jpg).

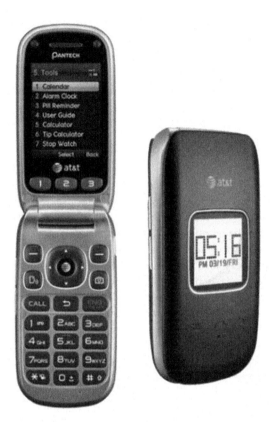

Figure 14.3 Pantech Breeze III (source: www.itechnews.net/2011/07/25/att-pantech-breeze-iii-clamshell-phone/).

accessibility challenges, mainly related to electromagnetic interference caused by the interaction of their hearing technology when digital mobile phones (and cordless phones) are brought close to the ear. This problem is generally reduced in the clamshell designs of feature phones (Federal Communication Commission 2016) that were popular before contemporary smartphones became dominant.

The United States Hearing Aid Compatibility Act (HAC Act) of 1988 required that telephones manufactured or imported for use in that country after August 1989 be hearing aid compatible. Compatibility means that phones are sufficiently shielded from electromagnetic interference caused by the proximity of phone receivers to hearing aids. The Federal Communications Commission (FCC) established new rules in 2003 extending these requirements to mobile phones. The 2003 rules required handset manufacturers and service providers to offer a minimum number of hearing aid compatible mobile phones that meet the American National Standards Institute (ANSI) rating for electromagnetic interference of M3 for acoustic coupling or T3 for telecoil coupling. The rules also required rating information on packaging, in the product manual, and on company websites. Despite these, a 2014 study showed that three-quarters of hearing aid users reported difficulty finding a mobile phone compatible with their hearing device; half reported dissatisfaction with the sound quality of their phones (Morris, Mueller, and Jones 2014)

14.2.3 Blind and low vision consumers

Mobile phones with simple numeric keypads were the most common type of device before the advent of the contemporary smartphone. Because of their simple layout, they were generally accessible to blind users for voice communications. Devices with keys that are raised above the surface of the dial pad, and that have a nub on the number five key, were particularly accessible. Most early mobile phones with robust text messaging and email capabilities were not accessible to blind and very low vision users. They did not come with pre-installed screen reading software such as TALKS (produced by Nuance) and Mobile Speak (by Code Factory). These applications, and their screen magnifier counterparts, were introduced in 2003 and 2004, respectively, and provided expensive accessibility solutions to blind and low vision consumers. Mobile phones running the Symbian OS operating system – mainly those manufactured by Nokia – were the first to allow the installation of third-party software, including the TALKS and Mobile Speak screen readers (Burton 2011). In 2011, facing declining cellphone market share and in search of a new operating system, Nokia partnered with Microsoft, making Windows Phone its primary smartphone operating system. Nokia ultimately abandoned the Symbian OS and in 2014 sold its handset business to Microsoft.

Microsoft was one of the early vendors to offer mobile phones that could run screen reading applications. Devices running Windows Mobile 5.0 (launched in 2005) and continuing through version 6.5 (launched in 2009) could install and run Mobile Speak, as well as Dolphin's Smart Hal screen reading software (Burton 2011). Microsoft's subsequent operating system, Windows Phone 7 was not compatible with Windows Mobile when it launched in 2010. It did not support screen readers. Nor did it have any built-in accessibility features (Schroeder and Burton 2010). Ultimately, Microsoft did offer screen reader capability on Windows Phone, but even as late as February 2013, the company was criticized for continuing "to offer very little in terms of accessibility for its Windows Phone devices" (Meddaugh 2013).

In 2010, Apple introduced its VoiceOver screen reader built into the iOS operating system, introduced on the iPhone 3GS. Available previously on the Mac OS X computer operating system, and later on the iPod Shuffle, which was launched in 2009. VoiceOver allowed iPhone users to navigate the touchscreen interface by drawing their finger across the screen and listening for the names of icons and elements in lists of contacts, songs, and other lists. VoiceOver was quickly embraced by blind and visually impaired consumers. Google subsequently offered Explore by Touch (which permits gesture-based inputs) with the launch of Android 4.0 in 2011. With Google's TalkBack, which offers spoken, audible, and vibration feedback and which originally required separate activation, users could use Explore by Touch to navigate the touchscreen interface (Figure 14.4). Later versions of Android combined the two accessibility features into TalkBack.

Google's quick response to Apple's VoiceOver and efforts to make Android accessible to people with visual impairment was recognized by professional reviewers in the visually impaired community. A July 2013 review of Android 4.2.2 running on the Nexus 4 smartphone and Nexus 7 Tablet observed that "the accessibility features of Google's Android OS have been considered less than stellar. The improvements that Google has made to their latest Android release, specifically for people with low vision, are now challenging that belief" (Rempel 2013). However, it still trails iOS in popularity among blind smartphone users, who overwhelmingly favored the iPhone over Android and other smartphones (Morris and Mueller 2014) (Figure 14.5).

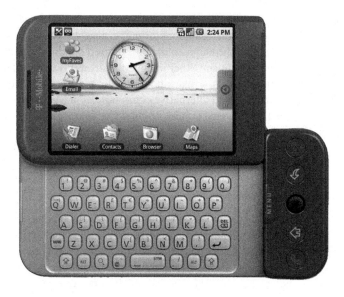

Figure 14.4 HTC Dream/T-Mobile G1 original Android smartphone (source: http://pocketnow.com/2015/02/04/consistent-ui).

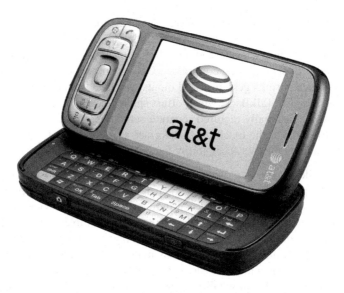

Figure 14.5 AT&T (HTC) Tilt with Windows Mobile 6 operating system (source: http://phonedb.net/img/gallery/big/att_tilt_open_angle.jpg).

14.2.4 Consumers with complex communications needs

Communication systems for people with complex communication needs (CCN) have experienced several transformations over the past 40 years (Shane et al. 2012). CCN can result from developmental and acquired conditions and injuries, including Down syndrome, autism, other intellectual disabilities, multiple sclerosis, amyotrophic lateral sclerosis, stroke, and traumatic brain injury. Some people with CCN use augmentative and alternative communication (AAC) methods and technologies based on graphic and textual symbols that represent objects, actions, and concepts (Bryen and Moolman 2015). These were initially analog systems. But dedicated AAC devices incorporating microprocessors became available in the 1980s. In the 1990s, dedicated AAC devices based on mainstream computer operating systems appeared, allowing access to additional activities such as word processing and internet browsing (Shane et al. 2012).

The advent of contemporary touchscreen smartphones and tablets represented an important advance for people who have difficulty with voice communication. As the first of the contemporary generation of touchscreen smart devices, Apple iOS-based products became especially popular among people with CCN, their families, therapists, and news media. This caused discomfort among some professionals because of concern over exaggerated claims of therapeutic progress among children with autism using iPads (Blank 2011). Despite caution, speech therapy professionals have supported the use of speech-generating apps on mainstream platforms when proper clinical techniques are used to assess patients and match them with the proper technology (Gosnell, Costello, and Shane 2011).

Mobile phones and tablets can be used for important activities of social, educational, and employment participation. Survey research conducted by the Rehabilitation Engineering Research Center for Wireless Technologies (Wireless RERC) found that adult AAC users own mobile phones at substantially lower rates than those with other disabilities. However, they own smartphones and tablets at similar or greater rates than others with disabilities (Wireless RERC 2014). Greater use of smart devices by AAC users requires that AAC and mainstream technology be even more accessible. As Shane et al. (2012) observed, "the rate at which some individuals create content or access information continues to be slow. The interfaces need to be easier to use, faster, more precise, and less fatiguing."

14.2.5 Consumers with mobility and dexterity limitations

Individuals with manual limitations can use a variety of low-tech and high-tech solutions to access wireless ICT devices, including non-slip skins, mounts for attaching devices to furniture and wheelchairs, as well as speech-to-text input (e.g., Dragon Naturally Speaking), voice control, and electronic personal assistants (Siri, Google Now, Cortana). In using ICT devices, people with more severe upper extremity limitations often confront accessibility and usability challenges like those with CCN. Accessibility solutions can include sip-and-puff controllers, head pointers, eye-gaze trackers, head switches mounted on wheelchairs, and other gesture inputs. This allows the user to navigate a keyboard, list, or set of commands by "scanning" rows and columns, and selecting the item. As with AAC, which often relies on similar switch-based scanning access, the process of creating content and accessing information can be slow and fatiguing.

Until recently, switch interfaces were separate pieces of assistive technology, provided by companies like AbleNet, Komodo OpenLab, and Zyrobotics. In 2013, Apple released iOS 7, which was the first of the major mobile ICT operating systems to offer built-in switch interface access, Switch Control. Android followed in 2014 with its built-in Switch Access functionality for the newly released Android 5.0 (Lollipop), and Samsung introduced Universal Switch when it launched the Galaxy S6 smartphones in 2015. The effectiveness of these solutions seems to be variable. The Android solution faces the substantial challenge of trying to function properly and consistently across many different devices from numerous manufacturers (Wandke 2017), and across many different mobile apps. Meanwhile, Apple's Switch Control has exhibited similar usability issues, including difficulty interacting with time-sensitive actions like answering phone calls, an excessive number of steps and screens to complete certain functions, and variable functioning across multiple apps with uneven levels of switch accessibility (Komodo OpenLab 2016). Still, the fact that the two leading operating systems and a major device manufacturer have developed built-in switch interfaces reflects substantial commitment by the industry to provide assistive and accessible technology. This is also reflected in the extensive list of built-in accessibility features in contemporary versions of iOS and Android operating systems (Table 14.1).

14.3 Legislation and regulation

The accessibility and assistive qualities of mobile wireless technology evolved in part under its own momentum – as technology became more sophisticated and helpful to people without disabilities, it also became more helpful to people with disabilities. Rehabilitation researchers, engineers, and assistive technology companies extended the usefulness and usability of these technologies to people with disabilities. But legislation and regulation also contributed substantially to the accessibility of these wireless technologies.

The Telecommunications Act of 1996 established the statutory foundation for accessibility requirements of ICT devices and services. Section 255 of the Telecommunications Act of 1996 states that: "A manufacturer of telecommunications equipment or customer premises equipment shall ensure that the equipment is designed, developed, and fabricated to be accessible to and usable by individuals with disabilities, if readily achievable." The same applies to services provided by telecommunications service companies. Telephone and cellphone accessibility in the United States is also regulated by other legislation and administrative rulemaking, particularly the Hearing Aid Compatibility Act (HAC Act) of 1988 and the 21st Century Communications and Video Accessibility Act of 2010 (CVAA).

As noted previously, the HAC Act requires that telephones manufactured or imported for use in the United States after August 1989 be hearing aid compatible. The HAC Act originally exempted "telephones used with public mobile services" (cellphones or mobile wireless phones). However, as a means to ensure that compatibility requirements kept pace with the ongoing development of telecommunications, the HAC Act also granted the Federal Communications Commission (FCC) the authority to revoke or limit this exemption. In 2003, the FCC determined that the complete exemption of mobile wireless telephones adversely affected hearing aid users and that limiting the exemption was achievable technologically. Consequently, the FCC established rules to require an increasing number of hearing aid compatible cellphones to be provided by manufacturers and service providers.

The CVAA was adopted to "keep up with the fast-paced technological changes that our society has witnessed over the past decade," according to the FCC, with "groundbreaking protections to enable people with disabilities to access broadband, digital and mobile innovations – the emerging 21st century technologies for

Table 14.1 Built-In Assistive/Accessibility Features of Leading Smartphones and Operating Systems

iOS 10.2	Android 7.1.2	Samsung (Galaxy S7 running Android 6.0.1)
Vision	**Services**	**Vision**
Voiceover	Talkback	Voice assistant help
Zoom	Switch access	Dark screen
Magnifier	Select to speak	Rapid key input
Display accommodations	**System**	Speak passwords
Speech	Captions	Text-to-speech
Larger text	Magnification gesture	Accessibility shortcut
Bold text	Font size	Voice label
Button shapes	Display size	Font size
Increase contrast	Click after pointer stops moving	High contrast fonts
Reduce motion	High contrast text	High contrast keyboard
On/off labels	Power button ends call	Show button shapes
Interaction	Auto-rotate screen	Magnifier window
Switch control	Speak passwords	Magnification gestures
AssistiveTouch	Large mouse pointer	Grayscale
Touch Accommodations	Mono audio	Negative colors
Keyboard	Accessibility shortcut	Color adjustment
Shake to undo	Text-to-speech output	**Hearing**
Vibration	Touch and hold delay	Sound detectors
Call audio routing	**Display**	Flash notification
Home button	Color inversion	Turn off all sounds
Reachability	Color correction	Hearing aids
Hearing		Samsung subtitles (CC)
Hearing devices		Google subtitles (CC)
TTY		Left/right sound balance
LED flash for alerts		Mono audio
Mono audio		**Dexterity and interaction**
Phone noise cancellation		Universal switch
Audio volume balance L/R		Assistant menu
Media		Easy screen turn on
Subtitles and captioning		Press and hold delay
Audio descriptions		Interaction control
Learning		**More settings**
Guided access		Direction lock
Accessibility shortcut		Direct access
		Notification reminder
		Single tap mode
		Manage accessibility

which the act is named." The law is comprised of two sections, the first covering "advanced communications services and equipment" and the second covering video programming. Under CVAA, the equipment and software offered for sale or distributed must be "accessible to and usable by individuals with disabilities, unless…not achievable." The same applies to services offered by communications service providers. Notably, any assistive technology needed to make communications technology accessible must be available at "nominal cost" under the CVAA.

The CVAA makes a distinction between assistive and accessible technology, by noting that manufacturers may satisfy the requirements to make their equipment accessible by either:

(A) ensuring that the equipment that the manufacturer offers is accessible to and usable by individuals with disabilities without the use of third-party applications, peripheral devices, software, hardware, or customer premises equipment; or

(B) if such a manufacturer chooses, using third-party applications, peripheral devices, software, hardware, or customer premises equipment that are available to the consumer at nominal cost and that individuals with disabilities can access them.

The CVAA adopted a more flexible approach than the HAC regulations to promote the accessibility of technology. Instead of prescribing a technical solution, CVAA puts the onus on industry to ensure that ICT equipment and services sold in the United States are "accessible, usable, and compatible," terms that are defined in the "Performance Objectives" section of the CVAA. These performance objectives are broadly defined, "more like the functional requirements in Section 508," according to The Paciello Group (Horton 2014). For instance, the objective "Non-interference with hearing technologies" requires technologies to "reduce interference to hearing technologies (including hearing aids, cochlear implants, and assistive listening devices) to the lowest possible level that allows a user to utilize the product." As The Paciello Group notes, relying on functional versus prescriptive requirements "makes the task of achieving accessibility more difficult for designers and manufacturers. […] but also leaves room to devise innovative approaches to achieving (the) performance objectives" (Horton 2014).

Apple's Made-for-iPhone (MFi) program provides a useful example of this functional versus prescriptive approach to regulating wireless ICT accessibility. The MFi program relies on Bluetooth pairing of the iPhone with Apple-certified hearing aids. Hearing aid settings are controlled directly on the iPhone, allowing users to switch between audiologist-prescribed preset configurations for different environments (indoors, outdoors, etc.). The Apple website lists dozens of certified hearing aid models produced by 23 different vendors (Apple 2017). The success of the MFi program and efforts by the hearing aid industry to leverage existing technologies for connecting to cell phones provide examples of industry efforts toward a desired outcome from a user experience perspective, rather than toward achieving mandated technical specifications for radio interference. Despite this success, in 2016, the FCC increased the number of hearing aid compatible handsets that service providers and manufacturers are required to offer. In this same Report and Order (FCC 16-103), the FCC stated: "we also reconfirm our commitment to pursuing 100 percent hearing aid compatibility to the extent achievable."

14.4 Wireless device ownership and activities

Access and use of mobile ICT have become essential to independent living, employment, and social participation. The ubiquity of technology in society and its increasing power and sophistication – especially the mobile kind – has made it ever more critical for communications, information access, entertainment, navigation/wayfinding, shopping, banking, and health monitoring. Data from the CTIA-The Wireless Association show over 355 million wireless service subscriptions in the United States (CTIA-The Wireless Association 2015). Survey data from the Pew Research Center show a steadily rising rate of cellphone ownership among the general population of American adults in recent years, from 73% in 2006 to 92% in 2015, with current smartphone ownership at 68%, and tablet ownership at 45% of American adults (CTIA-The Wireless Association 2015). In general, people with disabilities own and use consumer wireless technology at similar rates as the general population, according to data from the Survey of User Needs (SUN) conducted by the Wireless RERC and the Pew Research Center's ongoing surveys of consumer technology (Table 14.2). SUN data show that 84% of people with disabilities owned or used a cellphone or smartphone in 2012–2013, dropping to 82% in 2015–2016 (partly a result of sampling variability). Including tablet use raises the wireless device ownership rate for people with disabilities to 91% and 92% for the successive sampling periods.

Notably, smartphone ownership among people with disabilities rose from 57% to 72% from 2012–2013 to 2015–2016. Tablet ownership for people with disabilities rose from 35% to 50%. Meanwhile, ownership of simple "feature phones" dropped substantially over the same period to just 13% for the sample of people with disabilities. These results suggest that the more powerful "smart" devices offer critical features and functionality for people with disabilities.

Ownership rates are indicative of general access to ICT devices. However, what people with disabilities and the general population actually do with their devices reflects the degree to which they access and use the powerful features, functions, and electronic services available – particularly on smart devices. Survey research by the Wireless RERC and Pew Research Center provides data for comparing smartphone use by people with disabilities and the public. The focus on smartphones here is appropriate because their versatility (connectivity, size, and portability) and the growth of mobile software "apps" that run on a smartphone have

Table 14.2 Device Ownership by Adults with Disabilities (SUN) and in the General Population (Pew Research Center), 2012–2016

Device type	SUN 2012–2013	SUN 2015–2016	Pew 2013	Pew 2015
Basic phone (e.g., Motorola Razr, Pantech Breeze, Nokia 6350)	27%	13%	35%	24%
Smartphone (e.g., iPhone, Android phone, Windows phone)	57%	72%	56%	68%
Tablet (e.g., iPad, Kindle Fire, Galaxy Tab, Microsoft Surface)	35%	50%	34%	45%
Cellphone or smartphone ownership	84%	82%	87%	92%
Cellphone, smartphone, or tablet ownership	91%	92%	–	–

Sources: Wireless RERC, Survey of User Needs, 2012–2013; Survey of User Needs, 2015–2016. Pew Research Center, Cell Phone Activities 2013, www.pewinternet.org/files/old-media/Files/Reports/2013/PIP_Cell%20Phone%20Activities%20May%202013.pdf; Technology Device Ownership, www.pewinternet.org/2015/10/29/technology-device-ownership-2015/.

Table 14.3 Wireless Activities for Smartphone Users with Disabilities (SUN 2015–2016) and in the General Population (Pew Research Center 2015)

	SUN 2015–2016*	Pew 2015**
Texting	88%	97%
Email	85%	88%
Internet	81%	89%
Maps/GPS	74%	41%
Mobile apps	70%	N/A
Voice calling	67%	N/A
Social media	66%	75%
Video calling	39%	N/A

Sources: Wireless RERC, Survey of User Needs 2015–2016. Pew Research Center, US Smartphone Use in 2015 (data were collected in October 2014).

placed them at the center of many people's personal communications infrastructure and digital life.

The Wireless RERC survey identified eight core wireless activities for smartphones from its 2015–2016 Survey of User Needs, five of which are also included in Pew's 2015 survey on wireless device use (Table 14.3). For four of these activities (texting, email, internet, and social media), the Pew sample of the general population reported higher rates of use than the SUN sample of people with disabilities. However, both samples reported high rates of use for these activities, and the differences between the two samples were not greater than nine percentage points. Only for use of maps and GPS did the SUN sample exceed the Pew sample, and by a wide margin (74% and 41%, respectively). This might reflect the importance of maps and navigation to people with disabilities, especially people with vision, cognitive, and mobility limitations.

Except for the use of maps/GPS, the rank order of activities was similar for the two groups, with texting clearly the most common smartphone activity, followed by either email or mobile internet. Indeed, these three functions have become almost universally used by smartphone users in the general population and those with disabilities in recent years. Social media activity was considerably less common for both groups.

Two variables (income and age) can affect technology adoption, particularly for new technologies, which tend to be expensive and relatively unknown to the public. However, as technologies mature, prices go down and social acceptance expands. Ten years have passed since the iPhone was launched and almost 20 years since the first Blackberry devices with two-way messaging appeared. Additionally, the relative costs and benefits of competing technologies (landline phone service and personal computers) can drive the adoption of new technologies (smartphones and mobile service) by people with fewer financial resources – the phenomenon known as "wireless substitution" (Blumberg and Luke 2016).

Income and age might influence the smartphone activities of people with disabilities as well as the general population. However, the fact that smartphones can offer economical and robust assistive solutions may mitigate the impact of these variables. Smartphone features and functions like screen navigation by touch (e.g., VoiceOver on iOS and TalkBack on Android), speech-generating apps, mobile memory aids for people with cognitive deficits, and video calling for people with speech-hearing needs represent critical assistive technologies for these users. SUN data show that annual household income does indeed influence smartphone activities – respondents with higher income are more likely to use a range of smartphone features (Table 14.4). Most of the activities listed show moderate or strong positive relationships with household income, especially the use of mobile apps and social media. Email, video calling, and mobile internet show moderate positive relationships with household income.

SUN data support expectations that age is inversely related to the use of smartphone features and functions – younger smartphone owners with disabilities report higher rates of use than their older peers (Table 14.5). Use of the internet, mobile apps, social media, and video calling showed substantial differences between the youngest and oldest age cohorts of smartphone owners. For other activities – texting, email, and voice calling – the differences were much smaller but in the expected direction.

Table 14.4 Which Features and Functions Do You Use on Your Smartphone? (2015–2016, by Gross Annual Household Income)

	Less than $35,000 (n=246)	$35,000–$49,999 (n=80)	$50,000–$74,999 (n=137)	$75,000 or more (n=195)
Texting	86%	88%	91%	90%
Internet	78%	83%	85%	86%
Email	81%	85%	88%	90%
Mobile apps	63%	68%	72%	79%
Social media	66%	78%	76%	83%
Maps/GPS	66%	71%	66%	69%
Voice calling	70%	70%	59%	70%
Video calling	36%	41%	39%	45%

Source: Wireless RERC. Survey of User Needs 2015–2016.

Table 14.5 Which Features and Functions Do You Use on Your Smartphone? (2015–2016, by Age)

	18–29 (n=65)	30–49 (n=216)	50–64 (n=253)	65+ (n=152)
Texting	88%	91%	89%	84%
Internet	86%	88%	82%	68%
Email	86%	90%	85%	80%
Mobile apps	75%	78%	67%	63%
Social media	83%	79%	63%	48%
Maps/GPS	72%	81%	75%	62%
Voice calling	72%	74%	63%	65%
Video calling	51%	51%	34%	24%

Source: Wireless RERC. Survey of User Needs 2015–2016.

There are some notable differences in wireless activities between disability types (Table 14.6) that cut across income and age divides. The least surprising is that people with hearing and speaking difficulties use voice calling the least by a substantial margin in both the earlier and later periods. Perhaps more surprising is that people with seeing and hearing limitations use social media the least among the eight disability types listed in Table 14.6. One explanation is that these two disability types include low vision and hearing, which commonly result from aging-related decline in function. These results might be driven as much or more by age than disability. Areas of similarity in smartphone activities across disability types include core functions of text messaging, internet access, and email.

Table 14.6 Which Features and Functions Do You Use on Your Smartphone? (2015–2016, by Disability or Impairment)

	Thinking (n=144)	Anxiety (n=152)	Seeing (n=159)	Hearing (n=341)	Speaking (n=99)	Using arms (n=118)	Using hands, fingers (n=150)	Walking, climbing stairs (n=264)
Texting	87%	91%	88%	90%	88%	84%	87%	86%
Internet	85%	85%	79%	82%	80%	77%	80%	80%
Email	85%	88%	81%	88%	86%	81%	85%	83%
Mobile apps	71%	76%	74%	69%	68%	70%	69%	70%
Social media	71%	73%	55%	64%	71%	71%	71%	66%
Maps/GPS	74%	78%	75%	75%	74%	64%	67%	71%
Voice calling	77%	76%	77%	58%	50%	72%	75%	73%
Video calling	42%	42%	39%	33%	53%	37%	41%	36%

Source: Wireless RERC. Survey of User Needs, 2015–2016.

335

People with all disability types utilized these services at high rates. Furthermore, there was relatively little variation in use across disability types.

14.5 Internet of Things: Smart homes and wearable technology

The term "Internet of Things" (IoT) was coined in 1999 by Kevin Ashton, a British-born marketing executive for personal care products for Proctor & Gamble. Frustrated by the inability to track and adequately stock multiple colors of lipstick in retail outlets, Ashton helped create a global standard for low-cost, low-power radio frequency identification (RFID) tags for use in inventory management (Ashton 2009). IoT refers to "the network of physical objects that contain embedded technology to communicate and sense or interact with their internal states or the external environment" (Gartner 2018). IoT devices are those that until recently would not be expected to have an internet connection (e.g., thermostats, doorbells), and that can communicate with the network automatically, independent of human action. Personal computers, laptops, and smartphones, by this definition, are not generally considered IoT devices despite their numerous processors and sensors. For a detailed discussion of the many aspects of IoT, see the Institute of Electrical and Electronics Engineers white paper "Towards a definition of the Internet of Things (IoT)" (Minerva, Biru, and Rotondi 2015).

Wearable technology (activity trackers and smartwatches) and home automation (smart home hubs, thermostats, smart plugs, etc.) connected directly to Wi-Fi networks or to smartphones via Wi-Fi or Bluetooth, on the other hand, have come to represent key technologies in the consumer IoT constellation. IoT technologies offer substantial assistive and accessibility benefits to users, including multiple ways to collect, retrieve, view and process data, and control the environment using voice, touch, and gesture. Amazon, for instance, has been promoting the assistive and accessibility capabilities of the Amazon Echo smart home hub and Alexa smart assistant at disability conferences like the m-Enabling Summit and the CSUN Assistive Technology Conference. But usability challenges remain for the smart home/smart assistant. Controlling multiple smart home hubs (e.g., Amazon Echo and Amazon Echo Dot) can be confusing on a single mobile app. Having multiple connected devices in your smart home can make learning their "dialogue path" (e.g., "Alexa, ...") and names complicated and confusing for users, family members, and guests (Stinson 2017). It has been noted that Google Home cannot set reminders (Murnane 2017) – a key assistive function for people with difficulty remembering. One reviewer noted that a requested list of ingredients for a recipe was spoken too fast (even at the optional slower rate) to be useful (McGregor 2017). The Echo Dot does not offer the manual volume control found on the regular Echo, so changing the volume must be made vocally or less intuitively via a smartphone app.

Wearable technology, which is expected to grow from US$1.5 billion in 2014 to US$34 billion by 2020 (Lamkin 2016) and US$51.6 billion by 2022 (Wearable Technology Market 2017), also offers great promise and challenges for people with disabilities. Wearables offer automatic data capture of physical activity, as well as physical and emotional functioning, and can provide quicker access to information than a smartphone. One study on the feasibility of a coaching app for diaphragmatic breathing for people with post-traumatic stress was more effective and preferred on a smartwatch than a smartphone (Wallace and others 2017). The placement of wearable devices on specific parts of the body (typically on the wrist or forearm) can also produce more accurate readings of biological function and physical activity than mobile apps on a smartphone. These benefits of wearables are particularly useful to people with disabilities as they often have multiple secondary conditions needing regular monitoring. Combined with environmental sensor data, time, location, and other contextual information, physiological data can be used as inputs for artificial intelligence-based assistive technologies that anticipate user needs for things like environmental control and just-in-time access to information or assistance.

Despite expected growth in the wearables market over the coming years, the technology remains immature. A 2016 Gartner survey of the United States, United Kingdom, and Australia found that the adoption rates for smartwatches were still low – 12%, 9%, and 7%, respectively. Fitness trackers had higher but still modest rates of adoption – 23%, 15%, and 19%, respectively (Gartner 2016). Meanwhile, abandonment rates for smartwatches and fitness trackers remain high (29% and 30%, respectively, across the three countries), which, according to Gartner, is the result of the need for wearables to be more useful. Additionally, the accuracy of consumer technology trackers and wearable sensors remains in doubt. Marathon runners showed significant differences between distances recorded by mobile phones with a GPS-enabled app and GPS-enabled sports watches (Pobiruchin et al. 2017). Variable accuracy of inertial measurement units (IMUs) for measuring gait parameters such as gait speed, stance percent, swing percent, gait cycle time, stride length, cadence, and step duration has been noted (Washabaugh et al. 2017). Comparison of four consumer heart rate trackers (Fitbit, etc.) with gold standard ECG at rest and at 65% of maximum heart rate found variability in accuracy across the devices and for each device at different heart rates (Cadmus-Bertram 2017). A review conducted by the LiveWell RERC concluded that many commercial wearable devices just do not perform well or otherwise do not live up to manufacturer claims (Wallace 2016). Preliminary results of a survey of people with disabilities conducted by the LiveWell RERC found that usability and accessibility concerns of health and fitness tracking apps and devices were common

(LiveWell RERC 2017). Many respondents requested compatibility with existing AT or alternatives to manual keypad entry. Respondents with activity limitations requested diet and exercise apps that could more accurately measure activity levels (e.g., when using a wheelchair or other mobility aid) or allow for adjustments to diet/nutrition goals to suit their more limited caloric intake needs.

14.6 Future vision – "you are the product": Mass data intelligence, pervasive systems

Technology writer Walt Mossberg notes that we are in a "strange kind of lull" in which many technologies like smartphones and tablets are refined and reliable, while newer technologies are still emerging or yet to be available for general consumer use (Mossberg 2017). Smartphones and tablets generally offer solid accessibility features for people with disabilities. However, newly emergent technologies such as smart home hubs (Amazon Echo, Google Home) and wearables still need refinement for optimal use by people with disabilities. Just over the horizon, newer technologies – self-driving cars, virtual and augmented reality, and personal robots – will empower and liberate people of all abilities but will also need an extended period of deployment in the field to inform the refinements needed for equitable access and use.

Artificial intelligence (AI) will extend the power of these technologies by tying them all together and deeply integrating wireless ICT into many more areas of our lives, including: transportation and mobility; health, wellness and safety; education, training, and employment; commerce and shopping; entertainment and leisure; and environmental control at home and elsewhere. The data storage costs for such "mass data intelligence" have been dropping, while quantities of data stored have risen dramatically over the past several years (Meeker 2016). More and more of our lives will be processed and sorted by what we buy using credit and debit cards, where we go in our GPS-enabled cars (self-driving or not), what we say and how we sound to our smart assistants, who we take photos with, and how our bodies move or perform at any second on any day. The potential of AI to provide assistive solutions and enable technology access is considerable – our connected smart devices will be able to help us access what we want with ever greater accuracy and precise timing. However, the cost of such convenience and support in terms of privacy, manipulation, and ultimately autonomy could be considerable. In May 2017, *The Australian* newspaper uncovered a leaked confidential document prepared by Facebook showing that the company offered advertisers the opportunity to target 6.4 million younger users during moments of psychological vulnerability, such as when they felt "worthless," "insecure," "stressed," and "anxious" (Tiku 2017). Five years earlier, Facebook conducted a mass experiment that involved manipulating the emotions of nearly 700,000 users by deliberately feeding positive and negative content, the results of which were published in an academic journal (Kramer, Guillory, and Hancock 2014). Other examples abound: Google's Smart Reply feature for Gmail's computer vision to identify people, places, and things in photos and video; detection of emotional state by analyzing voice quality, and more. In short, the future of wireless ICT is full of potential from an assistive and accessible technology perspective, but those same capabilities will raise new, complex issues that will require considerable research and advocacy efforts to protect all individuals.

14.7 Discussion questions

1. Should we expect or hope smartphone adoption by people with disabilities to be 100% or at least in the 90% range as it is with the general population?
2. As technology gets ever more sophisticated and powerful, will accessibility by people with disabilities automatically improve?
3. Is the challenge of accessibility of wireless technology essentially solved?
4. What are the benefits and limitations of a prescriptive versus functional approach to regulating accessibility of wireless ICT (e.g., HAC regulations)?
5. What are the limitations of grouping people with any type of disabilities in the analysis of technology access and use?
6. As newer technologies emerge (e.g., wearables, home automation and control, voice assistants), will the accessibility of smartphones become less important?
7. Will the need for assistive technology solutions disappear as wireless ICT becomes eminently customizable to each user's needs and preferences?

Bibliography

Apple. "Use Made for iPhone Hearing Devices." Apple 2017, https://support.apple.com/en-us/HT201466.
Ashton, Kevin. 2009. "That 'Internet of Things' Thing." *RFID Journal* 22 (7): 97–114.
Blank, M. "Autism and Apps: An Open Letter to '60 Minutes.'" *Huffington Post*, last modified 2011, https://www.huffpost.com/entry/60-minutes-autism_b_1091378.
Blumberg, Stephen J. and Julian V. Luke. 2016. "Wireless Substitution: Early Release of Estimates from the National Health Interview Survey, January–June 2016." https://www.cdc.gov/nchs/data/nhis/earlyrelease/wireless201612.pdf.
Bryen, D. N. and E. Moolman. 2015. "Mobile Phone Technology for ALL: Towards Reducing the Digital Divide." Unpublished manuscript.
Burton, D. 2011. "Cell Phone Access: The Current State of Cell Phone Accessibility." *AFB AccessWorld Magazine* 6: 12.

Cadmus-Bertram, L. 2017. "Using Fitness Trackers in Clinical Research: What Nurse Practitioners Need to Know." *Journal for Nurse Practitioners* 13(1): 34–40.

CTIA-The Wireless Association. "Wireless Industry Summary Report, Year-End 2014." https://www.ctia.org/docs/default-source/default-document-library/ctia_survey_ye_ 2014_graphics.pdf?sfvrsn=2 (Accessed June 17, 2017).

Federal Communication Commission. "Twenty-First Century Communications and Video. Accessibility Act of 2010 - Pub. L. 111–260." Accessed 6/18, 2016, https://www.fcc.gov/ consumers/guides/21st-century-communications-and-video-accessibility-act-cvaa.

Furuki, K. and Y. Kikuchi. 2013. "Approach to Commercialization of Raku-Raku SMART PHONE." *Fujitsu Scientific & Technical Journal* 49(2): 196–201.

Gartner. "Gartner Glossary: Internet of Things (Iot)." Last modified 2018, https://www.gartner.com/en/information-technology/glossary/internet-of-things.

———. "User Survey Analysis: Wearables Need to Be More Useful." Last modified 2016, https://www.gartner.com/en/documents/3503017.

Gosnell, J., J. Costello, and H. Shane. 2011. "Using a Clinical Approach to Answer What Communication Apps Should We Use?" *Perspectives on Augmentative and Alternative Communication* 20: 87–96.

Horton, Sarah. 2014. "CVAA for Fostering Innovation and Change." The Paciello Group, https://developer.paciellogroup.com/blog/2014/04/cvaa-fostering-innovation-change/.

Komodo OpenLab. "The Tecla Shield 3 Interface for Users with Limited Mobility and Frail Elderly." Unpublished Research Report, National Research Council - Industrial Research Assistance Program (NRC-IRAP), Canada.

Kramer, A. D. I., J. E. Guillory, and J. T. Hancock. 2014. "Experimental Evidence of Massive-Scale Emotional Contagion through Social Networks." *Proceedings of the National Academy of Sciences* 111 (29): 8788–8790.

Lamkin, Paul. 2016. "Wearable Tech Market to Be Worth $34 Billion by 2020." *Forbes*. https://www.forbes.com/sites/paullamkin/2016/02/17/wearable-tech-market-to-be-worth-34-billion-by-2020/#6898c3413cb5.

LiveWell RERC. 2017. "Mobile Health Apps and the Needs of People with Disabilities: A National Survey." https://static1.squarespace.com/static/5698f3670ab377ee41d1ff0b/t/ 58c6c1f0f7e0ab65661a062b/1489420784728/mHealth+Survey+Report_2017-03-12.pdf.

Mann, W. C., S. Helal, R. D. Davenport, M. D. Justiss, M. R. Tomita, and B. D. Kemp. 2004. "Use of Cell Phones by Elders with Impairments: Overall Appraisal, Satisfaction, and Suggestions." *Technology and Disability* 16(1): 49–57.

McGregor, Jay. "An Honest Review of Google Home and Amazon's Alexa." *Forbes*, last modified 4/11/2017, accessed 6/12, 2017, https://www.forbes.com/sites/jaymcgregor/2017/04/ 11/an-honest-review-of-google-home-and-amazons-alexa/#3e057e715fd4.

Meddaugh, J. J. 2013. "2012: A Technology Year in Review." *AFB Access World Magazine* 14 (2). https://www.afb.org/aw/14/2/15840.

Meeker, M. 2016. "Internet Trends 2016." *Kpcb*. https://www.cs.rutgers.edu/~badri/552dir/ papers/intro/Meeker-2016.pdf.

Minerva, Roberto, Abyi Biru, and Domenico Rotondi. 2015. "Towards a Definition of the Internet of Things (IoT)." *IEEE Internet Initiative* 1: 1–86.

Morris, J. and J. Mueller. 2014. "Blind and Deaf Consumer Preferences for Android and iOS Smartphones." In *Inclusive Designing: Joining Usability*, edited by Accessibility and Inclusion, 69–79. London: Springer.

Morris, J., J. Mueller, and M. Jones. 2014. "Hearing Aid Compatibility of Cellphones: Results from a National Survey." *Journal on Technology and Persons with Disabilities* 2: 13–28.

Mossberg, Walt. 2017. "THE DISAPPEARING COMPUTER: Tech was Once Always in Your Way. Soon, it Will Be almost Invisible." *The Verge*. https://www.theverge.com/2017/5/25/ 15686870/walt-mossberg-final-column-the-disappearing-computer.

Murnane, K. 2017. "Alexa, Remind Google that Home Needs Reminders." *Forbes Magazine*, https://www.forbes.com/sites/kevinmurnane/2017/06/08/alexa-remind-google-that -home-needs-reminders/?sh=22dbb2916752.

Pew Research Center. 2015. "U.S. Smartphone Use in 2015." https://www.pewresearch.org/ internet/2015/04/01/us-smartphone-use-in-2015/.

Pobiruchin, M., J. Suleder, R. Zowalla, and M. Wiesner. 2017. "Accuracy and Adoption of Wearable Technology Used by Active Citizens: A Marathon Event Field Study." *JMIR Mhealth Uhealth* 5(2): e24.

Rempel, J. 2013. "Android's Big Step Forward: A Review of the Screen Enhancement Features of Android 4.2.2." *Access World Magazine* 14 (7).

Schroeder, P. W. and D. Burton. 2010. "Microsoft Backtracks on Accessibility in New Mobile Operating System." *Commits to Accessibility in Future Windows Phone Platform. Access World Magazine* 11 (8).

Shane, H. C., S. Blackstone, G. Vanderheiden, M. Williams, and F. DeRuyter. 2012. "Using AAC Technology to Access the World." *Assistive Technology* 24: 3–13.

Stinson, L. 2017. "Alexa is Conquering the World. Now Amazon's Real Challenge Begins." *Wired*.

Tiku, Nitasha. 2017. "Get Ready for the Next Big Privacy Backlash against Facebook." *Wired* 21. https://www.wired.com/2017/05/welcome-next-phase-facebook-backlash/.

Wallace, T. 2016. "Commercial and Experimental Biosensor Solutions for Use with Stress Management Apps on Smart Devices." *RERC for ICT Access* 2016 (1). https://static1. squarespace.com/static/5698f3670ab377ee41d1ff0b/t/58233c836b8f5b184ad1aeca/ 1478704261479/Biosensor+for+stress+management.final.pdf.

Wallace, T., J. T. Morris, S. Bradshaw, and C. Bayer. 2017. "BreatheWell: Developing a Stress Management App on Wearables for TBI & PTSD." *Journal on Technology and Persons with Disabilities* 5: 67–82.

Wandke, D. 2017. "Assistive Technology for Users with Mobility Disabilities: Android Switch Access." *Level Access*.

Washabaugh, E. P., T. Kalyanaraman, P. G. Adamczyk, E. S. Claflin, and C. Krishnan. 2017. "Validity and Repeatability of Inertial Measurement Units for Measuring Gait Parameters." *Gait* 55: 87–93.

Wearable Technology Market. "Wearable Technology Market by Product (Wristwear, Headwear/Eyewear, Footwear, Neckwear, Bodywear), Type (Smart Textile, Non-Textile), Application (Consumer Electronics, Healthcare, Enterprise & Industrial), and Geography - Global Forecast to 2022." Accessed 5/27, 2017, https://www.marketsand-markets.com/Market-Reports/wearable-electronics-market-983.html.

Wireless RERC. "2014 SUNspot (Number 01) - Augmentative and Alternative Communication Device Users and Mainstream Wireless Devices." *Georgia Tech*, last modified 2014, accessed 6/17, 2017, http://wirelessrerc.org/2014-sunspot-number-01-augmentative-and-alternative-communication-device-users-and-mainstream.

Chapter 15 Transportation access

A. Steinfeld and C. D'Souza

Contents

15.1 Chapter overview

Transportation is an important aspect of independent living and quality of life. Access to work is a key prerequisite to most forms of employment, so transportation barriers directly impact employability. Likewise, unimpeded mobility around one's community is a key indicator of equality and inclusion in society. Considerable advances have been made in accessible transportation as a direct result of various laws and regulations, but major barriers and inefficiencies remain.

DOI: 10.1201/b21964-18

Fortunately, there have also been recent advances in technology that can be leveraged by practitioners. While some options are designed for a specific need, many are mass-market products and systems. This is partly due to the obligation of public transit to serve *all* residents. Advances in smartphone and vehicle technology have also created new opportunities for leveraging mass-market solutions.

This chapter draws from the authors' experience and past research. Some content has been summarized from earlier publications (e.g., Giampapa et al. 2017c; Giampapa et al. 2017b; Giampapa et al. 2017a) and additional depth can be found in a dedicated book by this publisher (Steinfeld, Maisel, and Steinfeld 2017).

15.2 Pedestrian travel

Many people with disabilities prefer to live in neighborhoods favorable to daily travel along pedestrian rights of way (sidewalks). Being close to work, stores, and social activities dramatically reduces dependence on transportation service providers and enhances spontaneous travel. However, there are important factors to consider related to the built environment and wayfinding.

15.2.1 Accessible routes

Accessible routes in the context of transportation imply that any individual can get to their intended destination, bus stop, or transportation terminal unimpeded safely and efficiently. The beginning and end of a trip (i.e., what transportation planners call the "last mile problem" or "first mile problem") typically requires using built environment features such as sidewalks, street crossings and roundabouts at intersections, and curb cuts and access ramps to negotiate level changes. Compliance with the Americans with Disabilities Act (ADA) standards related to design and construction of these features alongside proper year-round maintenance (e.g., uneven sidewalk repairs, snow removal, replacing worn out or damaged tactile strips) are necessary and generally sufficient to ensure a barrier-free route for all users. However, deficiencies in the design and upkeep of the pedestrian environment impact users differently based on the type and severity of their impairment. For instance, uneven and cracked sidewalks, while a minor inconvenience to sighted ambulatory individuals, are a significant safety hazard for the frail, elderly and individuals with visual impairments. The roughness and cracks in sidewalks expose wheelchair users to whole-body vibrations, which over time can lead to harmful health effects to users, as well as breakdowns in the wheelchair itself (Duvall et al. 2016). City and metropolitan agencies tasked with the upkeep of the pedestrian environment face continued challenges due to funding shortages and aging infrastructure. Some cities are experimenting with crowdsourcing apps to help identify and prioritize problems in accessible routes.

15.2.2 Wayfinding and navigation

The popularity of smartphones has also led to a variety of pedestrian-oriented navigation tools, most notably the native Google and Apple map apps. Some of these include audio or tactile instruction. Grade elevation and avoidance of inaccessible pedestrian routes (e.g., lack of curb cuts at intersections) are often missing but progress is being made on this front. It is also possible for caregivers and advocates to markup electronic maps, but this often requires experience with certain software tools.

Software and products specifically designed for people who are blind or have low vision have a long history of development, especially systems offered by Sendero. However, the challenge of obtaining good maps and labeling of local features has been a recurring issue. New approaches are regularly developed in research groups so there is hope for next-generation systems that can perceive important details around the user (e.g., Coughlan and Manduchi 2018; NavCog 2017).

15.2.3 Bicycles and non-roadway vehicles

Cycling, as a form of active transportation (i.e., any self-propelled, human-powered mode of transportation) is an area of increasing attention due to its health benefits. Cycling can significantly expand independent mobility for both adults and children, particularly among groups that are currently unable or ineligible to drive. While bike-share programs can be found in most large cities and university campuses across the United States, few offer accessible options such as handcycles, e-bikes, tandem bicycles, recumbent bicycles, and adaptive tricycles for riders with special needs.

Besides physical strength, cycling also places demands on cognitive function. Limitations from cognitive and developmental disabilities (DD) manifested in a person's communication, socialization, attention, memory, focus, logical thinking, dynamic balance, and other higher-level cognitive functions can affect cycling performance. However, no predetermined boundaries on physical or cognitive capabilities exist that preclude individuals with DD from learning to ride bicycles. While research on this topic is limited, the consensus is that people with cognitive impairment generally take longer to learn bicycling but do eventually succeed.

Active transportation programs that focus on teaching children and young adults with DD to cycle more independently in their communities are rare. A recent study of one such program identified increased contact time, lower student-to-trainer ratio (three or four to one), careful assessment of cycling skills at baseline to customize the training goals and duration, and parental involvement in goal-setting and supporting the learning process as effective strategies to support cycle training in children and young adults with DD (Barros and D'Souza 2016). There is also an opportunity for designing technology interventions and training programs to increase the adoption of active transportation modes such as walking and bicycling in young adults with DD, which would greatly enhance their independent mobility, self-esteem, and health.

There are a variety of motorized vehicles designed for use on pedestrian rights of way. The most well-known is the Segway, which is large enough to create issues when entering buildings. At the other extreme are the Airwheel unicycle, hoverboard variations, and the Honda UNI-Cub β, the latter of which is used in a seated position. These compact platforms are usually smaller than a carry-on suitcase and are highly maneuverable. However, the size and maneuverability of these various platforms are offset by the need for good balance and the risk of falls. They may be a viable option for people who are not allowed to drive on streets but have the physical ability to manage these vehicles.

15.3 Automobiles

Travel in the United States is, and will likely continue to be, very focused on travel by automobile. While there are some vehicles specifically designed for people with disabilities, most vehicles are still intended to be driven by people without disabilities. This is partly due to market factors as well as payment and government policies. For example, accessible taxis are widespread in London, but harder to find in most US cities. New York City, for instance, mandates that a certain percentage of taxicabs be wheelchair accessible.

15.3.1 Ingress/egress

Entering and exiting the vehicle is a problem for many drivers and passengers. Strategically positioned grab bars may be adequate for individuals who have minor mobility limitations. A swivel seat can be used for individuals who are unable to maintain balance while stepping into the vehicle. Very few original equipment manufacturers (OEMs) provide factory-installed accessible ingress/egress features specifically aimed at improving access for users with impairments. For instance, the Toyota Sienna minivan offers an optional powered "Auto Access Seat" that rotates, extends out from the vehicle, and then lowers to a convenient transfer height, and upon the occupant transferring into the seat retracts back into the car with the occupant (Toyota Motor Co. 2017). However, this upgrade option is cost prohibitive and sales have been low.

Drivers or passengers who use wheelchairs as seating during travel rely on after-market installed lifts or ramps to aid entry to vehicles. Ramps are usually preferred because they allow more independence and minimize potential fall heights. The location of the ramp, either at the curbside or rear of the vehicle, dictates the path to the driver station. The turn required in a side-entry van set up to reach the driver station is often challenging. For self-propelled manual wheelchairs, the wheelbase is a key factor. For power wheelchairs, the turning radius is highly dependent on whether the device is a front, center, or rear wheel drive. At present, the MV-1 van from Mobility Ventures is the only multi-person vehicle designed from the ground up for wheelchair users, with a factory-installed curbside telescoping ramp, extra wide doors, and five-foot-high head clearance among other accessibility features.

15.3.2 Securement

A key challenge in in-vehicle occupant securement is to provide people who use wheelchairs as seating with a similar level of occupant protection to that of occupants traveling in conventional seating. The most common securement system is a four-point strap type tiedown with a vehicle-anchored seatbelt. A large majority of people are unable to secure their own wheelchair and apply the seatbelt alone and require assistance from a caregiver or transportation service provider. There are wheelchair self-docking systems that offer a higher level of independence while maintaining the needed crashworthiness for a passenger vehicle, but these often take several tries to engage and need added wheelchair hardware that decreases ground clearance. The Rehabilitation Engineering Association of North America (RESNA) has multiple published standards on wheelchair transportation safety and methods to test wheelchairs and related components when used as seats in automobiles. Example standards include the ANSI/RESNA WC18: Wheelchair Tiedowns and Occupant Restraint Systems, WC19: Wheelchair used as Seats in Motor Vehicles, and WC20: Wheelchair Seating. People with dexterity, range of motion, and vision deficits also have difficulty buckling, applying, and releasing conventional seatbelt systems.

15.3.3 Vehicle control

After-market modifications to private vehicles are possible so people with disabilities can drive or ride in them (van Roosmalen, Paquin, and Steinfeld 2010). Providing hand controls for the primary functions of acceleration and braking in lieu of foot pedals is one of the most popular categories of adaptive equipment in cars. Modified interfaces to the steering wheel include a simple spinner knob or a yoke to allow a secure hold for drivers who have minimal grip strength. In other instances, the primary control devices may need to be relocated to a position where they can be reached due to limitations in strength and range of motion. The National Mobility Equipment Dealers Association (NMEDA) has guidelines that cover many aspects of vehicle modifications, including best practices for accommodating people with specific needs and requirements while also ensuring structural integrity and compliance with federal motor vehicle safety standards. Functional assessments by a certified driver rehabilitation specialist (ADED 2017) and identifying suitable financing options are additional considerations in matching the right solution to an individual's needs.

15.3.4 Driver-vehicle interaction

Interaction with secondary vehicle controls remains a problem for many drivers with disabilities. Traditional mechanical controls require custom modification for drivers with significant motor impairments. However, their relative simplicity lowers barriers for people with cognitive disabilities. The current trend in vehicle design is moving toward increased use of multi-function touchscreen displays, even for heating and ventilation controls. Unfortunately, manufacturers have been slow to introduce alternate display modes for drivers who prefer reduced complexity and easier-to-read fonts and icons.

In-vehicle navigation systems and navigation apps on smartphones can be especially useful for people with memory or perception impairments. For example, it is not necessary to read the road names when given timely turn recommendations. Likewise, complex routes can be difficult for drivers of any ability to learn or remember.

Many modern vehicles now have additional interactions to support advanced vehicle control systems (e.g., backup cameras and blind spot warning systems, keyless entry and keyless ignition, adjustable pedals, and cruise control). Parking assistance, collision warning, and lane-keeping systems are increasingly common advanced and semi-autonomous vehicle control systems. All of these have value to populations with disabilities and should be considered on a case-by-case basis (Steinfeld 2008; van Roosmalen, Paquin, and Steinfeld 2010). Current market systems are not fully autonomous since drivers are still required to supervise key tasks (e.g., parking spot selection) and intervene when safety risks occur. It is important to remember that some implementations of these systems can create a risk of over-reliance and improper mental models of system performance.

Collision warning systems have promise for people with perception or cognition difficulties. Older drivers can encounter difficulty at night due to glare and other visual limitations. Forward-looking sensors can increase awareness of oncoming threats, theoretically leading to more advanced warning and time to react to danger. Adaptive cruise control has a similar value in that it can reduce the need for physical intervention. As with all advanced vehicle control systems, poor mental models can lead to dangerous scenarios. It is important to assess whether a driver understands a semi-autonomous feature before recommending use.

15.4 Mass transportation

Travel within mass transportation systems is often characterized by a sequence of stages. These modes rely on service delivery from people outside the traveler's immediate friends and family, thereby requiring additional stages like pre-planning, payment, and customer service. This section is organized around these elements.

An important aspect to be sensitive to is the choice between fixed-route transit and paratransit options. The latter is considerably more costly and far less spontaneous, so methods for encouraging the use of mainstream transit are desirable. As a result, there has been considerable interest in providing greater access to a fixed-route service (Thatcher and others 2013).

15.4.1 Pre-trip

Current methods for supporting independent use of mass transportation center around travel training and information resources. The former is comparable to methods used by orientation and mobility instructors to teach people who are blind or have low vision but will also include elements specific to the transportation service. Some transit agencies utilize mockups of fareboxes, seats, and other infrastructure during training sessions.

Payment has traditionally been a key focus for transit and paratransit training since people with disabilities often utilize special fares or payment models specific to the financial support they receive from the government or other organizations. This is becoming less complex with the steady introduction of smartcards, which are also valuable to people who encounter difficulty with managing and perceiving cash.

The widespread adoption of smartphones has created a wide range of information support options. Modern phones have the ability to pinpoint the user's location and orientation which, when paired with internet connections, provide the user with immediate access to location-aware information and schedules. Automatic vehicle location systems are becoming increasingly common, thereby enabling real-time arriving estimates for upcoming transit vehicles.

Assistance via phone calls has also improved in recent years. Some regions support the 511 phone number, which will often connect the user to an operator who can help with trip planning. Most demand-responsive providers (e.g., paratransit, taxis) also maintain call centers.

15.4.2 Wayfinding and navigation

Smartphones are particularly powerful tools for wayfinding and navigation during a trip. There are a plethora of mass transportation route planning apps, each with a different user interaction design and emphasis. For example, Livingstone-Lee et al. (2014) compared the wayfinding and navigation needs of people with cognitive disabilities against a selection of available apps. Unfortunately, there are very few apps specifically designed for people with disabilities and most developers do not utilize a universal design approach. In addition, good apps often disappear when startups are purchased or go out of business. Practitioners should periodically assess available options in their local market and advocate for accessible transit agency websites. The latter is important since the mobile version of an agency website is often adequate for many travelers (Figure 15.1).

A major limitation for most phone apps is reliable and scalable localization and navigation technology that will work in underground locations (e.g., transit stations). This is a recurring challenge for technology developers and the focus of multiple research groups. Pilot deployments of wireless beacon systems to address this challenge are being tested in several transit systems.

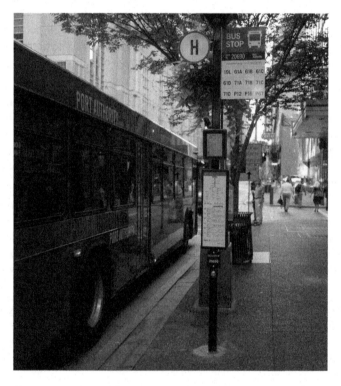

Figure 15.1 This bus stop in Pittsburgh includes high-contrast wayfinding information in a low-complexity layout, real-time arrival estimates, on-demand voice announcements, and a unique numerical label to use when seeking additional assistance about the stop. (Courtesy of Steinfeld.)

15.4.3 Ingress/egress

Similar to automobiles, a foremost challenge for persons with mobility and visual impairments when entering and exiting a transit vehicle involves negotiating a level change from grade or platform to the vehicle floor. However, additional concerns about causing delays to the vehicle (i.e., prolonged dwell time) and associated feelings of anxiety or embarrassment can make using public transit a very stressful experience for seniors and passengers with disabilities. The height of the door opening varies with curb height, and there are no standardized hand holds or audio cues to guide the passenger into the vehicle. People with mobility problems often use electromechanical lifts or folding ramps to aid entry to vehicles.

Low-floor buses are currently the most common type of bus design used in urban public transit (National Transit Database 2015). The lower bus floor coupled with a "kneeling" feature at bus stops contributes to a reduced step height and shorter dwell times (i.e., the amount of time a bus is stopped at the curb while passengers board and disembark; Figure 15.2). The reduced height also allows for using electromechanical ramps at the doorways while eliminating horizontal gaps between the bus floor and sidewalks, thereby improving access for wheeled mobility device users. Compared with platform lifts on high floor buses, access ramps have lower maintenance costs and do not require the bus driver to leave his/her seat to deploy and safely operate the ramp, resulting in substantially decreased dwell times. The use of platform lifts also draws unwanted attention to users making these less desirable compared with ramps.

Despite the advantages of access ramps, passengers using wheeled mobility devices experience a disproportionately higher rate of injuries on low-floor transit buses compared with their ambulatory counterparts. Further, they are 1.8 times more likely to experience an injury or mishap when entering and exiting low-floor buses than during transit or when the bus is stopped (Frost and Bertocci 2010). A recent study about access ramps on low-floor buses demonstrated that current US policies and guidelines on maximum allowable ramp gradients are inadequate and suggested a 7.1-degree (1:8) slope for safe unassisted ingress and egress (Lenker et al. 2016). Level boarding is the safest and most time-efficient option during ingress/egress. Newer bus rapid transit systems use level boarding by having a raised platform at the bus stop, solving the problem of the horizontal and vertical gap. Commuter rail systems have installed hinged folding or telescoping "bridge plates" on railcars that are manually operated by conductors or station personnel to address the gap issue (Figure 15.3).

15.4.4 On-board circulation

Accessibility of transit vehicle interiors is a multi-factorial problem influenced by the vehicle size, entry locations, fare payment system, seating arrangement,

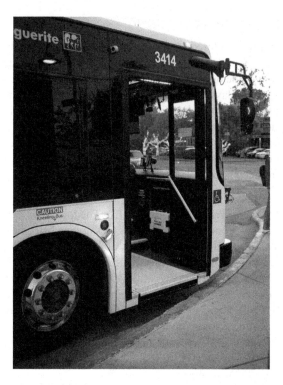

Figure 15.2 Example of an accessible low-floor transit bus showing the front doorway with a kneeling feature and folding access ramp. (Courtesy of Steinfeld.)

and assistive features such as hand holds and stanchions. A challenge to wheelchair accessibility is vehicle interior layouts that require turning maneuvers, often with other passengers in close vicinity (D'Souza et al. 2017; D'Souza et al. 2019). Pathways into a public transit or rail car that requires one or more 90-degree turns to reach the wheelchair station are not uncommon.

Similar to securement options in automobiles, the four-point tiedown system is the most common method of wheeled mobility device securement systems on transit buses. Tiedown systems often require significant driver assistance, which can impose additional delays and expose drivers to extreme postures while reaching around the wheelchair to the tiedowns. Passenger discomfort and reluctance, and inadequate training for drivers about how to secure the diverse designs of wheeled mobility devices, have resulted in the practice of wheelchair securement remaining low at around 33% (Buning et al. 2007). Newer securement systems designed for independent use such as the Q'Straint Quantum system, which uses two moving arms to hold the wheelchair in place and is operated at the push of a

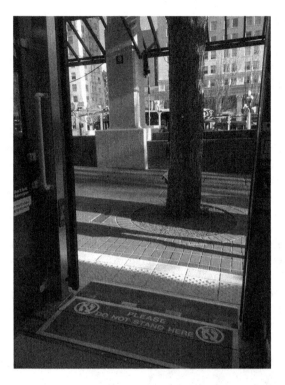

Figure 15.3 The TRIMET light rail system in Portland uses level boarding with folding bridge plates that extend out 15 inches and span a nominal two-inch horizontal and three-inch vertical gap between the low-floor rail car and boarding platform. Bridge plates ease boarding and exiting for people using mobility devices and are deployed for passengers upon request. (Courtesy of Steinfeld.)

button, combined with rear-facing wheelchair passenger stations, are proving to be a viable solution in low-g environments.

Safe and easy ingress, egress, and interior circulation is also challenging for those with visual impairments since doorway locations, seating configurations, and assistive features differ vastly by the transit agency. Availability of concise and situationally relevant information on the system's layout and its operation, as well as a helpful attitude of transit personnel, can enhance safety and accessibility for blind and visually impaired travelers. Orientation and mobility instructors provide a vital service in training individuals with visual impairments to use mass transit systems in a safe and efficient manner.

No one solution to vehicle interior circulation is optimal for the diverse spectrum of transit users, both with and without disabilities. Transit agencies would need to consider the local context, service goals, and ridership demographics to decide on the appropriate vehicle design. Unfortunately, economic considerations of increasing seating capacity often take precedence over improving accommodations and efficient on-board circulation for wheeled mobility and other large devices such as walkers, baby carriages, and shopping carts.

15.4.5 Human service

Information desks, kiosks, and two-way voice call systems remain a valuable form of receiving human assistance. Staffed desks are most prevalent at transit stations and mass transportation terminals due to the concentration of travelers and increased demand for customer service. Less busy stations often utilize a mixture of self-service kiosks and voice-based assistance. The latter can be very useful for people with visual or cognitive disabilities due to the accessibility barriers often present in touchscreen interfaces. In some cases, operators also have the ability to remotely control local infrastructure. Most service providers also offer customer service phone numbers but these are sometimes only in operation for part of the day. A small number of transit agencies reliably staff a Twitter account but only a portion of these provide customer service over Twitter (Figure 15.4).

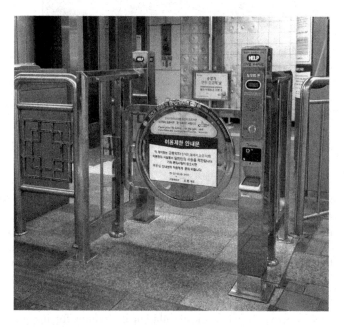

Figure 15.4 This fare gate in Seoul includes a smartcard reader and remote call assistance. (Courtesy of Steinfeld.)

Since taxi companies utilize call centers for dispatch, they have traditionally been an effective method for arranging an alternate mode of travel when encountering a service breakdown or accessibility barrier. However, taxis often do not support all users. As mentioned earlier, wheelchair-accessible taxis are rare in the United States. This has led to a variety of advocacy and legal actions, most notably in New York City.

The taxi industry is also encountering new competition from transportation network companies (TNCs) like Uber and Lyft. Unlike the long-regulated taxi industry, the exact legal responsibilities of TNCs to support people with disabilities are still in flux. As a result, practitioners will need to explore what rules and policies are in place for their local market. Both Uber and Lyft have very explicit policies supporting travel with service animals and prohibiting discrimination against passengers.

15.5 Future vision

Advances in technology, especially in mobile computing and autonomous systems, are occurring rapidly. These trends enable some potential advances that could lead to major improvements in spontaneous, independent travel. As with all disruptive future systems, policies and legal factors make specific predictions somewhat challenging.

Parts of this section summarize and mirror findings from Giampapa et al (2017a), which reviewed and assessed the potential for current technology research efforts to enhance accessible transportation in the reasonable future.

15.5.1 Connected vehicles and pedestrians

The US Department of Transportation has focused considerable attention on supporting real-time communication between vehicles, infrastructure, and pedestrians to help avoid collisions. Roadside infrastructure is unlikely to be in all locations, especially in suburban communities and mid-block areas. People with shorter stature due to height or wheelchair use are also at risk near residential driveways and in parking lots. Therefore, the ability to issue collision warnings directly between vehicles and smartphones has significant potential to reduce risk among pedestrians with disabilities. Likewise, drivers with disabilities may have reduced situation awareness for the rear and sides of their vehicles due to perceptual and neck motion impairments. Wu et al (2014) described a prototype system of this type and demonstrated use in clear line of sight and non-line of sight scenarios. Alerts were displayed for both the driver and pedestrian. Other research teams are using the same technology to tell a signal light that a specific pedestrian needs a longer walk phase when crossing.

15.5.2 Autonomous vehicles

In recent years, numerous teams have explored methods for vehicle autonomy, especially in urban and suburban areas. This is far more complex and unpredictable than highway driving, which has become considerably more automated as more advanced vehicles enter the market. Autonomous urban driving would dramatically increase access to spontaneous travel by people who cannot drive and create new options in regions poorly served by transit, paratransit, or other forms of mass transportation.

Larger market forces are motivating more capable urban and suburban autonomous driving but there is a risk that people with disabilities will be left behind. In most cases, when a person with a disability uses a transportation service, the driver or caregiver often facilitates the occupant's entry to the vehicle by deploying a wheelchair ramp, using a tiedown to secure the wheelchair, and assisting the passenger in donning the safety belt. The driver can assist further if the passenger has an emergency and they can request help. The driver can also communicate with the passenger regarding their destination. An autonomous car is useless if a person cannot enter it or tell it where they would like to go.

To be fully accessible, autonomous vehicles will need to directly perceive or seek explicit input from the passengers about what accommodations are needed. Research into automated wheelchair ramps capable of safe unsupervised deployment, and assistive robotics for wheelchair docking stations and belt-donning systems that meet high-g crash performance standards, could make it feasible and practical for occupants with disabilities to use autonomous vehicles for their transportation needs. Ensuring that the acceleration and deceleration profiles of autonomous vehicles are within ranges comfortable to the diverse spectrum of potential occupants is of particular concern.

Likewise, regulatory policies could limit the value of autonomous vehicles. For example, several states currently require a licensed driver behind the wheel of any autonomous vehicle. This is obviously a problem for people who cannot obtain a license and prohibits a shared vehicle from driving unmanned to pick up a suburban rider.

15.5.3 Guardian angel systems

The oncoming age wave and long-term focus on suburban planning within the United States will be increasingly problematic as seniors transition out of driving. Vehicle autonomy, TNCs, and other on-demand ride services may help mitigate this looming problem, but it will also be important to support and encourage shifts to non-driving modes. This will likely require a variety of technologies and services designed to coach users through unfamiliar transportation systems, inform users of options and alternatives in easy-to-understand ways, and act as a guardian angel in order to detect and warn users when they are about to make a mistake (e.g., take an outbound train instead of an inbound one). Caregiver tools for remote support will also likely be valuable since some barriers require immediate human assistance.

15.6 Opportunities for rehabilitation engineers in transportation

An understanding of transportation barriers and needs and preferences of the disability community can help rehabilitation engineers and therapists design, develop, prioritize, and implement rehabilitation interventions. As implied previously, there are numerous areas where a rehabilitation engineer can have a positive impact on independent travel by people with disabilities and older adults. This can occur either through direct support of the end user or through a service provider. For the former, opportunities center mostly on the development and maintenance of new technologies. There are very few options for key technologies, such as automated wheelchair securement systems, alternative vehicle controls, and transportation apps that meet the needs of people with severe disabilities. While software companies and automotive manufacturers frequently have internal accessibility teams, there are still many opportunities to expand the use of universal design and embedded accessibility features within mainstream products. There are an alarmingly low number of certified driver rehabilitation specialists, which will become an increasing problem as demand increases with an aging population. Travel trainers and orientation and mobility instructors will also need help with translating new technologies into practice. Rehabilitation engineers and therapists who recommend mobility-related device interventions to those who use public transportation will need to consider prevailing standards provisions and evolving technologies for wheeled mobility access and securement on transit vehicles in relation to the needs and capabilities of an individual client. The combined shortage of technology experts in these professions, coupled with the large changes underway in transportation technology, will put an increasing strain on therapists and specialists in these fields.

Rehabilitation engineers can also have an impact through transportation planning, construction, and service provision. Many service providers hire transportation engineers (frequently civil engineers) to support design and analysis of the built environment, vehicles, and service delivery plans. Transportation engineering firms often rely on contracted experts to help identify and resolve accessibility issues in their plans. Some larger firms employ such talent in-house.

At the service delivery level, larger providers typically have internal people or teams focused on accessibility. These experts often develop deep knowledge of the specifics of their industry and help ensure accessible services and technologies are specified, purchased, and maintained. It is also important for people in this role to plan and implement employee training due to the numerous accessibility breakdowns that occur due to a faulty understanding of policies or technologies.

15.7 Discussion questions

1. What features in a car are most useful to someone who uses a manual wheelchair, power wheelchair, or a cane? What about people who are deaf?
2. How can factors in the built environment influence independent travel? Are these factors positive, negative, or both? Provide examples.
3. What kinds of accessibility barriers could block someone from taking a bus from home to work?
4. Is the website of your local transit agency accessible? What kinds of travel training is offered by the agency?
5. How might a guardian angel system support public transit use by someone with a cognitive disability?

Bibliography

ADED. 2017. "The Association for Driver Rehabilitation Specialists." https://www.aded.net/default.aspx.

Barros, R. C. and C. D'Souza. 2016. "An Interview-Based Study of Cycle Trainings in Children with Cognitive Impairments." Washington, DC, June 2016.

Buning, Mary Ellen, C. A. Getchell, Gina E. Bertocci, and Shirley G. Fitzgerald. 2007. "Riding a Bus while Seated in a Wheelchair: A Pilot Study of Attitudes and Behavior Regarding Safety Practices." *Assistive Technology* 19 (4): 166–179.

Coughlan, James and Roberto Manduchi. 2018. "Camera-Based Access to Visual Information." In *Assistive Technology for Blindness and Low Vision*, edited by Roberto Manducki and Sri Kurniawan, 219–246. CRC Press.

D'Souza, Clive, Victor Paquet, James A. Lenker, and Edward Steinfeld. 2017. "Effects of Transit Bus Interior Configuration on Performance of Wheeled Mobility Users during Simulated Boarding and Disembarking." *Applied Ergonomics* 62: 94–106.

D'Souza, Clive, Victor L. Paquet, James A. Lenker, and Edward Steinfeld. 2019. "Self-Reported Difficulty and Preferences of Wheeled Mobility Device Users for Simulated Low-Floor Bus Boarding, Interior Circulation and Disembarking." *Disability and Rehabilitation: Assistive Technology* 14 (2): 109–121.

Duvall, Jonathan, Eric Sinagra, Rory Cooper, and Jonathan Pearlman. 2016. "Proposed Pedestrian Pathway Roughness Thresholds to Ensure Safety and Comfort for Wheelchair Users." *Assistive Technology* 28 (4): 209–215.

Frost, Karen L. and Gina Bertocci. 2010. "Retrospective Review of Adverse Incidents Involving Passengers Seated in Wheeled Mobility Devices while Traveling in Large Accessible Transit Vehicles." *Medical Engineering & Physics* 32 (3): 230–236.

Giampapa, Joseph Andrew, Aaron Steinfeld, Ermine Teves, M. Bernardine Dias, and Zachary Rubinstein. 2017a. "Accessible Transportation Technologies Research Initiative (ATTRI): Assessment of Relevant Research." *Report CMU-RI-TR-17-17, Robotics Institute*, Carnegie Mellon University.

———. 2017b. "Accessible Transportation Technologies Research Initiative (ATTRI): Innovation Scan." *Report CMU-RI-TR-17-16, Robotics Institute*, Carnegie Mellon University.

———. 2017c. "Accessible Transportation Technologies Research Initiative (ATTRI): State of the Practice Scan." *Report CMU-RI-TR-17-15, Robotics Institute*, Carnegie Mellon University.

Lenker, James A., Uma Damle, Clive D'Souza, Victor Paquet, Terry Mashtare, and Edward Steinfeld. 2016. "Usability Evaluation of Access Ramps in Transit Buses: Preliminary Findings." *Journal of Public Transportation* 19 (2): 7.

Livingstone-Lee, Sharon A., Ronald W. Skelton, and Nigel Livingston. 2014. "Transit Apps for People with Brain Injury and Other Cognitive Disabilities: The State of the Art." *Assistive Technology* 26 (4): 209–218.

National Council on Disability. 2015. *Transportation Update: Where We've Gone and What We've Learned*. National Council on Disability.

National Transit Database. 2017. "Federal Transit Administration: National Transit Database." https://www.transit.dot.gov/ntd.

NavCog. 2017. "Cognitive Assistance Lab." http://www.cs.cmu.edu/~NavCog.

Steinfeld, Aaron. 2008. "Smart Systems in Personal Transportation." In *The Engineering Handbook of Smart Technology for Aging, Disability, and Independence*, edited by Abdelsalam Helal, Mounir Mokhtari and Bessam Abdulrazak, 737–747.

Steinfeld, Aaron, Jordana L. Maisel, and Edward Steinfeld. 2017. *Accessible Public Transportation: Designing Service for Riders with Disabilities*. Routledge.

Thatcher, Russell, Caroline Ferris, David Chia, Jim Purdy, Buffy Ellis, Beth Hamby, Jason Quan, and Marilyn Golden. 2013. *Strategy Guide to Enable and Promote the Use of Fixed-Route Transit by People with Disabilities*. Transportation Research Board.

Toyota Motor Co. 2017. "Mobility Solutions: Auto Access Seat, Engineered by Toyota." http://www.toyotamobility.com/mobility_solutions.html.

van Roosmalen, L., G. J. Paquin, and A. M. Steinfeld. 2010. "Quality of Life Technology: The State of Personal Transportation." *Physical Medicine and Rehabilitation Clinics of North America* 21 (1): 111–125.

Wu, Xinzhou, Radovan Miucic, Sichao Yang, Samir Al-Stouhi, James Misener, Sue Bai, and Wai-hoi Chan. 2014. "Cars Talk to Phones: A DSRC Based Vehicle-Pedestrian Safety System." IEEE.

Chapter 16 Rehabilitation robotics

Michelle J. Johnson and
Rochelle Mendonca

Contents

16.1 Chapter overview

The World Health Organization estimates that approximately one billion people worldwide live with a disability, of which about 200 million experience considerable difficulties in functioning (World Health Organization 2011). As people age and survive diseases and traumas, the probability increases that they will live more of their lives with some type of disability. This chapter will discuss rehabilitation robotics, a special category of assistive technologies. Rehabilitation robots can support clinicians to treat and care for the aging population and those living

DOI: 10.1201/b21964-19

with various disabilities. This chapter will focus on providing a background on rehabilitation robots and provide a reason for why we need them. This chapter will define them and provide examples of their applications in adults and children with different diagnoses. Specifically, it will focus on therapy robots and assistive robots used in inpatient, outpatient, community, and/or home settings to support the recovery of motor and cognitive function. This chapter will first present examples of therapy robots designed to assist motor recovery in the lower and upper limbs. These robots assist in training the entire impaired limb or a specific joint and may be coupled with other physical modalities and imaging techniques to uncover how motor re-learning occurs. This chapter will also discuss current trends to provide more affordable therapy robots for home and community-based rehabilitation. In addition, examples of assistive robotics will be presented that provide personal service to elders by acting as companions, exercise coaches, and therapy guides. Finally, the chapter discusses a general framework for designing rehabilitation robots, describes a strategy for clinicians to prescribe and use them, and explains the strengths and limitations of robot technologies for rehabilitation, as well as speculates on what the future of the field may hold.

16.2 Need/motivation and definitions

Imagine what our world will be like in 2050. In 2050, 16.7% of the world's population (1.6 billion) will be 65 years and older. In high-income countries, these percentages are much higher. In the United States, the percentage is at about 22%, which represents a near doubling of the population from 48 million to 88 million (He, Goodkind, and Kowal 2016; Vincent and Velkof 2010), and in Japan, the current ratio of 26.7% of their 127 million population is expected to grow to 35.7% by 2050; that is, 1 in 2.8 persons will be over 65 (National Institute of Population and Social Security Research 2002). Although starker in high-income countries, the graying of the population is also seen in low- and middle-income countries. A rising number of elderly people means an increased prevalence of risk factors leading to adult disability. For example, the incidence of stroke increases as we age. Stroke is the leading cause of serious long-term disability with approximately 25.7 million people living with the effects of a stroke worldwide, including approximately five million in the United States, which will more than double by 2050 (Ovbiagele et al. 2013; World Health Organization 2018). At the same time, the projected number of physicians and rehabilitation clinical providers will be inadequate to meet the rehabilitation needs (Lin, Zhang, and Dixon 2015; Miller et al. 2010; Schoeb 2016; Zimbelman et al. 2010). Currently, in the United States, therapy is delivered by a rehabilitation team of professionals with the bulk delivered by 140,000 occupational therapists (OTs) and 185,000 physical therapists (PTs), with only 0.5% and 0.4% unemployment rates, respectively. From 2016 to 2026, it is projected that the employment of therapists will grow by 25% (Schoeb 2016; Zimbelman et al. 2010). This represents a ratio of 1.29 OTs and 3.62 PTs per 100 stroke patients. This is insufficient to meet stroke patient needs, much less the growing needs of the larger population with other disabilities. These disparities exist in larger numbers in low- and middle-income countries where ratios may range from 0 to 0.01 clinicians per 100 stroke patients.

The rehabilitation infrastructure worldwide is not prepared for these increasing numbers of adults with stroke and other disabilities (Demaerschalk, Hwang, and Leung 2010; Ovbiagele et al. 2013; Miller et al. 2010). Rehabilitation of an individual after injury or disease leading to impairment is necessary for a return to participation in his/her life. Despite the diversity of rehabilitation facilities in different parts of the world, a commonly evident observation is that very few individuals will receive intense, focused physical rehabilitation. Healthcare systems across the globe fail to meet rehabilitative needs for various reasons. In countries with privatized healthcare such as the United States, the third-party driven healthcare system greatly limits the number of physical/occupational therapy visits. In counties with public healthcare, there are limited therapists, limited access to advanced technologies, and/or limited systems in place to provide rehabilitation outside urban centers. Insufficient health insurance coverage, healthcare infrastructure challenges, and low ratios of rehabilitation practitioners to patients lead to poor health outcomes for individuals who require rehabilitation. Thus, in most countries across the world, the administration of physical rehabilitation is not sufficiently intense, structured, and comprehensive.

It is in this scenario that the need for rehabilitation robotics may be realized. A general definition of a robot is that it is an intelligent, computer-based mechanical system that can sense, think, and act to assist humans. With this definition, we define a rehabilitation robot as a reprogrammable, intelligent, multifunctional machine that is designed to function in an assistive or therapeutic capacity to aid persons with disabilities or diminished functional capacity. It does so by sensing its environment and thinking, that is, it processes sensor inputs coming from the environment to its microprocessors and decides on a course of action. For example, the action could manifest as the robot's body moving across the room or the robot's arm moving an attached limb or joint along a path. It is the hope that rehabilitation robotics technologies will bridge healthcare gaps (C. G. Kang et al. 2016; Keller et al. 2015; Reinkensmeyer and Dietz 2016; Technavio 2018). The rehabilitation robotics market is growing rapidly and is diverse in technology prescriptions. The global rehabilitation robotics market is expected to reach close to US$600 million by 2021 and possibly doubling by 2050 (Technavio 2018). Evidence suggests that these robots can improve functional outcomes, increase access to therapy and personal care, and supplement the shortage of trained rehabilitation staff. Engineers and roboticists' goals are to develop these technologies to support the aging and disabled population today and in 2050, our near future.

16.2.1 Target populations

Rehabilitation robots can be used in inpatient, outpatient, skilled nursing facilities, or laboratory environments. Therapy robots are currently not often seen in community-based or home environments due to their high cost. Assistive robots, on the other hand, are used in both hospital and community-based settings, including in nursing homes. Several populations have benefitted from the use of rehabilitation robots.

16.2.1.1 Stroke　A stroke or a cerebrovascular accident occurs when blood flow to the cerebral vasculature is blocked or cut off, resulting in a failure to supply oxygen to brain cells. This causes brain cells to die due to oxygen deprivation. A stroke may be hemorrhagic, a burst brain aneurysm or a blood vessel leak, or ischemic, which occurs when a blood vessel in the brain is blocked by a blood clot (World Health Organization 2018). Nearly 15 million people worldwide have a stroke each year with about five million people dying. It is one of the leading causes of long-term disability in the world (World Health Organization 2018). Stroke can have a wide variety of physical, sensory, and cognitive presentations such as weakness or paralysis on one side of the body, leading to difficulties in reaching, grasping, lifting, walking, vision problem, memory loss, and speech/language problems.

16.2.1.2 Traumatic brain injury　A traumatic brain injury (TBI) is typically caused by a bump, blow, jolt, or other head injuries that cause damage to the brain. Half of TBIs are caused by motor vehicle accidents, with other causes being falls and military-related causes. Approximately 69 million individuals sustain a TBI worldwide each year and TBI causes about 30% of all injury-related deaths (Dewan et al. 2018). A TBI can range from mild to severe, with symptoms ranging from headache, confusion, slurred speech, loss of coordination, weakness in upper and lower extremities, and numbness or tingling of the arms or legs.

16.2.1.3 Spinal cord injury　A spinal cord injury (SCI) impacts the vertebral column disrupting the signals between the body and the brain. The annual global incidence of SCI ranges from 13.1 to 163.4 per million new cases each year. The most common causes of SCI are vehicle crashes, falls, violent acts (such as gunshot wounds), and sports activities (Crewe and Krause 2009; Y. Kang et al. 2017). An SCI can be complete or incomplete. Complete SCI refers to the inability of the cord to send signals below the level of the injury, which results in paralysis (movement or sensation or both) below the level of the injury. In an incomplete injury, there might be some movement and sensation below the level of the injury.

16.2.1.4 Parkinson's disease　Parkinson's disease is a movement disorder that occurs when the brain nerve cells do not produce enough of a chemical called dopamine (Abbruzzese et al. 2016). It is estimated that about ten million people worldwide have Parkinson's disease and its prevalence is increasing. The most common symptoms are tremors of the hands, arms, legs, jaw, and face, stiffness of the arms, legs, and trunk, slowing down of movement, and poor balance and coordination. Over time, individuals with Parkinson's disease develop trouble with walking, talking, and doing simple activities of daily living (ADL) tasks.

16.2.1.5 Multiple sclerosis   Multiple sclerosis (MS) is a disorder of the nervous system that impacts the brain and the spinal cord by damaging the myelin sheath that surrounds and protects the nerve cells. This damage slows down or blocks messages between the brain and the body, leading to the symptomatology of MS such as muscle weakness, trouble with coordination and balance, visual disturbances, numbness, prickling, and cognitive issues. It is estimated that approximately 2.3 million people in the world live with MS (Browne et al. 2014).

16.2.1.6 Cerebral palsy   Cerebral palsy is a group of neurological disorders that appear in infancy or early childhood that affect body movement and muscle coordination caused by damage to the brain. According to the Centers for Disease Control and Prevention, about 2.9 in 1000 children worldwide have cerebral palsy (Dan and Paneth 2017). Symptoms can vary depending upon the part of the brain that is injured. Typical presentation includes problems with movement and posture, intellectual disability, seizures, impaired vision or hearing, and speech and language difficulties (Krigger 2006).

16.2.1.7 Elders   The population of older adults is growing around the world. There were 962 million individuals aged 60 and older in 2017 and this number is expected to increase to 2.1 billion by 2050, especially due to the aging of the baby boomer generation (He, Goodkind, and Kowal 2016). As individuals age, they become vulnerable to a number of age-related disabilities such as generalized weakness, sensory changes, cognitive changes, falls, cardiovascular diseases, difficulty completing daily living tasks, and fatigue, in addition to specific diagnoses such as arthritis, stroke, and Parkinson's disease to name a few (Jaul and Barron 2017).

Therapy robots targeting the upper extremity are often used with the stroke population, however, a number of robots have now been applied to children and adults with cerebral palsy and adults with other challenges such as MS (Kwakkel, Kollen, and Krebs 2008; Maciejasz et al. 2014; Reinkensmeyer and Dietz 2016). Therapy robots targeting the lower extremity are often used in gait recovery with stroke and spinal cord injured patients (Y. Kang et al. 2017; Keller et al. 2015). For assistive robots targeted for personal care and service, the most extensive work has been done with the elderly population.

16.3 Therapy robots

Technology-assisted therapy using robotics was birthed in the early 1990s with a focus on making the lives of people with disabilities better. A general design strategy encourages three key features. Therapy robots should deliver autonomous or semi-autonomous therapy to the body (e.g., arm, leg, finger, ankle), assess the level of disability and impairment in the given body part(s), and be adaptive to support motor recovery induced during training. In general, an effective therapy robot should reduce motor impairment, increase function, and be able to demonstrate clinically significant outcomes. When coupled with an imaging modality such as computed tomography (CT) scans or magnetic resonance imaging (MRI), evidence of training-induced brain re-organization should be seen. Typically, in developing therapy robots, engineers play with several parameters such as the context for therapy, the activities trained, the level of assistive and resistive forces, and the type of feedback given to the patient. These parameters may influence how therapy is delivered to the body part, the frequency and intensity of the therapy, how the therapy impacts recovery, and how engaged the patient is during the exercises. All these factors may be key criteria for motor learning leading to neuroplasticity (Kwakkel, Kollen, and Krebs 2008; Maciejasz et al. 2014; Mehrholz et al. 2015; Mehrholz, Thomas, and Elsner 2017).

Therapy robots can be classified by the control mechanism of the device or by the design of the user interface (Kwakkel, Kollen, and Krebs 2008; Maciejasz et al. 2014; Mehrholz et al. 2015; Mehrholz, Thomas, and Elsner 2017). Control mechanisms may be active or passive. Active systems have an actuator to assist an impaired limb. Passive systems offer non-powered assistance with elastic bands or springs to support a limb during movement. The classification of robots by user interface may be either end-effector based or exoskeletal. End-effector robots are attached to the user's hand or forearm or leg at a single point of contact, and are typically adjustable, but do not control movement at individual joints. Exoskeletal robots, on the other hand, are "wearable" devices, and typically have separate torque control applied to each joint. There may be hybrid systems that are both. Therapy robots can have one or more degrees of freedom (DOF), operate in and out of the plane, and provide feedback to the user via a variety of methods such as vibration, sound, visual, and force feedback. For example, haptic robot therapy devices interact with the user through a sense of touch and provide force feedback to the user via tactile sensations.

16.3.1 Lower limb therapy robots

The early lower limb therapy robots attempted to mimic aspects of therapy and focused on reducing the physicality of rehabilitation and the burden, as well as the fatigue, present in the retraining process. The focus of these robots is to assist patients in the recovery of gait and walking in the community (Hesse et al. 2000; Hidler et al. 2011; Hidler and Wall 2005; Keller et al. 2015; Mehrholz et al. 2015; Mehrholz, Thomas, and Elsner 2017; Reinkensmeyer and Dietz 2016; Schmidt et al. 2005; Sicari et al. 2011; Straudi et al. 2016; Aurich-Schuler et al. 2015; C. G. Kang et al. 2016). For example, 54–80% of stroke survivors have gait disturbance, which leads to the loss of independence and compromised mobility (C. G. Kang et al. 2016). A classic lower limb example of lower limb gait training that inspired the development of lower limb gait training robots is body weight-supported treadmill gait training where two to three therapists support a patient's impaired lower limbs to move in the gait patterns needed for independent gait (Figure 16.1). Here, it was envisioned that if a robot can be developed to deliver the guiding forces to the two legs while supporting the weight of the patient, then only one therapist would be needed to direct the overall "high-level" process of therapy. The other therapist would then be free to treat other patients, and both therapists would be spared the potential injury inherent in the more physical treatment method.

This strategy was probably used to develop end-effector and exoskeletal gait training robots such as the Lokomat (Hocoma, Ltd) and the Gait Trainer GTII (Reha-Stim). The Lokomat is one of the first commercial exoskeletal gait training robot (Aurich-Schuler et al. 2015; C. G. Kang et al. 2016; Mehrholz, Thomas, and Elsner 2017; Reinkensmeyer and Dietz 2016; Straudi et al. 2016; Keller et al. 2015; Figure 16.2a). Used with children and adults with moderate to severely impaired gait, the Lokomat features two exoskeleton robots with two DOF, one for moving the knee joint and one for moving the hip joint, connected by a hip mechanism and an overhead harness that provides body weight support. The patients are strapped

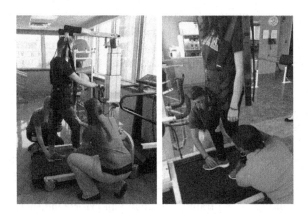

Figure 16.1 Body-weight supported treadmill training with two therapists. Permission from Chad E Cook PT, MBA, PhD, FAPTA at https://medspace.mc. duke.edu/concern/documents/6q182k57v?locale=en

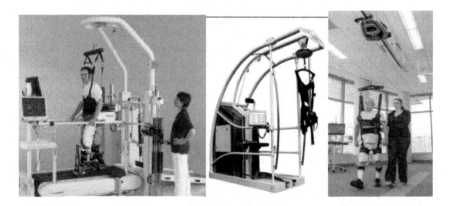

Figure 16.2 Three therapy robots: (a) Lokomat (Aurich-Schuler et al. 2015; Straudi et al. 2016); (b) Gait Trainer GII (Hesse et al. 2000; Schmidt et al. 2005); and (c) the ZeroG (Hidler et al. 2011). Permission received from Lokomat and Andago (www.hocoma.com/media-center/media-images/).

into the system and suspended above an integrated treadmill. The therapist then directs the gait activities via a graphical user interface (GUI), which allows them to modify training parameters including time, duration, and gait speed to name a few. In contrast, the first commercial end-effector gait training robot was the Gait Trainer GTII, inspired by the Gangtrainer GT1 and the haptic walker developed in Germany (Schmidt et al. 2005; Hesse et al. 2000). This gait training system also uses two robots each with three DOF, one for each leg, and provides a contact with patients at the sole of the feet. The body weight of the patient is also adaptively supported.

Studies comparing training within one or more of these two contrasting robot-assisted training paradigms with conventional gait therapy show that robot-assisted gait retraining is possible and that training within these systems, especially in end-effector systems, leads to increased walking velocity and walking capacity (C. G. Kang et al. 2016; Mehrholz, Thomas, and Elsner 2017; Straudi et al. 2016). The review also suggests that for people in the subacute phase of recovery, the odds of experiencing independent walking increase when they are trained using these systems. The benefits of training in the chronic phase are still unclear (C. G. Kang et al. 2016; Mehrholz, Thomas, and Elsner 2017). Some suggest that the method of recovery is not close enough to natural gait, that is, the muscles being activated are not typical of normal walking (Hidler et al. 2011; Hidler and Wall 2005). These criticisms have led to designs of new robots focused on encouraging a more natural gait and training through gait error. One such system is the ZeroG Robot Gait and Balance Trainer which focuses on overground walking and provides body weight support and force-feedback via a one-DOF robot suspended on a track above the user (Figure 16.2c). The unloading mechanism can support

300 lbs. (136.4 kg) in static support and 150 lbs. (68.2 kg) in dynamic walking using series elastic actuators to control the cable forces (Hidler et al. 2011). In truth, it seems reasonable to expect that more severely impaired patients with severe paralysis and weakness in their legs would first use Lokomat that supports the entire leg, and as they improve, progress to a ZeroG environment.

In general, many clinicians see the benefit of using these systems. Kang and colleagues surveyed a total of 100 physiatrists and 100 physical therapists from 38 hospitals in Korea about robot-assisted gait training (C. G. Kang et al. 2016). Many believed that gait-training robots serve to improve gait treatment effects (28.5%), help standardize treatment (19%), help to motivate patients (17%), and improve patients' self-esteem (14%). They report that the subacute period (one to three months poststroke onset) was the preferred period for the use of these devices with the preferred model being the treadmill type (47.5%) versus the overground walking type (40%). The typical robot-assisted gait therapy period was 30–45 min, three times a week.

Given the constraints on time for therapy in modern settings, a relatively recent trend is to build therapy robots to provide patients with additional opportunities for more training and provide engagement in gait therapy outside the inpatient hospital setting. The exoskeletal robots, ReWalk (Argo Ltd) and Ekso (Ekso Bionics), were born from the idea of having robots that provide both therapy and assistive device benefits (Brenner 2016; Esquenazi et al. 2012; Naro et al. 2017). The ReWalk robot is a powered exoskeleton that allows individuals with thoracic or lower-level motor-complete or incomplete SCI (C7-T12) to walk independently (Figure 16.3). ReWalk is a six-DOF system that has bilateral hip and knee joint motors, ankle double-action orthotic joints with limited motion and spring-assisted dorsiflexion, rechargeable batteries, and a computerized control system carried in a backpack. A tilt sensor determines the angle of the torso and generates a preset hip and knee displacement (angle and time) that results in a step (Esquenazi et al. 2012). The EksoGT-powered exoskeleton robot is a four-DOF system that has bilateral hip and knee joint motors, with computer-controlled assistance. Indicated mainly for stroke and SCI patients, patients must be <220 lbs. (100 kg) and between 150 cm and 187.5 cm. The system now incorporates functional electrical stimulation (FES) to support muscle activation during overground walking (Babaiasl et al. 2016; Brenner 2016).

Both systems require significant upper arm strength and are most frequently used with patients with spinal cord injury. Clinicians usually have patients first practice standing and ambulating in the device with the use of a front-wheeled walker, then onto Loftstrand forearm crutches (FC) or other specialized crutches that use pressure sensors in the arm and footpad to trigger a step in the contralateral leg when placed on the ground. These systems are considered safe and effective for training overground walking. Patient users with a spinal injury, previously

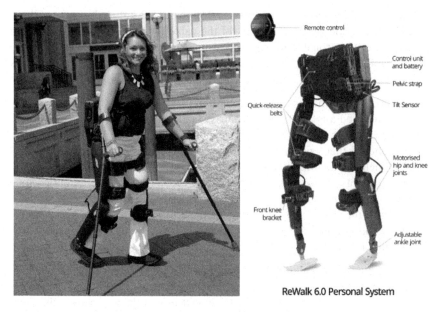

Figure 16.3 ReWalk (Brenner 2016). Permission received from ReWalk: http://rewalk.com/gallery-2/.

limited to a wheelchair, typically report increases in the emotional benefits of being able to see the world eye-to-eye and other positive effects such as a reduction of spasticity and pain (Brenner 2016).

16.3.2 Upper limb therapy robots

Like the lower limb therapy robots, the early upper limb therapy robots mimicked aspects of therapy and focused on reducing the physicality of rehabilitation and the burden, as well as the fatigue, present in the retraining process (Amirabdollahian et al. 2007; Babaiasl et al. 2016; Brokaw et al. 2014; C. G. Burgar et al. 2011; C. Burgar, Lum, and Shor 2000; Colomer et al. 2013; Fasoli et al. 2003; Fluet et al. 2009; Hartwig 2014; Hesse L. et al. 2005; Hesse et al. 2003; Johnson et al. 2006; Kim, Rivera, and Stein 2015; Klamroth-Marganska et al. 2014; Krebs et al. 1998; Krebs et al. 2009; Lambercy et al. 2007; Lambercy et al. 2011; Liao et al. 2012; Lo et al. 2009; Loureiro et al. 2003; Lum et al. 2002; Nathan, Johnson, and McGuire 2009; Nef, Mihelj, and Riener 2007; Page, Hill, and White 2013; Rahman et al. 2000; Reinkensmeyer and Housman 2007; Riener et al. 2011; Bouzit et al. 2002; Rosier et al. 1989; Schulz et al. 2015; Theriault, Nagurka, and Johnson 2014; Timmermans et al. 2014; Towery, Machek, and Thomas 2017; Wagner et al. 2011; Wolf et al. 2015). The design of the upper limb therapy robots presents a more difficult challenge given the large variety of activities that can be performed by the arm and hand such as cooking, cleaning, fishing, and so on. The left and right arm and hand can be engaged in symmetric and asymmetric bilateral or unilateral activities. Upper limb therapy robots most often focus on reaching and/or grasping activities in virtual or real contexts. Simpler upper limb therapy robots with fewer DOFs often use video games as the context for therapy delivery. We present examples of upper limb therapy robots that span the field in terms of degrees of freedom, control strategy, training context, and user interface. They are single or multi-DOF robot manipulators for training the impaired arm of the stroke patient, guiding the person through therapeutic exercises from point-to-point reaching to real activities.

Two of the earliest systems were the MIT-Manus robot, which later spawned the commercial InMotion Arm™ robot, and the Mirror-Image Motion Enabler (MIME; Figure 16.4). Both systems were for stroke patients and were multi-DOF end-effector robots and implemented reaching tasks using impedance-based control strategy. The InMotion system focused on using a custom robot to move the impaired arm in 2D space, while the MIME robot system focused on using a modified commercial robot to move the impaired arm in 3D space by capitalizing on the movement of the less-impaired arm. In both systems, the patient is typically seated in a wheelchair or custom chair at a height adjustable table and their forearm(s) and hand(s) are supported in an orthosis attached to the end of the robot. The InMotion Arm is the most widely researched upper extremity rehabilitation robot system and has been shown to benefit populations such as adults and children with stroke and cerebral palsy and has been extended to populations with MS (Wagner et al. 2011; Fasoli et al. 2003; Krebs et al. 1998; Krebs et al. 2009; Lo et al. 2009). It was developed at the Neuman Laboratory for Biomechanics and Human Rehabilitation at the Massachusetts Institute of Technology, Cambridge. It is a planar, two DOF end-effector robot that primarily supports movements at the shoulder and elbow. In addition, there is a wrist module that can be operated as a standalone unit or mounted to the end of the shoulder-elbow robot. The patient grasps a joystick and moves their upper extremity to play reaching games on a screen in front of them. Tasks are practiced in 2D space. An impedance control mode provides assistance or resistance as needed by the patient to facilitate movement, strength, coordination, and speed.

In contrast, the MIME was developed via a collaboration with the Department of Veterans Affairs Palo Alto Health Care System and Stanford University (Brokaw et al. 2014; C. G. Burgar et al. 2011; C. Burgar, Lum, and Shor 2000; Lum et al. 2002) and primarily tested in the stroke population. The MIME robot is an active, end-effector robot, consisting of a six-DOF PUMA 560 robot that allows the practice of shoulder and elbow movements in a 3D space. The system has 12 trajectories of reaching movements to real targets and four modes of practice: passive,

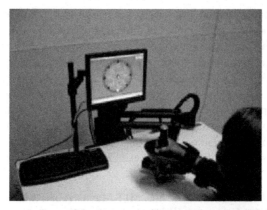

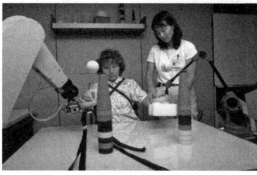

Figure 16.4 InMotion Arm robot-basic module (top; Fasoli et al. 2003; Krebs et al. 1998; Krebs et al. 2009; Lo et al. 2009; Wagner et al. 2011) and MIME (bottom; Brokaw et al. 2014; C. G. Burgar et al. 2011; C. Burgar, Lum, and Shor 2000; Lum et al. 2002).

active assisted, active resisted, and bimanual training, where the unaffected upper extremity guides movement of the affected upper extremity.

Pilot studies evaluating the efficacy of robot-assisted therapy with the MIT-Manus and MIME have generally shown gains in function and strength for individuals with chronic stroke in assessments such as the Fugl-Meyer Assessment (Gladstone, Danells, and Black 2002), the Motor Status Scale (Ferraro et al. 2002), the Functional Independence Measure (FIM) (Hamilton et al. 1987; Heinemann et al. 1994), and motor power both in the short and long term. Training sessions vary from 15 to 24 sessions and are typically 60 minutes in duration. Some have examined therapy robots with respect to conventional therapy and have varied time, dosage, and intensity to understand their impact. Meta-analyses and clinical trials primarily with the InMotion robot show that rehabilitation outcomes with robots are comparable to standard and intensity-matched stroke rehabilitation and significantly improve functional outcomes in terms of motor control with low to modest improvements in ADL function (Babaiasl et al. 2016; Brenner 2016; Fasoli et al. 2003). The use of robotic therapy has demonstrated promise in potential cost savings and efficient use of therapists' time throughout the labor-intensive and long-term process of stroke rehabilitation. Lo et al. showed that after 36 weeks, a robot-therapy platform for stroke was just as effective in reducing motor impairment as an intensity-matched regime with similar healthcare costs (Krebs et al. 2009; Lo et al. 2009). The main complaint with these systems is that their impact on independent functioning is not as robust as desired.

To improve ADL functional outcomes, several versions of therapy robots have been proposed. One thought was that the practice of purposeful tasks involving both reach and grasping of virtual objects or real objects may be a solution. The use of the commercial Haptic Master robot (MOOG, Inc) was incorporated into several robot-assisted therapy strategies (Figure 16.5). The Gentle(s) (Amirabdollahian et al. 2007; Loureiro et al. 2003), Activities of Daily Living Exercise Robot (ADLER) (Johnson et al. 2006), and NJIT-RAVR (Fluet et al. 2009) robot systems were all developed with the goal of training stroke survivors to complete reaching and grasping tasks in more purposeful environments and 3D space either in virtual or real contexts. The Haptic Master is a six-DOF end-effector robot with three active DOF for positioning and three for the orientation of the gimbal. Typically, the user sits at a workstation with the arm supported by the gimbal through an elbow or forearm splint, which allows for supination, pronation, and wrist flexion and extension. An admittance force control is employed with the haptic master robot, which allows larger forces (>100 N) to be produced at the end-effector, which can support whole arm movement under assistance or resistance with minimal friction. In the Gentle/s system, users wore a separate hand robot to assist with opening and closing of the hand, while in the ADLER system, users could practice tasks with or without a custom functional electrical stimulation glove designed to support grasping (Nathan, Johnson, and McGuire 2009). Like the MIME and InMotion systems, to determine their effectiveness, training in these robot systems was contrasted with a control group. Participants practiced tasks such as drinking from a cup, combing hair, choosing a bottle, or taking money from a purse. Results demonstrated that participants in the experimental showed a significant improvement over time on the Action Arm Research Test (ARAT), and participants in both groups improved on the Motor Activity Log (MAL) and the results were maintained at six months after training. However, there were no between-group differences in any of the outcome measures (Fugl-Meyer, ARAT, and MAL) (Brokaw et al. 2014). Again, these results suggest improvement can occur, but the training is not consistently significantly different from dosage and intensity matched conventional rehabilitation care. The carry-over to functional activities still fell short of expectations.

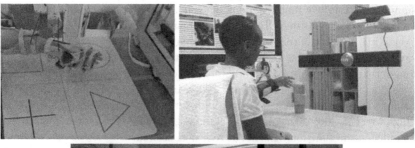

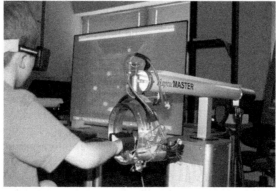

Figure 16.5 Three ADL focused therapy robots: (a) Gentle/s (Amirabdollahian et al. 2007; Loureiro et al. 2003), (b) ADLER (Nathan, Johnson, and McGuire 2009); and C. NJIT-RAVR (Qiu et al. 2009).

Another strategy to improve the ability of robot-assisted therapy of the upper limb to improve ADL function was to propose exoskeletal systems that would be able to train individual joints and not just the whole arm. This thought spawned several systems leading to ArmIn, which later became the commercial system ArmeoPower (Hocoma; Klamroth-Marganska et al. 2014; Nef, Mihelj, and Riener 2007; Riener et al. 2011) and the T-Wrex, which later became the commercial product ArmeoSpring (Hocoma; Colomer et al. 2013; Reinkensmeyer and Housman 2007). The ArmIn was developed by ETH Zurich (Klamroth-Marganska et al. 2014) and is an exoskeletal robot that provides "patient-directed" levels of assistance, which means that the robot only gives assistance as needed. It has a low impedance system with seven DOF that supports movements at the shoulder, elbow, forearm, wrist, and hand to provide intensive and task-specific training of the upper extremity (Figure 16.6). The patient can practice various games and activities of daily living in a virtual environment such as kitchen activities and ball games. The system provides haptic, visual, and auditory feedback to the patient during use. In contrast, the T-Wrex was developed by the University of California, Irvine (Reinkensmeyer and Housman 2007). The

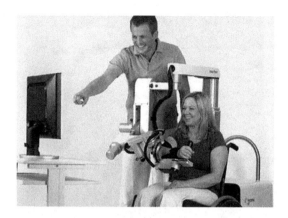

Figure 16.6 Armeo Power (Klamroth-Marganska et al. 2014). Permission received from Armeo (www.hocoma.com/media-center/media-images/)

clinical version known as ArmeoSpring is a passive, body-powered orthosis that has easily adjustable elastic bands to support the limb and allow an active range of motion and reach. The system allows the user to engage in virtual games such as moving things in a supermarket. The T-Wrex and ArmeoSpring support the impaired arm against gravity, however, they cannot assist the patient with the completion of movements, while the ARMinIII can apply and control torques at each joint individually and provide customized assistance. Studies have compared therapy with the ARMinIII robot to conventional therapy in patients with chronic stroke. One study with 77 chronic stroke patients, who were training in 24 to 45 sessions over eight weeks on either the ARMinIII or with conventional therapy found that patients in the robotic group had greater improvements on the Fugl-Meyer at post-assessment (Klamroth-Marganska et al. 2014). This strategy also did not result in clear carry-over superiority over dose and intensity matched conventional therapy.

More recent trends suggest that the issue is one of dosage and there is a need for upper limb therapy robots that can be used in the community and home environments. The MyoPro Myoelectric robot is an example of a wearable upper extremity exoskeleton device that assists outside of the hospital environment and supports elbow, wrist, and finger movements. It uses a surface electromyography control mechanism to detect and amplify signals from the biceps and triceps. The amount of force generated by Myomo is based on the amplitude of the EMG signal, which proportionally produces assistance (Rahman et al. 2000). Stroke patients training with the Myomo exoskeleton in clinics and/or at home experienced significant improvements and increased independence (Kim, Rivera, and Stein 2015; Page, Hill, and White 2013). The system functions as a therapy and assistive device (Figure 16.7).

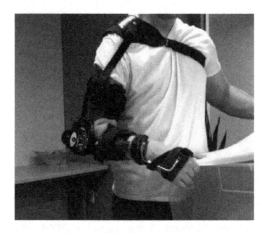

Figure 16.7 MyoPro (Rahman et al. 2000). Permission received directly from Dr. Sam Kesner (www.myomo.com).

16.3.3 Simpler and more affordable therapy robots

Most commercial robot-assisted therapy devices are expensive with costs of more than US$50,000–US$200,000 for a single unit. This cost is prohibitive for the home and community-based rehabilitation settings, where space, money, and human resources limit the ability to acquire and use expensive robotic technology or provide intensive rehabilitation. Rehabilitation services and innovative solutions are thus also needed to augment health service delivery so as to enable more therapy outside of hospital environments.

One of the earliest lower cost upper limb therapy robot systems was the Bi-Manu Trak, a system designed for bilateral rehabilitation of the upper extremity by training movements at the wrist and forearm. The system enables mirror-like practice, with three modes of practice: passive-passive, where both arms are controlled by the robot; active-passive, where the non-affected arm drives the affected side; and active-active, where both arms actively move against resistance. One advantage of this system is that it is simple using one DOF robots and providing haptic feedback (Hesse L. et al. 2005). Bi-Manu-Trak improves motor function and arm activity, and a decrease in spasticity in stroke survivors (Liao et al. 2012; Hesse et al. 2003). More recent commercial affordable robots are focused on retraining the hand and fingers to improve carry-over to real activities. Examples are the haptic knob, a two DOF end-effector robot that can be adapted to different hand sizes, finger orientations, and people with right or left-sided impairments of the hand. Differently shaped fixtures can be attached to the interface to train different hand functions, including power grasp, pinch, and lateral pinch. It can generate up to 50 N of assistive or resistive forces in opening and closing of the hand and up to 1.5 Nm of torques in pronation and supination (Lambercy et al. 2007; Lambercy et al. 2011). Other devices that work on retraining hand function include Rutgers Master II (Bouzit et al. 2002), Hand Mentor Pro (Motus Nova (Wolf et al. 2015), Tyromotion's Amadeo and Pablo (Hartwig 2014), among others. Some of these robot systems focus on exercising one joint such as the wrist or elbow or shoulder. Others are specific for finger or hand exercise movements. Technologies such as Armeo Senso (Hocoma: US$4800) and Rapael Smart Glove (Neofect: US$16,000; Wolf et al. 2015) typically target moderate to high functioning stroke patients in that they do not apply large adaptive forces but use motion and pressure sensing technologies to measure arm, hand, and/or finger position for game-based exercise. Many of these lower costs systems do not support the more severely impaired stroke survivor. In response, a more recent low-cost system, the haptic Theradrive, is a one DOF robot to support shoulder and elbow exercises and is capable of supporting stroke survivors with a severely impaired arm with up to 40–45 Nm at its crank arm (Theriault, Nagurka, and Johnson 2014). A prototype of this robot exists with some pilot evidence, however, clinic-based testing is still needed.

16.4 Assistive robots

Assistive rehabilitation robots are most frequently used with elderly patients and patients with SCI. Assistive robots are defined as robots that serve humans by augmenting their current function. Typically, these robots are used after remediation of impairment is completed. As such, they may be designed to (1) perform the activities users still have difficulty completing, (2) replace the function of an amputated limb or one that is permanently paralyzed and weakened, and (3) monitor and be a companion to a user.

For SCI patients who have high-level quadriplegia and cannot move arms and legs independently, robot arms can be used to support the manipulation of the environment. One class of assistive robots is called wheelchair-mounted robot arms. Often, these robot arms are mounted onto powered wheelchair bases or mobile robot wheelchair bases. For example, the Manus is a wheelchair-mounted robotic arm originally developed in the Netherlands in the early 1990s (Driessen, Evers, and van Woerden 2001; Hagan et al. 1997; Kwee 1998; Rosier et al. 1989; Schulz et al. 2015; Towery, Machek, and Thomas 2017). It is a six DOF robot manipulator with a two-fingered gripper, which has passive canting mechanisms for secure three-point grasping action of most objects. The Manus robot can be controlled via a modular control system for steering it to a desired location. A simple user interface can be configured by the user or the therapist to allow control of the robot via teach pendent or voice or visual servo. After evolution of 20 years, Manus is a commercially available product called iARM (Exact Dynamics) and is one of the few wheelchair-mounted robot arms being prescribed for users in places such as the Netherlands and France. It has been shown to increase independence and support patients' return to work (Driessen, Evers, and van Woerden 2001). Another more recent example is the JACO manipulator (Clearpath robotics), which is lightweight (3 kg) and designed to be mounted on a powered wheelchair. It has 6DOF and a three-fingered hand. Through a joystick and button, users can toggle control modes to move the robot hand position, orient the hand, and then open the hand. It is able to reach 1 m in all directions and lift up to 2.5 kg (Beaudoin et al. 2018; Campeau-Lecours et al. 2016; Routhier et al. 2014; Figure 16.8). These robots can complete a variety of activities such as reaching to open a door, scratching the face, or providing the user with a drink. The system was able to improve independent living and social participation of elders (Routhier et al. 2014).

With elder users, assistive robots—often called personal care or social robots—are designed to do a variety of service tasks in the home and community (Breazeal 2002; Gallagher 2007; Goher, Mansouri, and Fadlallah 2017; Schulz et al. 2015; Sefcik et al. 2018). These robots can take on a variety of forms, humanoid, animaloid, or other. For example, in home activities such as fetching and carrying objects, the CARE-O-BOT, an autonomous mobile robot with a manipulator, was one of the first systems developed for such use (Graf, Hans, and Schraft 2004). For elder patients with cognitive impairments, many assistive robots often provide reminders and monitor health by tracking biometrics (Goher, Mansouri, and Fadlallah 2017; Johnson et al. 2017a), as well as providing companionship and social interaction. The Paro, a seal-like robot, has been used to improve mental health and social connectedness with elders in a nursing home (Hebesberger et al. 2016; Shibata and Wada 2011; Wada and Shibata 2007; Figure 16.9). The Paro is a fully responsive and learning seal robot that can remember the direction of voices and words such as its name, greetings, and praise, petting actions, and interacting with elders in a realistic pet-like manner. It is capable of these behaviors because of tactile, light, audition, temperature, and posture sensors that allow it to perceive people and its environment. An embedded control algorithm allows it to learn and

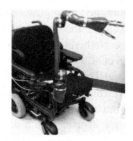

Figure 16.8 ACO (Kinova) for wheelchair manipulators (Beaudoin et al. 2018; Campeau-Lecours et al. 2016; Routhier et al. 2014).

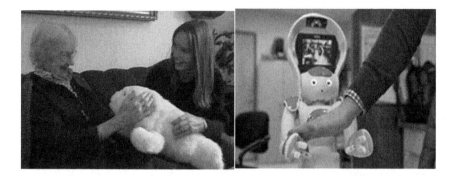

Figure 16.9 (a) Paro (Hebesberger et al. 2016; Wada and Shibata 2007) [Permission granted by AIST, Japan] and (b) Nao social robots (Gouaillier et al. 2009; Miskam et al. 2013).

act based on sensor activation and history of interaction. It is currently an eighth-generation design that has been in use in Japan and Europe. More recent systems use advanced machine learning techniques to allow these types of robots learn and adapt to individual patients in order to provide more patient-specific care.

To provide therapeutic exercise, the Nao (Softbank), a 58 cm tall humanoid robot, has been used to demonstrate exercise activities and invite older adults to follow along (Gouaillier et al. 2009) (Figure 16.9b). The Nao is a fully responsive humanoid robot that can walk, talk, grasp objects, be taught to mimic movements, and so on. Once programmed, it can be made to execute a variety of tasks autonomously (Miskam et al. 2013). The Nao robot functions as both an assistive robot and a therapy robot. Another example is Bandit, which can guide elderly patients and brain-injured patients in enjoyable therapeutic exercise in nursing homes and hospitals (Fasola and Mataric 2012; Matarić et al. 2007). Bandit, a non-contact social and therapy agent provided not only active guidance, feedback, and task monitoring, but also instructed and steered the task, hence it was instrumental in achieving physical exercise for older adults. Bandit provided elders with personalized praise and empathized with failed attempts and it was effective in increasing motivation to exercise even in the absence of a therapist. Another example is the Baxter, a commercial humanoid robot with two arms, which has been used in physical-social interactive tasks such as hand clapping and other novel interactive games (Fitter et al. 2018). In contrast to the therapy robots described previously, these assistive robots for therapy (also known as socially assistive robots or SAR) can deliver therapy with or without physical contact with the patient. The robot acts as a social agent and invites patients to engage in therapeutic exercise; they guide the exercise activity with behaviors designed to make exercise more enjoyable (speech, facial expressions, gestures, or movements of the robot arms) and monitor the patient's resulting movements for accuracy. Assistive robots monitor upper or lower limb activities with a variety of methods such as accelerometers, body sensors, and visual 3D motion tracking with Kinect or stereo cameras and provide encouragement (praise and empathetic noises), reminders, and guidance when needed.

16.5 Clinical considerations

There are several advantages to using rehabilitation robots. First, robotic systems provide objective measurement of users' performance such as measurements of kinematics, kinetics, physiological changes, and degrees of movement. These systems can measure minute changes in function that are often not detectable by clinical measurements. Robots are also capable of consistently applying forces and assisting or resisting movement or engaging tirelessly. Unlike humans, robots do not feel fatigued. Especially in cases where high intensity and high levels of repetitive practice are required, robotic systems have advantages over human therapists. In terms of personal care, given sensors and monitoring tools, they can provide clinicians with information about patients at a distance and stand in the gap when the clinician's physical presence is not always possible.

A rehabilitation robot is an advanced tool to be used under the therapist's direction. Clinical decisions to employ and use rehabilitation robots should be managed by the rehabilitation team. How to use the robot for care should be carefully planned so that the patient is matched to the right system. Ideally, the therapist should use the rehabilitation robots to off-load repetitive tasks that require more than a few reps and labor-intensive training, and are suitable for a robot to do ethically. There are several barriers that clinicians face when considering how best to integrate the technology or technologies into their rehabilitation settings. One barrier is technical comfort. Clinicians often do not have the technical expertise to set up or troubleshoot technology, especially high-end technology like robots, however, with appropriate training, it has been shown that it is entirely possible to use rehabilitation robots for clinical interventions. Additionally, as the field evolves, there is a move toward increasing the usability of these systems for easier integration into clinical settings. Another barrier is cost. Robotic systems are expensive, however, when comparing the initial cost of a rehabilitation robot to the potential clinical potential of integrating a robot into therapeutic settings, there are definite advantages in terms of time or consistency of interventions; these advantages will be clearer in hospital-based rehabilitation settings where resources are more plentiful. Rehabilitation settings such as nursing homes and daycare centers may not have the money to purchase these systems or the space to host them. The trend toward creating affordable robotic systems for home and community-based settings should ultimately address this limitation. Lastly, there are ethical barriers. Many clinicians are still resistant to the use of robots because it diminishes human-human contact. However, there is a significant amount of research exploring patient-therapist interactions and models to improve human-robot interactions that would ethically serve all patients in the face of impending shortages (Mohan, Mendonca, and Johnson 2017; Sharkey and Sharkey 2012).

Often a challenge for therapists in the use of rehabilitation technology is choosing the systems that will best match the setting and the client population. The general rule of thumb in rehabilitation is to provide the appropriate amount of support and challenges to patients to encourage them to achieve maximum functional capability. For example, if the patient is higher functioning, the system should provide less assistance and possibly more resistance, and if the patient is lower functioning, the system should provide more assistance. Highly adaptable systems can be used in a wider range of settings and with a wider diversity of patients. When deciding which robotic system to use, it is necessary for therapists to understand which system targets the function that needs training in the population the system will be used with. These systems must have a way of quantifying functional change or change in the level of impairment. Often, it is useful to use a human-centered design approach such as the human, activity, assistive technology (HAAT) model to understand the appropriateness of a device for a setting (Cook and Polgar 2014).

16.6 Robot design considerations

There are several accepted design methodologies, such as universal design and human-centered design, which place the patient/human user at the center of the product design process and increase the probability that rehabilitation robots are useful for clinical settings (Cook and Polgar 2014; Smith et al. 2018; Story 1998). The analysis of user needs is a critical first phase and includes a consideration of the following: (1) the real clinical problem; (2) all the human users; and (3) the user activity context and goals. In the assessment of disabled user needs, a systematic approach is recommended such as the HAAT model (Cook and Polgar 2014). As described in more detail in Chapter 14, this HAAT model asks the designer/engineer to critically assess the following: (1) human stakeholders (e.g., patient, caregiver, therapist); (2) the activity or activities the human desires the device to do; and (3) the context/environment in which the human desires to do these activities. Typically, the robot device requirements will be implied after assessing humans, activity, and context. Applying the universal design principles provides another systematic approach. The seven universal design principles guide product development (Story 1998). Products should be useful for a diverse group (1: equitable in use) and be designed for people of diverse abilities (2: flexible in use). In the case of rehabilitation robots, where possible, robots should provide the same benefit and function to all users as well as be usable to a wide functional range of individuals. For example, an assistive robot that is usable and appeals to all family members and not just the elders would better achieve these principles. Products should be easy to understand, regardless of the user's experience, knowledge, language skills, or current concentration level (3: simple and intuitive to use) as well as communicate necessary information effectively to the user, regardless of ambient conditions or the user's sensory abilities (4: perceptible information). Products should be designed to avoid the adverse consequences of accidental or unintended actions (5: ensure tolerance for error) and maximize the user's efficiency and minimize fatigue (6: require low physical effort). Clearly, if rehabilitation robots were designed with rules four to six in mind, the robot would be easier to set up and use in the rehabilitation setting. Finally, how to approach, reach, and manipulate the product's physical interface should be considered to ensure that users with varying body sizes, posture, and mobility can be accommodated (7: size and space to approach and use). Current robots are not always designed with the HAAT model or with universal design principles. Consequently, engineers risk increasing user frustration with the system, diminishing user enthusiasm and acceptance of the system, and thus, slowing the adoption into clinical settings.

To better integrate robots into clinical and community-based environments, engineers should ensure that the systems are easy to set up, easy to use, and easy to maintain. Clinicians may abandon these devices if setting up takes more than 10% of the typical 30 to 45 minutes they are allotted for each patient's therapy because the user interface is complicated and non-intuitive and if the system breaks frequently. Designers can minimize abandonment by ensuring that the design process involves all the stakeholders. Surveys, focus groups, show and tell, immersion of the team in the target environment, and rapid prototyping can be beneficial processes for querying stakeholders.

Safety and efficacy are extremely important. It is necessary to design the robots so that they can be easily customized to the diverse needs of the patients and their caregivers, including family and clinicians. Patient needs range from high to low functioning, impairments in upper or lower extremities, robots for social interaction, and the ability to train gross or fine motor function. Contra-indications should be clear, so clinicians are aware of how and who can interact with or be trained using robots.

16.7 Future directions

A quick review of current activities in the rehabilitation field shows that artificial intelligence, specifically machine learning, brain computing interfaces, new "soft" materials for robots, and affordability provide the next frontier in rehabilitation robot device development. Machine learning offers increasing potential to improve the ability of both therapy and assistive robots to accurately perceive, predict, and act to control the environment (Boquete et al. 2005; Montemerlo et al. 2002). Use cases are emerging that suggest that future robots will be able to quickly recognize faces and predict health failures in patients, as well as predict user control intent for a wheelchair robot to ease the burden of using them. Brain computing interfaces and imaging techniques such as electroencephalography (EEG) and electrocorticography (ECOG), coupled with new frontiers in implantable electrodes for the brain, suggest that in the foreseeable future, there will be thought-controlled and neural-controlled therapy and assistive robots (Galan et al. 2008; Scherer et al. 2012). Our desire to interact closer and safer with robots has seen the emergence of soft robots for rehabilitation. These robots are often able to be in close contact with patients due to the use of novel deformable materials. Examples of exoskeletal soft robots for the body and hands are harbingers of wearable robots that are transparent, not bulky or heavy, and are able to be worn all day to augment healthy or impaired limbs (Radder et al. 2016; Xiloyannis et al. 2016). Given the knowledge of a worldwide need for rehabilitation technology solutions that are not only appropriate for developed countries, and developing countries, we anticipate an expansion of the scope and populations using rehabilitation robots and the development of low-cost robot systems that can be used in group-based robot training environments where one therapist can oversee four or more patients. Circuit training and group therapy in robot gyms and group exercise and play with social robots are emerging as cost-effective solutions for developing and low-resource environments (Bustamante Valles et al. 2016; Johnson et al. 2017b). Recently, in their statement entitled "Rehabilitation 2030: A call for action," the World Health Organization placed the need for accessible and affordable rehabilitation front and center in achieving Sustainable Development Goal (SDG) 3, "Ensure healthy lives and promote well-being for all at all ages" (World Health Organization 2017).

16.8 Discussion questions

Problem 1: What is the ratio of severely disabled people per therapist in the United States and Mexico? Is this appropriate? Assume a 52-week year and 40 h/week for each clinician. How many seconds could they allow for each severely disabled person in the United States?

Problem 2: Which populations are currently benefitting from the use of therapy robots? How are they the same or different from those who typically benefit from assistive robots?

Problem 3: How are exoskeletal robots the same and different from endoskeletal robots? Explain similarities and differences using an example of each.

Problem 4: How are therapy robots different from assistive robots? Explain differences using an example of each type.

Problem 5: How is conventional gait therapy different from therapy using gait therapy robots? What are the pros and cons of each type?

Problem 6: Describe challenges to implementing rehabilitation robots in today's clinical environments. How can these challenges be ameliorated?

Problem 7: Describe key features for rehabilitation robots that improve their acceptance by patients and therapists.

Problem 8: Ethical concerns act as a potential barrier to the implementation and acceptance of rehabilitation robots in today's clinics. Discuss them and how they may be resolved.

Problem 9: Universal design and HAAT model are two design techniques that have been used with rehabilitation robots. How are they different? How are products in general and rehabilitation robots improved using these processes?

Problem 10: Consider the following case: Jane is a 12-year-old female who was diagnosed with hemiplegic cerebral palsy at the age of two. She lives in Philadelphia in a two-bedroom apartment with her parents and an older brother. She goes to a school for children with disabilities and is in Grade 5. She has moderate functioning in terms of motor and cognition and is described as easily distractible. Jane is left hand dominant. She uses a manual wheelchair that must be pushed by a caregiver. She is weak in both limbs. Her caregiver desires her to strengthen her limbs to the point that she would be able to help. She would like to be able to push herself. Based on an upper limb test, she is able to use her right limb to pick up 30 blocks, while the left arm can only pick up three in one minute.

  a. Use the HAAT model to determine the optimum rehabilitation robot's key requirements?
  b. What should the caregiver's retained role be?
  c. Identify an appropriate rehabilitation robot. Justify your answer.
  d. Describe how the rehabilitation team would interact to provide support for Jane to integrate the device into her daily life.
  e. What would be different if Jane was now in a developing country such as in Malawi?

Problem 11: Consider this case: Gladwin is an 83-year-old woman who immigrated from Jamaica (low-resource) to New York City (high-resource) 33 years ago. She is in relatively good health for her age—but has mild issues with mobility and right-side weakness, as well as mild, aging-related vision loss and dementia. She lives independently and can complete basic self-care ADLs—but gets easily fatigued and struggles with some more tiresome activities, like grocery shopping or banking. She has two children and two grandchildren that live two hours away from her. They try to visit regularly to check up on her. At her most recent physician's visit, Gladwin's physician found that she needs to drink more water (even though she claims to never be thirsty) and maintain a more active lifestyle. Gladwin currently uses a walker for mobility outside the home.

- a. Use the HAAT model to determine the optimum rehabilitation robot's key requirements.
- b. What should be the caregiver's retained role?
- c. Identify an appropriate rehabilitation robot. Justify your answer.
- d. Describe how the rehabilitation team would interact to provide support for Gladwin to integrate the device into her daily life.
- e. What would change in your design if Gladwin went back to live in Jamaica?

Bibliography

Abbruzzese, G., R. Marchese, L. Avanzino, and E. Pelosin. 2016. "Rehabilitation for Parkinson's Disease: Current Outlook and Future Challenges." *Parkinsonism and Related Disorders* 22: S60–S64.

Amirabdollahian, Farshid, Rui Loureiro, Elizabeth Gradwell, Christine Collin, William Harwin, and Garth Johnson. 2007. "Multivariate Analysis of the Fugl-Meyer Outcome Measures Assessing the Effectiveness of GENTLE/S Robot-Mediated Stroke Therapy." *Journal of Neuroengineering and Rehabilitation* 4: 4.

Aurich-Schuler, T., B. Warken, J. V. Graser, T. Ulrich, I. Borggraefe, F. Heinen, A. Meyer-Heim, H. J. van Hedel, and A. S. Schroeder. 2015. "Practical Recommendations for Robot-Assisted Treadmill Therapy (Lokomat) in Children with Cerebral Palsy: Indications, Goal Setting, and Clinical Implementation within the WHO-ICF Framework." *Neuropediatrics* 46 (4): 248–260.

Babaiasl, Mahdieh, Seyyed Hamed Mahdioun, Poorya Jaryani, and Mojtaba Yazdani. 2016. "A Review of Technological and Clinical Aspects of Robot-Aided Rehabilitation of Upper-Extremity after Stroke." *Disability and Rehabilitation: Assistive Technology* 11 (4): 263–280.

Beaudoin, Maude, Josiane Lettre, François Routhier, Philippe Archambault, Martin Lemay, and Isabelle Gélinas. 2018. "Long-Term Use of the JACO Robotic Arm: A Case Series." *Disability and Rehabilitation: Assistive Technology* 14: 1–9.

Boquete, Luciano, Rafael Barea, Ricardo GarcÃa, Manuel Mazo, and Miguel-Angel Sotelo. 2005. "Control of a Robotic Wheelchair Using Recurrent Networks." *Autonomous Robots* 18: 5–20.

Bouzit, M., G. Burdea, G. Popescu, and R. Boian. 2002. "The Rutgers Master II-New Design Force-Feedback Glove." *IEEE/ASME Transactions on Mechatronics* 7 (2): 256–263.

Breazeal, Cynthia. 2002. "Towards Sociable Robots." *Robotics and Autonomous Systems* 42 (3–4): 167–175.

Brenner, Lisa. 2016. "Exploring the Psychosocial Impact of Ekso Bionics Technology." *Archives of Physical Medicine and Rehabilitation* 97: e113–e113.

Brokaw, Elizabeth B., Diane Nichols, Rahsaan J. Holley, and Peter S. Lum. 2014. "Robotic Therapy Provides a Stimulus for Upper Limb Motor Recovery after Stroke that is Complementary to and Distinct from Conventional Therapy." *Neurorehabilitation and Neural Repair* 28 (4): 367–376.

Browne, V. P., J. D. Chandraratna, J. C. Angood, J. H. Tremlett, J. C. Baker, J. B. Taylor, and J. A. Thompson. 2014. "Atlas of Multiple Sclerosis 2013: A Growing Global Problem with Widespread Inequity." *Neurology* 83 (11): 1022–1024.

Burgar, Charles G., Peter S. Lum, A. M. E. Scremin, Susan L. Garber, der Loos H.F. Machiel, Deborah Kenney, and Peggy Shor. 2011. "Robot-Assisted Upper-Limb Therapy in Acute Rehabilitation Setting Following Stroke: Department of Veterans Affairs Multisite Clinical Trial." *Journal of Rehabilitation Research & Development* 48 (4): 445–458.

Burgar, Charles, Peter Lum, and Peggy Shor. 2000. "Development of Robots for Rehabilitation Therapy: The Palo Alto VA/Stanford Experience." *Journal of Rehabilitation Research and Development* 37 (6): 663–673.

Bustamante Valles, Karla, Sandra Montes, Maria de Jesus Madrigal, Adan Burciaga, Maria Elena Martinez, and Michelle J. Johnson. 2016. "Technology-Assisted Stroke Rehabilitation in Mexico: A Pilot Randomized Trial Comparing Traditional Therapy to Circuit Training in a Robot/Technology-Assisted Therapy Gym." *Journal of NeuroEngineering and Rehabilitation* 13 (1): 83.

Campeau-Lecours, Alexandre, Vã© Maheu, Sã© Lepage, Hugo Lamontagne, Simon Latour, Laurie Paquet, and Neil Hardie. 2016. "JACO Assistive Robotic Device: Empowering People with Disabilities through Innovative Algorithms." *Conference: Rehabilitation Engineering and Assistive Technology Society of North America (RESNA)*, 2016.

Colomer, C., A. Baldoví, S. Torromé, M. D. Navarro, B. Moliner, J. Ferri, and E. Noé. 2013. "Efficacy of Armeo® Spring during the Chronic Phase of Stroke. Study in Mild to Moderate Cases of Hemiparesis." *Neurologia (Barcelona, Spain)* 28 (5): 261–267.

Cook, A. M. and J. M. Polgar. 2014. *Principles of Assistive Technology: Introducing the Human Activity Assistive Technology Model.* 4th ed., 1–15. St. Louis, MO: Elsevier/Mosby.

Crewe, N. M. and J. S. Krause. 2009. "Spinal Cord Injury." In *Medical, Psychosocial and Vocational Aspects of Disability*, edited by M. G. Brodwin, F. W. Siu, J. Howard and E. R. Brodwin, 3rd ed., 289–304. Athens, Greece: Elliot & Fitzpatrick Inc.

Dan, Bernard and Nigel Paneth. 2017. "Making Sense of Cerebral Palsy Prevalence in Low-Income Countries." *The Lancet Global Health* 5 (12): e1174–e1175.

Demaerschalk, B. M., H.-M. Hwang, and G. Leung. 2010. "US Cost Burden of Ischemic Stroke: A Systematic Literature Review." *American Journal of Managed Care* 16 (7): 525–533.

Dewan, Michael C., Abbas Rattani, Saksham Gupta, Ronnie E. Baticulon, Ya-Ching Hung, Maria Punchak, Amit Agrawal, et al. 2018. "Estimating the Global Incidence of Traumatic Brain Injury." *Journal of Neurosurgery* 1: 1–18.

Driessen, B. J. F., H. G. Evers, and J. A. van Woerden. 2001. "MANUS - A Wheelchair-Mounted Rehabilitation Robot." *Proceedings of the Institution of Mechanical Engineers, Part H: Journal of Engineering in Medicine* 215 (3): 285–290.

Esquenazi, Alberto, Mukul Talaty, Andrew Packel, and Michael Saulino. 2012. "The ReWalk Powered Exoskeleton to Restore Ambulatory Function to Individuals with Thoracic-Level Motor-Complete Spinal Cord Injury." *American Journal of Physical Medicine & Rehabilitation* 91 (11): 911–921.

Fasola, J. and M. J. Mataric. 2012. "Using Socially Assistive Human–Robot Interaction to Motivate Physical Exercise for Older Adults." *Proceedings of the IEEE* 100 (8): 2512–2526.

Fasoli, Susan E., Hermano I. Krebs, Joel Stein, Walter R. Frontera, and Neville Hogan. 2003. "Effects of Robotic Therapy on Motor Impairment and Recovery in Chronic Stroke." *Archives of Physical Medicine and Rehabilitation* 84 (4): 477–482.

Ferraro, Mark, Jennifer Hogan Demaio, Jennifer Krol, Chris Trudell, Keren Rannekleiv, Lisa Edelstein, Paul Christos, et al. 2002. "Assessing the Motor Status Score: A Scale for the Evaluation of Upper Limb Motor Outcomes in Patients after Stroke." *Neurorehabilitation and Neural Repair* 16 (3): 283–289.

Fitter, N. T., M. Mohan, K. J. Kuchenbecker, and M. J. Johnson. 2018. "Exercising with Baxter: Design and Evaluation." *Journal of NeuroEngineering and Rehabilitation* 17 (1).

Fluet, Gerard G., Soha Qinyin Qiu, Diego Saleh, Sergei Ramirez, Donna Adamovich, Heta Kelly, and Heta Parikh. 2009. "Robot-Assisted Virtual Rehabilitation (NJIT-RAVR) System for Children with Upper Extremity Hemiplegia." New York: IEEE Publishing, 06.

Galan, Ferran, Marnix Nuttin, Eileen Lew, G. Vanacker, Johan Philips, and Jose del R. Millan. 2008. "A Brain-Actuated Wheelchair: Asynchronous and Non-Invasive Brain-Computer Interfaces for Continuous Control of Robots." *Clinical Neurophysiology* 119 (9): 2159–2169.

Gallagher, Shaun. 2007. "Social Cognition and Social Robots." *Pragmatics & Cognition* 15: 435–453.

Gladstone, David J., Cynthia J. Danells, and Sandra E. Black. 2002. "The Fugl-Meyer Assessment of Motor Recovery after Stroke: A Critical Review of its Measurement Properties." *Neurorehabilitation and Neural Repair* 16 (3): 232–240.

Goher, Khaled, Naz Mansouri, and S. Fadlallah. 2017. "Assessment of Personal Care and Medical Robots from Older Adultsâ€™ Perspective." *Robotics and Biomimetics* 4 (1): 5.

Gouaillier, David, Vincent Hugel, Pierre Blazevic, Chris Kilner, J Monceaux, Pascal Lafourcade, Brice Marnier, Julien Serre, and Bruno Maisonnier. 2009. Mechatronic Design of NAO Humanoid. *Proceedings – IEEE International Conference on Robotics and Automation.*

Graf, Birgit, Matthias Hans, and Rolf Schraft. 2004. "Care-O-Bot II – Development of a Next Generation Robotic Home Assistant." Autonomous Robots 16: 193–205.

Hagan, K., M. Hillman, S. Hagan, and J. Jepson. 1997. The Design of a Wheelchair Mounted Robot. *IEE Colloquium on Computers in the Service of Mankind: Helping the Disabled*, pp. 6/1–6/6.

Hamilton, B. B., C. V. Granger, F. S. Sherwin, M. Zielezny, and J. S. Tashman. 1987. "A Uniform National Data System for Medical Rehabilitation." In *Functional Evaluation of Stroke Patients*, edited by M. J. Fuhrer, 137–147. Baltimore: PH Brooks.

Hartwig, Maik. 2014. "Modern Hand- and Arm Rehabilitation: The Tyrosolution Concept." *Neurology & Rehabilitation* 2: 111–116.

He, Wan, Daniel Goodkind, and Paul Kowal. 2016. "An Aging World: 2015 International Population Reports." *Aging* 165.

Hebesberger, D., T. Koertner, C. Gisinger, P. Juergen, and C. Dondrup. 2016. "Lessons Learned from the Deployment of a Long-Term Autonomous Robot as Companion in Physical Therapy for Older Adults with Dementia A Mixed Methods Study." *Eleventh ACM/IEEE International Conference on Human Robot Interaction (HRI '16)*, 27–34. IEEE Press.

Heinemann, A., J. Linacre, B. Wright, B. Hamilton, and C. Granger. 1994. "Prediction of Rehabilitation Outcomes with Disability Measures." *Archives of Physical Medicine and Rehabilitation* 75 (2): 133–143.

Hesse, S., C. Werner, M. Pohl, S. Rueckriem, J. Mehrholz, and M. Lingnau. 2005. "Computerized Arm Training Improves the Motor Control of the Severely Affected Arm after Stroke: A Single-Blinded Randomized Trial in Two Centers." *Stroke* 36 (9): 1960–1966.

Hesse, Stefan, Gotthard Schulte-Tigges, Matthias Konrad, Anita Bardeleben, and Cordula Werner. 2003. "Robot-Assisted Arm Trainer for the Passive and Active Practice of Bilateral Forearm and Wrist Movements in Hemiparetic Subjects 1 1 an Organization with Which 1 or More of the Authors is Associated has Received or Will Receive Financial Benefits from a Co." *Archives of Physical Medicine and Rehabilitation* 84 (6): 915–920.

Hesse, Stefan, Dietmar Uhlenbrock, Cordula Werner, and Anita Bardeleben. 2000. "A Mechanized Gait Trainer for Restoring Gait in Nonambulatory Subjects." *Archives of Physical Medicine and Rehabilitation* 81 (9): 1158–1161.

Hidler, J. M., David Brennan, Iian Black, Diane Nichols, Kathy Brady, and Tobias Nef. 2011. "ZeroG: Overground Gait and Balance Training System." *Journal of Rehabilitation Research and Development* 48: 287–298.

Hidler, J. M. and A. E. Wall. 2005. "Alterations in Muscle Activation Patterns during Robotic-Assisted Walking." *Clinical Biomechanics* 20 (2): 184–193.

Jaul, Efraim and Jeremy Barron. 2017. "Age-Related Diseases and Clinical and Public Health Implications for the 85 Years Old and Over Population." *Frontiers in Public Health* 5: 355.

Johnson, M. J., K. J. Wisneski, J. Anderson, D. Nathan, and R. O. Smith. 2006. "Development of ADLER: The Activities of Daily Living Exercise Robot." IEEE.

Johnson, Michelle J., Megan A. Johnson, Justine S. Sefcik, Pamela Z. Cacchione, Caio Mucchiani, Tessa Lau, and Mark Yim. 2017a. "Task and Design Requirements for an Affordable Mobile Service Robot for Elder Care in an All-Inclusive Care for Elders Assisted-Living Setting." *International Journal of Social Robotics* 12: 989–1008.

Johnson, Michelle Jillian, Roshan Rai, Sarath Barathi, Rochelle Mendonca, and Karla Bustamante-Valles. 2017b. "Affordable Stroke Therapy in High-, Low- and Middle-Income Countries: From Theradrive to Rehab CARES, a Compact Robot Gym." *Journal of Rehabilitation and Assistive Technologies Engineering* 4: 2055668317708732.

Kang, Chang Gu, Min Ho Chun, Min Cheol Chang, Won Kim, and Kyung Hee Do. 2016. "Views of Physiatrists and Physical Therapists on the Use of Gait-Training Robots for Stroke Patients." *Journal of Physical Therapy Science* 28 (1): 202–206.

Kang, Y., H. Ding, H. Zhou, Z. Wei, L. Liu, D. Pan, and S. Feng. 2017. "Epidemiology of Worldwide Spinal Cord Injury: A Literature Review." *Journal of Neurorestoratology* 6: 1–9.

Keller, U., S. Schölch, U. Albisser, C. Rudhe, A. Curt, R. Riener, and V. Klamroth-Marganska. 2015. "Robot-Assisted Arm Assessments in Spinal Cord Injured Patients: A Consideration of Concept Study." *PLoS ONE* 10 (5): e0126948–e0126948.

Kim, Grace J., Lisa Rivera, and Joel Stein. 2015. "Combined Clinic-Home Approach for Upper Limb Robotic Therapy after Stroke: A Pilot Study." *Archives of Physical Medicine and Rehabilitation* 96 (12): 2243–2248.

Klamroth-Marganska, Verena, Javier Blanco, Katrin Campen, Armin Curt, Volker Dietz, Thierry Ettlin, Morena Felder, et al. 2014. "Three-Dimensional, Task-Specific Robot Therapy of the Arm after Stroke: A Multicentre, Parallel-Group Randomised Trial." *Lancet Neurology* 13 (2): 159–166.

Krebs, Hermano, Neville Hogan, Mindy Aisen, and Bruce Volpe. 1998. "Robot-Aided Neurorehabilitation." *IEEE Transactions on Rehabilitation Engineering: A Publication of the IEEE Engineering in Medicine and Biology Society* 6: 75–87.

Krebs, Hermano, Barbara Ladenheim, Christopher Hippolyte, Linda Monterroso, and Joelle Mast. 2009. "Robot-Assisted Task-Specific Training in Cerebral Palsy." *Developmental Medicine and Child Neurology* 51 Suppl 4: 140–145.

Krigger, K. W. 2006. "Cerebral Palsy: An Overview." *American Family Physician* 73 (1): 91–100.

Kwakkel, Gert, Boudewijn J. Kollen, and Hermano I. Krebs. 2008. "Effects of Robot-Assisted Therapy on Upper Limb Recovery after Stroke: A Systematic Review." *Neurorehabilitation and Neural Repair* 22 (2): 111–121.

Kwee, H. H. 1998. "Integrated Control of MANUS Manipulator and Wheelchair Enhanced by Environmental Docking." *Robotica* 16 (5): 491–498.

Lambercy, O., L. Dovat, R. Gassert, E. Burdet, T. Chee Leong Teo, and T. Milner. 2007. "A Haptic Knob for Rehabilitation of Hand Function." *IEEE Transactions on Neural Systems and Rehabilitation Engineering* 15 (3): 356–366.

Lambercy, Olivier, Ludovic Dovat, Hong Yun, Seng Kwee Wee, Christopher W. K. Kuah, Karen S. G. Chua, Roger Gassert, Theodore E. Milner, Chee Leong Teo, and Etienne Burdet. 2011. "Effects of a Robot-Assisted Training of Grasp and Pronation/Supination in Chronic Stroke: A Pilot Study." *Journal of NeuroEngineering and Rehabilitation* 8 (1): 63.

Liao, Wan-wen, Ching-yi Wu, Yu-wei Hsieh, Keh-chung Lin, and Wan-ying Chang. 2012. "Effects of Robot-Assisted Upper Limb Rehabilitation on Daily Function and Real-World Arm Activity in Patients with Chronic Stroke: A Randomized Controlled Trial." *Clinical Rehabilitation* 26 (2): 111–120.

Lin, Vernon, Xiaoming Zhang, and Pamela Dixon. 2015. "Occupational Therapy Workforce in the United States: Forecasting Nationwide Shortages." *PM R* 7 (9): 946–954.

Lo, Albert C., Peter Guarino, Hermano I. Krebs, Bruce T. Volpe, Christopher T. Bever, Pamela W. Duncan, Robert J. Ringer, et al. 2009. *Multicenter Randomized Trial of Robot-Assisted Rehabilitation for Chronic Stroke: Methods and Entry Characteristics for VA ROBOTICS*. Vol. 23. Newbury Park, CA: Sage Publications.

Loureiro, Rui, Farshid Amirabdollahian, Michael Topping, Bart Driessen, and William Harwin. 2003. "Upper Limb Robot Mediated Stroke Therapy–GENTLE/s Approach." *Autonomous Robots* 15 (1): 35–51.

Lum, Peter S., Charles G. Burgar, Peggy C. Shor, Matra Majmundar, and Machiel Van Der Loos. 2002. "Robot-Assisted Movement Training Compared with Conventional Therapy Techniques for the Rehabilitation of Upper-Limb Motor Function after Stroke." *Archives of Physical Medicine and Rehabilitation* 83 (7): 952–959.

Maciejasz, Pawel, Jörg Eschweiler, Kurt Gerlach-Hahn, Arne Jansen-Troy, and Steffen Leonhardt. 2014. "A Survey on Robotic Devices for Upper Limb Rehabilitation." *Journal of Neuroengineering and Rehabilitation* 11 (1): 3.

Matarić, Maja, Jon Eriksson, David Feil-Seifer, and Carolee J. Winstein. 2007. "Socially Assistive Robotics for Post-Stroke Rehabilitation." *Journal of NeuroEngineering and Rehabilitation* 4: 5.

Mehrholz, Jan, Marcus Pohl, Thomas Platz, Joachim Kugler, and Bernhard Elsner. 2015. "Electromechanical and Robot-Assisted Arm Training for Improving Activities of Daily Living, Arm Function, and Arm Muscle Strength after Stroke." *The Cochrane Database of Systematic Reviews* 2015 (11): D006876.

Mehrholz, Jan, Simone Thomas, and Bernhard Elsner. 2017. "Treadmill Training and Body Weight Support for Walking after Stroke." *The Cochrane Database of Systematic Reviews* 8 (8): CD002840.

Miller, Elaine L., Laura Murray, Lorie Richards, Richard D. Zorowitz, Tamilyn Bakas, Patricia Clark, and Sandra A. Billinger. 2010. "Comprehensive Overview of Nursing and Interdisciplinary Rehabilitation Care of the Stroke Patient: A Scientific Statement from the American Heart Association." *Stroke* 41 (10): 2402–2448.

Miskam, Mohd, Mohd Hamid, Hanafiah Yussof, Syamimi Shamsuddin, Norjasween Malik, and Siti Basir. 2013. "Study on Social Interaction between Children with Autism and Humanoid Robot NAO." *Applied Mechanics and Materials* 393: 573–578.

Mohan, M., R. Mendonca, and M. J. Johnson. 2017. "Towards Quantifying Dynamic Human-Human Physical Interactions for Robot Assisted Stroke Therapy." *IEEE International Conference on Rehabilitation Robotics*. Jul 2017: 913–918.

Montemerlo, Michael, Joelle Pineau, Nicholas Roy, Sebastian Thrun, and Vandi Verma. 2002. "Experiences with a Mobile Robotic Guide for the Elderly." *Eighteenth National Conference on Artificatial Intelligence. American Association for Artificial Intelligence*, 587–592.

Naro, A., A. Bramanti, P. Bramanti, and R. S. Calabrò. 2017. "Motor Recovery after Stroke: The Role of Overground Exoskeletons in Shaping Brain Plasticity." *Italian Journal of Anatomy and Embroyology* 122: 154–154.

Nathan, D. E., M. J. Johnson, and J. R. McGuire. 2009. "Design and Validation of Low-Cost Assistive Glove for Hand Assessment and Therapy during Activity of Daily Living-Focused Robotic Stroke Therapy." *Journal of Rehabilitation Research and Development* 46 (5): 587–602.

National Institute of Population and Social Security Research. 2002. "Population Projections for Japan: 2001–2050."

National Institutes of Health. "What Are the Common TBI Symptoms?" https://www.nichd.nih .gov/health/topics/tbi/conditioninfo/symptoms.

Nef, Tobias, Matjaz Mihelj, and Robert Riener. 2007. "ARMin: A Robot for Patient-Cooperative Arm Therapy." *Medical & Biological Engineering & Computing* 45: 887–900.

Ovbiagele, Bruce, Larry Goldstein, Randall T. Higashida, Virginia J. Howard, S. Claiborne Johnston, Olga A. Khavjou, Daniel T. Lackland, et al. 2013. "Forecasting the Future of Stroke in the United States: A Policy Statement from the American Heart Association and American Stroke Association." *Stroke* 44 (8): 2361–2375.

Page, Stephen J., Valerie Hill, and Susan White. 2013. "Portable Upper Extremity Robotics is as Efficacious as Upper Extremity Rehabilitative Therapy: A Randomized Controlled Pilot Trial." *Clinical Rehabilitation* 27 (6): 494–503.

Parkinson's Foundation. "Statistics." https://www.parkinson.ca/about-parkinsons/

Qiu, Q., D. A. Ramirez, S. Saleh, G. G. Fluet, H. D. Parikh, D. Kelly, and S. V. Adamovich. 2009. "The New Jersey Institute of Technology Robot-Assisted Virtual Rehabilitation (NJIT-RAVR) System for Children with Cerebral Palsy: A Feasibility Study." *Journal of NeuroEngineering and Rehabilitation* 6: 40. doi: 10.1186/1743-0003-6-40

Radder, Bob, Gerdienke Prange, Anke Kottink, Liesbeth Gaasbeek, Johnny Holmberg, Thomas Meyer, Alejandro Melendez-Calderon, Johan Ingvast, Jaap Buurke, and Johan Rietman. 2016. "A Wearable Soft-Robotic Glove Enables Hand Support in ADL and Rehabilitation: A Feasibility Study on the Assistive Functionality." *Journal of Rehabilitation and Assistive Technologies Engineering* 29(3): 2055668316670552.

Rahman, Tariq, Whitney Sample, Rahamim Seliktar, and Michael Alexander. 2000. "A Body-Powered Functional Upper Limb Orthosis." *Journal of Rehabilitation Research and Development* 37 (6): 675–680.

Reinkensmeyer, David J. and Volker Dietz. 2016. *Neurorehabilitation Technology*, 2nd ed. Cham: Springer International Publishing.

Reinkensmeyer, David and Sarah Housman. 2007. "If I Can't Do It Once, Why Do It a Hundred Times?: Connecting Volition to Movement Success in a Virtual Environment Motivates People to Exercise the Arm after Stroke." *Virtual Rehabilitation* 2007: 44–48.

Riener, R., M. Guidali, U. Keller, A. Duschau-Wicke, V. Klamroth, and T. Nef. 2011. "Transferring ARMin to the Clinics and Industry." *Topics in Spinal Cord Injury Rehabilitation* 17 (1): 54–59.

Rosier, J. C., J. A. van Woerden, L. W. van der Kolk, H. H. Kwee, J. J. Duimel, J. J. Smits, A. A. Tuinhof de Moed, G. Honderd, and P. M. Bruyn. 1989. "The MANUS Wheelchair-Mounted Manipulator: System Design and Implementation." *IEEE/ASME Transactions on Mechatronics* 19: 225–237.

Routhier, F., P. S. Archambault, M. Cyr, V. Maheu, M. Lemay, and I. Glinas. 2014. "Benefits of JACO Robotic Arm on Independent Living and Social Participation: An Exploratory Study." *RESNA Conference 2014*.

Scherer, R., P. Grieshofer, C. Enzinger, and G. Muller-Putz. 2012. "Predicting Functional Stroke Rehabilitation Outcome by Means of Brain Computer Interface Technology: The BCI4REHAB Project." *Neurorehabilitation and Neural Repair* 26: 772–772.

Schmidt, H., S. Hesse, R. Bernhardt, and J. Krüger. 2005. "HapticWalker---A Novel Haptic Foot Device." *ACM Transactions on Applied Perception (TAP)* 2 (2): 166–180.

Schoeb, Veronika. 2016. *Non-Communicable Diseases are the Biggest Challenges of the 21st Century: What is the Physiotherapist's Role in Global Health?* Rochester, NY: Elsevier BV.

Schulz, Richard, Hans-Werner Wahl, Judith T. Matthews, Annette De Vito Dabbs, Scott R. Beach, and Sara J. Czaja. 2015. *Advancing the Aging and Technology Agenda in Gerontology.* Vol. 55. Oxford, UK: Oxford University Press.

Sefcik, J. S., M. J. Johnson, M. Yim, T. Lau, N. Vivio, C. Mucchiani, and P. Z. Cacchione. 2018. "Stakeholders' Perceptions Sought to Inform the Development of a Low-Cost Mobile Robot for Older Adults: A Qualitative Descriptive Study." *Clinical Nursing Research* 27 (1): 61–80.

Sharkey, A. and N. Sharkey. 2012. "Granny and the Robots: Ethical Issues in Robot Care for the Elderly." *Ethics of Information Technology* 14: 27–40.

Shibata, Takanori and K. Wada. 2011. "Robot Therapy: A New Approach for Mental Healthcare of the Elderly – A Mini-Review." *Gerontology* 57: 378–386.

Sicari, M., S. Cavazza, Pia Marchi, C. Pampolini, L. Balugani, L. Lutzoni, A. Santagata, Erika Giannotti, Marina Manca, and Nino Basaglia. 2011. "Muscle Activation Pattern during Gait Versus Robotic-Assisted Gait Training in Hemiplegic Subjects." *Gait & Posture - GAIT POSTURE* 33 (1): S65.

Smith, R. O., M. J. Scherer, R. Cooper, D. Bell, D. A. Hobbs, C. Pettersson, N. Seymour, et al. 2018. "Assistive Technology Products: A Position Paper from the First Global Research, Innovation, and Education on Assistive Technology (GREAT) Summit." *Disability and Rehabilitation: Assistive Technology* 13 (5): 473–485.

Story, M. F. 1998. "Maximizing Usability: The Principles of Universal Design." *Assistive Technology* 10: 4–12.

Straudi, S., C. Fanciullacci, C. Martinuzzi, C. Pavarelli, B. Rossi, C. Chisari, and N. Basaglia. 2016. "The Effects of Robot-Assisted Gait Training in Progressive Multiple Sclerosis: A Randomized Controlled Trial." *Multiple Sclerosis* 22 (3): 373–384.

Technavio. 2018. *Global Rehabilitation Robots Market 2018–2022.* Technavio.

Theriault, Andrew, Mark Nagurka, and Michelle J. Johnson. 2014. "Design and Development of an Affordable Haptic Robot with Force-Feedback and Compliant Actuation to Improve Therapy for Patients with Severe Hemiparesis." *IEEE Transactions on Haptics* 7 (2): 161–174.

Timmermans, Annick, Ryanne Lemmens, Maurice Monfrance, Richard Geers, Wilbert Bakx, Rob Smeets, and Henk Seelen. 2014. "Effects of Task-Oriented Robot Training on Arm Function, Activity, and Quality of Life in Chronic Stroke Patients: A Randomized Controlled Trial." *Journal of Neuroengineering and Rehabilitation* 11 (1): 45.

Towery, N. D., E. Machek, and A. Thomas. 2017. *Technology Readiness Level Guidebook.* Washington, DC: US Department of Commerce, Economics and Statistics Administration, US Census Bureau.

United Nations. "Ageing." https://www.un.org/development/desa/ageing/.

Vincent, Grayson K. and Victoria A. Velkof. 2010. *The Next Four Decades: The Older Population in the United States: 2010 to 2050 – Population Estimates and Projections.* Washington, DC: US Department of Commerce, Economics and Statistics Administration, US Census Bureau.

Wada, K. and Takanori Shibata. 2007. "Living with Seal Robots - Its Sociopsychological and Physiological Influences on the Elderly at a Care House." *IEEE Transactions on Robotics* 23: 972–980.

Wagner, Todd H., Albert C. Lo, Peter Peduzzi, Dawn M. Bravata, Grant D. Huang, Hermano I. Krebs, Robert J. Ringer, et al. 2011. "An Economic Analysis of Robot-Assisted Therapy for Long-Term Upper-Limb Impairment after Stroke." *Stroke* 42 (9): 2630–2632.

Wolf, Steven L., Komal Sahu, R. C. Bay, Sharon Buchanan, Aimee Reiss, Susan Linder, Anson Rosenfeldt, and Jay Alberts. 2015. "The HAAPI (Home Arm Assistance Progression Initiative) Trial: A Novel Robotics Delivery Approach in Stroke Rehabilitation." *Neurorehabilitation and Neural Repair* 29 (10): 958–968.

World Health Organization. 2017. *Rehabilitation 2030: A Call to Action.* World Health Organization.

———. 2018. "Stroke, Cerebrovascular Accident." Retrieved from http://www.who.int/topics /cerebrovascular_accident/en/.

———. 2011. *World Report on Disability.* World Health Organization.

Xiloyannis, Michele, Leonardo Cappello, Dinh Binh Khanh, Chris Wilson Antuvan, and Lorenzo Masia. 2016. "Preliminary Design and Control of a Soft Exosuit for Assisting Elbow Movements and Hand Grasping in Activities of Daily Living." *Journal of Rehabilitation and Assistive Technologies Engineering (RATE)* 4: 557–561.

Zimbelman, Janice L., Stephen P. Juraschek, Xiaoming Zhang, and Vernon W. -H Lin. 2010. "Physical Therapy Workforce in the United States: Forecasting Nationwide Shortages." *PM R* 2 (11): 1021–1029.

Chapter 17 Universal interfaces and information technology

Gregg Vanderheiden and
Jutta Treviranus

Contents

17.1 Chapter overview

The viewpoint of this chapter is that people do not have disabilities – they experience them when their abilities do not match the requirements of the world as it is designed.

In fact, many of us experience disabilities or functional limitations due to circumstances in daily life. For instance, in a very noisy environment, an individual who ordinarily has no trouble hearing may have great difficulty or find it impossible

DOI: 10.1201/b21964-20

to hear the auditory output from a device such as a cell phone or ticket vending machine. While driving a car, one often needs to operate devices without using vision. Others may find themselves in an environment where it is dark or may be without their glasses and be unable to see controls or labels.

Figure 17.1 describes a simple cause-effect flow that helps highlight the roles that impairment, circumstance, and design can play in creating what is perceived as a disability. One can also see that "reduced ability" does not need to lead to disadvantage if the "inability to access" is reduced.

Table 17.1 provides some parallels between individuals with disabilities and individuals without disabilities who may find themselves experiencing environmental or task-induced constraints. When all of these people are considered, as well as individuals experiencing a wide range of temporary disabilities, it is useful to note that "those with disabilities" are not a small portion of the population. And when people are considered across their lifetime (rather than looking at a snapshot of the population at any point in time), the result is that all people will acquire disabilities as they age.

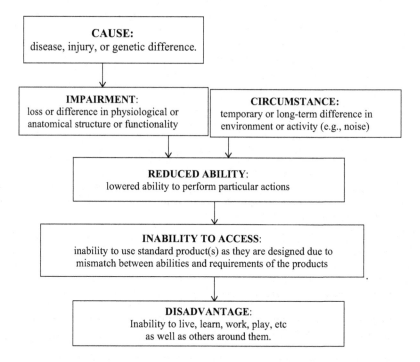

Figure 17.1 Cause-effect model shows the role that both impairment and design play in "disability," as well as the parallel role that conditions or circumstances can play.

Table 17.1 Parallel Chart – Disability versus Situation

Requirement	Disability related need	Situation related need
Operable with low vision	People with visual impairment	• Using a small display or in a high glare or dimly lit environment
Operable without vision	People who are blind	• People whose eyes are busy (e.g., driving a car or phone browsing) • People in a room without light
Operable with limited hearing	People who are hard of hearing	People in noisy environments
Operable with no hearing	People who are deaf	• In very loud environments In forced silence (library or meeting)
Operable with limited manual dexterity	People with a physical disability	People in a space suit or chemical suit or who are in a bouncing vehicle
Operable with limited cognition	People with a cognitive disability	People who are distracted • or panicked • or under the influence of alcohol
Operable without reading	People with a cognitive disability	• can't see the display well enough • don't know the language displayed • are visitors • left reading glasses behind

17.1.1 We will all experience disabilities – if we live long enough

Everybody hopes to live well into their 70s, 80s, and beyond. Unfortunately, an ever-increasing percentage of people will acquire functional limitations as they age. In fact, all of us will acquire disabilities – unless we die first. Figure 17.2 provides a glimpse of this effect by plotting the percentage of individuals with functional limitations as a function of age. If this series is continued, it will reach 100% as one increases in age. These disabilities may include physical, visual, hearing, and cognition. In addition, people acquire multiple disabilities as they age. Unfortunately, those who are designing the world in which we must live are usually the youngest, most able, and most technically oriented. It is ironic that although the majority of the wealth is held by those who are older, the majority of products are designed with the young as the target audience.

17.2 Spectrum of user interface needs

There are many different ways of looking at user needs. One way is to explore the needs of disability. This is the approach originally taken in studying consumer

Disability as a Function of Age

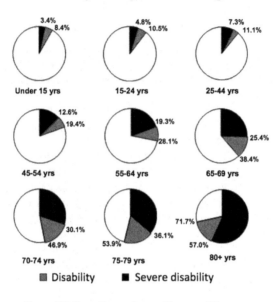

Source: U.S. Census Bureau, Survey of Income and Program
Participation: June – September 2002.

Figure 17.2 Pie charts show the percentage of people who have a disability as a function of age (Steinmetz 2006).

product accessibility guidelines (Nyamcenterforhistory.org 2018), Guide 71,* and many others that are organized by disability or limitations. However, a more useful approach for designers might be to examine user needs by interface component, or interface dimension, across disabilities. That is, examine the different parts or functions of the human interface individually and look at the impact or barriers experienced by individuals with different disabilities. This is how product designers approach their products – and the approach allows cross-disability interface strategies to be more easily identified and understood. Unlike the design of assistive technologies, the design of mainstream technologies is best approached not by looking at the product one disability at a time, but by looking at the product functions and identifying strategies that will work across disabilities or functional limitations and exceptional abilities at the same time. This is particularly important for designing access into mainstream and public devices, where the interface must be usable by all.

---

* ISO/IEC Guide 71:2001 Guidelines for standards developers to address the needs of elderly persons and persons with disabilities.

The Trace Center developed a user needs profile based on basic access/use essentials. It should be noted that these are not just essentials for individuals who have disabilities, but essential components that must be there for *anyone* to be able to effectively use an interface. Everyone must be able to *perceive*, *operate*, and *understand* a product interface in order to use the product. It must also be *compatible* with anything that is part of their person (glasses, clothes, or, for people with disabilities, any assistive technologies they must use while using the product).

The basic essentials are summarized in the following sections.

(1) Perceive

In order to use a product, users:

(1a) must be able to *perceive any information that is displayed.*

- This includes information that is displayed passively (labels, instructions) or actively (on displays).
- It includes both visually displayed information and information delivered in auditory form (usually speech).
- Includes labels, signs, manuals, text on the product, and information conveyed by symbols on displays, alerts, alarms, and other output.

(1b) must be able to *perceive the existence and location of actionable components.*

- Buttons, controls, latches, etc.
- Must be able to find them and re-find them easily.
- Must be able to perceive the status of controls and indicators.
- Includes progress indicators and the status of any switches, dials, or other controls, real or virtual.

1c) must be able to *perceive any feedback* from operation.

- Includes not only programmed feedback but natural feedback such as machine sounds that are important for safe and effective use of the device.

(2) Operate

In order to use a product, users:

(2a) must be able to *invoke and carry out all functions* via at least one mode of operation.

- Including daily maintenance and setup expected users.
- Preferably all of maintenance and setup.

(2b) must be able to *complete all actions and tasks within the time allowed.*

- By life competition, productivity requirements, etc.

(2c) must be able to *operate without accidentally activating actions.*

(2d) must be able to *recover from errors.*

- Physical or cognitive errors.

(2e) must have equivalent *security and privacy.*
- – If alternate modes are needed, they need to provide equivalent security and privacy.

(2f) must be able to use *without causing* personal risk.
- – For example, seizures, physical injury.

(3) Understand

In order to use a product, users

(3a) must be able to *understand how to use the product.*
- – Including discovery and activation of any access features needed.

(3b) must be able to *understand the output* or displayed material.
- – Even after they have perceived it accurately.

(4) Compatible with personal technologies

In order to use a product, users

(4a) must be able to *use the product in conjunction with any personal technologies.*
- – For example, glasses, wheelchairs, and hearing aids.
- – For some, it would be more efficient if they could use their own personal interface devices with the products they encountered.
- – For others, the only way they would be able to use products would be to use specialized input devices that they would bring with them since it would be impractical to have them built into the products they encounter.

These basic principles were expanded into a user needs profile that includes the different problems with different components of the interface by individuals with various types, degrees, and combinations of disabilities. In 2005, these were submitted to the Joint Technical Committee, ISO-IEC Special Working Group on Accessibility (ISO/IEC JTC1 SWGA) where they underwent review, comment, and revision process, resulting in the ISO/IEC technical report TR 29138-1 and eventually ISO/IEC (Table 17.2).

17.3 Strategies for addressing user needs

17.3.1 General approaches

If someone is not able to use the environment and devices they encounter in daily life effectively, there are three approaches to intervention:

1. *Change the individual,* so that they can use the world better as they find it.
2. *Adapt or provide adapters to individual products after manufacture* to make them usable for the person.
3. *Change the world,* so that people can use it with the abilities they have.

Table 17.2 User Needs Summary Trace Center, University of Wisconsin-Madison

Basic users need to be able to *perceive* all information presented by the product	Problems using products	User needs
Perceive static displayed info • labels • signs • manuals • text • etc.	**People who are blind** • Cannot see (to read) • printed labels on keys, controls, slots, etc. • printed signs near the device or instructions printed on the device • manuals or other printed material provided with the product • Cannot access information presented (only) via graphics • Cannot find public devices (cannot see where the device is or see signs giving location) **People with low vision** • Cannot see (to read) signs and labels: • if text is too small for them • if contrast with the background is too low • if text is presented as small, raised letters (same color as the background) • if information is coded with color only (color deficiency). • if there is glare (intensity) — if they have light sensitivity • if there is surface (reflective) glare • (Many problems same as blindness) **People with physical disabilities** • Often cannot re-position themselves to see information if not in easy sightline • May not be able to see due to glare/reflections (and cannot re-position enough)	**Some users with disabilities...** • ...need to have all static text information required for use provided via speech output or large raised text • Note 1: Braille is also very useful to people who know where it is practical to put it on the product. But it would be in addition to speech not instead since most people who are blind do not know braille, including those who acquire it late in life and those who have diabetes that takes away sensation in the fingertips. • Note 2: Speech output is also important for those with cognitive disabilities (see "UNDERSTAND") • Note 3: Raised text would need to be approx. 3/4 inch high. • ...need to have visual cues provided in auditory form. • ...need to have sufficient contrast between all printed information and its background. • ...need to have text presented in large easy-to-read fonts. • ...need to avoid surface (reflective) glare. • ...need to have information within viewable range of people in wheelchairs and those of short stature. • ...need to have any information presented in color (other than color) be also presented in a way that does not depend on color perception.

(Continued)

399

Table 17.2 (Continued) User Needs Summary Trace Center, University of Wisconsin-Madison

Basic users need to be able to *perceive* all information presented by the product	Problems using products	User needs
Perceive info presented via dynamic displays,	**People who are blind**	**Some users with disabilities...**
• screens	• Cannot see what is displayed on visual display units (all types)	• ...need to have all DYNAMIC visual information required for use also provided via speech output
• alerts	• Cannot determine current function of soft keys (where the key function is dynamic with the label shown on dynamic display like LCD.)	• Note 1: Dynamic braille displays are very expensive and impractical for inclusion in devices.
• alarms	**People with low vision**	• Note 2: Speech output also important for those with cognitive disabilities (see "UNDERSTAND")
• other output	• Same problems as static text (size, contrast, color) – (see above)	• Note 3: Raised text won't work for dynamic information.
	• glare – from the environment or too bright a screen	• ...need a means for identifying all keys and controls via speech.
	• miss information presented temporarily where they are not looking	• ...need sufficient contrast between all display information (audio or visual) and its background.
	• sometimes cannot track moving/scrolling text	• ...need to have text presented in large easy-to-read fonts.
	People who are deaf	• ...need to avoid surface (reflective) glare.
	• Cannot hear information presented through	• ...need to avoid brightness glare.
	• Speech	• ...need to have information within viewable range of people in wheelchairs and those of short stature.
	• Tones	• ...need to have all auditory information required for use also available in visual and/or tactile form
	• Natural machine sounds	• Note 1: Tactile presentation only useful for products that will always be in contact with user's body.
	People who are hard of hearing	• ...need to have auditory events, alerts, etc. be multi-frequency so that they can hear it.
	• May miss any information presented auditorily:	• ...need sufficient volume (preferably adjustable) for audio output.
	a. At a frequency they can't hear	• ...need to have any information presented in color (other than color) be also presented in a way that does not depend on color perception.
	b. Background noise blocks it or interferes with it (including echoes)	
	c. Too soft	
	d. Poor quality speech	
	e. Speech too fast – and user can't slow it down	
	f. Presented as two different tones that can't be distinguished.	
	g. information is presented that requires stereo hearing	
	People with physical disabilities	
	• Cannot maneuver to see display or avoid glare	

(Continued)

Table 17.2 (Continued) User Needs Summary Trace Center, University of Wisconsin-Madison

Basic users need to be able to *perceive* all information presented by the product	Problems using products	User needs
	People with cognitive disabilities	• ...need to be able to control the colors in which information is presented.
	• Distracted by dynamic movements on screen	• ...need to be able to control the pitch of information presented auditorily.
		• ...need to have audio information conveyed by sound pattern not frequency.
		• ...need to have audio information conveyed by vibration to use patterns not frequency or strength.
		• Stereo information available in monaural form.
		Some users with disabilities...
Perceive existence and location of actionable components	**People who are blind**	• ...need a means to access all product functionality via tactilely discernable controls.
• buttons	• Cannot determine number, size, location, or function of controls on touchscreens	• ...need controls to be locatable without activating control or nearby controls.
• controls	• flat membrane keypads	• ...need sufficient landmarks (nibs, groupings, spacing) to be able to locate controls easily tactilely once they have identified them (per above)
• latches	• Cannot find controls in a large featureless group; cannot be relocated easily even if known to be there	• ...need to have controls visually contrast with their surroundings so they can be located with low vision.
• etc.	• Switch or control in an obscure location may not be discoverable even if visible	• ...need to have any keyboard be operable without site.
(find them and re-find them)	• Might touch tactilely sensitive controls while exploring with hands	• ...need to have controls be in places where they can be easily found with poor and with no sight.
	• Can be fooled by phantom buttons (tactile) – (things that feel like buttons but are not, e.g., a logo, a round flat raised bolt head, a styling feature)	• ...need to have pointing cursors (on screen) be large enough to be visible with low vision.
	• Cannot type on a non-touch typeable keyboard	• ...need to have logos, and other details do not look like or feel like buttons or controls.
	People with low vision	• ...need to have controls where they can be seen by people of short stature and those using wheelchairs.
	• Cannot find buttons that don't contrast with the background (won't feel where nothing is visible or expected)	
	• Phantom buttons (visual) (logos, styling that looks like a button when blurred)	
	• Cannot locate where the cursor is on the screen	

(Continued)

Table 17.2 (Continued) User Needs Summary Trace Center, University of Wisconsin–Madison

Basic users need to be able to *perceive* all information presented by the product	Problems using products	User needs
Perceive status of controls and indicators includes PROGRESS indicators	**People with physical disabilities** • Often cannot re-position themselves to see controls if not in easy sightline **People with cognitive disabilities** • Do not recognize stylized control as a control **All disabilities** • Cannot tell state if the same alternative is provided for different signals **People who are blind** • Cannot tell status of visual indicators (LEDs, on-screen indicators, etc.) • Cannot tell the status of switches or controls that are not tactilely different in different states (or where tactile difference is too small) **People with low vision** • Cannot read visual indicators with low vision if the indicator is not bold • Cannot distinguish between some colors used to indicate status • Cannot see or read small icons for status • Cannot see cursors unless large and high contrast. Static harder than dynamic to spot **People who are deaf** • Cannot hear audio indicators of status • Cannot hear natural sounds (e.g., machine running, stalled, busy) **People who are hard of hearing** • May not hear status sounds due to volume, frequency used, background noise, etc. **People with physical disabilities** • May not have a good line of sight to indicators • May not have tactile sensitivity to detect tactile status indications. **People with cognitive disabilities** • May not recognize or understand different indicators	**Some users with disabilities…** • …need an auditory or tactile equivalent to any visual indicators or operational cues, synthetic or natural. • …need a visual or tactile indicator for any auditory indicators or operational cues, synthetic or natural. • …need visual or auditory alternative to any subtle tactile feedback. • …need visual indicators to be visible with low vision. • …need all indications that are encoded (or presented) with color to be encoded (marked) in a non-color way as well. • …need large high contrast pointer cursors. • …need sufficient volume and clarity for audio cues. • …need alternatives that are different, when different signals are used (e.g., different ring tones, or tactile or visual indicators). • …need indicators and cues to be obvious or explained. • …need to have controls and indicators located where they can be seen by people of short stature and those using wheelchairs.

(Continued)

Table 17.2 (Continued) User Needs Summary Trace Center, University of Wisconsin-Madison

Basic users need to be able to *perceive* all information presented by the product	Problems using products	User needs

Perceive feedback from operation
(be able to OPERATE the product)
	All disabilities
	• Cannot tell state if the same alternative is provided for different signals
	People who are blind
	• Cannot see visual feedback of operation
	People with low vision
	• Cannot see visual feedback of operation unless large, bold
	  a. Often have hearing impairments as well so cannot always count on audio
	People who are deaf
	• Cannot hear auditory feedback of operation
	People who are hard of hearing
	• Often cannot hear auditory feedback of operation due to
	  a. Volume
	  b. Frequency used
	  c. Background noise
	  d. Speech feedback not clear or repeatable.
	People with physical disabilities
	• May not be able to feel tactile feedback due to insensitivity or impact of hand or use of artificial hand, stick, splint, etc. to operate the control
	People with cognitive disabilities
	• Feedback to subtle or not directly tied to action
		Some users with disabilities…
		• …need visual feedback that is dramatic (Visual from 10 ft).
		• while others need it to be audio or tactile feedback.

(Continued)

Table 17.2 (Continued) User Needs Summary Trace Center, University of Wisconsin-Madison

Basic users need to be able to *perceive* all information presented by the product	Problems using products	User needs

Be able to invoke and carry out all functions (via at least one method)	**People who are blind**
	• Cannot use controls that require eye–hand coordination
	  a. Pointing devices including mice, trackballs, etc.
	  b. Touchscreens of any type
	• Cannot use devices with touch-activated controls (can't explore tactilely)
	• Can't use products that require the presence of iris or eyes (e.g., for identification)
	
	People with low vision
	• Difficult to use the device with eye-hand coordination.
	
	People who are deaf
	• Many cannot use if speech input is the only way to do some functions
	• Cannot operate devices where actions are in response to speech (only)
	
	People with physical disabilities
	• Cannot operate devices if operation *requires* (i.e., no other way to do function)
	  a. Too much force
	  b. Too much reach
	  c. Too much stamina (including long operation of controls with arm extended or holding the handset to head for a long period unless able to prop or rest arm)
	  d. Contact with body (so that artificial hands, mouth sticks, etc. cannot be used)
	  e. Simultaneous operation of two parts (modifier keys, two latches, etc.)
	  f. Tight grasping
	  g. Pinching
		Some users with disabilities…
		• …need to be able to operate all functionality using only tactilely discernable controls coupled with audio or tactile feedback/display (no vision required).
		  a. Not require a pointing device.
		• …need to not have touch sensitive or very light touch controls where they would be touched while tactilely finding keys, they must use to operate the device.
		• …need alternate identification means if biometrics are used for identification.
		• …need an alternate method to operate any speech-controlled functions.
		• …need to be able to access all computer software functionality from the keyboard (or keyboard emulator).
		• …need a method to operate product that does not require
		  a. simultaneous actions,
		  b. much force,
		  c. much reach,
		  d. much stamina,
		  e. tight grasping,
		  f. pinching,
		  g. twisting of the wrist, or
		  h. direct body contact.

(Continued)

Table 17.2 (Continued) User Needs Summary Trace Center, University of Wisconsin-Madison

Basic users need to be able to *perceive* all information presented by the product	Problems using products	User needs

	h. Twisting of the wrist
	i. Fine motor control or manipulations (i.e., can't operate with a closed fist).
	• Cannot use products that require the presence of fingerprints or other specific body parts or organs (e.g., for identification)
		Some users with disabilities…
		• …need to have all messages either stay until dismissed or have a mechanism to keep the message on screen or easily recall it.
		• …need to have the ability to either
		  a. Have no timeouts or
		  b. Have the ability to turn off timeouts,
		  c. Be able to set timeouts to ten times the default value, or
		  d. Be warned when timeout is coming and be provided with the ability to extend timeouts
		except where it is impossible to do so.
		• …need to have a way to turn off or freeze any moving text.

Be able to complete actions and tasks within the time allowed (by life, competition, productivity requirements, etc.)	**People who are blind** • must use non-visual techniques that are often slower, requiring more time than usual to read/listen to output, explore and locate controls, etc. **People with low vision** • often take longer to read text and locate controls **People who are deaf** • may be reading information in a second language (sign language being first) • may be communicating (or operating phone system) through a relay/interpreter that introduces delays **People who are hard of hearing** • may have to listen more than once to get audio information. **People with physical disabilities** • may take longer to read (due to head movement), position themselves, reach, or operate controls **People with cognitive disabilities** • may take longer to remember, look things up, figure out information, and operate the controls All of these can cause problems if • Information or messages are displayed for a fixed period and then disappear • Users are only given a limited amount of time to operate device before it resets or moves on • Text moves on them while they are trying to read it	

(Continued)

405

Table 17.2 (Continued) User Needs Summary Trace Center, University of Wisconsin-Madison

Basic users need to be able to *perceive* all information presented by the product	Problems using products	User needs
Won't accidentally activate functions	**People who are blind** • Might touch "touch sensitive" controls or screen buttons while tactilely exploring • Might miss warning signs or icons that are presented visually • Might bump low activation force switch(es) while tactilely exploring **People with low vision** • Might bump low-contrast switches/controls that they do not see **People who are deaf or hard of hearing** • May not detect alert tone and operate the device when unsafe **People with physical disabilities** • Might activate functions due to extra body movements (tremor, chorea) • Might activate functions when resting arm while reaching **People with cognitive disabilities** • Might not understand the purpose of control (or control changes due to softkey).	**Some users with disabilities...** • ...need to have products designed so they can be tactilely explored without activation. • ...need products that can't cause injury with spasmodic movements. • ...need to have products that don't rely on users seeing hazards or warnings in order to use products safely. • ...need to have products that don't rely on users hearing hazards or warnings in order to use products safely. • ...need to have products where hazards are obvious and easy to avoid and hard to trigger.
Be able to recover from errors (physical or cognitive errors)	**People who are blind or have low vision** • May not detect an error if the indication is visual • May not be able to perceive contextual cues (if visual only) to know they did something wrong or unintended (when not an "error" to the device). **People who are deaf** • Will not hear auditory "error" sounds. **People who are hard of hearing** • May not hear auditory "error" sounds or be able to distinguish between them. **All disabilities** • User may not be able to figure out how to go back and undo the error.	**Some users with disabilities...** • ...need a mechanism to go back and undo the last thing(s) they did – unless impossible. • ...need good auditory and visual indications when things happen so that they can detect errors. • ...need to be notified if the product detects errors made by the user. • ...need clear unambiguous feedback when an error is made and what to do to correct it.

(Continued)

Table 17.2 (Continued) User Needs Summary Trace Center, University of Wisconsin-Madison

Basic users need to be able to *perceive* all information presented by the product	Problems using products	User needs
Have equivalent, security, and privacy	**People with all disabilities** • Do not have privacy when human assistance is required **People who are blind** • Have more difficulty detecting people looking over shoulder • If no headphone or handset – information is broadcast to others via speaker **People with low vision** • Larger print makes it easier for others to look over shoulder **People who are deaf** • May not detect sensitive information being said aloud **People who are hard of hearing** • Louder volume may allow eavesdropping – even with headphones. a. Use may not realize volume of audio **People with physical disabilities** • In a wheelchair, body doesn't block view of sensitive information like someone standing. **People with cognitive disabilities** • Less able to determine when information should be kept private.	**Some users with disabilities…** • ….need the ability to listen privately. • ….need to have the product designed to help protect privacy and security of their information even if they are not able to do the "expected" things to protect it themselves.

(Continued)

Table 17.2 (Continued) User Needs Summary Trace Center, University of Wisconsin–Madison

Basic users need to be able to *perceive* all information presented by the product	Problems using products	User needs
Not cause health risk (e.g., seizure)	**People who are blind** • Cannot see to avoid hazards that are visual • Cannot see warning signs, colors, markers, etc. • If using headphones – they are less aware of surroundings (and not used to it). **People who are deaf or hard of hearing** • May miss auditory warnings or sounds that indicate device failure **People with physical disabilities** • May hit objects harder than usual and cause injury • May not sense when they are injuring themselves **People with photosensitive epilepsy** • May have seizures triggered by provocative visual stimuli. **People with allergies and other sensitivities** • May have adverse reactions to materials, electro-magnetic emissions, fumes, and other adverse aspects of products they touch or are near	**Some users with disabilities...** • ...need products that don't assume body parts will never stray into openings or that only gentle body movements will occur around the products (unless required by task). • ...need to have products that take into account their special visual, physical, chemical, etc. sensitivities so that they are not prevented from using products except when the nature of the product or task would prevent them (e.g., not by product design).
Be able to efficiently navigate product (be able to UNDERSTAND)	**People who are blind** • Often have to wait for unnecessary audio before getting to the desired information **People with low vision** • Have trouble tracking cursors on screen **People with physical disabilities** • Have trouble with navigation requiring many repeated actions to navigate **People with cognitive disabilities** • Have trouble with hierarchical structures	**Some users with disabilities...** • ...need to have alternate modes of operation that are efficient enough to allow them to be able to compete in education and employment settings • ...need to control speech output rate • ...need the ability to preserve their access settings

(Continued)

408

Table 17.2 (Continued) User Needs Summary Trace Center, University of Wisconsin-Madison

Basic users need to be able to *perceive* all information presented by the product	Problems using products	User needs
Understand how to use product (including discovery and activation of any access features needed)	**All disabilities** • May have trouble understanding how to turn on special access features they need • May have trouble understanding how to operate it if different than standard users **People who are blind (or have low vision)** • Have a more difficult time getting a gestalt since they cannot see the overall visual layout or organization. • Complex layouts can behave like a maze for someone navigating with arrow keys **People who are deaf** • English (or the spoken/written language used on the product) may be different than their natural (first) language (e.g., if it is sign language). **People with cognitive disabilities** • Have trouble remembering the organization of a product, its menus, etc. • Have a harder time with any hierarchical structures • Cannot read labels, signs, manuals, etc. due to reading limitations • May have trouble understanding directions — especially if printed • May have trouble remembering steps for use • May have trouble getting it turned on — and therefore active • May be confused by options, buttons, and controls that they do not need or use • Icons and symbols may not make sense to them — and they don't remember • Product may differ from real-life experience enough to leave them at a loss. • might have trouble with products that operate in non-standard ways (user need: 13-3)	**Some users with disabilities...** • ...need a way to get an overview and orient themselves to product and functions/parts without relying on visual presentation or markings on a product. • ...need products to operate in predictable (standard or familiar) ways. • ...need a way to understand a product if they don't think hierarchically very well. • ...need to have clear and easy activation mechanisms for any access features. • ...need interfaces that minimize the need to remember. • ...need to have language used on products to be as easy to understand as possible given the device and task. • ...need to have printed text read aloud to them. • ...need to have steps for operation minimized and clearly described. • ...need information and feedback to be "salient," and "specific" rather than subtle or abstract in order to understand it. • ...need keys that don't change function. • ...need cues to assist them in multistep operations. • ...need to have simple interfaces that only require them to deal with the controls they need (advanced or optional controls removed in some fashion).

(Continued)

Table 17.2 (Continued) User Needs Summary Trace Center, University of Wisconsin–Madison

Basic users need to be able to *perceive* all information presented by the product	Problems using products	User needs
Understand the output or displayed material (even after they perceive it accurately) see also "perceive"	**People who are blind** • Output often only makes sense visually. Reading it is confusing (e.g., "select item from list at the right" when they get to it by pressing down arrow) • Have difficulty with any simultaneous presentation of audio output and audio description of visual information (e.g., reading of screen information while playing audio) **People who are deaf** • Reading skills – English may not be the primary language (ASL) • Can have difficulty with simultaneous presentation of visual information and (visual) captions of auditory information **People with cognitive disabilities** • May not be able to read information presented in text • Language may be too complex for them • Long or complex messages may tax their memory abilities. • Use of idiom or jargon may make it hard to understand. • Structures, tabular or hierarchical information may be difficult.	**Some users with disabilities...** • ...need descriptions, instructions, and cues to match audio operation – not just visual operation • ...need to have any printed material be worded as clearly and simply as possible. • ...need to have any printed material read to them. • ...need to have audio generated by access features do not interfere with any other audio generated by the device. • ...need to have visual information generated by access features (such as captions) not occur simultaneously with other visual information they must view (and then disappear before they can read the captions).

(Continued)

410

Table 17.2 (Continued) User Needs Summary Trace Center, University of Wisconsin-Madison

Basic users need to be able to *perceive* all information presented by the product	Problems using products	User needs
Ability to use their AT to control the product (not always possible with public devices but common with personal or office workstation technologies) Note: to replace built-in access, AT must allow all of the above basics to be met.	**All disabilities** • Cannot use their AT to access products if a. Product is in public and they will not have their technology with them b. They do not have permission to use their AT with the product • e.g., cannot install AT software on Library systems a. **They are not able to connect their AT to it** • Cannot use their AT if the device interferes with it • Cannot use their AT if they are not easily able to find the connection mechanism given their disability • AT is not available for new technologies when they come out **People who are blind** • Would need all visual information to be available to their AT in machine readable form via a standard connection mechanism • Would need to be able to activate all functionality from their AT (or from tactile controls on the product) **People with low vision** • Would need all visual information to be available in machine readable form to their AT via a standard connection mechanism so that the AT could enlarge it or read it. **People who are deaf** • Would need all auditory information to be available to their AT in machine readable form via a standard connection mechanism. **People who are hard of hearing** • Would need all audio information to be available via a standard connection mechanism that is compatible with their assistive listening devices (ALDs). a. Need a standard audio connector to plug their ALD b. Something held up to the ear should be T-Coil compatible	**Some users with disabilities…** • …need to not have product interfere with their AT. • …need to be able to connect their AT. • …need to have full functionality of product available through their AT if they have to use their AT to access the product. a. …need to have software use standard system-provided input and output methods. b. …need to have all displayed text made available to their AT.…need to have full functionality of the product available to them via their AT. c. …need information about user interface elements including the identity, operation, and state of the element to be available to assistive technology. d. All controls need to be operable from AT. • …need to be able to access all computer software functionality from the keyboard (or keyboard emulator). • …need to have all controls work with them at manipulators, artificial hands, pointers, etc. • …need to have new technologies be compatible with their AT when the new technologies are released.

(Continued)

Table 17.2 (Continued) User Needs Summary Trace Center, University of Wisconsin-Madison

Basic users need to be able to *perceive* all information presented by the product	Problems using products	User needs
	People with physical disabilities • Cannot use products that aren't fully operable with an artificial hand, stick, stylus, etc. • Need connection point that allows operation of all controls **People with cognitive disabilities** • Would need all information to be available in machine readable form to their AT via a standard connection mechanism	
Cross cutting issues	**All disabilities** • Accessibility is not available in new technologies when they come out • Support services are not accessible (no training or proper communication equipment)	**Some users with disabilities...** • ...need to have new technologies be accessible when they are released. • ...need to have support and training services that are accessible.

The first approach, *changing the individual*, is based on a medical model and is a very important strategy. It seeks to increase the basic abilities of the individual through both medical and other rehabilitation strategies. It may include surgery and rehabilitation therapy, but also includes training, the learning of techniques from peers, and in many cases, equipping the individual with personal assistive technologies such as glasses, hearing aids, prostheses, splints, and wheelchairs. Today, individuals (both with and without disabilities) carry around with them specialized interface technologies or devices that are tuned to the individual's needs and could act as their personal interfaces to the devices around them. These *personal assistive technologies* stay with, and are available to, the individual as they encounter the world, and are thought of as extensions of the individual. Smartphones are the most common form of this.

The second approach, *adapt or provide adapters to individual products after manufacture*, has been around as long as there have been inventive people with disabilities and/or inventive friends. This approach basically focuses on custom adapting the devices to the individual so that they are operable by the individual. This includes, for example, adding tactile markings to a stove or microwave or putting grab bars near the toilet. Adaptations for information and communication technology include special keyboards, screen readers, and enlargers. This category includes products that are developed on a custom basis for individuals, as well as commercially available adaptive assistive technologies used with mainstream products to make the mainstream products more accessible and usable by individuals with particular disabilities. These bridging or adaptive technologies are especially important for individuals with severe and/or multiple disabilities, where building sufficient accessibility into mainstream products is not practical or not yet practical. It is also important in employment settings where the employee with a disability must be able to access a product and use it efficiently enough to be competitive and productive so a tight fit to devices at the worksite is required.

The third approach, *changing the world, so that people can use it with the abilities they have*, has many names. "universal design" (UD), "design for all" (DFA), "accessible design," "barrier-free design," and "inclusive design." "User-based design" (Wobbrock et al. 2018) is also related but can be used for the design of products for individuals or groups as well as for mainstream products.

The term "universal design" has had many definitions. The term universal design was originally coined by Ron Mace, an architect and Director of the Center for Universal Design at North Carolina State University. He defined it as follows: "Universal design means simply designing all products, buildings and exterior spaces to be usable by all people to the greatest extent possible" (Broetz et al. 2010).

This definition has served well as a reference point but has raised concerns among some designers because it sets no practical limits. What is possible is not necessarily commercially viable. As UD/DFA moved from a goal to appear in social legislation, designers began to fear the implications of such an ideal goal ("designing things that everyone can use") if the term was used in a requirements context. For example, building a $2,000 Braille display into every electronic device with a visual display is not generally practical. As a result, some designers began to fight the movement rather than embrace or explore the basic concept.

A debate also surfaced as to whether UD/DFA included compatibility with assistive technology, which may view as being key to being able to use mainstream technologies. This is particularly true with regard to personal assistive technologies, as discussed earlier.

To address these issues and create a practitioner's definition of universal design (or design for all), a companion definition was proposed:

(commercial) universal design (or design for all).
The *process* of designing products so that they are usable by the widest range of people operating in the widest range of situations as is commercially practical. It includes making products directly accessible and usable (without the need for any assistive technology) and making products compatible with assistive technologies for those who require them for effective access.

(Shindo et al. 2011; emphasis added)

It is important to note the word "process" in the above definition. UD/DFA is a process, not an outcome. *There are no "universal designs."* That is, there are no designs that can be used by everyone, no matter how many or how severe their disabilities. Universal design is not the process of creating products that *everyone* can use. It is a process of insuring that designs can be used by as many people as is practical, and then constantly moving that line as new approaches are discovered, and new technologies become available. For some products, this might result in a very narrow range of users if they have extremely high user demands (e.g., jet fighters). For other products, it can have an extremely wide range of users. Fare machines, information kiosks, and even voting systems have been designed that can be used by individuals who have low vision, are blind, hard of hearing, or deaf, have almost no reach, cannot read, or have various cognitive, language, and learning disabilities. (Rayegani et al. 2014, 137–151; Deafblind.com 2018). Moreover, they do not require multiple modes of operation, but rather options for operation in the same way that both the keyboard and mouse can be used to navigate windowing environments. Yet no matter how good the universal designs, there are individuals who will not be able to operate products directly without the need for some type of assistive technology or alternate interface. Hence, the importance of compatibility with assistive technology to complement direct access.

414

Today, the term "inclusive design" is more common – and less often misunderstood – and is the recommended terminology of the authors.

17.3.2 Pluggable user interfaces

The idea of pluggable user interfaces has been around for some time, and there are even international standards for pluggable user interfaces. A five-part ISO standard (ISO 24752, adopted in January 2008) describes a standard method for mainstream products to expose their functionality so that they can be directly controlled from personal alternate interface devices. This represents a breakthrough in the ability to design products that can be used by a much broader range of users as they encounter them.

Figure 17.3 shows the typical way an individual interacts with a product. The product has certain needs for information and/or commands from the user. A television, for example, needs to know the channel that the user wants to be watching, the volume that the user wants to set, the various color tints and settings to be selected, the source of the signal (cable, DVD, etc.), and so on. It does not care whether it gets the information by having the user push a button, turn a dial, or pick an item from a menu. However, the television comes with a built-in interface that takes its general device requirements (volume, channel, etc.) and changes them into specific actions that a user must perform. These actions may or may not be easy to perform for an individual with a disability.

Figure 17.4 shows the same device, except that an interface socket has been added that allows the individual to plug a different interface into the device to provide the television with the various types of information it needs, but this time using an interface of the user's choosing. An individual who is blind may choose an

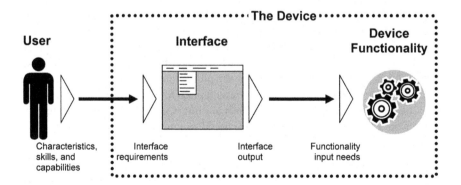

Figure 17.3 Typical interface where the only access to the device's functionality is through the interface built into the product with its particular assumptions and requirements regarding the user's abilities (Jordan and Vanderheiden 2017).

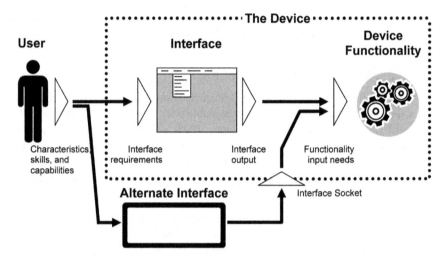

Figure 17.4 By adding an alternate interface connection point to the device in Figure 17.3, it is possible for a user to connect an alternate interface that better matches their abilities (Jordan and Vanderheiden 2017).

all-auditory interface, while an individual with a physical disability may choose an interface that only requires sipping and puffing, and so on.

The interface socket provides all of the information necessary for the user's personal interface to be able to construct and present an interface to the user for each device they encounter. Whenever the user encounters a device (that supports this standard) in their environment, their personal interface can discover it and download all of the information about the product functions and any commands or settings needed to operate the device. Optionally, the device can also provide hints as to how an interface should be structured. The user's personal interface can then construct an interface for the product that meets the user's needs. If they were blind, it might be auditory. If they have severe paralysis, it might be voice controlled. For a user who is deaf-blind, it might be a Braille-based interface. It should be noted that the pluggable user interface may connect to products without the need for any physical plug. Merely coming near a product may be all that is necessary for an alternate interface to link up to an interface socket on a product, allowing the individual to control the product using their alternate interface.

Key to this approach is the Universal Remote Console (URC) standards (ANSI-INCIT 2005-389 to 393 and ISO-24752). Unlike products controlled by universal remote controls that need to be programmed, products implementing the URC standards automatically provide all of the information needed by a URC to construct an interface for a user. In this way, an individual could approach an unknown device and their URC would be able to automatically construct an interface for this device that met the user's needs and preferences.

Personal pluggable user interfaces like this that the user would carry about with them would be examples of both a type one (change the user) and type three (change the world) strategy working together. It could also be used for a type two (adapt the individual products encountered by the person to make them usable to the person) but that would be less common since it is rarely possible for anyone besides the manufacturer to create an interface socket for a product. It can be seen, however, how the approaches are blending together as technologies advance.

The major barrier to date for personal pluggable interfaces has been the reluctance of manufacturers to provide interface sockets on their products, for fear that the products' functionality will become commoditized. They fear that users will only remember the interface they are looking at and not the product being controlled. If the user operates their TV through say Apple TV or Amazon TV, when it comes time to replace the TV, their identification and loyalty will be to the device they use to interface to their screen – and not the manufacturer of their screen. The screen will be commoditized and will be viewed by users are easily replaced by any other screen. Pluggable user interfaces have therefore been of limited impact to date. Market and technology pressures however may cause a shift in the future. If this were to happen, it could have profound effects on the ability of users to have their own personal interfaces that they can use with the products around them. This is already happening somewhat today as products provide smartphone interfaces to their products – which allow users with disabilities to control a wide range of products from their phone – via special interfaces to their phone. And with the Internet of Things making more and more devices in our environment controllable from our phones, this trend will continue.

17.3.3 Working together, blending together

All of these techniques (change the person, adapt the environment, and change the environment) need to work together in order to accommodate individuals with the full range of abilities and limitations. In general, individuals with less severe disabilities can be accommodated through universal design/design for all. This includes a large percentage of individuals who are aging. For individuals with more severe and/or multiple disabilities, it may be more difficult to build interfaces into mainstream products that will work effectively for them. Either adaptive assistive technology, or perhaps personal assistive technology that connects through pluggable user interface sockets, may provide them with effective access. We do not expect that inclusive design will ever eliminate the need for wheelchairs or braille displays. But more flexible, inclusive design of mainstream products can significantly reduce the number of people who need to buy special assistive technologies by designing mainstream interfaces that are flexible enough to allow them to use them directly.

Thus, a combination of inclusive design and assistive technologies will likely be required for the foreseeable future.

17.3.4 Specific strategies to address needs

Previously, an extremely wide range of specific techniques that can be used for addressing needs was outlined. Table 17.3 provides a summary of the basic strategies organized in parallel with the essentials of "perceivable," "operable," "understandable," and "compatible." A more comprehensive listing of strategies as well as specific techniques that can be useful when implementing them on different technologies can be found at www.trace.wisc.edu/designtools.

As always, these strategies may be employed in the design of the mainstream product itself or may be made possible by allowing the connection of adaptive assistive technologies or personal assistive technologies.

17.4 Priorities in implementation

In looking at accessibility-usability features, it is important to prioritize because of the multi-dimensional nature of disability (vision, hearing, physical, cognitive) and the large number of individual design techniques or strategies that might be implemented for each dimension. When examining a number of design strategy collections, between 200 and 300 different strategies were identified for making products more accessible to people with disabilities (and this did not include the large number of different strategies documented in general usability literature). Without a means to prioritize, two behaviors have been observed in interactions with industry.

First, product designers become overwhelmed with the sheer number of different techniques and strategies. Just contemplating building over 100 different strategies into a product causes many to walk away or approach feature selection (focusing of their efforts) in a somewhat random fashion. Usability tests by themselves are not a solution to the problem of being overwhelmed since they quickly generate a long list of problems that, in turn, point back to an even longer list of potential solution strategies.

The second behavior observed is a poor prioritization in efforts where features that were first thought of or easiest to implement are chosen rather than strategies or features that are more important. The result is a product that has multiple low priority features (which are helpful but not essential for access) while lacking key

Table 17.3 Basic Strategies for Access to Electronic Products and Documents

Basic access guideline	Why	How (general)
Make **all information** (including status and labels for all keys and controls) **perceivable** • Without vision • With low vision and no hearing • With little or no tactile sensitivity • Without hearing • With impaired hearing • Without reading (due to low vision, learning disability, illiteracy, cognition, or other) • Without color perception • Without causing seizure • From different heights • Note: Other aspects of cognition covered below	Information that is presented in a form that is only perceivable with a single sense (e.g., only vision or only hearing) is not accessible to people without that sense. **Note:** This includes situations where some of the information is only presented in one form (e.g., visual) and other information is only presented in another (e.g., auditory). **In addition:** Information that cannot be presented in different modalities would not be accessible to those using mobile technologies, for example: • Visual only information would not be usable by people using an auditory interface while driving a car. • Auditory-only information would not be usable by people in a noisy environment	**For information:** Make all information available either in a) **Presentation independent form** (e.g., electronic text) that can be presented (rendered) in any sensory form (e.g., visual-print, auditory-speech, tactile-braille). **OR** b) **Sensory parallel form** where redundant and complete forms of the information are provided for different sensory modalities (synchronized) (e.g., a captioned and described movie — including e-text of both). **For products:** Provide a mechanism for presenting all information (including labels) in visual, enlarged visual, auditory, enhanced auditory (louder and if possible better signal-to-noise ratio), and (where possible), tactile form. **Note:** This includes any information (semantics or structure) that is presented via **text formatting or layout**.

(Continued)

419

Table 17.3 (Continued) Basic Strategies for Access to Electronic Products and Documents

Basic access guideline	Why	How (general)
Provide at least one mode (or set of different modes) for all product features that **is operable:** • Without pointing • Without vision • Without requirement to respond quickly • Without fine motor movement • Without simultaneous action • Without speech • Without requiring presence or use of particular biological parts (touch, fingerprint, iris, etc.)	Interfaces that are input device or technique specific cannot be operated by individuals who cannot use that technique (e.g., a person who is blind cannot point to a target in an image map; some people cannot use pointing devices accurately). **In addition:** Technique-specific interfaces may not be accessible to users of mobile devices. For example, people using voice to navigate may not be able to "point." Many individuals will not be able to operate products, such as workstations with sufficient efficiency to hold a competitive job if navigation is not efficient.	**Provide at least one mode (set of modes) where….** a) All functions of the product are controllable via tactiley discernable controls and both visual and voice output is provided for any displayed information required for operation including labels. **AND** b) There are no timeouts for input or displayed information, OR allow user to freeze timer or set it to a long time (five times default or range), OR offer extended time to the user and allow ten seconds to respond to the offer. **AND** c) All functions of the product operable with: • No simultaneous activations • No twisting motions • No fine motor control required • No biological contact required • No user speech required • No pointing motions required 1. **AND** d) If biological techniques are used for security, have at least two alternatives with one preferably a non-biological alternative unless biological-based security is required. **AND** e) Allow users to jump over blocks of undesired information (e.g., repetitive info – or jump by sections if large document), especially if reading via sound or other serial presentation means. f) Make actions reversible or request confirmation. *(Continued)*

Table 17.3 (Continued) Basic Strategies for Access to Electronic Products and Documents

Basic access guideline	Why	How (general)
Facilitate understanding of operation and content • Without skill in the language used on the product (poor language skills or it is a second language for them) • Without good concentration, processing • Without prior understanding of the content • Without good memory • Without background or experience with the topic	Many individuals will have trouble using a product (even with alternate access techniques) if the **layout/organization** of the information or product **is too difficult to understand.** People with cognitive or language difficulties (or inexperienced users) may not be able to use devices or products with complex language.	a) Make overall organization understandable (e.g., provide overview, table of contents, site maps, description of layout of device). b) Don't mislead/confuse. (Be consistent in the use of icons or metaphors. Don't ignore or misuse conventions.) c) Consider having different navigation models for novice vs expert users. d) Use the simplest, easiest to understand language and structure/format as is appropriate for the material/site/situation. e) Using graphics to supplement or provide alternate presentations of information. f) If phrases from a different language (than the rest of the page) are used in a document, either identify the language used (to allow translation) or provide a translation to the document language.
Provide compatibility with assistive technologies commonly used by people • With low vision • Without vision • Who are hard of hearing • Who are deaf. • Without physical reach and manipulation • Who have cognitive or language disabilities	In many cases, a person coming up to a product will have assistive technologies with them. If the person cannot use the product directly, it is important that the product be designed to allow them to use their assistive technology to access the product. (This also applies to users of mobile devices people with glasses, gloves, or other extensions to themselves.)	a) Do not interfere with the use of assistive technologies • Personal aids (e.g., hearing aids) • System-based technologies (e.g., OS features) b) Support standard connection points for • Audio amplification devices • Alternate input and output devices (or software) c) Provide at least one mode where all functions of the product are controllable via human understandable input via an external port or a network connection.

421

high priority features that are needed to make the product (or key functions of the product) accessible for the same disability group. This is equivalent to changing the plush carpet in the entire building to a tighter nap to make it easier for wheelchairs to get around, but leaving the steps at the front door and having no elevators to get off of the ground floor.

The purpose is to map out the dimensions of complexity involved and then to develop simplified and straightforward (as possible) techniques and procedures for addressing or accommodating them. The advice of Albert Einstein is appropriate to remember here:

"Everything should be made as simple as possible. But no simpler."

Hence the goal is to make this as simple as possible, but not to simplify where that leads to inaccuracy or poor decisions.

17.4.1 First dimension for prioritization: Accessibility/usability

In looking at the usability of a product to different people, there is a continuous range that runs all the way from:

- people who have no problems at all in using all of the functions of a product (usually a small number of people), through
- people who have little difficulty with all, to
- people who have difficulty with some features, to
- people who have trouble with most features, to
- people who are unable to use the product at all.

Even the features vary in importance to the overall use of the product. Some features are essential, while others are merely convenient.

To address this, it was found useful to evaluate the importance of product features, as follows:

Essential – features which, if they have not been implemented, will cause a product to be unusable for certain groups or situations.

Important – features which, if not implemented, will make the product very difficult to use for some groups or situations.

Improving usability – features which, if they are implemented, will make the product easier to use but do not make a product usable or unusable (except for individuals who are just on a margin due to other factors and this small amount of usability pushes them over the threshold).

In looking at this dimension, however, it is important to note that features that may just improve the usability for some people may be essential to allow use by others. This is especially true for people with cognitive, language, and learning disabilities.

17.4.2 The second dimension affecting prioritization: Independence vs. co-dependence

In addition to the accessibility/usability dimension, there is a second dimension that deals with independence versus co-dependence. Everybody depends on others for some aspects of life. Few people know how to repair a car and television set. Some do not know how to change printer cartridges or clear paper jams or reformat hard drives. In daily life, there are some things people need to be able to do independently and some things that they can depend on others for. In setting usability priorities, this independence/co-dependence can be taken into account to facilitate decisions regarding the expenditure of effort.

For example, it is more important that an individual be able to load their work into the input hopper on a copier and operate the controls to get the required number and type of copies than it is for them to be able to change the toner or clear a paper jam. In fact, in many offices, only people trained in clearing paper jams are allowed to do so. Loading new reams of blank paper into the copier generally falls somewhere in between. Similarly, it is more important for an individual to be able to launch and operate programs than it is for them to be able to configure their modem settings. This importance stems not from the technical difficulty of the two tasks but from the fact that one is an activity that is required continuously as a part of their daily operation, whereas the other is something that needs to only be done once or which can be planned for and scheduled when there is someone to assist.

Figure 17.5 shows a rough hierarchy based on the need for independence versus the ability to deal with co-dependence. The exact ordering of the items will vary for different types of products and different environments (e.g., the availability of the co-dependent facilitator), but the general ordering can be seen. This can then be used to set priorities in a resource-constrained or time-constrained product design program.

17.4.3 The third dimension affecting prioritization: Efficiency and urgency requirement

The third dimension of prioritization deals with the need for *efficiency*. If a task is performed only once a day and there is no particular time constraint on its accomplishment (e.g., the person is not trying to disarm an alarm before it goes off), then the relative efficiency of operation is not as critical as in the case of a function that must be used continuously throughout the day. For example, if it takes

1. Functions/features needed for basic use of the product
2. Unpredictable, but typically user-serviceable (by "average" user) maintenance or recovery operations
3. Unpredictable service, maintenance or recovery, typically corrected by support personnel
4. Predictable or schedulable maintenance that can be delegated to others
5. Unpacking and initial setup
6. Repair

NOTE: The location and availability of support personnel (e.g. in a home office) affect this dimension.

Figure 17.5 Priority based on the need for a person to be able to independently accomplish tasks.

an individual five times longer to operate the "on" switch on their computer than the average worker, it will not have a major impact on their productivity or effectiveness. In fact, turning the on switch is such a small part of booting a computer that the total time it takes for them to turn the computer on is likely to be only negligibly longer than the time for anyone else to boot their computer. If it takes an individual five times as long to type characters on their computer, however, and they spend the bulk of their day entering information into their computer, the difference in efficiency could be catastrophic. If it took them five days to get an average day's worth of work done, it would be hard for them to compete in either an educational or work environment. Thus, for the on/off switch, level one accessibility may be all that is required. However, for data entry, levels one, two, and three may all be critical on an individual's workstation.

A close parallel to efficiency is the *urgency* issue. If there are situations where a user must do something within a particular time constraint in order to avoid an adverse situation, then, even if it is rarely done, it may be important to strive for level two or level three usability in order to allow the individual to be able to carry out the activity within the time allowed.

The importance that is attached to this dimension is the function of at least three factors.

1. The reversibility of the action.
2. The severity of the consequence for failure.
3. The ability of the person to adjust the time span to meet their increased reaction times.

Situations where the result is not reversible or is dire in nature, and is also of a type that does not allow for user adjustment or extension (as in some security-related situations), would create the highest priority for providing not only an accessible but a highly usable interface for the group or situation.

17.4.4 A pseudo-priority dimension: Ease of implementation

In setting priorities for the implementation of usability features in products, a factor that is often used to select features is the ease with which they can be implemented in the product. In this context, "ease" may have many different characteristics, including cost in dollars, cost in time, ease in getting clearance from supervisors, minimized impact on other features, minimized impact on testing, minimal impact on documentation, and so on. Often referred to as "low-hanging fruit," such features are often very tempting when compared with features that are much more difficult to implement. Although it is always good to look at this dimension, there is great danger as well. Often this strategy leads one to believe that five low-hanging fruit features must be better than one that is more difficult to achieve. This can lead to the implementation of multiple "usability" features instead of key "essential" accessibility features. Often this occurs with features intended to benefit the same disability group, so that a product may have usability features for a disability group that cannot, in fact, use the product.

Within the "essential" accessibility features, however, one will also often find either a low-hanging fruit or features that would have such mass-market appeal that their "costs" are offset by their market benefit.

17.4.5 Cognitive constraints: A unique dimension

In looking at the dimensions, it is important to note that the cognitive dimension is unique with respect to the other dimensions. It is possible to make most products usable to individuals with no vision or no hearing and even with no physical ability. However, there are very few products, if any, that are usable by individuals with no cognitive abilities. This is due to the fact that it is possible to translate most types of information between sensory modalities and most types of activities between physical interface techniques, but there is no mechanism for transferring cognitive processing into another domain. While it is true that there are some activities and types of information for which good strategies do not exist for providing access to individuals with severe or total visual limitation, severe or total hearing limitations, or severe or total physical limitations, the number of devices and activities that are excluded are much smaller than for severe or total cognitive limitations. For this reason, strategies for "enabling access" for people with cognitive disabilities basically look like techniques to "facilitate" with each technique, which "facilitates" pushing a few more people over the threshold into the category of individuals who "can use" a product.

It is also important to note that there are a number of dimensions that are often lumped in with cognitive disabilities where products can be made accessible. For example, there are strategies that can allow individuals who think clearly but are completely unable to read for some reason to be able to effectively use a wide variety of products. In this case, the difficulty is not in general cognitive processing or memory, but rather in a specific skill, which is decoding printed information on a page.

The point is just now being reached where there is the computing power and language processing knowledge needed to begin to effectively tackle some of these areas. While some of this specialized cognitive processing may not be appropriate for mainstream devices, approaches like pluggable user interfaces may allow users to carry cognitive orthoses with them.

In the meantime, there is much that can be done to mainstream products to make them easier for people with cognitive language and learning disabilities to use and make them easier to use by everyone else as well.

17.4.6 Setting priorities

The suggestion overall therefore is to focus on what is important to people with the full range of disabilities and order one's list in that order – rather than cost or difficulty. Then work from the top doing what can be done and looking for opportunities where "difficult or expensive" solutions become possible due to other events or discoveries.

Ordering options by difficulty often results in unimportant or even useless (by themselves) features being added (e.g., only half of the provisions needed for access for each disability are included, resulting in a product no one can use).

It is also important to remember that what is a usability feature for one, may be required for another to be able to use a product, process, or service.

17.5 Discussion questions

1. How does an individual's environment influence disability? Does this remain constant across different environments? Why or why not?
2. What basic needs has the Trace Center identified to achieve optimal device usability?
3. What is the impact of implementing universal design?

4. For which devices would you prioritize certain features over others? Why did you prioritize them in that manner?
5. How does feature prioritization change for different populations?
6. How can one device meet the needs of different populations and obtain optimal functioning?

Bibliography

Broetz, Doris, Christoph Braun, Cornelia Weber, Surjo R. Soekadar, Andrea Caria, and Niels Birbaumer. 2010. "Combination of Brain-Computer Interface Training and Goal-Directed Physical Therapy in Chronic Stroke: A Case Report." *Neurorehabilitation and Neural Repair* 24 (7): 674–679.

Deafblind.com. "The Braille Page." Accessed 4/23, 2018, http://www.deafblind.com/braille.html.

Jordan, J. Bern and Gregg C. Vanderheiden. 2017. *Towards Accessible Automatically Generated Interfaces Part 1: An Input Model that Bridges the Needs of Users and Product Functionality.* Springer.

Nyamcenterforhistory.org. "Pieter Adriaanszoon Verduyn I Books, Health and History." Last modified 2018, accessed 4/30, 2018.

Rayegani, S. M., S. A. Raeissadat, L. Sedighipour, I. Mohammad Rezazadeh, M. H. Bahrami, D. Eliaspour, and S. Khosrawi. 2014. "Effect of Neurofeedback and Electromyographic-Biofeedback Therapy on Improving Hand Function in Stroke Patients." *Topics in Stroke Rehabilitation* 21 (2): 137–151.

Shindo, Keiichiro, Kimiko Kawashima, Junichi Ushiba, Naoki Ota, Mari Ito, Tetsuo Ota, Akio Kimura, and Meigen Liu. 2011. "Effects of Neurofeedback Training with an Electroencephalogram-Based Brain–Computer Interface for Hand Paralysis in Patients with Chronic Stroke: A Preliminary Case Series Study." *Journal of Rehabilitation Medicine* 43 (10): 951–957.

Steinmetz, Erika. 2006. *Americans with Disabilities, 2002.* US Department of Commerce, Economics and Statistics Administration.

Wobbrock, Jacob O., Krzysztof Z. Gajos, Shaun K. Kane, and Gregg C. Vanderheiden. 2018. "Ability-Based Design." *Communications of the ACM* 61 (6): 62–71.

Chapter 18 AAC in the 21st century

The outcome of technology: Advancements and amended societal attitudes

H. Shane, J. Costello, J. Seale, K. Fulcher-Rood, K. Caves, J. Buxton, E. Rose, R. McCarthy, and J. Higginbotham

Contents

DOI: 10.1201/b21964-21

18.1 Chapter overview

Wikipedia (2017) defines augmentative and alternative communication (AAC) as follows:

> the communication methods used to supplement or replace speech or writing for those with impairments in the production or comprehension of spoken or written language. AAC is used by individuals across a wide range of significant speech, language and motoric impairments and across the lifespan.

This chapter will overview this unique rehabilitation approach that in only a few decades has provided efficient and inventive ways for many of the most disabled people on the planet to better understand and to be understood. In particular, the chapter will discuss the historical, research, and technological aspects of AAC and their relevance to the clinical practice of rehabilitation engineers (RE).

18.1.1 Social history

Imagine a world in which its inhabitants are almost motionless or wander aimlessly in restricted, barren spaces unable to express ailments or pain, request assistance, talk about feelings, or simply ask for things they want or need. In this bizarre setting, their helplessness stems from one or several factors, including an intellectual challenge, impoverished language models, or idle and unattended muscles that are not able to control movement or speech. Overseers, known as caretakers, aids, or attendants, police almost every aspect of their existence. While this backdrop might be fitting for an inspired horror movie, it regrettably portrays the conditions endured by countless people who resided in state-sponsored institutions that spanned the United States and other parts of the world throughout most of the 20th century. The inhabitants were adults who aged here or babies and children abandoned by unwitting parents who acquiesced to a prevailing attitude that out-of-sight and out-of-mind was best for their family and society at large. Institutionalization was essentially a life sentence, although no crime had been committed.

Now, imagine a world where people of all ages who evidence these same conditions can express themselves, access information from the internet, move across a room, or traverse the country – to live more independently. The remarkable shift from institutional to community life was the result of a perfect storm where a growing humane and progressive attitude met advancing technologies head-on, and the result transformed the lives of countless people living with a disabling condition. For the first time in human history, persons with significant communication disorders stemming from congenital conditions such as cerebral palsy were not just put away and forgotten but became the beneficiaries of life-changing innovations. Similarly, persons with acquired conditions such as brain injury or amyotrophic lateral sclerosis (ALS) also profited from this technological renaissance.

With deinstitutionalization came the indisputable certainty that technology could improve the communication ability of those with congenital as well as acquired conditions. This led to the need for a new breed of professionals who aimed to not only improve or restore function, but also invent "machines" and interfaces that could augment (or replace) biological speech, voice, and language mechanisms. The emergent reality of such man-machine connectivity spawned the engineering specialty that became known as rehabilitation engineering.

The early history of communication devices is mainly a chronicle of equipment built by engineers – some seasoned and some students – who were inspired by a person with much to say and little means of expressing it – at least independently. These projects were often focused on persons with cerebral palsy who had strong language abilities but restricted speech and movement. For example, in the late 1960s, the Communicator was designed by this chapter author, Shane, and constructed by electrical engineering students at the University of Massachusetts. Haig Kafafian (1973, 1974) of Washington, DC-based Cybernetics Research Institute received a 1974 patent for the Cybertype, a communication system that drove a typewriter without requiring the specificity of movement generally needed to create text. Richard Foulds (1972), an engineering student at Tufts University, built the Tufts Interactive Communicator (TIC), and at the same time, Gregg Vanderheiden at the University of Wisconsin designed the Autocom. When ALS struck a family member, Walt Waltosz, an aeronautical engineer, created a computer-based communication system controlled by a single movement. Recognizing the importance of that inventive work, Waltosz went on to establish Words +, a commercial company mainly serving those with ALS. Bruce Baker, a linguist, had an extraordinary idea called Minspeak and worked with Barry Romich, an engineering student at Case Western Reserve, who earlier had founded a commercial communication company, Prentke-Romich, based on a student communication project. Minspeak was a departure from traditional spelling and symbol construction based on traditional English syntax that could only become a reality because of the evolving power and flexibility of computers.

The technology revolution was the genesis of inventive communication options never before available, and as the technologies expanded in functionality, so too did the feature set that led to the inclusion of more people with extraordinary communication needs. With respect to communication technology, it was indeed fortuitous that the confluence of deinstitutionalization and the advent of the personal computer led to the creation of a multitude of communication breakthroughs for society's most disabled citizens.

18.2 Research

Research and development (R&D) in AAC has been conducted for over 60 years, first with anecdotal and individual case studies (as noted earlier), models of augmented communication, and small group observational investigations. As a field, most research studies during this time have been applied, that is, focused on finding solutions for the significant problems found in the field, with a significant portion of the work directed to developing and assessing AAC technologies. Systematic progress in the AAC field has been challenging due to the historically low number of researchers (with technical and clinical backgrounds) versus the large problem space that these researchers have had to address (e.g., communication and interaction, literacy and education, access, internet and the web), as well as due to the diverse set of disorders underlying individual communication problems (e.g., cerebral palsy, autism, ALS, aphasia, head injury). As a consequence, the production of high-quality studies focused on specific problems has been sparse. As many published systematic reviews have pointed out, clear results are often mitigated by substantial differences in research methods and diversity of participant groups. In this section, three areas of AAC research and development will be presented, including AAC access, interfaces and devices, and social interaction This will be followed by a short discussion on the implication of research results for the practicing rehabilitation engineer in the AAC field.

18.2.1 AAC access research: Efficiency and production rates

Most models of AAC in the 20th century were based on the information-theory/sender-receiver model, which focused on the linguistic information characteristics of communication (Coleman et al., 1980).

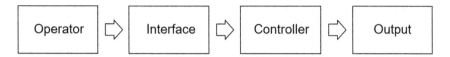

Figure 18.1 Sender-receiver model of communication (adapted from Coleman et al., 1980).

As shown in Figure 18.1, the model is decomposable into several parts: the operator, interface, controller, and output, allowing quantitative assessment of communication efficiency, measured in terms of switch selection and keystroke savings. Further, output production rates can be determined by comparing the physical actions of the operator given the access interface and controller against the information output of the device (D. J. Higginbotham, 1992; Koester & Arthanat, 2018). Later versions of this model included the communication partner as well as being adapted for multiple communication modes.

Early work in the access area established the basic switch, switch mount systems and positioning and access protocols used for the last 30 years, with more recent work focusing on mobile technology access strategies and self-adaptive access systems (e.g., Koester). Higginbotham (1992) analyzed the keystroke savings of several contemporary text-based AAC systems, finding that these technologies varied significantly, with the best achieving keystroke savings of approximately 40–50%, which is still accurate for contemporary AAC systems (D. J. Higginbotham et al., 2012). Surprisingly, cognitive demands due to display complexity, task, and interaction demands appear to diminish many of the potential benefits of technology advances (D. J. Higginbotham et al., 2007, 2012).

18.2.2 Access

Lesher et al. (1998) evaluated the switch savings of 14 different scanning* configurations and character/word prediction algorithms across a number of test texts. They found significant (34%) savings of time, using a frequency arranged alphabet matrix with additional increases (up to 39%) using character and word prediction. Needless to say, deviations from alphabetic or QWERTY organizations must be learned, and any dynamic component (prediction, dynamic keyboard) provides additional cognitive loads during use. Examples of alphabetic and time-optimized scanning arrays are shown in Figure 18.2.

In a recent systematic review of seven text interfaces (Koester & Arthanat, 2018), automatic speech recognition, standard on-screen keyboard (OSK), cursor OSK,

---

* Scanning is a historically important access strategy in AAC. Essentially, it refers to the control (i.e., start, stop, direction) of an indicator (cursor) that enables a person with limited movement to point out the location of desired content in the form of letters, words, symbols, and so on.

A	B	C	D	Sp	.	-
E	F	G	H	,	"	'
I	J	K	L	M	N	(
O	P	Q	R	S	T	,
U	V	W	X	Y	Z	;
Sh	Ret	0	1	2	3	4
Bk	:	5	6	7	8	9

Sp	E	A	R	D	F	V
T	O	N	L	G	K	J
I	S	U	Y	B	X	Z
H	C	P	Q	'	0	2
M	W	,	"	1	3	4
Sh	.	-	9	5	6	7
Bk	Ret	:	8	(	)	;

Figure 18.2 Scanning arrays. (a) Alphabetic scanning array. (b) Frequency and time-optimized scanning array.

and scanning OSK, based on more than 30 reviewed studies apiece, produced a text entry rate averaging 15.4, 12.5, 4.2, and 1.7 words per minute (WPM), respectively. Morse code and brain-computer interface (BCI) results, based on less than four studies apiece, showed text entry rates at 12.5 (2-switch Morse), 5.0 (1-switch Morse), and 0.7 (ASR) WPM. Using automated data logging, Smith et al. (2006) analyzed the communication output of seven individuals using direct-selection AAC devices during daily living activities. Production rates averaged seven WPM but varied considerably depending on the type of interface (text versus icon) and the manual dexterity and typing experience. Using advanced language models, Roark, Fried-Oken, and Gibbons (2015) demonstrated production rates for BCI substantially higher than previously reported research, averaging five WPM for 16 non-impaired participants and two WPM for one individual with locked-in syndrome.

Despite the potential advantages afforded by AAC technology, the cognitive and social interaction demands related to device use significantly shape the potential usefulness of specific AAC features. Simulation by Koester and Levine (1996) found that the time needed to visually scan a word prediction display effectively mitigates whatever potential speed advantages offered by word prediction. Higginbotham and Wilkins (1999) found a three-fold increase for one augmented speaker using a word and letter board (19 WPM) versus a computer-based word predictor, due largely to the time needed to review the prediction list and delays in the dynamic display screen updates.

Higginbotham et al. (2009) studied a group of non-impaired adults using advanced word prediction systems across several different communication tasks. Communication speeds were significantly impacted by differences in task demands (high versus low social interaction demands), but not the sophistication of the word prediction system. Moreover, there was a 15% reduction in keystroke savings between participants' actual AAC use compared with a reanalysis of the same text output performed in optimal conditions. That is, participants frequently ignored the prediction list while typing.

18.2.3 Interaction in time with technology

Early research in the area of AAC and social interaction focused on documenting the interaction patterns of AAC users using low-tech systems, finding that their utterances are often collaboratively constructed – a letter or word at a time – with the communication partner repeating or rephrasing the AAC user's selection (Buzolich & Wiemann, 1988; D. J. Higginbotham, 1989; Light et al., 1985). Many AAC users were also found to be responsive, rather than initiative in their interactions, with communication partners exerting a disproportionate amount of control in the interactions (D. R. Beukelman & Yorkston, 1982; Farrier et al., 1985). Starting in the mid-1980s, research began to focus on evaluating the impact of new technologies on perception, comprehension, and interaction. Lower quality speech synthesis was found to detrimentally impact the intelligibility and comprehension of the spoken message (K. Drager & Reichle, 2001; D. J. Higginbotham et al., 1994; Kim, 2001). Furthermore, the coding and symbolic interfaces used in new high-tech systems differentially impacted learning and interaction (Light et al., 1990). A series of studies by John Todman and colleagues (Todman, 2000; Todman et al., 2008) explored the use of utterance-based systems that allowed AAC users to produce utterances at speeds approximating 50 WPM or better. Todman (2000) found that AAC users and their partners demonstrated a marked preference for this faster AAC approach. Some of these advances have since found their way into the InterAACT system, available from the Tobii Dynavox company (DynaVox InterAACt, n.d.).

Recently, researchers have begun to explore how the AAC user and their conversational partners collaborate through, with, and around AAC technology in order to successfully interact with one another. Higginbotham and Wilkins (1999) examined the role of social time constraints on social interaction. Research by Bloch and Wilkinson (2004) identified the "Out of Context Problem" that results when the communication time to complete an utterance is so delayed that the augmented speaker's interactants forget. Wilkinson, Bloch, and Clarke (2011) have explored the ways in which materials in the communication context are involved in an interaction. Recent research has also focused on improving utterance intelligibility and interaction through a variety of multimodal supplementation strategies (Hanson et al., 2013); the use of visual scenes (D. R. Beukelman et al., 2015; McKelvey et al., 2010); and semantic-pragmatic frame-based AAC systems (D. J. Higginbotham & Wilkins, 2006; McCoy et al., 2011; Todman et al., 2008). This work has led to the recognition that AAC-mediated interaction occurs in time, is heavily multimodal (speech, intonation, gestures, body movement, object in the environment), contextually framed, and occurs for a purpose.

Specific properties of different communication technologies (phone, video chat, texting, email, AAC device) have a powerful shaping effect in that they communicate, depending on their interaction requirements (e.g., face-to-face, voice only, text; permanence of message, immediate or delayed response; Chapanis et al., 1972; Clark et al., 1991; D. J. Higginbotham & Caves, 2002). Higginbotham et al. (2016) propose three timeframes in which augmented speakers and their partners interact that significantly impact device use and communication success. Most augmented speakers and their partners prefer interacting in Now-Time, by producing immediately responsive expressions through speech, vocalizations, and gestures. Currently, most AAC devices do not support Now-Time communications and, in fact, impede it by requiring extended typing sequences to produce any word or utterance. Near-Time expressions can be accomplished with well-designed AAC systems that allow individuals to express themselves with one or two selections. Delayed-Time communications refer to utterance compositions that take many seconds and sometimes up to several minutes to produce. These Delayed-Time communications can result in frequent misunderstandings due to the communication partner's lapses in attention, forgetfulness, and distractibility. Delayed-Time utterances are often constructed letter-by-letter, word-by-word over the course of minutes. Higginbotham et al. (2016) recommend several ways in which technologies can be improved including alternative or amplified views expressive gestures, rapid access to pragmatically useful phrases, quick access to one's communication history, and shared communication interfaces. Pullin, Trevaranus, Patel, and Higginbotham (2017) discuss the implications of AAC design on identity, social interaction, and inclusion.

18.2.4 Integrating research findings into practice: Responsibilities of the rehabilitation engineer

As a rehabilitation engineer, tasks in the AAC field may involve recommending, installing, fitting, and maintaining AAC devices. Being knowledgeable about current R&D in the field is essential to ethical and competent outcomes. We offer several suggestions for the practicing rehabilitation engineer.

- Rely on high-quality evidence whenever possible. This includes the use of clinical practice guidelines, systematic reviews, and meta-analyses published by scientific and professional associations such as the American Speech-Language and Hearing Association (ASHA), the Rehabilitation Engineering Society of North America (RESNA), and the Occupational Therapy Associations within specific countries (e.g., AOTA in the United States and CAOT in Canada). Systematic reviews can also be found in the Campbell Collaborations (n.d.), as well as PubMed (n.d.).
- Study/consider the investigative quality of the article. For example, the scoping review of speech supplementation strategies by Hanson et al. (2013) excludes large numbers of randomized treatment experiments but provides a careful analysis of available evidence from the field. Make certain the study adequately examines the data in ways relevant to your needs.
- In applying research information to your practice, reflect on your personal investment and possible biases, so that you are serving the best interest of the client. To this end, The Oxford Center for Evidence-Based Medicine (www.cebm.net/ocebm-levels-of-evidence/) provides current information on evaluating research study quality. They also offer practical guidelines to help practitioners make decisions based on available evidence. These include:
- Is your client sufficiently similar to the participants in the research study?
- Does the recommended behavioral or technology intervention have clinically relevant benefits that outweigh its drawbacks?
- Given your client's values and circumstances, may another approach be more appropriate?
- Are you actually asking the right question?

18.3 Synthetic speech

The development of computer-generated speech or synthetic text-to-speech, approximating the clarity and richness of the authentic human voice, has been a goal of developers since the early 20th century. The VODER (Voice Operated Demonstrator), produced in 1939 by Homer Dudley, was the first device that could electronically transduce key presses into continuous human speech (Dudley et al., 1939). Even before that, as far back as the second half of the 18th century, efforts were made to mechanically create human speech sounds (Von Kempelen, 1791). Yet, it was the innovations of computer technology in the 1970s that ushered in commercial text-to-speech and speech synthesis products (Klaat, 1987).

The most important qualities of a speech synthesis system are naturalness and intelligibility (Taylor, 2009). While the early electronic speech synthesis was robotic and frequently barely intelligible, contemporary speech synthesis much more closely approximates the sound and clarity of natural speech. Despite this, speech synthesis continues to remain distinguishable from authentic human speech.

The first commercial application of speech synthesis technologies included Texas Instruments' Speak 'n Spell toy in the late 1970s, and Kurzweil Reader, the first text-to-speech reader for the blind in 1976. During the early 1980s, there were lower-cost versions of commercial synthesizers, such as the Echo, using an algorithm developed by the Naval Research Labs (Morris, 1979), and the Votrax Type 'n Talk (Gagnon, 1978). Notably, the Votrax Type 'n Talk censored language by replacing the spoken output of curse words, with *sanitized* language. While these synthetic speech options were more affordable for the augmentative communication market, their intelligibility was quite poor and highly robotic in nature.

In 1979, Allen, Hunnicut, and Klatt introduced the MITalk (pronounced "MY Talk"), a project that influenced the theory and practice of speech synthesis by converting English text-to-speech signals (Karjalainen, 1988; Klaat, 1987). Dennis Klatt continued to improve the source code and in 1982 introduced the Klattalk software, which was then licensed to the Digital Equipment Corporation (DEC) and commercialized as DECtalk in 1983. DECtalk was the first commercially available speech synthesis technology to provide multiple voice options across gender and age. With continued improvements in the technology, DECtalk was able to provide gender and age-matched voices to people with disability who rejected a voice that did not match their identity. Similarly, research studying of effects of synthesized speech intelligibility showed DecTalk to be more intelligible, comprehensible, and preferred to other speech synthesizers available in the late 20th century (K. D. Drager et al., 2010; K. Drager & Reichle, 2001; Gorernflo et al., 1994; D. J. Higginbotham et al., 1994).

Realizing Klatt's vision for special applications of DECTalk, in 1991, DEC established a partnership with the Institute of Applied Technology at Children's Hospital Boston to develop and distribute the MultiVoice, the first speech synthesizer developed expressly for persons with disabilities using the high-quality DECtalk speech (H. C. Shane, personal communication, 2017), which was prominently featured in the "Information Age: People, Information and Technology" interactive exhibit at the Smithsonian Institution in Washington, DC (Mergen, 1992).

Since the introduction of DECTalk speech, there has been an eruption of speech synthesis options, offered in dozens of languages with many options for gender and age. Voices have been created by companies worldwide including ATT Natural Voices, Ivono, Cepstral, Loquendo, and Acapela. Much like DECTalk's "Perfect Paul" voice being engineered using a voice sampling of Dennis Klatt's own voice recordings (*Klatt's Last Tapes: A History of Speech Synthesizers*

Video, 2013), these new synthesis options have at their foundation voice actors who, in a controlled sound studio environment, record a large script. This script is developed to represent a complete sampling of co-articulated speech sounds of the language. Some of these synthetic voices are standard options with specific augmentative communication speech generating devices (SGD), while a different SGD technology may offer a different selection of voices. This variability in default voice options in SGDs is likely related both to the cost of licensing agreement with the voice company as well as the linguistic and age demographic of voices provided by the specific SGD manufacturer. For example, a manufacturer with a product marketed to a pediatric population is more likely to license voices from a company that offers child voices as well as adult voices, supporting the end user to have a voice that matures along with them through the ages.

Perhaps there is no clearer demonstration of the intelligibility of current speech synthesis than the successful control of voice recognition technologies used for home automation through synthetic speech commands (Medcalf, 2017). Popular voice-controlled devices such as the Amazon Alexa Echo system or Google Home voice control can be used to activate music, make web-based phone calls, and control integrated home automation. They can be activated with synthetic speech commands from many speech synthesizers. Much like the naturally spoken command with the human voice, failed recognition is often due to the rate of speech and pause time between the activation word and the command.

18.3.1 Speech synthesis and personal identity

As intelligibility and naturalness of speech synthesis have continued to improve, R&D has shifted to the personalization of voice and the impact on the communication and comprehension of intent with one's personal voice (D. J. Higginbotham, 2010). In his work focused on capturing and preserving banked messages of people at risk of losing the ability to speak (Message Banking), Costello (2017) suggested that one's voice is an acoustical fingerprint. He asks:

> How many times have you heard someone say "It is so good to hear your voice!"? Through authentic voice, we are able to provide comfort, establish personal connection and bring the spectrum of emotions to people around us through our voice and our unique intonation, prosody and passion.

Portnuff, an augmented speaker with ALS asserted, "I want to be able to be sensitive or arrogant, assertive or humble, angry or happy, sarcastic or sincere, matter of fact or suggestive and sexy" (Portnuff, 2006).

The capability to express emotion and tone easily and in the moment with synthetic speech remains difficult to date, although companies such as Loquendo do offer voices that can be manipulated to reflect emotion. As indicated by

439

Pullin (2015) "Tone of voice is such an elusive and intangible quality: difficult for even phoneticians to define, let alone AAC users and carers to discuss in the context of their everyday lives." Some AAC technologies, such as Predictable (*Therapy Box*, 2017), allow the user to mark their message with emotional intent by creating emotion "tags" that produce a sound such as laughter, throat clearing, sobbing, and so on when placed at the end of a typed-out message. A recent article by Euphony Inc. reflected on the economic benefit for industry creating emotive synthetic speech (Euphony Inc., 2017). They report "In many cases, emotive synthetic voice is a better alternative than hiring voice actors or using audio banks, because it allows quick, cost-effective changes and the ability to overlay emotion on a voice." Recent research by Székely et al. (2011, 2012, 2014) has demonstrated ways of generating low-cost emotive voices and explored ways of triggering appropriate emotive expressions triggered by facial expressions. While currently in a pre-commercial research phase, the hope is that corporate investment in emotive synthetic speech will ultimately benefit people with severe speech impairments who rely on speech-generating devices to be their voices and spoken identity.

18.3.2 Voice banking

Voice banking is a process by which a person who is at risk of losing the ability to speak due to motor neuron disease, laryngectomy, or other medical conditions or interventions may create a personal synthetic voice. There are multiple options to create a personal voice including ModelTalker (*Model Talker*, 2017), Acapela My Own Voice (Acaplea Group, 2017), CereProc Voice Me (CereProc, 2017), and VocalID Vocal Legacy (*VocalID*, 2017). From the consumer's perspective, a major difference in these approaches relates to recording effort and time, cost, and quality. In terms of recording time, most require the speaker to enroll in an online recording process requiring the production of up to 1600 sentences to produce a synthesized voice. VocalID also offers a different service called BeSpoke Voice (*VocalID*, 2017), whereby a personalized digital voice is created using several seconds of the recipient's vocalization and combined with a voice model selected from a voicebank of several thousand voices (Mills et al., 2014). Currently, costs for developing a personalized voice range from US$100 (ModelTalker) to approximately US$2400 to record and engineer the synthetic voice. An additional distinguishing feature is that some services will create the voice and the consumer may then choose to purchase it after assessing the quality while others require payment prior to creating and premiering the voice.

Testimony to the rapid progress in speech synthesis development, at the time of this writing, Acapela announced Acapela Deep Neural Network (DNN), which will allow for custom voice creation with an average of 10–15 minutes of clean audio recordings and the associated text transcription of the audio samples. In addition, for persons at risk of losing their ability to speak and who have participated in message banking and have at least 30 minutes of high-quality recordings, those authentic messages may be used to "double dip," and create an Acapela DNN synthetic voice from those messages while also having the authentic messages recorded with emotion and intonation also available in the speech-generating device.

18.4 Alternative access technologies for AAC

The purpose of this section is to explore augmentative and alternative communication (AAC) strategies and the spectrum of technologies used to support aided communication. Just as we determine "what" low-, mid-, or high-tech system or systems a person will use to augment communication, "how" a person *accesses* or interacts with a device must also be addressed. *Alternative access technologies* allow a person to interact with assistive technology, which in turn enables greater participation and independence in mobility, communication, recreation, leisure, vocational, and activities of daily living (ADLs).

18.4.1 Access defined

A human–computer interaction includes an array of access tools such as mice, keyboards, and touchscreens. Alternative access solutions provide the ability to interact with all levels of technology despite physical, cognitive, and visual limitations. Access can be divided into three components or parts:

1. *Input device.* The control interface that the user interacts with in order to connect with a device, for example, keyboards, switches, or joysticks.
2. *Symbol selection set.* The symbol system or set used to represent a choice, for example, letters, words, phrases, pictures, or symbols represented in a visual, auditory, or tactile format.
3. *Selection method.* The method by which the user makes selections using the input device. Selection methods can be divided into direct access and indirect access.
   - *Direct access.* Users may access the control interface directly using their hands, fingers, toes, light pointers, head pointers, eye point, and so on. This *direct access method* is typically faster and requires less cognitive skill but necessitates greater motor control.
   - *Indirect access.* Because of physical limitations, intermediary methods categorized as "scanning" or "encoding" are used to facilitate access.
     - Scanning: arrays of choices are systematically arranged in rows and columns and then scanned over by an auditory and/or visual

indicator. The user makes a section with their input device (e.g., switch).

- Encoding: a pre-coded display is presented and the user indicates affirmative responses in a sequence (e.g., select a number and then a color grouping to indicate an item within a particular display).

Cook and Hussey (1995) introduced the Human Activity Assistive Technology (HAAT) model in the first edition of *Assistive Technology Principles and Practice*. In the fourth edition, Cook and Polgar (2015) commented that the HAAT model "describes someone (human) doing something (activity) in a context using AT." This basic definition is worded specifically to point out that the provision of AT occurs after the person, the activity, and the context have been identified. Higginbotham, Shane, Russell, and Caves (2007) helped to contemporize the definition of AAC access to better identify it as "a collection of features and techniques that an individual can use to control an AAC system."

18.4.2 Assessment of alternative access technologies

The assessment process for determining access to a speech-generating device is a dynamic one and must account not only for the user's strengths, abilities, and limitations but also for the requirements of the task or activity and the contextual setting. A feature-matching model is utilized to identify alternative access technologies and methods that are best suited to the individual and their unique needs and limitations. Once potential access technologies are identified, systematic trials help to determine the ideal option for a particular user functioning in a specified setting and for a specific task.

People with complex communication needs (CCN) demonstrate unique physical abilities and limitations due to abnormal tone and reflexes, spasticity and variability in motor control, range of motion, and strength. These characteristics can affect the ability to produce voluntary and consistent movements. Limitations in any of these physical abilities interfere with the person achieving "consistent, reliable non-fatiguing physical access to AAC technologies" (D. J. Higginbotham et al., 2007). Assessment should consist of a holistic approach to address all aspects of the user's disability profile.

A *physical assessment* will help identify both the selection method and choice of input device and should include a consideration of the following areas when trying to identify the most effective access method:

- Controlled voluntary movement
- Fine and gross motor control
- Range of motion

- Strength
- Fatigue

Efforts to avoid the following should be taken:

- Movements that are dominated by abnormal reflex patterns
- Movements that cause a significant increase in abnormal tone, for example, total body extension (straightening and stiffening of the body)
- Movements that are abnormal movement patterns such as excessive internal rotation of the arm (i.e., the arm turned inward and wrist deviation; Cook & Polgar, 2015)

The *sensory assessment* helps determine display features including the need for visual and/or auditory feedback. Identifying the cognitive and intellectual skills of the individual will help focus decisions regarding language and literacy, memory, sequencing, and the complexity of displays and technologies.

The contextual settings in which the individual will access the technologies continue to remain important, and aspects such as mounting of the device, lighting, portability, and positioning will help to determine optimal access methods and technologies.

To ensure successful implementation of AT and AAC, the individual must be able to access their technology and often this requires mounting systems – the physical attachment of the (assistive technology device/speech generating device [ATD/SGD]) to a tabletop, wheelchair arm, or tray (Cook & Hussey, 1995).

18.4.3 Exploring alternative access technologies

The following are examples of traditional and innovative alternative access technologies.

18.4.3.1 Direct access methods   Traditional input devices should first be considered such as mice, trackpads, trackballs, and joysticks controlled by a hand, foot, or mouth. External input devices can connect to computers, mobile devices, and SGDs through Bluetooth, wires, Wi-Fi, or infrared technologies. Each of these external input devices needs to be mounted appropriately to ensure the person has consistent and reliable access.

When traditional mainstreamed interface options are not viable, alternative access technologies that interpret body movements are often pursued. The body movements and actions required to access these interfaces directly include:

- Pointing (head, hands, fingers, toes)
  - Traditionally, if the user can use their hands or fingers to point directly to a touchscreen (iPad with AAC app or SGD), this method

443

is generally adopted, as it is the most natural. For many AAC users who do not have functional use of upper extremities, feet and toes are sometimes effective means of accessing touchscreens.

- Tracking (head and eye and body parts)
  - Eye tracking: cameras mounted to the ATD/SGD emit infrared signals that bounce off the retina and can be translated into cursor movements.
  - Head tracking: through the use of a reflective dot worn on the forehead, a camera mounted to the ATD/SGD translates the user's head movements directly into cursor movements.
  - Gesture tracking: the technology also exists to use cameras to capture an algorithm of the user's face (or finger, nose, chin, etc.) and translate these body movements into cursor movements.

For all of these methods, individual selections of content are made through a pause (i.e., dwelling over a target area), blinking, smiling, or activating a switch when the cursor is located on the preferred location (item) on the screen. A wide range of SGDs now incorporates these alternative access technologies (Fager et al., 2012).

Over the past few years, integrated wheelchair control systems allow the user to use their power wheelchair drive systems (such as joysticks, pneumatic sip and puff controls, and switches) to control cursor movement. This access method is often overlooked but the reader is cautioned to consider secondary access methods for when the user is in their manual wheelchair, bed, or other positioning device (stander, gait trainer, couch, bean bag) and requires access to their ATD/SGD.

18.4.3.2 Indirect access methods Adaptive switches allow a person to activate assistive technology devices in their environment. A switch acts as an interface between the user and a computer, toy, environmental control unit, or other device. The individual uses a volitional, repeatable, suppressible, and yet intentional action to activate the switch. It allows the user to indicate a choice by the use of motor responses.

18.4.3.2.1 Switch interface options Switches may be single, double, multiple, or joystick types. A particular user may need specific levels of:

- Sensitivity
- Adjustability
- Degree of surface area
- Height
- Amount of travel
- Sensory feedback – the user must have some signal that the switch has been activated. This can be in a visual, auditory, or tactile form.

- Mounting – the switch may need to be positioned or mounted to a specific site to allow easy access for the user.

18.4.3.2.2 Switch activation methods   Switches can be made to respond to a variety of user actions including:

- Pressure difference
- Pneumatic
- Proximity
- Motion detection (mercury)
- Light sensitivity
- Sound sensitivity
- Myoelectric (muscle)
- Brain Activity

18.4.3.2.3 Scanning   Scanning is an indirect selection method in which an array of choices is presented and sequentially and systematically scanned by a cursor or light, and optionally an auditory preview or cue. The user makes a selection by activating the switch. In order to increase the efficiency of the scanning method, consideration should be made for the layout of the selection set and the frequency of targets/items used.

- Single switch scanning – the array of choices is offered automatically and the user activates the switch to indicate a choice at the correct timing that the choice is offered.
- Two switch step scanning – the user advances the cursor or scanning indicator one item group at a time. Choice selection is then made by activating a secondary switch.

18.4.4 Switch skill progression

People with CCN often present with such complex motor profiles that identifying switch access body sites can be challenging. Often, the user's abnormal tone and reflexes may impede consistent and reliable action by the user. Continued assessment and trials with a variety of switches at a variety of switch sites should be examined before a final switch site is determined. Once a switch site is determined, depending on the developmental, intellectual, and/or motor profile, activities targeted at improving switch access behaviors will allow for even greater automaticity. Once the movement pattern becomes a learned motor response, the user will be able to focus on the cognitive and language aspects of the activity. A typical switch skill progression includes cause and effect switch activities, then learning to maintain switch activation, then timing the release of the switch, and then automatic and single switch scanning (Bean, 2011).

18.4.5 The future of alternative access technologies

We now face a new demand for tools that are context-specific, user-created, data-driven, nimble, wearable, embeddable, networked, and device agnostic (Crosslan et al., 2016). Innovative alternative access technologies, which help to lessen the digital divide and allow for increased independence and participation of people with CCN (Gray et al., 2010), continue to be created as the field of rehabilitation engineering continues to grow.

- New developments in user interfaces and input options continue to be developed and are awaiting the technology transfer from the research venues to the end user. Examples include motion-capture and gesture-based gaming, such as Sony PlayStation Move and Xbox Kinect.
- BCIs: the non-invasive BCI access method relies on sensors placed in contact with the scalp and invasive BCI involves surgically placing electrodes on the motor cortex – these electrodes in both scenarios are connected to a computer that translates the brain activity to control signals.
- New developments in user interfaces and input options (e.g., touch screens, gesture recognition, brain interfaces, haptic feedback).
- Brain Sensors that can transform brain signals into human language.

18.5 Low- and mid-technology options

Low-tech AAC includes object-based, picture-based, symbol-based, and text-based communication without voice output. This may consist of objects, photographs, or picture communication symbols, a letter/word board, a communication board with many photograph/symbol options, or a multi-page communication book in which each page contains photograph/symbol options. Users can access aided non-electronic systems through a variety of techniques including direct touch, pointers, low-tech gaze, scanning, partner-assisted techniques, and so on. Photographs/symbols may be presented in a variety of formats. Figure 18.3a illustrates a few essential phrases (i.e., yes, no, and I need help) attached to a wheelchair tray for portable and immediate access. The user is able to point to or look at the symbols to answer a question or request assistance. Photographs and symbols may also be presented by a single topic display, which consists of a variety of words and phrases related to a single topic or activity, as shown in Figure 18.3b. A multi-page picture communication book provides more extensive vocabulary by flipping through the pages of a categorically organized book (see Figure 18.3c). For individuals with literacy skills, a letter board may be used to spell out partial or full words or sentences (see Figure 18.3d). All communication methods should be personalized to fit each individual's unique communication needs.

Figure 18.4 displays two word and letter boards designed by their adult users for conducting a face-to-face conversation. The first, designed by Hal F. Roe in

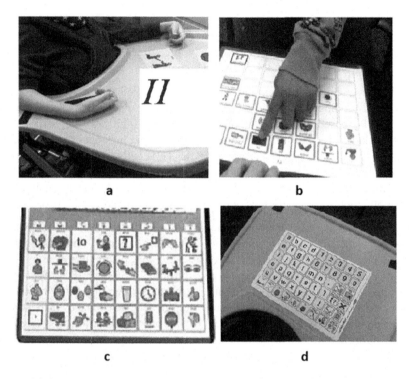

Figure 18.3 Examples of low-tech-AAC systems. (a) Wheelchair tray with symbols for essential messages ("yes, no," and "I need help"). (b) Topic display board – which provides several vocabulary words associated with a single activity or subject. (c) Example of a Flip 'n Talk communication book. (d) Letter cueing board.

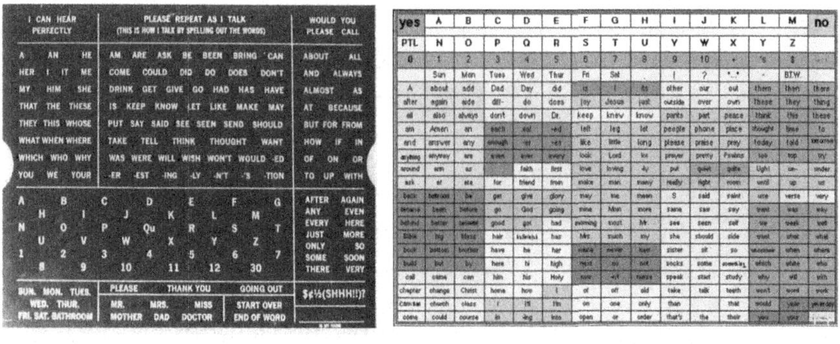

Figure 18.4 Word and letter boards.

the late 1940s and early 1950s, contains many strategic features for competent communication. The second device was used by its owner to reliably produce utterances at over 20 WPM, approximately three times faster than her use of her high-tech word prediction device (D. J. Higginbotham & Wilkins, 1999).

Mid-tech AAC includes communication aids that are electronic but are typically not overtly computer based. They consist of single or sequenced message devices and overlay-based digitized speech output devices. Digitized voice output typically includes premade phrases, music, words, or other messages that are directly recorded and then played back when the device is activated. Through digitized speech output, mid-tech AAC provides increased multi-sensory feedback for learning and applying language. Speech output can also be used to gain someone's attention across a distance or convey messages to multiple individuals.

A *single message device* produces a single digitized message upon activation. It may be located near the communicator (e.g., on a desk), transported by the communicator to different locations, or placed within the environment in which the messages would typically be used, as illustrated in Figure 18.5a. *Sequenced message devices* consist of a single button but can be programmed to play a series of recorded messages. Each time the user activates the device face, the next message plays. In this way, users can access many messages (e.g., different greetings while walking down a hallway at school), have back-and-forth conversations, and participate in other multi-utterance situations, such as telling a story or a joke (Figure 18.5b).

An *overlay-based voice output device* consists of replaceable static overlays, each comprised of multiple messages that can be individually accessed. By manually inserting a different pre-programmed overlay, the device can be repurposed for a different communication task (e.g., game, going to the store) or for a different

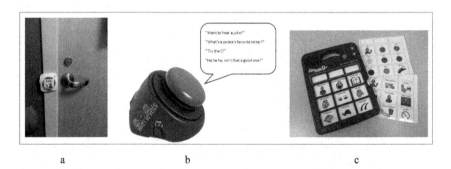

a   b   c

Figure 18.5 Examples of mid-Tech AAC devices. (a) Single message system. (b) Sequenced/multiple message device (LITTLE Step-by-Step Communicator). (c) Overlay-based device (The GoTalk 9+).

individual. These devices vary by manufacturer, though most permit recordings of several overlays saved on different "levels" of the device (Figure 18.5c).

18.5.1 Benefits and limitations of low-tech and mid-tech AAC

Low-tech and mid-tech AAC offer several benefits. These systems may be more immediately available and ready to implement, as some may only require a printer or a collection of objects to construct the device. They also require less technical expertise and are significantly less expensive than high-tech communication devices. Low-tech systems may be more portable and may be a better match for specific environments (e.g., the use of a communication board at the pool as opposed to an electronic device). Furthermore, low- and mid-tech systems may offer a tool for fundamental communication skill development that can translate to more robust future communication abilities.

Low-tech and mid-tech AAC also possess several significant limitations. First, low-tech AAC produces no audible output, therefore it cannot be used to secure or maintain a partner's attention through sound. Second, these systems lack an extensive vocabulary, and accessing prepared extended vocabulary may be slow and cumbersome (e.g., flipping through multiple pages of a book to locate a word, changing a device overlay). Third, the creation and maintenance of these systems can also be labor intensive and time consuming, as vocabulary may need to be updated on a regular basis by the supporting practitioner. Specialized software, such as Boardmaker, is often required to select picture communication symbols for use on these systems. Finally, some evidence suggests that some AAC users, their families, their educational/vocational support teams, and the community strategies do not value low and mid-tech AAC compared with high-tech AAC systems (Romski & Sevcik, 2005). Ultimately, an individual's unique skills and needs must be carefully considered when determining the tools and strategies to support a total communication approach.

18.6 High-technology communication options

High-technology AAC devices (high-tech AAC) consist of a diverse group of computerized options for individuals with AAC needs, including dedicated systems, computer applications, specialized accessories, and mobile technologies. With high-tech AAC, individuals can store large amounts of content (e.g., words, phrases, stories, songs, videos) for display and output via synthesized speech. In addition, some high-tech AAC can provide environmental controls (e.g., turn on lights, change the TV channel, answer the phone), as well as access to the internet and computer applications (e.g., games, web browsers, word processors).

449

High-tech AAC also affords individuals with complex physical needs a variety of sophisticated uni- and multimodal access options, including scanning, head pointing, eye gaze, and pen and gesture recognition.

18.6.1 Types of high-tech AAC

High-tech AAC can be divided into three general types of technology: *dedicated*, *non-dedicated*, and *mobile*. Although similar (both utilize dynamic touch-responsive display screens, digitized and synthesized speech output, etc.), dedicated and mobile high-tech AAC differ from each other in some important ways. Dedicated high-tech AAC is manufactured specifically for AAC purposes and support spoken or typed communication output but restrict access to the internet and other computer features. Once purchased, dedicated high-tech AAC can be "unlocked" for internet and application access by paying an additional fee to the manufacturer. Prices for dedicated high-tech AAC usually range between US$6000 and US$12000, and in the United States are frequently approved for purchase by insurance companies, Medicaid and Medicare. Non-dedicated high-tech AAC consists of computer applications and peripheral devices that can be used with standard desktop and laptop computer systems. These include, but are not limited to, word prediction software with speech synthesis options, symbol-based communication software, and head and eye-tracking hardware peripherals. Non-dedicated high-tech AAC can provide a lower-cost alternative to dedicated high-tech AAC and can be tailored for specific purposes and locations. However, non-dedicated high-tech AAC often lacks personal manufacturer support, which is important for setting up and troubleshooting.

Unlike dedicated AAC, mobile, high-tech AAC (i.e., cell phones, tablets) can provide a plethora of applications for web browsing, email, texting, social networking, word processing, and so on. Mobile high-tech AAC provides an attractive alternative to dedicated high-tech AAC because of its low cost (< US$1000), size and weight, availability of education, and productivity and entertainment software, as well as being indistinguishable from any other mobile technology used by one's peers. As noted in the next section, these differences have significantly altered the AAC industry as well as service delivery. The following sections are a description of the features and options available for most high-tech AAC.

18.6.2 Display options

Literate individuals are often successful at using on-screen QWERTY, or alphanumeric keyboards (Figure 18.6a,b). Spelling communication techniques afford individuals with significant vocabulary possibilities, limited only by the individual's spelling knowledge and/or prediction dictionary. In addition to literacy, this method of communication requires intact cognitive-linguistic skills. For individuals who spell messages letter-by-letter, most high-tech AAC options offer

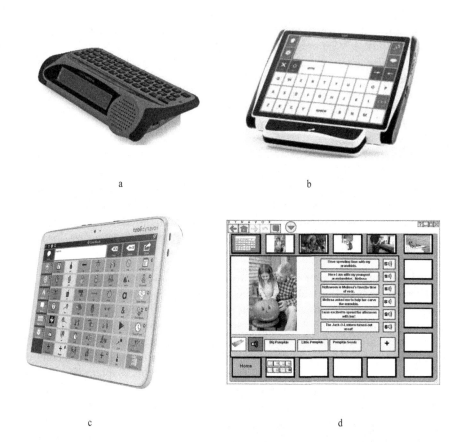

Figure 18.6 Examples of high-tech AAC devices. (a) Lightwriter portable communication device. (b) Tobii-C15 Communication aid (with eyEtracking). (c) Tobbi Dynavox Indi with Communicator 5 software. (d) Visual Scenes Display.

word prediction features, which aim to reduce keystrokes for AAC users (Trnka et al., 2009). Letter-by-letter message communicators also benefit from a means for saving and retrieving texts (e.g., announcement, joke, presentation, story, vital information) that can be used later, thereby saving on typing time and effort.

Other individuals with complex communication needs who have impaired literacy and/or cognitive-linguistic skills (e.g., aphasia) may use graphic symbols for language access. Many high-tech AAC displays are organized in a traditional grid display, with individual icons, words, and/or phrases arranged in a series of squares, spaced evenly in a grid (Figure 18.6c).

In contrast to the traditional grid display, visual scenes display (VSD) represents another visual display approach that can reduce the cognitive-linguistic load for individuals who have difficulty using traditional grid layouts (D. R. Beukelman

451

et al., 2015; D. J. Higginbotham et al., 2007; K. M. Wilkinson et al., 2012; Figure 18.6d). A VSD uses highly relevant, contextualized pictures to represent a specific event/activity and related vocabulary. Research has shown that VSD systems can benefit both young children during the early phases of language and interaction development, as well as individuals with aphasia and closed head injury who may struggle with the abstract symbols of current AAC devices (D. R. Beukelman et al., 2015; Light & Drager, 2007).

18.6.3 Physical access options

To control and interact with high-tech AAC devices, individuals can make device selections through touch, eye, and head movements, as well as using a switch attached to the device. Both dedicated and mobile high-tech AAC can provide a variety of built-in adjustments to optimize direct and indirect access for individual use.

Head tracking allows an individual to operate the screen cursor to access an on-screen keyboard or make selections on an AAC application. Similar to head tracking, eye tracking uses eye movements to control the device's screen cursor. Both forms of high-tech AAC utilize an infrared camera to track an individual's head or eye movements (Fitzgerald et al., 2009; D. J. Higginbotham et al., 2007). Individuals may also use scanning to operate their high-tech AAC, a technique that was covered in the research and access sections of this chapter.

18.7 Service delivery

Changes in societal attitudes (embodied in legislation and activist movements) and technological advancements have dramatically shaped service delivery models in AAC. Historically, models of service delivery were based on current trends in the field (e.g., behavior modification, language and cognitive development), each approach emphasizing different areas of expressive communication and placing restrictions with respect to candidacy for AAC services. Thankfully, candidacy restrictions gave way to more inclusive ways of thinking, and as a part of current best AAC practice, there are no clinical prerequisites for an individual to receive AAC services and products (D. Beukelman & Mirenda, 2013).

18.7.1 Participation and feature matching models

18.7.1.1 Participation model Currently, two complementary models of assessment and service delivery are considered to be best practice. They are the participation model and the feature matching model. The participation model focuses on providing the individual with access to relevant language and communication

452

to successfully engage in activities important for daily living and social participation (i.e., accomplishing school, work, leisure; D. Beukelman & Mirenda, 2013; Blackstone et al., 2007). To perform an evaluation, the practitioner first determines the individual's personal and social communication needs, their current natural communication skills, their ability to use AAC technologies, and the current supports, barriers, and potential opportunities for successful social participation. As can be seen in Figure 18.7, a number of specific assessments are typically conducted, some focusing on the individual's potential and barriers to accessing AAC technology given their current abilities, as well as determining what external circumstances (institutional policy, as well as practitioner practice, skill, knowledge, and attitude) enhance or impede communication performance. Based on this information, the practitioner (and team) plan immediate and long-term AAC interventions. The outcome, or success, of the implementation of this model is contingent on evaluating the individual's participation patterns (i.e., are they participating more) after implementing AAC treatment.

18.7.1.2 Feature matching model   Imagine a room filled with the latest and most effective low-, mid-, and high-tech devices along with a growing collection of peripherals such as symbol sets, switches, mounting hardware, and so on. This assembly of products in the hands of informed clinicians has the potential to enhance the communication capability of those who are non-speaking. The availability of this body of equipment, however, is no guarantee that the appropriate equipment will be selected for a particular candidate. Moreover, as the volume of technology and related peripherals multiplies so too does the complexity of assigning which device, display, symbol set, and so on is best suited for a particular individual with a particular set of communication challenges and needs. Shane and Costello (1994) offered a framework to help remedy this clinical challenge. They proposed a process whereby a candidate's capability in critical areas such as motor control, cognition, language, and sensory (visual and hearing) function when matched to the characteristics of available technology (low, mid, high) could lead to a more successful clinical outcome. Finally, they argue that feature matching is not a recipe for how to assess the non-speaking person, but rather a framework for what to assess and how to apply the resulting clinical data to maximize the person–machine interface, which, in turn, maximizes communication capacity.

18.7.2 Changes to service delivery models in the last decade

The field continues to undergo dramatic shifts in service delivery approaches in response to technological advancements, improved knowledge of the communication process, and changing societal awareness of AAC, or technology-mediated

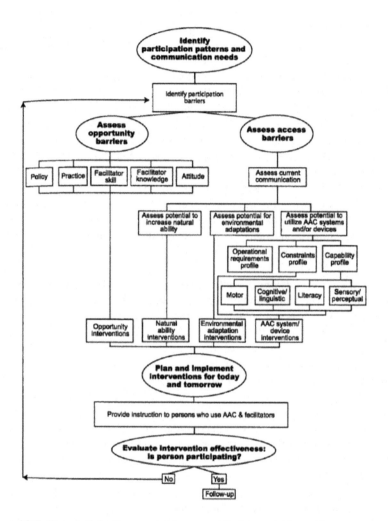

Figure 18.7 The participation model for augmentative and alternative communication (AAC) (Beukelman & Mirenda 2013).

communication (D. J. Higginbotham et al., 2007; Light & McNaughton, 2012; Romski & Sevcik, 2005). Now, more people are receiving AAC services that promote practical language treatments that allow for aided and unaided language use in natural environments.

Parent and consumer advocacy movements have led to more appreciation for cultural and individual family characteristics being more widely considered. As a result, individuals with CCN, families, and caregivers are being viewed as valuable information providers and considered an integral part of the AAC acquisition and learning process. Although speech-language pathologists continue to serve as the primary gatekeepers for accessing AAC technology that is approved by funding providers (i.e., insurances, vocational rehabilitation, schools), the increased availability of low-cost mobile high-tech AAC has enabled consumers and families into a more independent and empowered role in AAC device selection and training. For example, low-cost mobile high-tech AAC devices and AAC applications are often purchased prior to the evaluation of AAC applications, thus undermining participation and feature matching assessments by forcing practitioners to find ways of making consumer-selected devices work, despite potentially contradictory evaluation results. Complicating matters further is the reluctance of funding agencies to purchase mobile technologies and software.

18.8 Conclusion

This chapter provides the nascent rehabilitation engineer an overview of the current state of knowledge with respect to the burgeoning field of augmentative and alternative communication, or AAC. In order to appreciate the full measure of present-day AAC advancements, a historical perspective of what past generations of individuals with developmental disabilities had to endure after confinement in residential institutions, while receiving little to no services, has been included. The mention of the abhorrent conditions these unwitting individuals routinely suffered was not intended to rouse moral outrage, but rather to highlight how humane societal acceptance and the digital revolution coalesced in a way that bolstered the possibilities of AAC at just the right time in human history. Had either the digital age or this age of enlightenment toward disabled citizens not taken place, it is unlikely there would be a need for this chapter.

It is essential that current and future rehabilitation engineers understand the current AAC options for persons with physical and intellectual differences that affect their ability to engage in written and spoken communication. That said, AAC is not just about high-tech devices. It is also about the proper application of different levels of communication technology, ranging from the most sophisticated to more mid-range and low-tech options. Equally important are the technological innovations that allow an individual with a physical impairment to be able to control (or interface with/access) the communication option/s most suited for that individual. Importantly, the chapter explains a feature matching approach that attempts to select particular AAC devices or systems based on a careful consideration of a range of human factors such as psycholinguistic knowledge and capability, which reveals symbolic potential as well as physical abilities that portend how an AAC device will need to be accessed. Without some ordered approach, the complex task of assigning communication hardware, software, and peripherals would follow an unruly trial and error approach. Furthermore, the selection process needs to take into consideration the growing body of research that examines rate of communication and the ideal layout of content in an effort to improve overall communication efficiency. And while past studies are essential to the process of selecting AAC options, careful research should also be part of a design process for those rehabilitation engineers who will strive to create the next generation of AAC technologies. As part of this inventive process, these authors believe it is important to keep in mind the adage "if people read more, they would discover less." Finally, because providing a voice for those unable to speak is emblematic of the AAC discipline, the reader has been provided with a historical perspective on computer-generated voices. This narrative describes the evolution of machine-generated voices that were robotic and at times unintelligible to the more contemporary quest for voices that are natural and gender specific or even capture the essence of a person's own voice and speech characteristics.

18.9 Discussion questions

1. What aspects of AAC systems contribute to delayed-time experienced by participants in augmented interactions? Identify at least three and propose potential solutions or existing solution designs that have not yet proven effective.
2. Name two types of physical access options currently available to individuals who use AAC. Describe a profile of an individual who might use the access methods you identify.
3. What are the social benefits and drawbacks of using a lower-tech communication system in an increasingly tech-centered world?
4. What is the participation model and how is it used? How does it relate to the process of feature matching?
5. Why should the rehab engineer understand the roles of the other professionals involved in the evaluation, prescription, setup, and support of AAC for individuals with CCN?

References

Acaplea Group. (2017). *Acapela my own voice* (Vol. 2017, Issue May 24). http://www.acapela-group.com/voices/voice-replacement/my-own-voice-partners/.

Bean, I. (2011). *Switch progression roadmap, Inclusive Technology, Oldham* (Vol. 2017, Issue April 30). www.inclusive.co.uk/Lib/Doc/pubs/switch-progression-road-map.pdf.

Beukelman, D., & Mirenda, P. (2013). Supporting participation and communication for beginning communicators. *Augmentative and Alternative Communication*, 225–254.

Beukelman, D. R., Hux, K., Dietz, A., McKelvey, M., & Weissling, K. (2015). Using visual scene displays as communication support options for people with chronic, severe aphasia: A summary of AAC research and future research directions. *Augmentative and Alternative Communication*, *31*(3), 234–245.

Beukelman, D. R., & Yorkston, K. M. (1982). Communication interaction of adult communication augmentation system use. *Topics in Language Disorders*, 2(2), 39–53.

Blackstone, S. W., Williams, M. B., & Wilkins, D. P. (2007). Key principles underlying research and practice in AAC. *Augmentative and Alternative Communication*, 23(3), 191–203.

Bloch, S., & Wilkinson, R. (2004). The understandability of AAC: A conversation analysis study of acquired dysarthria. *Augmentative and Alternative Communication*, 20(4), 272–282.

Buzolich, M. J., & Wiemann, J. M. (1988). Turn taking in atypical conversations: The case of the speaker/augmented-communicator dyad. *Journal of Speech, Language, and Hearing Research*, 31(1), 3–18.

CereProc. (2017). (Vol. 2017, Issue May 19). https://www.cereproc.com/en/products/cerevoiceme.

Chapanis, A., Ochsman, R. B., Parrish, R. N., & Weeks, G. D. (1972). Studies in interactive communication: I. The effects of four communication modes on the behavior of teams during cooperative problem-solving. *Human Factors*, 14(6), 487–509.

Clark, H., Brennan, S., Resnick, L., Levine, J., & Teasley, S. (1991). *Grounding in communication perspectives on socially shared cognition* (pp. 127–149). Washington, DC: American Psychological Association.

Coleman, C. L., Cook, A. M., & Meyers, L. S. (1980). Assessing non-oral clients for assistive communication devices. *Journal of Speech and Hearing Disorders*, 45(4), 515–526.

Cook, A., & Hussey, S. (1995). *Assistive technologies: Principles and practices*. St. Louis, MO. Mosby-Year Book.

Cook, A., & Polgar, J. (2015). *Assistive technologies: Principles and practice*. 4th ed. St. Louis, MO: Mosby-Year Book.

Costello, J. (2017). *ALS augmentative communication program: Message banking* (Vol. 2017, Issue April 4). http://www.childrenshospital.org/alsmessagebanking.

Crosslan, A., Ruedel, K., Gray, T., Wellington, D., Reynolds, J., & Perrot, M. (2016). *Future ready assistive technology: Fostering state supports for students with disabilities*. Washington, DC: American Institutes for Research.

Drager, K., & Reichle, J. (2001). Effects of age and divided attention on listeners' comprehension of synthesized speech. *Augmentative and Alternative Communication*, 17(2), 109–119.

Drager, K. D., Reichle, J., & Pinkoski, C. (2010). Synthesized speech output and children: A scoping review. *American Journal of Speech-Language Pathology*, 19(3), 259–273.

Dudley, H., Riesz, R., & Watkins, S. (1939). A synthetic speaker. *Journal of the Franklin Institute*, 227(6), 739–764.

DynaVox InterAACt. (n.d.). (Vol. 2018, Issue May 5). http://www.dynavoxtech.com/interaact/.

Euphony Inc. (2017). *Simulations that need emotive speech synthesis* (Vol. 2017, Issue May 22). https://medium.com/@EuphonyInc/5-simulations-that-need-emotive-synthetic-speech-1d9303dc70f8

Fager, S., Beukelman, D. R., Fried-Oken, M., Jakobs, T., & Baker, J. (2012). Access interface strategies. *Assistive Technology*, 24(1), 25–33.

Farrier, L., Yorkston, K., Marriner, N., & Beukelman, D. (1985). Conversational control in nonimpaired speakers using an augmentative communication system. *Augmentative and Alternative Communication*, 1(2), 65–73.

Fitzgerald, M. M., Sposato, B., Politano, P., Hetling, J., & O'Neill, W. (2009). Comparison of three head-controlled mouse emulators in three light conditions. *Augmentative and Alternative Communication*, 25(1), 32–41.

Foulds, R. (1972). *The Tufts interactive communicator*. Washington, DC: ERIC Clearinghouse, 16–24.

Gagnon, R. (1978). Votrax real time hardware for phoneme synthesis of speech. *ICASSP '78. IEEE International Conference on Acoustics, Speech, and Signal Processing 3*, 175–178.

Gorernflo, C. W., Gorernflo, D. W., & Santer, S. A. (1994). Effects of synthetic voice output on attitudes toward the augmented communicator. *Journal of Speech, Language, and Hearing Research, 37*(1), 64–68.

Gray, T., Silver-Pacuilla, H., Overton, C., & Brann, A. (2010). *Unleashing the power of innovation for assistive technology.* Washington, DC: American Institutes for Research.

Hanson, E. K., Beukelman, D. R., & Yorkston, K. M. (2013). Communication support through multimodal supplementation: A scoping review. *Augmentative and Alternative Communication, 29*(4), 310–321.

Higginbotham, D., Fulcher, K., & Seale, J. (2016). Time and timing in interactions involving individuals with ALS, their unimpaired partners and their speech generating devices. In *The silent partner* (pp. 199–229). Havant, UK: J&R Press Ltd.

Higginbotham, D. J. (1989). The interplay of communication device output mode and interaction style between nonspeaking persons and their speaking partners. *Journal of Speech and Hearing Disorders, 54*(3), 320–333.

Higginbotham, D. J. (1992). Evaluation of keystroke savings across five assistive communication technologies. *Augmentative and Alternative Communication, 8*(4), 258–272.

Higginbotham, D. J. (2010). Humanizing vox artificialis: The role of speech synthesis in augmentative and alternative communication. In *Computer synthesized speech technologies: Tools for aiding impairment* (Vol. 1–Book, Section, pp. 50–70). Hershey, PA: IGI Global.

Higginbotham, D. J., Bisantz, A. M., Sunm, M., Adams, K., & Yik, F. (2009). The effect of context priming and task type on augmentative communication performance. *Augmentative and Alternative Communication, 25*(1), 19–31.

Higginbotham, D. J., & Caves, K. (2002). AAC performance and usability issues: The effect of AAC technology on the communicative process. *Assistive Technology, 14*(1), 45–57.

Higginbotham, D. J., Drazek, A., Kowarsky, K., Scally, C., & Segal, E. (1994). Discourse comprehension of synthetic speech delivered at normal and slow presentation rates. *Augmentative and Alternative Communication, 10*(3), 191–202.

Higginbotham, D. J., Lesher, G. W., Moulton, B. J., & Roark, B. (2012). The application of natural language processing to augmentative and alternative communication. *Assistive Technology, 24*(1), 14–24.

Higginbotham, D. J., Shane, H., Russell, S., & Caves, K. (2007). Access to AAC: Present, past, and future. *Augmentative and Alternative Communication, 23*(3), 243–257.

Higginbotham, D. J., & Wilkins, D. (1999). Slipping through the timestream: Social issues of time and timing in augmented interactions. *Constructing (in) Competence: Disabling Evaluations in Clinical and Social Interaction, 2*, 49–82.

Higginbotham, D. J., & Wilkins, D. P. (2006). The short story of Frametalker: An interactive AAC device. *Perspectives on Augmentative and Alternative Communication, 15*(1), 18–22.

Kafafian, H. (1973). *Study of man-machine communications systems for the handicapped. C/R/I second report, volumes I and II.* Washington, DC: Cybernetics Research Institute.

Kafafian, H. (1974). *Cybertype* (Patent No. 3.831.147). Google Patents.

Karjalainen, M. (1988). Review of from text to speech: The MITalk system (Cambridge studies in speech science and communication) by Jonathan Allen, M. Sharon Hunnicutt, and Dennis Klatt, with Robert C. Armstrong and David Pisoni. Cambridge University Press 1987. *Computational Linguistics, 14*(2), 76–77.

Kim, K. E. (2001). *Effect of speech rate on comprehension.* Buffalo, NY: University at Buffalo.

Klaat, D. H. (1987). Text to speech conversion. *Journal Acoustical Society of America, 82*(3), 737–793.

Klatt's last tapes: A history of speech synthesizers video. (2013). BBC Radio 4. www.bbc.co. uk/programmes/b03775fy: http://communicationaids.info/history-speech-synthesisers/.

Koester, H. H., & Arthanat, S. (2018). Text entry rate of access interfaces used by people with physical disabilities: A systematic review. *Assistive Technology, 30*(3), 151–163.

Koester, H. H., & Levine, S. (1996). Effect of a word prediction feature on user performance. *Augmentative and Alternative Communication, 12*(3), 155–168.

Lesher, G., Moulton, B., & Higginbotham, D. J. (1998). Techniques for augmenting scanning communication. *Augmentative and Alternative Communication, 14*(2), 81–101.

Light, J., Collier, B., & Parnes, P. (1985). Communicative interaction between young nonspeaking physically disabled children and their primary caregivers: Part II— Communicative function. *Augmentative and Alternative Communication, 1*(3), 98–107.

Light, J., & Drager, K. (2007). AAC technologies for young children with complex communication needs: State of the science and future research directions. *Augmentative and Alternative Communication, 23*(3), 204–216.

Light, J., Lindsay, P., Siegel, L., & Parnes, P. (1990). The effects of message encoding techniques on recall by literate adults using AAC systems. *Augmentative and Alternative Communication, 6*(3), 184–201.

Light, J., & McNaughton, D. (2012). The changing face of augmentative and alternative communication: Past, present, and future challenges. *Augmentative and Alternative Communication, 28*(4), 197–204.

McCoy, K. F., Hoag, L., & Bedrosian, J. (2011). Next generation utterance-based systems: What do pragmatic studies tell us about system design? *Perspectives on Augmentative and Alternative Communication, 20*(2), 57–63.

McKelvey, M. L., Hux, K., Dietz, A., & Beukelman, D. R. (2010). Impact of personal relevance and contextualization on word-picture matching by people with aphasia. *American Journal of Speech-Language Pathology, 19*(1), 22–33.

Medcalf, L. (2017). *5 ways to utilize your Amazon echo—Assistive technology easter seals crossroads* (Vol. 2018, Issue May 5). http://www.eastersealstech.com/2017/01/11/5-ways-utilize-amazon-echo/.

Mergen, B. (1992). Information age: People, information and technology. *The Journal of American History, 79*(1), 219–225.

Mills, T., Bunnell, H. T., & Patel, R. (2014). Towards personalized speech synthesis for augmentative and alternative communication. *Augmentative and Alternative Communication, 30*(3), 226–236.

Model Talker. (2017). (Vol. 2017, Issue May 13). https://www.modeltalker.org.

Morris, L. (1979). A fast FORTRAN implementation of the US Naval Research Laboratory algorithm for automatic translation of English text to VOTRAX parameters. *ICASSP, 4*, 907–913.

Portnuff, C. (2006). Augmentative and alternative communication: A user's perspective. *Lecture Delivered at the Oregon Health and Science University, 18*.

Pullin, G., & Hennig, S. (2015). 17 ways to say yes: Toward nuanced tone of voice in AAC and speech technology. *Augmentative and Alternative Communication, 31*(2), 170–180.

Pullin, G., Treviranus, J., Patel, R., & Higginbotham, J. (2017). Designing interaction, voice, and inclusion in AAC research. *Augmentative and Alternative Communication, 33*(3), 139–148.

Roark, B., Fried-Oken, M., & Gibbons, C. (2015). Huffman and linear scanning methods with statistical language models. *Augmentative and Alternative Communication, 31*(1), 37–50.

Romski, M., & Sevcik, R. A. (2005). Augmentative communication and early intervention: Myths and realities. *Infants & Young Children, 18*(3), 174–185.

Shane, H., & Costello, J. (1994). Augmentative communication assessment and the feature matching process. In mini-seminar presented at the Annual Convention of the American Speech-Language-Hearing Association, New Orleans, LA.

Shane, H. C. (2017). [Personal communication].

Smith, L. E., Higginbotham, D. J., Lesher, G. W., Moulton, B., & Mathy, P. (2006). The development of an automated method for analyzing communication rate in augmentative and alternative communication. *Assistive Technology*, *18*(1), 107–121.

Székely, É., Ahmed, Z., Hennig, S., Cabral, J. P., & Carson-Berndsen, J. (2014). Predicting synthetic voice style from facial expressions. An application for augmented conversations. *Speech Communication*, *57*, 63–75.

Székely, E., Cabral, J. P., Cahill, P., & Carson-Berndsen, J. (2011). Clustering expressive speech styles in audiobooks using glottal source parameters. In *Twelfth Annual Conference of the International Speech Communication Association*. INTERSPEECH 2011. Florence, Italy, August 27–31.

Székely, E., Kane, J., Scherer, S., Gobl, C., & Carson-Berndsen, J. (2012). Detecting a targeted voice style in an audiobook using voice quality features. *012 IEEE International Conference on Acoustics, Speech and Signal Processing (ICASSP)*, 4593–4596.

Taylor, P. (2009). *Text-to-speech synthesis*. Cambridge, UK: Cambridge University Press.

Therapy Box. (2017). https://www.therapy-box.co.uk/predictable.

Todman, J. (2000). Rate and quality of conversations using a text-storage AAC system: Single-case training study. *Augmentative and Alternative Communication*, *16*(3), 164–179.

Todman, J., Alm, N., Higginbotham, J., & File, P. (2008). Whole utterance approaches in AAC. *Augmentative and Alternative Communication*, *24*(3), 235–254.

Trnka, K., McCaw, J., Yarrington, D., McCoy, K. F., & Pennington, C. (2009). User interaction with word prediction: The effects of prediction quality. *ACM Transactions on Accessible Computing (TACCESS)*, *1*(3), 1–34.

VocalID. (2017). (Vol. 2017, Issue May 28). https://www.vocalid.co/products.

Von Kempelen, W. (1791). *Mechanismus der menschlichen Sprache*. Degen.

Wikipedia. (2017). *Augmentative and alternative communication*. https://en.wikipedia.org/w/index.php?title=Augmentative_and_alternative_communication&oldid=785317918.

Wilkinson, K. M., Light, J., & Drager, K. (2012). Considerations for the composition of visual scene displays: Potential contributions of information from visual and cognitive sciences. *Augmentative and Alternative Communication*, *28*(3), 137–147.

Wilkinson, R., Bloch, S., & Clarke, M. (2011). On the use of graphic resources in interaction by people with communication disorders. In J. Streeck, C. Goodwin and C. LeBaron (eds), *Embodied interaction: Language and body in the material world* (pp. 152–168). Cambridge, UK: Cambridge University Press.

Chapter 19 Cognitive technologies

C. Bodine and V. Haggett

Contents

19.1 Chapter overview

Although many practitioners have used assistive technologies and created adaptations for a wide range of mainstream technologies to address the needs of persons with cognitive impairments over the years, a more general recognition of the importance and need for cognitive technologies is a fairly recent phenomenon.

DOI: 10.1201/b21964-22

This chapter seeks to provide relevant information on a range of cognitive disabilities along with an overview of where we are today in our development and application of technologies to facilitate independence. The chapter is composed of sections that detail the demographics of cognitive impairments and their potential causes, along with an overview of the most common technologies and applications currently available. Within these descriptions, the sections are divided into the applications of these various technologies for activities of daily living, training or therapeutic interventions, workplace, and educational applications. The chapter concludes with a discussion of the promise of cognitive technologies of the future.

19.2 Introduction: Background

19.2.1 Cognitive disability statistics

This is an exciting and highly dynamic time to be engaged in work surrounding cognitive technologies, due in large part to the fact that we are becoming a nation heavily populated by older adults ("2010 Census Data," 2014; "AOA Administration on Aging," 2014; "Taskforce on the Aging of the American Workforce," 2008; Thornton, 2002). There is a quickly growing recognition that technology has the potential to facilitate community independence and improved health outcomes and healthcare for seniors, including those with cognitive impairments (Boger & Mihailidis, 2011; Demers, 2007; Helal, Mokhtari, & Abdulrazak, 2008; Mosner, 2003; Pew & Hemel, 2004). There is also a quickly growing recognition that we must develop technology solutions to support care providers as well as those living with cognitive disabilities (Bodine, 2007; Boger & Mihailidis, 2011; Demers, 2007; Hammel, 2000; Hammel et al., 2008; Lindenberger, Lovden, Schellenbach, Li, & Kruger, 2008).

In 2009, persons 65 or older in the United States numbered 39.6 million, representing 12.9% of the US population (one in every eight Americans; "2010 Census Data," 2014). By 2030, it is projected there will be about 72.1 million older persons—growing to 19% of the population (Christensen, Doblhammer, Rau, & Vaupel, 2009). In a prevalence study completed by Plassman et al. (2008), they estimated the prevalence of dementia among individuals aged 71 and older at 13.9%, comprising about 3.4 million individuals in the United States (Plassman et al., 2008). Dementia prevalence increased with age, from 5% in ages 71–79 years to 37.4% of those 90 and older (Plassman et al. 2008, 427–434).

In addition, more infants with cognitive and other significant disabilities are surviving worldwide and living a full life span. From 1990 to 2012, the world's neonatal mortality rate fell from 33 deaths to 21 deaths per 1000 live births (Christensen et al., 2009). The overall result was a reduction in neonatal deaths globally from 4.6 million in 1990 to 2.9 million in 2012. While this is good news, the reality is that many of the infants who do survive have significant cognitive and other disabilities. In the United States alone, about 40,000 babies a year are born prematurely (< 24 weeks' gestation; "2010 Census Data," 2014). Survival odds of infant boys born between 22 and 24 weeks' gestation are 69%; with 50% experiencing severe impairments. Females of the same age and weight have survival odds of 86% with a 23% chance of severe impairment. Almost all will live a full lifespan ("2010 Census Data," 2014; Fanaroff et al., 2007; Wilson-Costello, Friedman, Minich, Fanaroff, & Hack, 2005).

Medicine is not only helping infant survival rates. It is also helping trauma victims, many with cognitive insults, to survive. Of the more than 2.3 million American veterans of the Iraq and Afghanistan wars, at least 20% have post-traumatic stress disorder (PTSD) and/or depression. Nineteen percent of veterans are estimated to have traumatic brain injury (TBI) (Fischer, 2010). In the United States alone, 1.7 million civilians experience a TBI annually with a significant number retaining permanent disability. In the United States, direct medical costs and indirect costs for TBI, such as lost productivity, are annualized to an estimated US$60 billion (Finkelstein, Corso, & Miller, 2006; Langlois, Rutland-Brown, & Wald, 2006).

Additionally, the number of adults with intellectual/developmental disabilities (IDD) age 60 years and older living in the United States is projected to double from 641,860 in 2000 to 1.2 million by 2030 (Walsh, Heller, Schupf, & Van Schrojenstein Lantman-de Valk, 2001). IDD is defined as a disability that occurs before age 18. It includes individuals who experience significant limitations in two main areas: (a) intellectual functioning and (b) adaptive behavior. An estimated 4.6 million Americans are identified as having an IDD; although prevalence studies may not identify all people because this data is gathered from multiple sources such as Medicaid/Medicare/Social Security, and not everyone with an IDD is necessarily receiving benefits (Kim, Larson, & Charlie Lakin, 2001).

19.2.2 Cognitive disability

Cognition encompasses perception (taking in information visually, auditorily, and through our touch sensors, or kinesthesia); memory, learning, judgment, abstract reasoning, and problem solving; using language both expressively and receptively, and planning. Interestingly, all of these skillsets often occur simultaneously. Our brain also interacts with every other system in our body including respiratory, circulatory, motor, digestive, and many others. Yet, we are rarely aware of everything that is going on inside our brain (Robinson-Riegler & Robinson-Riegler, 2016).

What happens when injury, illness, or a congenital disorder affects the brain? Cognitive impairments can occur due to all sorts of brain issues such as closed head injuries, infections, exposure to neurotoxins (i.e., substances that are toxic to the brain), genetic factors, tumors, strokes, and disease. The specific type of cognitive impairment someone develops depends on the part of the brain that is impacted. Figure 19.1 provides a brief reminder of the various components of the brain and their primary functions.

The following paragraphs will briefly describe some of the many causes and influences of injury, disease, illness, or genetic factors on cognition.

Brain disorders due to traumatic injuries can result from a single major head trauma (such as a blow to the head due to a fall) or from a repeated series of head injuries, such as those sustained by football players. The degree and nature of cognitive impairment due to head trauma depend on the location and severity of the injury. People with this type of injury may experience amnesia (an inability to learn and recall new information and/or remember previously learned information or past events), persistent memory loss, irritability and other emotional lability, problems sustaining attention, depression, apathy, and other personality changes. This type of injury is most common among young men who engage in high-risk behaviors such as riding a motorcycle without a helmet or driving while intoxicated (Dams-O'Connor et al., 2017).

A blunt head trauma, or closed head injury, describes an injury to the head that does not result in an open wound. Concussions (when the brain bounces against

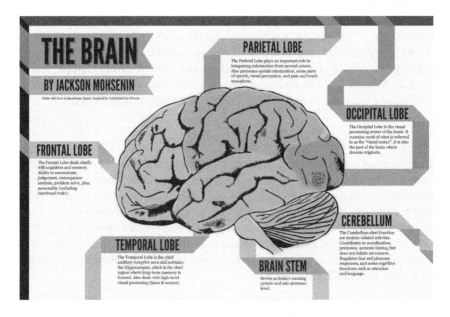

Figure 19.1 The brain (courtesy of Jackson Mohsenin).

the skull), hematomas (brain bruises or bleeding), and traumatic brain injuries are all types of closed head injuries. The severity and type of cognitive impairment caused by closed head injuries depend on where and how the brain was struck (Quayle, Holmes, & Kuppermann, 2014).

Disruptions in the blood supply to the brain are one of the most common causes of brain damage. Strokes are caused by blockages to blood vessels (ischemic strokes) or by the bursting of a blood vessel (a hemorrhagic stroke). The risk factors for stroke include age, family history, heart disease, uncontrolled diabetes, high blood pressure, and smoking. Common cognitive effects of stroke include impaired memory, language difficulties, and paralysis, but again, they depend on the part of the brain that is affected (Kelly-Hayes et al., 1998).

Infections can also cause cognitive disorders. Both bacteria and viruses can cause significant problems in how the brain functions and how well it recovers. Meningitis is one of the most common forms of brain infection. It results due to an inflammation (swelling) of the protective covering that surrounds the brain and the central nervous system. Typically, it is caused by a bacterial or viral infection of the fluid surrounding the brain and spinal cord. Other causes include injuries, cancer, certain drugs, and other types of infection. Physicians treating meningitis vary their treatment based on the specific cause of the infection. Someone with this illness may develop deafness, cognitive impairment, and in severe cases, death (Too, Ball, McGregor, & Hunt, 2014)

Some cognitive impairments are inherited. For instance, individuals with Down syndrome have an extra 21st chromosome. People with this syndrome often have intellectual functioning that is significantly below average, combined with an impaired ability to adapt to the demands of everyday functioning. Fragile X syndrome is an X-linked dominant disorder. It is the number one form of inherited intellectual disability with one in approximately 4000 males affected. Individuals with fragile X have intellectual impairments that range from a mild learning disability and a normal IQ to severe intellectual disability and autistic behaviors (Cornish, Turk, & Hagerman, 2008; Garber, Visootsak, & Warren, 2008).

Repeated and/or significant exposure to toxic chemicals (neurotoxins) such as metals (e.g., lead, mercury), drugs (e.g., cocaine, alcohol), or other substances (e.g., paint, glue) can also cause cognitive impairment. The type of cognitive impairment created by neurotoxins depends on the type of toxin, the degree of exposure (how much was taken in, and for how long), and when the exposure occurred (whether the person affected was an infant, child, or adult). Typically, young children exposed to neurotoxins are more likely to develop cognitive disorders (because their brains are experiencing more rapid development) than adults (Burstein, Zhang, Levy, Aoki, & Brin, 2014). Tumors are masses of cells that grow and infiltrate the body. These masses of cells can be either benign (i.e., they can be removed and stop growing at that point) or malignant (i.e., they are

465

difficult to remove and will continue to grow and spread). Both benign and malignant tumors in the brain can cause impaired cognitive functioning, depending on their size and location. The surgery required to treat either type can cause brain damage in and of itself. Those with malignant tumors will experience varying degrees of cognitive deficits as the cell mass presses on and destroys healthy tissue in the brain and spinal cord, blocks the fluid that flows around and through the brain, and/or causes swelling due to accumulation of fluid. Malignant tumors are often lethal (Zülch, 2013).

Diseases that cause cognitive disorders can result from any one or more of the disorders discussed earlier. For instance, Huntington's disease is a disorder that affects thinking, emotions, and movement. Multiple sclerosis is a movement disorder created when the body attacks the lining of brain cells, called myelin, decreasing the brain's ability to deliver messages quickly and efficiently. Both of these diseases have a strong genetic component. In contrast, Parkinson's disease, also a movement disorder, and epilepsy, or seizures, can be the result of multiple factors including defective genes, brain infections, tumors, trauma, and a host of other causes (Bates, Tabrizi, & Jones, 2014; Blake & Bodine, 2002; Lotharius & Brundin, 2002).

The word dementia is an umbrella-like term referring to any brain syndrome that causes multiple cognitive deficits. In other words, saying someone has dementia is similar to saying that someone has a fever; you are not specifying the exact cause of the symptoms. Someone diagnosed with dementia may experience a myriad of disorders including impaired orientation, or not knowing where he or she is, who he or she, or someone else is, or what time it is. The ability to make decisions about personal issues and financial or medical concerns can be severely impacted. The ability to remember recent events or newly learned information is also limited. Executive functioning, or the ability to plan and carry out daily tasks and make rational decisions is particularly debilitating. Individuals with some form of dementia may also have impaired language skills—meaning a decreased ability to communicate with others (expressive language) or being able to understand what is being communicated to them (receptive language; M. Prince et al., 2013).

While there are over 50 categories of dementia, the most prevalent are Alzheimer's disease, which accounts for 50–70% of all dementia cases; Lewy body disease—up to 20% of cases; and vascular disease—15–20% of all dementia cases, including stroke. Other medical conditions that can also cause dementia include HIV/AIDS, head trauma, Parkinson's disease, Huntington's disease, Pick's disease, Creutzfeldt-Jakob disease, normal pressure hydrocephalus, and Wernicke–Korsakoff syndrome. According to the National Institutes on Aging, the cost of caring for those living in the United States with dementia is about US$100 billion every year. Worldwide, approximately 46.8 million people are living with dementia, with Alzheimer's disease accounting for 70–75% of these cases. This number is projected to almost double every 20 years, reaching 74.7 million in 2030 and 131.5 million in 2050. There are over 9.9 million new cases of dementia each year worldwide, implying one new case every 3.2 seconds. The risk of developing AD increases dramatically with age; almost 50% of individuals over 85 are coping with this disorder (M. J. Prince, 2015).

19.2.3 Overview of design and development considerations

Cognitive technology development for individuals with disabilities takes place on a spectrum between universal design and complete customization. Universal design provides standard assistance intended for most people with a disability. Complete customization provides more personalization based on the individual needs of the person. While complete customization is ideal, it is important to consider the trade-offs of costs, training, and maintenance necessary when designing with customization settings versus incorporating some universal design applications (Agree, 2014).

Convergence is a design application where the integration of different types of cognitive technologies provides multiple types of assistance on the same device or platform. People with cognitive disabilities often have comorbidities and other accessibility needs beyond the needs of their primary disability. For example, many individuals with cognitive impairments also experience communication disorders and benefit from augmentative/alternative communication devices (Chapter 18). Others struggle with sensory impairments (Chapter 20); motor difficulties (Chapters 12 and 16); transportation (Chapter 15); and congenital or acquired limb loss (Chapter 21). Developing accessible technology to accommodate these secondary needs is a great challenge for the clinicians and engineers researching and developing technologies for this population. It is critical to understand the design considerations necessary for integrating multiple types of assistance or allowing for the integration of other assistive technologies in order to make products easier to use and operate (Agree, 2014). As you read the following sections on the various types of cognitive technologies and applications, consider the design characteristics or requirements needed to make them effective for persons with a range of cognitive disorders.

19.3 Mobile technologies

Prompting technologies or software are one of the most frequently prescribed technologies for persons with cognitive impairments to support memory and overall cognition. They can be programmed to offer assistance in the form of linear sequences, non-linear sequences, and context-aware technology that can learn and adapt with the user. Linear sequencing is one of the simplest ways to program technology, where assistance is given on a device, typically tablet or phone-based, as sequential steps to complete tasks. Non-linear sequencing is more adaptable, in that the steps to complete a task can be different depending on the situation. This allows for broader applications and opportunities for skipping steps during learning. Other opportunities to make the technology even more adaptable include making the device smarter, or more context-aware, by detecting tasks/steps with the ability to anticipate; tracking the task itself; the person's location in relationship to the task; and, based on time, what should be happening. Using these parameters, the system can detect any problems and deliver appropriate assistance within a set of tasks (Gomez, 2014).

Personal and handheld devices are any portable device that a person with cognitive disabilities uses to compensate for their disability. Some of the most common include smartphones, tablets, personal data assistants (PDAs), electronic handheld writing interfaces, recording devices, and pagers (Gomez, 2014; Jamieson, Cullen, McGee-Lennon, Brewster, & Evans, 2014; Rispoli, Machalicek, & Lang, 2014). These devices can be combined with software and other applications that use prompting technology and task assistance software or applications in order to improve functionality for people with cognitive disabilities. They also have the advantage of being portable and subtle, and often have the ability to be integrated into personal technology someone already owns (Leopold, Lourie, Petras, & Elias, 2015; Rispoli et al., 2014).

19.3.1 Activities of daily living

People with memory impairments due to an acquired brain injury or degenerative disease can greatly benefit from personal devices that assist them in completing tasks through prompting or providing instructions to complete a task. Personal devices can also aid this population in compensating for memory loss through voice recording or providing pictures or videos with people or information they frequently forget (Jamieson et al., 2014). Additionally, people with intellectual disabilities can benefit from mobile technology by using it to help interact and communicate with others (den Brok & Sterkenburg, 2015).

AmICog (Gomez, 2014) is one example of a prompting technology that has been applied for assistance in activities of daily living. *AmICog* utilizes smartphones and QR codes placed in the environment to detect a task the user wants to complete and the user's position in order to help with task completion. QR codes are one technology development consideration that eliminates problems with global positioning system (GPS) tracking for indoor environments, where distances may be too short to pick up and obstacles prevent the user from taking the suggested shortest route. *AmICog* has not been tested with real users yet, but it is practical and promising in the use of an easily accessible smartphone and QR codes as an alternative to GPS.

Online calendars accessed through mobile technology have also proven useful as a tool for people with cognitive disabilities (Leopold et al., 2015; McDonald et al., 2011; Rispoli et al., 2014). McDonald et al. (2011) showed that Google Calendar was more effective in appointment and task management for people with cognitive disabilities than a standard paper calendar. A randomized controlled study of 12 people with acquired brain injury was completed using a five-week baseline phase and two five-week intervention phases. The interventions used either Google Calendar or a paper calendar to assist in the completion of targeted daily activities, with family and caregivers monitoring completion success. Google Calendar was more effective and generally preferred due to the reminder prompts that increased success and independence (McDonald et al., 2011).

Evald (2015) reported that most people with TBI use applications and features of a smartphone as their primary assistive technology to help them with activities of daily living. An intervention was completed in 13 people with TBI who lived in a community setting and received six weeks of training with a smartphone to use the features that could assist them with memory and activities of daily living. Following this intervention, the participants were asked about their satisfaction. They liked the audio and visual reminders but did not like that they depended on battery life. Overall, ten of the 13 participants decided to keep using the device as a memory aid, indicating that the advantages of using smartphone features to assist in activities of daily living outweighed the disadvantages (Evald, 2015). Furthermore, devices with built-in, programmable timers and alerts are often used by people with TBI to compensate for memory deficits. This can include pill bottles with timers on them for medications, as well as alarms and alerts that are programmed into smartphones and other personal devices (Chu, Brown, Harniss, Kautz, & Johnson, 2014).

People with intellectual disabilities and, in particular, autism spectrum disorder, can benefit from technology that assists them in behaviors of daily living so they can better interact with others and learn skills (den Brok & Sterkenburg, 2015). Much of the prompting technology used on handheld and personal devices consists of instructional and prompting videos and pictures on personal devices. Personal devices are an advantageous vehicle for this kind of assistive technology as the technology can be developed as an application that can work on many devices. In addition, it is portable and can generally be used more independently (den Brok & Sterkenburg, 2015; Mechling & Savidge, 2011).

One study using three middle school students with autism spectrum disorder evaluated the use of a personal digital assistant (PDA) for assisting with task completion. The participants had training and a baseline test of task completion using a task strip prior to the intervention. The intervention included the use of a PDA that had four different activity-based tasks with reinforcement provided following completion of each task. All students were able to complete more tasks correctly and better transition between tasks when using the PDA that assisted in prompting. This study supports the use of prompting technology in task assistance for children and teens with autism spectrum disorder, but additional information should be gathered from more students to identify settings to best fit this population (Mechling & Savidge, 2011).

Older adults who have mild Alzheimer's disease or other cognitive impairments have a harder time using technology in general than their peers. One study used 39 adults with Alzheimer's disease and 28 adults with mild cognitive impairment to see if technology use affected the performance of activities of daily living. Results from this study showed that older adults with Alzheimer's disease or mild cognitive impairments experienced more difficulty using technology when they had a lowered ability for processing activities of daily living. For older adults with mild cognitive impairments, there was a stronger relationship between motor ability and difficulty in using technology (Ryd, Nygard, Malinowsky, Ohman, & Kottorp, 2015). Therefore, it is important that personal and handheld cognitive technologies can adapt to fit the level of disease progression when used to assist this population in activities of daily living. It is also important that the design of cognitive technologies for older adults have accessible features for motor, vision, or hearing impairments that may worsen with age.

19.3.2 Workplace

Personal and handheld devices are most commonly used in the workplace to assist in disability management and job function using prompting, scheduling, and task-based instruction software (Gomez, 2014; Gunther, Sliker, & Bodine, 2017; Rispoli et al., 2014). Typical concerns of employers of people with cognitive disabilities in the workplace include problems with task execution and workplace efficiency. Mobile technologies in the workplace aim to compensate for these deficiencies (Gomez, 2014). Figure 19.2 shows an example of how a mobile tablet might be used to give on-the-job instructions and feedback.

Warehouse navigation assistance is an application of mobile technology designed to assist the user in the workplace. Gunther et al. (2017) utilized ultra-high frequency radio frequency identification (UHF RFID) technology for tracking purposes in order to design a system that could determine the real-time position and provide environmental feedback to a mobile device. This technology has the advantage of only needing a one-time setup with "tags" that are read by the antennae to determine the location in order to provide feedback in the form of navigation to assist the user in finding items in a warehouse. This system was tested in a group of seven people without disabilities, where the participants had to get the system running by themselves with a set of instructions and navigate to three different destinations. Participants were monitored for task completion

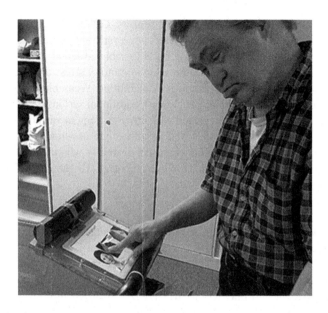

Figure 19.2 A person with a cognitive disability uses an augmented job coach.

using time on task and number of errors. Most errors occurred when setting up the software, which would usually not be completed by a user with a disability, and few errors occurred in the navigation tasks. Furthermore, the accuracy of the cart location was within 0.5 meters. Though there are still improvements to be made to the algorithm for it to perform optimally and additional testing with the intended users, this method of navigation is promising in aiding individuals with cognitive disabilities to work more independently in a warehouse setting (Gunther et al., 2017).

PDAs and other devices with programmable calendars and alarm settings have also proved useful in assisting people with acquired brain injury in the workplace. These devices can help manage calendars and appointments, as well as provide task alerts and assist with task completion (Hartmann, 2010; Rispoli et al., 2014). In a case study of an adult male with a mild brain injury, it was found that a proper evaluation of assistive technology could improve work productivity and satisfaction. Though this should be tested over a larger population, it is one example of how an individualized, accessible environment can improve independence and opportunities in the workplace for people with cognitive disabilities (Hartmann, 2010).

Wearables have been shown to be practical for work, as smart watches and other wearables are available to the public and priced for the average consumer. Sensors that are, or could be, integrated into wearables include accelerometers,

471

gyroscopes, thermometers, light and UV sensors, GPS, and sensors that monitor variables of health. Sensors that can detect heart rate, blood pressure, and perspiration can be used to identify health-related variables, such as stress and arousal. These variables can be used in combination to monitor stress and provide behavioral feedback for people with cognitive disabilities. Wearable devices can also be used to monitor vital signs of people with additional serious health conditions. Additionally, GPS tracking integrated with other movement variables can be used to provide task completion and schedule adherence assistance to improve the quality of work for someone with a cognitive disability who may have a memory or processing impairment (Dibia, Trewin, Ashoori, & Erickson, 2015).

19.3.3 Training/therapy

Children with autism spectrum disorder can benefit from handheld cognitive technologies (Escobedo et al., 2012; Wass & Porayska-Pomsta, 2014). Escobedo et al. (2012) created *MOSOCO*, which is a mobile application that can be used to recognize when another user is in the area and help facilitate and encourage social engagement and interaction. *MOSOCO* was tested in a group of 12 children between the ages of eight and 11 years old, three with autism spectrum disorder and nine typically developing peers who were identified as "potential interaction partners." Video analysis was done during lunch breaks and recess when the interactions took place, followed by interviews about the experience using *MOSOCO*. Overall, the response to using *MOSOCO* was positive, and findings showed that the students with autism spectrum disorder spent less time in "social missteps," defined as behavioral issues, when using *MOSOCO*. While this worked well in a school setting, other tests would have to be done and adaptations made to the device in order to use this technology outside of a more contained environment (Escobedo et al., 2012). This type of mobile platform can work well for children with autism spectrum disorder because people with autism spectrum disorder generally report enjoying technology because it is predictable and secure. Additionally, mobile cognitive technology that can be used in real-life can help bridge the gap between exercises done for therapeutic purposes and real-life interactions (Wass & Porayska-Pomsta, 2014).

19.4 Computer-driven software

Just as personal and handheld devices can be uploaded with applications or have software integrated into them to assist someone with a cognitive disability, computers can be uploaded with software and applications to do the same. Many times, this takes the form of video and picture manual-type instructions that assist in completing a task or training someone to complete a task in a safe environment (den Brok & Sterkenburg, 2015). Computer-driven software can be more useful than just building a novel device because software is generally easier and cheaper to update and customize. It also has the benefit of being easier and cheaper to fix, with no real device maintenance (Agree, 2014).

Adults with cognitive disabilities are less likely to use the internet than those without cognitive disabilities, likely due to inequalities in internet access and accessibility of online content. Furthermore, adolescents with cognitive disabilities are less likely to use the internet than their peers due to restrictions put on them by guardians who are worried about the possible consequences of internet access (Agree, 2014). Therefore, it is important to consider internet safety concerns when developing software and applications for populations with cognitive disabilities.

19.4.1 Activities of daily living

Personal computers can host calendar applications, e-mail, and organization software that people with TBI have reported can help them organize their daily lives and compensate for short-term memory loss (Chu et al., 2014). Additionally, computers can be programmed with prompting software to assist people with cognitive disabilities to complete tasks of daily living. O'Neill, Best, Gillespie, and O'Neill (2013) implemented prompting technology in an inpatient and home setting for an adult male with a severe cognitive impairment in order to help him complete his morning routine more independently. This computer software, *Guide*, acted as an alarm that then gave audible prompts with steps that required a "yes" or "no" response. If a "no" response was given, *Guide* would then attempt to assist in problem solving before moving on to the next step. In the inpatient setting, *Guide* assisted the man with a severe cognitive impairment in completing his morning routine independently 50% of the time versus almost no independence in the morning routine without *Guide*. However, when the system was moved into the home, he was only able to complete his morning routine independently with *Guide* 18.18% of the time. While this type of technology in the home may not allow someone with a cognitive disability to be completely independent, it may serve as a useful tool to assist caregivers as well as possibly encourage rehabilitation in populations with acquired brain injury and should be tested in a larger group of individuals with cognitive disabilities (O'Neill et al., 2013).

19.4.2 Training/therapy

Prompting through computer programs using videos has demonstrated usefulness in training for task performance of people with intellectual disabilities. This mode can work well as there is the option to personalize training and therapeutic interventions. It is important to have the option to change the training environment through the computer and make training stimulating for each individual (den Brok & Sterkenburg, 2015; Van Laarhoven, Kraus, Karpman, Nizzi, & Valentino, 2010). Even though computers can be useful in task performance for this population, research shows that people with intellectual disabilities still may need prompting in real-life situations outside of simulated training through the computer. In one study, two 13- and 14-year-old students with autism spectrum disorder and mild to moderate intellectual disabilities were taught a skill using picture prompts and a different skill using video prompts, both on a computer, following pretests that were used to identify different skills to use for testing. This study concluded that both types of prompting worked well, but video prompting worked slightly better when measuring efficiency. This type of system worked well for the two individuals in this study, and future research on a larger population could further fine-tune prompting technology to be helpful for teens with cognitive disabilities (Van Laarhoven et al., 2010). Computer software can also be programmed as assistive technology and act as a memory aid for people who have TBI. In addition to prompting, computer software can be useful in providing question-and-answer training with abilities to answer through computer text or through a voice recorder (Leopold et al., 2015).

Inexpensive technology can be integrated with computer software to help provide therapy. Integrating computer software with the Microsoft Kinect is one example of how therapy can be provided outside of the clinic. It can be used to demonstrate and correct exercises while providing physical rehabilitation therapy (Chang, Chen, & Huang, 2011; Deb, 2015; Gonzalez-Ortega, Diaz-Pernas, Martinez-Zarzuela, & Anton-Rodriguez, 2014). Additionally, it can be used to provide cognitive therapy through 3D movement tracking, providing instructions and feedback for rehabilitation and training purposes. The Kinect can easily connect to a computer using a USB port and customized software can be developed using Microsoft's Kinect Software Development Kit. Using the Kinect, body movement and facial expressions can be tracked to provide instruction and/or feedback. Gonzalez-Ortega et al. (2014) used these functions to create a rehabilitation platform for left-right confusion, which is a cognitive disability where people are not able to identify left and right parts or sides of objects and people. Rehabilitation exercises were determined and delivered through a video and monitored through the integrated Kinect and computer software, and then saved to a patient file for progress tracking by therapists. Therapists could then modify the sequence and number of exercises to suit the patient's needs. Preliminary testing completed with this technology in ten healthy individuals, two individuals with frontal lobe injury, and three individuals with mild dementia was promising. It was successful 96.28% of the time it correctly monitoring tasks, although researchers found that improvements needed to be made in identifying movements toward the ear and compensating for any moving or turning of the head. Furthermore, two individuals with dementia said they would want assistance while using the program. More research and development of this application needs to be done, but it shows that human movement tracking with the Kinect device could be used for cognitive therapeutic applications with the benefit of having an inexpensive, off-the-shelf device that can provide and track therapy outside of the therapist's office (Gonzalez-Ortega et al., 2014).

Computer-driven software can also be used to assist as a different mode of therapy for children with autism spectrum disorder (Bauminger-Zviely, Eden, Zancanaro, Weiss, & Gal, 2013; Wass & Porayska-Pomsta, 2014). Bauminger-Zviely et al. (2013) used a computer program to teach social conversation to 22 children with an autism spectrum disorder. Children in this study showed improvements in concept clarification, problem-solving ability, and some improvements in social engagement. Software also has the benefits of being modifiable and creating outputs to provide feedback to therapists, who can then change the training or therapy to fit the individual better. Other computer-based interventions for children with autism spectrum disorder have also been shown to be useful for social skill development. However, training children regarding emotion and face recognition and social skills has proven to be more of a challenge, as success in the training through computer software does not always translate to those skills presenting in real-life situations (Wass & Porayska-Pomsta, 2014).

19.4.3 Education

Computer-driven software to assist with learning in an educational setting can be extremely helpful for children and young adults with learning disabilities who can benefit from customization and strategies aimed at maintaining engagement (Weng, Maeda, & Bouck, 2014). Additionally, students with disabilities can benefit from features within an e-learning environment that can adapt to their needs and assist in learning. The ideal educational computer technology or software not only provides accessible content, it also is accessible in the design and function of the computer or software. This includes functions for people with visual or hearing impairments, such as screen reading or closed captioning. It also includes personalization functions for people with other cognitive or mobility impairments, including preference changes for larger buttons or text, control settings, and compatibility with other assistive technology that allows users with cognitive impairments to interact with accessible learning content (Laabidi, Jemni, Jemni Ben Ayed, Ben Brahim, & Ben Jemaa, 2014). For educational purposes, computer-driven software should use proven instructional methods with adaptive preferences for personalization, be aimed at maintaining attention and engagement, and provide useful feedback, either to an instructor or a student (Weng et al., 2014).

One example of how assistive technology is applied to education is $Moodle^{Acc+}$, developed by Laabidi et al. (2014) using the e-learning platform, Moodle. $Moodle^{Acc+}$ was developed with a "Learner Assistance Tool," where the user can choose their disability and edit preferences to personalize settings based on the needs of their impairments. Based on the preferences and disability information provided, the "Accessible Course Generation Tool" then adapts the content of the e-learning material. An "Author Assistance Tool" allows for further personalization and addition of alternative modes to relay the information. The overall goal of this adapted e-learning platform was to create better access to content for people with a variety of disabilities who have different needs. Although this research is ongoing and has not yet been tested with individuals with disabilities, it is important to consider alternative and accessible features to make electronic or online educational content fully accessible to those with cognitive disabilities.

Children with learning disabilities generally need assistance and adaptations in the classroom in order to succeed in an educational environment. Sometimes this can be a difficult task for teachers when there are different levels of disability and levels of learning in a single classroom. Computer-based software can be a useful form of cognitive technology that has the ability to adjust to the differing levels of ability and engagement of children with learning disabilities. One example of computer-based software proven helpful in an educational setting is *Strategic Reader.*

Strategic Reader is a digital reading environment that assists in maintaining engagement while reading to learn with preferences that can be changed to adapt teaching to the needs of each individual child. Children can read books that a teacher assigns while answering questions and being encouraged to use learning strategies throughout the reading. Additionally, *Strategic Reader* has an integrated assessment tool that the teacher can assign at any time to monitor a child's learning progress. This tool was implemented in 14 middle school classrooms with ten teachers, 307 students total, 73 students with disabilities, and 64 of those with learning disabilities to test the functionality and applicability of *Strategic Reader.* All students were split into two treatment groups with one group using the online *Strategic Reader* and the other group using a pencil and paper format with the same reading content. Students were tested pre- and post-intervention using a standardized reading comprehension test to track progress. Students were also surveyed at the end of the study, and teachers were interviewed about their experience using this tool. All students had a significant improvement in reading comprehension scores with both the online and offline versions of the program. However, children with learning disabilities benefitted the most from the online learning environment with a significant increase in reading comprehension scores using *Strategic Reader* online as compared with no significant increase in reading comprehension scores for students with learning disabilities in the offline group. When implemented in an actual classroom setting, teachers were able to better personalize and track learning, and students showed significant improvement when using *Strategic Reader.* Furthermore, the adaptive online environment and feedback were particularly beneficial for middle school students with learning disabilities (Hall, Cohen, Vue, & Ganley, 2015).

In addition to using Microsoft's Kinect device for training and therapy, it can also be used as an educational tool to aid learning in children with disabilities. Deb (2015) designed software for the Kinect device for children to draw and identify objects. The camera would identify an object for a child to draw, for example, a shape. Then the voice recorder would pick up the word that the child named it. The system would assess for accuracy by having the child do this for each object more than one time. This is a strategy a child could use to practice drawing shapes, numbers, letters, and so on in a more interactive environment. The system was tested in four children with cognitive disabilities. All subjects were taught content with traditional textbook learning with a test following the lesson. A few days later, they were taught the same content using the Kinect system and took a test again. When learning through this mode versus textbook learning, the children with disabilities used to test this system scored much higher on tests following the teaching of content through learning with the Kinect software. However, children were taught the same content and the order of interventions was not randomized. Although this is a promising educational environment for more interactive learning, more tests need to be done in a larger group with randomized treatment conditions.

19.5 Virtual reality

Virtual reality (VR) is a technology that can be used for training and rehabilitation in a computer-generated environment. This virtual environment creates a space for users to interact with the environment and simulate experiences that might happen in their daily lives. This gives users an opportunity to train and rehabilitate in a safe setting and continually work on the same skills (Joseph, Mazaux, & Sorita, 2012; Klinger, 2013; Rispoli et al., 2014). VR can run on a computer that uses a joystick or other controller for movement in a 3D environment or can involve a headset that immerses a person in a virtual world, where physical tracking of the person lets them act in that virtual world (Joseph et al., 2012; Wass & Porayska-Pomsta, 2014). An example of a VR headset that can be used with a simple mobile phone to view videos, things, places, and so on is shown in Figure 19.3.

19.5.1 Training/therapy

VR can be particularly useful in re-training for people who have an acquired brain injury where people can experience and react to simulated activities of daily living, such as appointment visits, shopping, banking, and driving

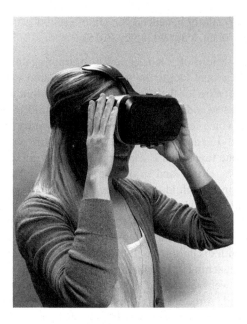

Figure 19.3 VR technology used as a headset.

(Cox et al., 2010; Joseph et al., 2012; Rispoli et al., 2014). VR can provide a way to practice different skills without fear of running into problems in the real world or as a way to practice skills when someone may not yet be ready to start rehabilitation. A person with acquired brain injury can simulate real-world experiences using different controllers, such as a computer keyboard or joystick, when they are not yet mobile (Joseph et al., 2012).

AGATHE is a project that uses VR to assist therapists to create customizable simulated activities of daily living for rehabilitation purposes, specifically for people with acquired brain injury. AGATHE can present predetermined tasks to patients while monitoring activity in real-time so therapists can assess the patient. The predetermined tasks and VR experiences were co-designed with therapists and doctors to provide applicable VR experiences for rehabilitation. Only two pilot tests have been done so far, but they indicate that therapists were able to customize experiences to assist in rehabilitation based on the needs of patients with acquired brain injury. Research is ongoing, but AGATHE is a promising example of an application of VR that can help customize therapy for individuals with acquired brain injury (Klinger, 2013).

VR can provide a safe space for people with intellectual disabilities to practice important situations of daily living that not only assist them in interacting with others in social situations, but also simulate situations that can teach them how to keep themselves safe (den Brok & Sterkenburg, 2015). In addition, VR can create a reinforcing environment to practice different task completion strategies with assistance (Joseph et al., 2012). VR has also been used as a mode of therapy to train people with autism spectrum disorder on how to react in real-world situations. This VR practice can make them more comfortable and perhaps help them to stay safe in real-world situations. Children with autism spectrum disorder can also benefit from therapy interventions using VR to simulate virtual people, where the child can decide how to interact with the person and the therapist can adjust different aspects and emotions of the virtual person (Wass & Porayska-Pomsta, 2014).

19.6 Social assistive robots

Social assistive robots (SARs) are robots that interact with a person with cognitive disabilities in order to provide a more engaging mode of assistance, therapy, or assessment. SARs have been used to assist in activities of daily living for older adults with cognitive impairments and also provide stimulation (Drake, 2012; Granata et al., 2013). SARs can assist with therapy, specifically with children, to encourage learning of social interaction and processing and aid in progression inside and outside of standard therapy (Kozyavkin, Kachmar, & Abilkova, 2014; Malik, Yussof, & Hanapiah; Shamsuddin et al., 2012). Additionally, SARs can have built-in assessment features to aid clinicians in progress assessment for children with cognitive disabilities, who may need greater stimulation and engagement for an accurate assessment (Encarnacao et al., 2014; Malik et al.).

19.6.1 Activities of daily living

SARs can be one form of cognitive technology used to assist older adults with cognitive impairments to complete or engage in activities of daily living. Granata et al. (2013) tested the usability of a robot called Kompaï that was specifically intended to assist older adults with daily living ("Kompai Robotics: Help for frail people and caregivers,"). Granata et al. (2013) specifically tested the usability of the shopping list and agenda functions of Kompaï with 11 older adults who had mild cognitive impairments and 11 healthy older adults. Even though the older adults with cognitive impairments took longer and made more errors, both groups were able to use the functions with minimal help and performance improved with practice.

Additionally, SARs can provide interaction and entertainment for people with cognitive disabilities when a caregiver cannot always be available to entertain someone who may be home- or care-facility bound. When someone with cognitive disabilities may not have the capacity to be able to care for an animal, an interactive robotic animal could take the place of a pet. Therefore, SARs can also provide stimulation and sense of purpose for people with cognitive disabilities (Drake, 2012).

19.6.2 Training/therapy

Social assistive robots can function as a training tool that can be used for people with intellectual disabilities and serve as a form of interactive teaching for deficits in processing and social communication. Most robots are used with the intent to engage the user in play and encourage interaction in an appealing way. This can be done by allowing control of the robot or having the robot respond to visual or verbal cues (den Brok & Sterkenburg, 2015). Figure 19.4 shows a child interacting with a SAR intended to introduce play to a therapy session.

Children with autism spectrum disorder can benefit from therapy using SARs, as robots are predictable, which people with autism spectrum disorder often prefer. SARs also bring an element of play into therapy for children. SARs can be programmed to mirror and react in ways that can help teach children with autism spectrum disorder how to share, which can hopefully translate to the concept of sharing with their peers (Wass & Porayska-Pomsta, 2014).

SARs are particularly useful for children as they are like using a toy for training exercises and therapy (Malik et al.). One example is the *CosmoBot*, which can be controlled by both the therapist and the child. The *CosmoBot* was used in physical therapy in a study with six children between the ages of four and six years old with cerebral palsy who used the *CosmoBot* in therapy for 16 weeks. Therapists reported that the robot was easy to use and created a play atmosphere for therapy that children enjoyed. All six children were motivated by therapy with this SAR,

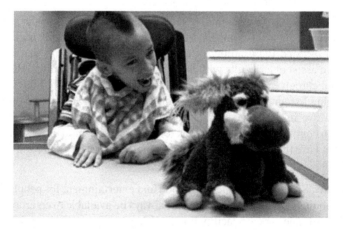

Figure 19.4 Child interacting with a SAR during therapy.

and at the end of the intervention period, four of the six children showed improvements in upper extremity strength and three children showed improvements in coordination. This study was done on a small group of children, but it suggests that SARs can be a fun way to deliver therapy for young children with cerebral palsy (Brisben, Safos, Lockerd, Vice, & Lathan).

KineTron is another SAR that was pre-programmed with movements and noises based on how the child communicated with the robot. This study also used six children with cerebral palsy to test the use of this SAR, and children were between four and nine years old. *KineTron* was used in physical therapy for all children for five to seven sessions for 20 minutes. Again, a study with the SAR reported that all children involved were motivated by engaging with the SAR during rehabilitation therapy. However, there were no clinical outcomes that were used in this study, so it can only suggest that a SAR can create a play environment for young children that can help keep them engaged in therapy (Kozyavkin et al., 2014).

A case and pilot study on the response of a ten-year-old boy with autism spectrum disorder to a SAR was done to test how a child with autism could benefit from using a SAR for therapeutic purposes. The SAR used five different modules that encouraged interaction during a therapy session. The child's autistic behavior was suppressed, and more eye contact was made with the robot than was usually made with the therapist. Although this was a case study that only applied to one child, it suggests that SARs may be a useful therapeutic tactic to encourage social interaction in children with autism spectrum disorder (Shamsuddin et al., 2012).

19.6.3 Assessment

SARs can also have integrated assessment functions (Encarnacao et al., 2014; Malik et al.). Current cognitive assessments may not be completely accurate for children with severe motor and/or communication impairments, as they involve question-and-answer through pointing or eye gaze. Children may have a hard time staying engaged and interested with this type of assessment, leading to an underestimation of their abilities (Encarnacao et al., 2014).

NAO is an example of a SAR that has been tested on two children with cerebral palsy for an eight-week intervention. *NAO* is intended to provide engagement in encouraging therapeutic exercises and is intended to assess the common test measurements of gross motor function, time up and go, and comprehensive trail making. Therapists validated the exercises that *NAO* provided as suitable to assess the intended measures. Both children were able to do the therapy exercises with the robot through imitation learning. However, scores for comprehensive trail making and time up and go tasks only changed minimally. Though testing to improve clinical outcomes is still ongoing, this study suggests that a SAR can help deliver therapy in a fun way for young children (Malik et al.).

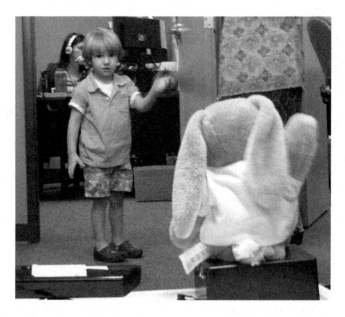

Figure 19.5 Child mirroring a SAR.

Encarnacao et al. (2014) used play activities with a virtual SAR to try to better assess children with cognitive disabilities by sustaining engagement and using play. Twenty typically developing children and nine children with cerebral palsy between the ages of 2.5 and 5.5 years old participated in this study. The virtual robot was used because, as a software version, it was cheaper and easier to maintain and update than a real robot. A virtual robot also has the advantage of having software preferences to make the environment more interesting for each individual child. They were able to create play activities for four different skill development assessments and tested the difference between these activities with an actual robot versus the virtual robot. They found that children were able to perform similarly in the same assessment activities with the virtual robot and the physical robot, suggesting that a virtual robot may be a good alternative when a therapist does not have access to or technical expertise for a physical SAR. In addition to providing a stimulating way to provide therapy to children with cognitive disorders, it can provide therapists with an additional assessment tool to help track progress. Figure 19.5 shows a child mirroring movements that might typically be completed during therapy as a tool to help with assessment.

19.7 Smart home technology

Smart home technology can be useful in helping to manage the daily activities of people with cognitive disabilities in order to improve independence. Smart home

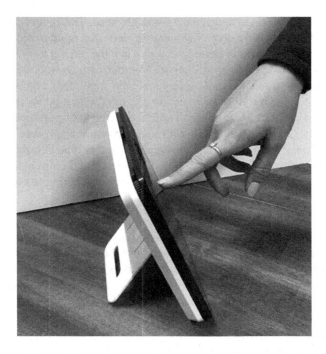

Figure 19.6 Smart home technology to consolidate functions of the home.

technology can include various motion, temperature, electrical, water use, and sound sensors throughout a living space. These sensors can be used to collect information and provide audible feedback to people in the home if water, lights, appliances, and so on are left on or if other daily patterns are out of the ordinary. Smart home technology can also include control panels that allow people with cognitive and mobility disabilities to perform different functions throughout their living space in a more accessible way (Boman, Lindberg Stenvall, Hemmingsson, & Bartfai, 2010; Drake, 2012; Giroux et al., 2015; Rispoli et al., 2014). Additionally, smart home cognitive technology can provide 24-hour access to assistance, which can help to supplement and reduce the costs of caregivers for people with cognitive disabilities (Drake, 2012). Figure 19.6 shows a smart home device designed to link with and control other smart technology throughout the home at the touch of a finger.

19.7.1 Activities of daily living

Boman et al. (2010) used electronic memory aids in an apartment setting, utilizing a main computer, control panels or doors, windows and the TV, and a variety of kitchen alarms. The main computer assisted with scheduling and the general

483

organization of information that a person might need. The control panels served to prompt the user when a door or window was left open or unlocked or a TV was left on. The kitchen alarms alerted the user when the refrigerator or freezer was left open or the stove or water was left on. Fourteen patients who were recovering from a stroke or traumatic brain injury and who were medically stable enough to stay alone in the training apartment for five days were used for this study. An occupational therapist assessed the use of the apartment by participants throughout the study. Overall, participants with acquired brain injury were able to learn to use the "smart" apartment, and it indicated that this type of technology could not only keep those with acquired brain injury safer and more independent but could also serve as a way to provide training in remembering to complete tasks on their own.

Giroux et al. (2015) created a community living lab for people with TBI with integrated smart home technology to assist with activities of daily living and independence. The living lab had sensors and interactive technology throughout the living space for ten people. One feature of the living lab was a cooking assistant intended to provide assistance and feedback to the residents with TBI to improve autonomy and assure safety during meal preparation. The evaluation of the effectiveness and usefulness of this living lab is currently ongoing, and future case studies are the intended next step to try to personalize prompting systems for activities of daily living for people with TBI.

Smart home technology can also be helpful for older adults who are developing cognitive impairments or Alzheimer's disease to remain in their homes longer with more independence. Prompting technology fed by sensors can help with reminders and task completion in the home to keep older adults independent and safe (Lapointe et al., 2013). Lapointe et al. (2013) used a test smart apartment to evaluate different smart home technologies for people with cognitive impairments. Preliminary data was collected from an unknown number of subjects. This data suggests that in a smart home setting, people with cognitive impairments should be familiarized with the smart home technology and prompting technology should provide an alert prompt to gain attention before providing task assistance. Additionally, it suggested that video prompting with sound was the most effective method of prompting for smart home technology. Although this study is ongoing, the preliminary data is promising to suggest that smart home technology can be effective for task completion assistance for people with cognitive disabilities.

19.8 Future vision

As discussed in the introduction to this chapter, cognitive technologies provide a new and often unique approach to facilitating the lives of persons with cognitive impairments. Much of the work is still in early stage development and there is obviously a great deal of research and development needed across these promising technologies before any real conclusions can be drawn.

However, the aging demographics around the world have captured the attention of both mainstream and assistive technology developers. This market force will serve to drive the development of untold numbers of readily accessible and cognitively friendly devices and services over the next several decades. This benefits both children and adults with cognitive disabilities. For example, as simplified interfaces for mainstream products such as microwave ovens, entertainment systems, and so on become more usable for seniors (simpler text/fewer buttons, more visible icons, etc.), these technologies will also become more usable by persons of all ages with cognitive impairments.

It is highly possible to imagine a future, not too far away, where smart homes can work to the advantage of persons with a traumatic brain injury, stroke, or autism. Social engagement can be supplemented or supported through the use of socially assistive robots or immediate access to another person through face-to-face interaction technologies.

As we continue to learn more about how the brain functions, and how to support therapeutic cognitive interventions, technology will play a key role. Untold millions of individuals around the world will require access to cognitive interventions and there simply will not be enough personnel to provide individual one-on-one treatment. Supplemental interventions to support clinical treatment will be a critical and identified need in the decades to come.

The projected increases in the aging population and the need for persons aging with cognitive disabilities to continue to live at home will also place unbearable stress on our current healthcare system. Smart home technologies personalized to the individual's cognitive and healthcare needs are a robust and emerging market. It too will continue to expand over the coming years.

As our population ages and individuals acquiring or born with cognitive disabilities live a typical lifespan, we will experience an expanded workforce that includes older adults and working-age adults with disabilities. This will require a need for workplace accommodations and tools that are readily accessible for those who need them to be competitive in the workplace.

Thirty years ago, little recognition was given to supporting persons with cognitive impairments through technology. In fact, when Section 508 of the Americans with Disabilities Act was published (1990), requiring reasonable accommodations for persons with disabilities, cognitive access was completely overlooked because of its perceived difficulty and the many biases prevalent in the mainstream community. Today, we recognize we must work to create assistive and commercial technologies that have the potential to improve the lives of this very worthy population.

19.9 Discussion questions

1. What differences in cognitive functioning might you see between a twelve-year-old with autism and an eighty-year-old who has early stage dementia?
2. What are the potential differences between someone who is born with a congenital cognitive disability and someone who acquires a cognitive disability as an adult? What differences in learning, experiential knowledge, and independence might you see?
3. Why is cognitively accessible technology so important for persons with cognitive impairments?
4. How can we improve current designs to facilitate human-computer interactions for persons with cognitive disabilities?
5. What types of smart home technologies and features can you envision for the future?
6. What are some features that should be included in social assistive robots to enable persons with cognitive impairments to learn?
7. How would you feel about working side-by-side with someone who has a cognitive disability? Would it make you uncomfortable? Would it impact your performance at work?
8. Why is there even a need to create additional technologies for persons with cognitive disabilities?
9. How can current computer- and tablet-based applications be improved for persons with cognitive impairments? Children? Adults? Seniors?
10. How should we evaluate the success or failure of cognitive technologies?
11. What makes research and development of technologies designed for persons with cognitive impairments so challenging?
12. What makes research and development of cognitive technologies so rewarding?

Bibliography

2010 Census Data. (2014). Retrieved from http://factfinder2.census.gov.

Agree, E. M. (2014). The potential for technology to enhance independence for those aging with a disability. *Disability and Health Journal*, 7(1 Suppl), S33–39. doi:10.1016/j.dhjo.2013.09.004.

AOA Administration on Aging. (2014). Retrieved from http://www.aoa.gov.

Bates, G., Tabrizi, S., & Jones, L. (2014). *Huntington's disease*. Oxford, UK: Oxford University Press.

Bauminger-Zviely, N., Eden, S., Zancanaro, M., Weiss, P. L., & Gal, E. (2013). Increasing social engagement in children with high-functioning autism spectrum disorder using collaborative technologies in the school environment. *Autism, 17*(3), 317–339. doi:10.1177/1362361312472989.

Blake, D. J., & Bodine, C. (2002). An overview of assistive technology for persons with multiple sclerosis. *Journal of Rehabilitation Research and Development, 39*(2), 299.

Bodine, C. (2007). Aging well: The use of assistive technology to enhance the lives of elders. In *Universal Acess in Human Computer Interaction. Coping with Diversity*, 861–867.

Boger, J., & Mihailidis, A. (2011). The future of intelligent assistive technologies for cognition: Devices under development to support independent living and aging-with-choice. *NeuroRehabilitation, 28*(3), 271–280.

Boman, I. L., Lindberg Stenvall, C., Hemmingsson, H., & Bartfai, A. (2010). A training apartment with a set of electronic memory aids for patients with cognitive problems. *Scandinavian Journal of Occupational Therapy, 17*(2), 140–148. doi:10.3109/11038120902875144.

Brisben, A. J., Safos, C. S., Lockerd, A. D., Vice, J. M., & Lathan, C. E. (2005). *The CosmoBot™ system: Evaluating its usability in therapy sessions with children diagnosed with cerebral palsy*. Cambridge, MA: MIT.

Burstein, R., Zhang, X., Levy, D., Aoki, K. R., & Brin, M. F. (2014). Selective inhibition of meningeal nociceptors by botulinum neurotoxin type A: Therapeutic implications for migraine and other pains. *Cephalalgia, 34*(11), 853–869.

Chang, Y. J., Chen, S. F., & Huang, J. D. (2011). A Kinect-based system for physical rehabilitation: A pilot study for young adults with motor disabilities. *Research in Developmental Disabilities, 32*(6), 2566–2570. doi:10.1016/j.ridd.2011.07.002.

Christensen, K., Doblhammer, G., Rau, R., & Vaupel, J. W. (2009). Ageing populations: The challenges ahead. *The Lancet, 374*(9696), 1196–1208. doi:10.1016/S0140-6736(09)61460-4.

Chu, Y., Brown, P., Harniss, M., Kautz, H., & Johnson, K. (2014). Cognitive support technologies for people with TBI: Current usage and challenges experienced. *Disability and Rehabilitation: Assistive Technology, 9*(4), 279–285. doi:10.3109/17483107.2013.823631.

Cornish, K., Turk, J., & Hagerman, R. (2008). The fragile X continuum: New advances and perspectives. *Journal of Intellectual Disability Research, 52*(Pt 6), 469–482. doi:10.1111/j.1365-2788.2008.01056.x.

Cox, D. J., Davis, M., Singh, H., Barbour, B., Nidiffer, F. D., Trudel, T., … Moncrief, R. (2010). Driving rehabilitation for military personnel recovering from traumatic brain injury using virtual reality driving simulation: A feasibility study. *Military Medicine, 175*(6), 411–416.

Dams-O'Connor, K., Mellick, D., Dreer, L. E., Hammond, F. M., Hoffman, J., Landau, A., … Pretz, C. (2017). Rehospitalization over 10 years among survivors of TBI: A National Institute on Disability, Independent Living, and Rehabilitation Research Traumatic Brain Injury Model Systems Study. *The Journal of Head Trauma Rehabilitation, 32*(3), 147–157.

Deb, S. S., & Bhattacharya, P. (2015). Blended interaction for augmented learning - An assistive tool for cognitive disability. Paper presented at the *12th International Conference on Cognition and Exploratory Learning in Digital Age (CELDA)*. Maynooth, Ireland.

Demers, L., Jutai, J. W., Fuhrer, M. J., Lenker, J. A., & DeRuyter, F. (2007). Advancing assistive technology outcomes research in aging. Paper presented at the *Festival of International Conferences on Caregiving, Disability, Aging and Technology*, Toronto, ON.

den Brok, W. L., & Sterkenburg, P. S. (2015). Self-controlled technologies to support skill attainment in persons with an autism spectrum disorder and/or an intellectual disability: A systematic literature review. *Disability and Rehabilitation: Assistive Technology, 10*(1), 1–10. doi:10.3109/17483107.2014.921248.

Dibia, V., Trewin, S., Ashoori, M., & Erickson, T. (2015). Exploring the potential of wearables to support employment for people with mild cognitive impairment. *ASSETS 2015 Proceedings of the 17th International ACM SIGACCESS Conference on Computers & Accessibility.* 401–402. doi:10.1145/2700648.2811390.

Drake, M. (2012). Cognitive and assistive technologies in care practice: A view from the delivery end. Paper presented at the *EUCogIII*, University of Sussex.

Encarnacao, P., Alvarez, L., Rios, A., Maya, C., Adams, K., & Cook, A. (2014). Using virtual robot-mediated play activities to assess cognitive skills. *Disability and Rehabilitation: Assistive Technology, 9*(3), 231–241. doi:10.3109/17483107.2013.782577.

Escobedo, L., Nguyen, D. H., Boyd, L., Hirano, S., Rangel, A., Garcia-Rosas, D., … Hayes, G. (2012). MOSOCO: A mobile assistive tool to support children with autism practicing social skills in real-life situations. *CHI 2012 Proceedings of the SIGCHI Conference on Human Factors in Computing Systems*, 2589–2598. doi:10.1145/2207676.2208649.

Evald, L. (2015). Prospective memory rehabilitation using smartphones in patients with TBI: What do participants report? *Neuropsychological Rehabilitation, 25*(2), 283–297. doi:1 0.1080/09602011.2014.970557.

Fanaroff, A. A., Stoll, B. J., Wright, L. L., Carlo, W. A., Ehrenkranz, R. A., Stark, A. R., … Poole, W. K. (2007). Trends in neonatal morbidity and mortality for very low birthweight infants. *American Journal of Obstetrics and Gynecology, 196*(2), 147.e141–147. e148. doi:10.1016/j.ajog.2006.09.014.

Finkelstein, E. A., Corso, P. S., & Miller, T. R. (2006). *The incidence and economic burden of injuries in the United States.* New York: Oxford University Press.

Fischer, H. (2010). *U.S. military casualty statistics: Operation new dawn, operation Iraqi freedom, and operation enduring freedom.* Washington, DC: Congressional Research Service.

Garber, K. B., Visootsak, J., & Warren, S. T. (2008). Fragile X syndrome. *European Journal of Human Genetics: EJHG, 16*(6), 666.

Giroux, S., Bier, N., Pigot, H., Bouchard, B., Bouzouane, A., Levasseur, M., … Le Pévédic, B. (2015). Cognitive assistance to meal preparation: Design, implementation, and assessment in a living lab. Paper presented at the *Ambient Intelligence for Health and Cognitive Enhancement, AAAI Spring Symposium.* Paolo Alto, CA.

Gomez J. X. A. M. G. T. J. C. (2014). AmICog--mobile technologies to assist people with cognitive disabilities in the work place. *Advances in Distributed Computing and Artificial Intelligence Journal, 1*(4), 9–17. doi:10.14201ADECAIJ201317917.

Gonzalez-Ortega, D., Diaz-Pernas, F. J., Martinez-Zarzuela, M., & Anton-Rodriguez, M. (2014). A Kinect-based system for cognitive rehabilitation exercises monitoring. *Computer Methods and Programs in Biomedicine, 113*(2), 620–631. doi:10.1016/j.cmpb.2013.10.014.

Granata, C., Pino, M., Legouverneur, G., Vidal, J. S., Bidaud, P., & Rigaud, A. S. (2013). Robot services for elderly with cognitive impairment: Testing usability of graphical user interfaces. *Technol Health Care, 21*(3), 217–231. doi:10.3233/THC-130718.

Gunther, E. J., Sliker, L. J., & Bodine, C. (2017). A UHF RFID positioning system for use in warehouse navigation by employees with cognitive disability. *Disability and Rehabilitation: Assistive Technology, 12*(8), 832–842. doi:10.1080/17483107.2016.1274342.

Hall, T. E., Cohen, N., Vue, G., & Ganley, P. (2015). Addressing learning disabilities with UDL and technology. *Learning Disability Quarterly, 38*(2), 72–83. doi:10.1177/0731948714544375.

Hammel, J. (2000). Assistive technology and environmental intervention (AT-EI) impact on the activity and life roles of aging adults with developmental disabilities: Findings and implication for practice. *Aging and Developmental Disability, 18*(1), 37–58.

Hammel, J., Jones, R., Smith, J., Sanford, J., Bodine, C., & Johnson, M. (2008). Environmental barriers and supports to the health, function, and participation of people with developmental and intellectual disabilities: Report from the State of the Science in Aging with Developmental Disabilities Conference. *Disability and Health Journal, 1*(3), 143–149.

Hartmann, K. D. (2010). Assistive technology: A compensatory strategy for work production post mild brain injury. *Work, 36*(4), 399–404. doi:10.3233/wor-2010-1048.

Helal, A., Mokhtari, M., & Abdulrazak, B. (Eds.). (2008). *The engineering handbook of smart technology for aging, disability and independence.* Hoboken, NJ: John Wiley & Sons.

Jamieson, M., Cullen, B., McGee-Lennon, M., Brewster, S., & Evans, J. J. (2014). The efficacy of cognitive prosthetic technology for people with memory impairments: A systematic review and meta-analysis. *Neuropsychological Rehabilitation, 24*(3–4), 419–444. doi:1 0.1080/09602011.2013.825632.

Joseph, P. A., Mazaux, J. M., & Sorita, E. (2012). Virtual reality for cognitive rehabilitation: From new use of computers to better knowledge of brain black box? Paper presented at the *9th Intl Conf Disability*, Laval, France.

Kelly-Hayes, M., Robertson, J. T., Broderick, J. P., Duncan, P. W., Hershey, L. A., Roth, E. J., ... Trombly, C. A. (1998). The American Heart Association stroke outcome classification. *Stroke, 29*, 1274–1280.

Kim, S., Larson, S. A., & Charlie Lakin, K. (2001). Behavioural outcomes of deinstitutionalisation for people with intellectual disability: A review of US studies conducted between 1980 and 1999. *Journal of Intellectual and Developmental Disability, 26*(1), 35–50. doi:10.1080/13668250020032750.

Klinger, E., Kadri, A., Sorita, E., Le Guiet, J.-L., Coignard, P., Fuchs, P., Leroy, L., Du Lac, N., Servant, F., & Joseph, P.-A. (2013). AGATHE: A tool for personalized rehabilitation of cognitive functions based on simulated activites of daily living. *IRBM, 34*(2), 113–118. doi:10.1016/j.irbm.2013.01.005.

Kompai Robotics: Help for frail people and caregivers. Retrieved from https://kompai.com/.

Kozyavkin, V., Kachmar, O., & Abilkova, I. (2014). Humanoid social robots in the rehabilitation of children with cerebral palsy. *REHAB, Pervasive Health 2014 Proceedings of the 8th International Conference on Pervasive Computing Technologies for Healthcare,* 430–431.

Laabidi, M., Jemni, M., Jemni Ben Ayed, L., Ben Brahim, H., & Ben Jemaa, A. (2014). Learning technologies for people with disabilities. *Journal of King Saud University - Computer and Information Sciences, 26*(1), 29–45. doi:10.1016/j.jksuci.2013.10.005.

Langlois, J. A., Rutland-Brown, W., & Wald, M. M. (2006). The epidemiology and impact of traumatic brain injury: A brief overview. *The Journal of Head Trauma Rehabilitation, 21*(5), 375–378.

Lapointe, J., Bouchard, J., Verreault, A., Potvin, A., Bouchard, B., & Bouzouane, A. (2013). How to maximize the effectiveness of prompts in assistive technologies according to the particular cognitive profile of people with Alzheimer's disease? *International Journal of Smart Home, 7*(5), 19–38. doi:10.14257/ijsh.2013.7.5.03.

Leopold, A., Lourie, A., Petras, H., & Elias, E. (2015). The use of assistive technology for cognition to support the performance of daily activities for individuals with cognitive disabilities due to traumatic brain injury: The current state of the research. *NeuroRehabilitation, 37*(3), 359–378. doi:10.3233/NRE-151267.

Lindenberger, U., Lovden, M., Schellenbach, M., Li, S. C., & Kruger, A. (2008). Psychological principles of successful aging technologies: A mini-review. *Gerontology, 54*(1), 59–68.

Lotharius, J., & Brundin, P. (2002). Pathogenesis of Parkinson's disease: Dopamine, vesicles and [alpha]-synuclein. *Nature Reviews. Neuroscience, 3*(12), 932.

489

Malik, A. N., Yussof, H., & Hanapiah, F. A. Potential use of social assistive robot based rehabilitation for children with cerebral palsy. 2016 *2nd IEEE International Symposium on Robotics and Manufacturing Automation (ROMA)*, pp. 1–6. University of Teknologi MARA.

McDonald, A., Haslam, C., Yates, P., Gurr, B., Leeder, G., & Sayers, A. (2011). Google Calendar: A new memory aid to compensate for prospective memory deficits following acquired brain injury. *Neuropsychological Rehabilitation*, *21*(6), 784–807. doi:10.1080/09602011.2011.598405.

Mechling, L. C., & Savidge, E. J. (2011). Using a personal digital assistant to increase completion of novel tasks and independent transitioning by students with autism spectrum disorder. *Journal of Autism and Developmental Disorders*, *41*(6), 687–704. doi:10.1007/s10803-010-1088-6.

Mosner, E., Spiezle, C., and Emerman, J. (2003). *The convergence of the aging workforce and accessible technology*. Seattle, WA: Microsoft Corporation.

O'Neill, B., Best, C., Gillespie, A., & O'Neill, L. (2013). Automated prompting technologies in rehabilitation and at home. *Social Care and Neurodisability*, *4*(1), 17–28. doi:10.1108/20420911311302281

Pew, R., & Hemel, S. (2004). *Technology for adaptive aging*. Washington, DC: National Academies Press.

Plassman, B. L., Langa, K. M., Fisher, G. G., Heeringa, S. G., Weir, D. R., Ofstedal, M. B., … Wallace, R. B. (2008). Prevalence of cognitive impairment without dementia in the United States. *Annals of Internal Medicine*, *148*(6), 427–434. doi:10.7326/0003-481 9-148-6-200803180-00005

Prince, M., Bryce, R., Albanese, E., Wimo, A., Ribeiro, W., & Ferri, C. P. (2013). The global prevalence of dementia: A systematic review and metaanalysis. *Alzheimer's & Dementia*, *9*(1), 63–75. e62.

Prince, M. J. (2015). *World Alzheimer report 2015: The global impact of dementia: An analysis of prevalence, incidence, cost and trends*. London, UK: Alzheimer's Disease International.

Quayle, K. S., Holmes, J. F., & Kuppermann, N. (2014). Epidemiology of blunt head trauma in children in US emergency departments. *New England Journal of Medicine*, *371*(20), 1945–1947.

Rispoli, M., Machalicek, W., & Lang, R. (2014). *Assistive technology for people with acquired brain injury*. 21–52. New York: Springer Publishing. doi:10.1007/978-1-4899-8029-8_2.

Robinson-Riegler, B., & Robinson-Riegler, G. L. (2016). *Cognitive psychology: Applying the science of the mind*. Boston, MA: Pearson.

Ryd, C., Nygard, L., Malinowsky, C., Ohman, A., & Kottorp, A. (2015). Associations between performance of activities of daily living and everyday technology use among older adults with mild stage Alzheimer's disease or mild cognitive impairment. *Scandinavian Journal of Occupational Therapy*, *22*(1), 33–42. doi:10.3109/11038128.2014.964307.

Shamsuddin, S., Yussof, H., Ismail, L. I., Mohamed, S., Hanapiah, F. A., & Zahari, N. I. (2012). Initial response in HRI - A case study on evaluation of child with autism spectrum disorders interacting with a humanoid robot NAO. *Procedia Engineering*, *41*, 1448–1455. doi:10.1016/j.proeng.2012.07.334.

Taskforce on the Aging of the American Workforce. (2008). *Report on the taskforce on the aging of the American workforce*. Retrieved from http://www.doleta.gov/reports/FINAL_Taskforce_Report_2-11-08.pdf.

Thornton, J. E. (2002). Myths of aging or ageist stereotypes. *Educational Gerontology*, *28*(4), 301–312. doi:10.1080/036012702753590415.

Too, L., Ball, H., McGregor, I., & Hunt, N. (2014). A novel automated test battery reveals enduring behavioural alterations and cognitive impairments in survivors of murine pneumococcal meningitis. *Brain, Behavior, and Immunity, 35,* 107–124.

Van Laarhoven, T., Kraus, E., Karpman, K., Nizzi, R., & Valentino, J. (2010). A comparison of picture and video prompts to teach daily living skills to individuals with autism. *Focus on Autism and Other Developmental Disabilities, 25*(4), 195–208. doi:10.1177/1088357610380412.

Walsh, P. N., Heller, T., Schupf, N., & Van Schrojenstein Lantman-de Valk, H. (2001). Healthy ageing – Adults with intellectual disabilities: Women's health and related issues. *Journal of Applied Research in Intellectual Disabilities, 14*(3), 195–217. doi:10.1046/j.1468-3148.2001.00070.x.

Wass, S. V., & Porayska-Pomsta, K. (2014). The uses of cognitive training technologies in the treatment of autism spectrum disorders. *Autism, 18*(8), 851–871. doi:10.1177/1362361313499827.

Weng, P. L., Maeda, Y., & Bouck, E. C. (2014). Effectiveness of cognitive skills-based computer-assisted instruction for students with disabilities: A synthesis. *Remedial and Special Education, 35*(3), 167–180. doi:10.1177/0741932513514858.

Wilson-Costello, D., Friedman, H., Minich, N., Fanaroff, A. A., & Hack, M. (2005). Improved survival rates with increased neurodevelopmental disability for extremely low birth weight infants in the 1990s. *Pediatrics, 115*(4), 997–1003. doi:10.1542/peds.2004-0221.

Zülch, K. J. (2013). *Brain tumors: Their biology and pathology.* New York: Springer-Verlag.

Chapter 20 Technology for sensory impairments (vision and hearing)

J. A. Brabyn, H. Levitt,
and J.A. Miele

Contents

DOI: 10.1201/b21964-23

20.1 Chapter overview

This chapter aims to provide relevant information on sensory impairments, specifically vision and hearing. The chapter is composed of two sections, which will focus on vision and hearing technologies separately. Detailed descriptions of vision and hearing characteristics and an overview of some of the most common technologies and applications that are currently available are also explored. Overall, this chapter seeks to provide readers with an overview of past and present developments and the application of technologies to promote independence.

20.2 Introduction: Historical overview

Since the inception of what we now know as rehabilitation engineering, perhaps the majority of the field has been devoted to addressing physical disabilities. However, impairments of a sensory nature – mainly vision and hearing – can be equally disabling and efforts to address them through the application of technology have an equally long history. Spectacle lenses, sticks to detect obstacles, and ear trumpets to augment sounds have existed since time immemorial, but the growth of sensory assistive technology as we know it today is mostly a post-World War II phenomenon. The Veterans Administration at that time developed and adopted formalized procedures for use of the long cane by blind pedestrians, which carried the art of orientation and mobility well beyond the traditional carrying of a stick.

The invention of the transistor and the advent of modern electronics triggered the development of a wide variety of portable sensory enhancement and sensory substitution devices for both visual and hearing deficits. These included an array of ultrasonic and other sensory systems to aid blind mobility, as well as the first practical hearing aids. As analog electronics were augmented and to a large extent eclipsed by digital electronics and personal computing, the scope for sensory technology increased exponentially – with much of it aimed at giving blind individuals access to digital computers and deaf people access to communications. As the digital age has become the information age, much of the challenge is to give the sensory-impaired population access to the resulting blizzard of information of all types that unimpaired people take for granted.

20.3 The visually impaired population: User characteristics and needs

Based on Health Interview Surveys, the prevalence of visual impairment among American adults has been estimated at up to 9.3% (19.1 million people, including

0.7 million with blindness; Ryskulova et al. 2008), with more conservative estimates in the seven million range (Erickson, Lee, and Von Schrader 2017). The most accurate available quantitative estimates (Congdon et al. 2004), using measured binocular visual acuity rather than surveys, estimated that nearly one million Americans older than 40 years of age were legally blind (bilateral corrected acuity 20/200 or worse) and an additional 2.4 million were bilaterally visually impaired for a total of 3.3 million Americans with significant visual impairment. The National Eye Institute recently estimated that the number of US residents with blindness or visual impairment (in this case defined by worse than 20/40 or the customary level required to get a driver's license) will double by 2050 (Varma et al. 2016). Increasingly, blindness and visual impairment are often associated with co-existing sensory, motor, and/or cognitive impairments.

In infants and children, the most outstanding and increasing problem is cortical visual impairment (CVI), mainly caused by premature births associated with perinatal hypoxia resulting in brain damage – leading to a wide range of vision loss from severe to near-normal acuity but with other perceptual problems (Good 2007). Children with CVI often have other associated conditions such as cerebral palsy and developmental delay. In the adult population, older individuals make up a steadily increasing proportion of the population, and even "normal" aging results in significantly impaired vision that has practical impacts on independent living. Brabyn et al. (2007) showed that many elders with visual impairments have multiple other impairments, especially hearing deficits that affect the ability to communicate.

In general, loss or partial loss of vision can hamper many tasks in modern life including reading, travel, operation of tools and appliances, and access to various types of information such as graphics, maps, and videos. The following sections summarize available rehabilitation engineering and assistive technology solutions that aim to address these problems.

20.4 Impact of emerging visual prostheses and new medical treatments

While details are outside the scope of this chapter, there are many projects around the world to develop retinal, optic nerve, or cortical implants to restore a degree of vision in totally blind subjects. Most involve implanting arrays of electrical stimulators in the retina; perhaps the most well-known being the Argus system developed by Second Sight, and approved by the FDA in 2013 (e.g., see Mills, Jalil, and Stanga 2017). These technologies require a functional optic nerve pathway and are targeted primarily at patients who are totally blind from retinitis pigmentosa. Rehabilitation professionals will now be meeting clients who have been implanted with such prostheses, which effectively provide a type of "low vision," presenting the recipient and the professional with unique challenges in training and rehabilitation. Meanwhile, there is a race between the implant technologies and the development of medical treatments for blinding diseases, as evidenced by the recent emergence of drugs that can slow or reverse the visually disabling impacts of age-related maculopathy (Spooner et al. 2019). These medical developments are changing the nature of the blind and visually impaired population, with far fewer individuals developing the dense scotomas (blind spots) that previously characterized this condition.

20.5 Vision measures and assessment

The usual way of measuring vision is "visual acuity," a measure of resolution, expressed as a fraction of "normal" or standard resolution. For example, a person with 20/200 acuity needs a magnification of ten (or needs to be ten times closer) to resolve a high contrast letter as well as a "normally sighted" person. In the United States, this level of resolution, or a visual field extent of fewer than 20 degrees, corresponds to "legally blind," a very misleading phrase, and is mainly useful because it is the legal threshold at which individuals qualify for government aid.

Acuity from approximately 20/70 to about 20/1000 is termed "low vision"; with suitable magnification, most people in this range can read and perform many other tasks visually. At lower levels than this, vision is less useful, and the individual is often functioning as a blind person.

Visual acuity measures resolution for the small central zone of the visual field, but many common eye conditions affect other areas of the field. Retinitis pigmentosa causes a narrowing of the visual field or "tunnel vision," even though acuity in the center may be quite good for a long time. Glaucoma also causes impairments in the outer or peripheral visual field. A stroke can sometimes cause a "hemianopia," in which the individual can only see one half (left or right) of the visual field. In age-related macular degeneration, blind spots develop in or near the center of the field but are usually irregular in shape and location. Standard visual field tests may be able to map these "scotomas" crudely but testing by a skilled low vision practitioner can obtain a more accurate assessment of scotoma size, shape, and position.

It is important to note that visual acuity numbers refer only to the ability to recognize small high contrast (black on white) targets in ideal lighting. In most visually disabling diseases and pathologies, performance under less-than-ideal conditions (low contrast, low light, glare, etc.) is affected much more than standard acuity, often leading to an underestimate of the problem (J. Brabyn et al. 2004). Accordingly, the use of low contrast vision measures such as contrast sensitivity or low contrast acuity is to be encouraged in order to obtain a better understanding of real-world vision function (Figure 20.1).

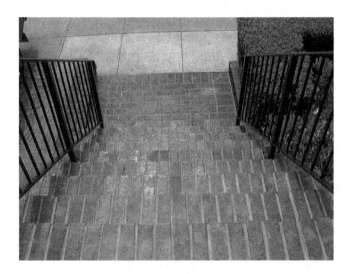

Figure 20.1 Importance of contrast: steps like this are very hard to see for anyone with reduced contrast sensitivity (due to cataracts or many other causes), even if their acuity is relatively good. Painting contrasting stripes on the edges helps tremendously (Courtesy of Roger O. Smith).

Patients with significantly reduced vision that cannot be corrected by glasses, contacts, surgery, or medical treatments should be referred to a low vision specialist, who is normally an optometrist or ophthalmologist with special expertise and resources to assess and help make the best use of the remaining vision. Low vision clinics may also include low vision therapists, teachers, or occupational therapists trained in low vision rehabilitation, who work with the client on training and using assistive technology.

20.6 Technology for reading, writing, and note taking

Reading machines. Stand-alone reading machines and optical character recognition software for computers and CCTV magnifiers are available to enable printed material to be scanned and read aloud in synthetic speech. An example of a handheld version of this technology is the KNFB Reader (knfbreader.com) now available as a smartphone app.

20.6.1 Audio recordings

Listening to audio recordings provides one way for blind and visually impaired individuals to access many publications. "Talking books" have progressed from vinyl records to cassette tapes to CDs to downloadable digital media. The "Daisy" (Digital Accessible Information System) consortium has established standards for digital recordings of books and other publications, and numerous different Daisy-compatible players are now available. For more information see http://daisy .org. Recorded newspapers and magazines are also available, for example, via the National Federation of the Blind "Newsline" service, which provides access to 400 newspapers and magazines via telephone and iPhone and iPad downloads.

20.6.2 Braille reading and writing technology

Listening to audio recordings has drawbacks for many types of materials including technical or math, and Braille provides a more active, interactive experience more closely akin to visual reading and writing. Braille literacy is almost universal among employed blind individuals (Ryles 1996). For Braille writing, the simple, highly portable slate and stylus and the mechanical Perkins Brailler are still in use, but portable electronic Braille writers and notetakers are also available. For use in conjunction with a computer, Braille translation software and personal Braille embossers have become more affordable and provide thousands of blind persons with Braille material on demand. Electronic paperless or "refreshable" Braille displays mechanically present a line of Braille characters at a time, and larger "full-page" Braille displays are nearing commercial production. Compact devices incorporating a six-key Braille keyboard for input, and speech and/or single line refreshable braille displays for output, have also become popular, providing much of the functionality that a standard notebook computer gives a sighted individual.

20.6.3 Optical low vision aids

A large array of optical magnifiers, often with built-in lighting, is available for reading. For low magnifications (two or three times), handheld or stand-mounted magnifiers can be used. "Reading telescopes" with a spectacle-type frame can facilitate comfortable posture with the head a normal distance from the reading material. If higher magnifications are needed, a strong positive lens mounted in or clipped on one spectacle lens allows the reading material to be held an inch or two away from the face, providing eight to ten times magnification compared with a normal reading distance of 16 inches.

20.6.4 "CCTV" magnifiers

Larger magnification (up to about 60 times) can be obtained with electronic systems that use cameras that display a magnified image on a visual computer or TV-type monitor. Numerous brands and variants are available, including low-cost versions with a camera that connects to the user's existing TV monitor. At the higher end, systems with features such as optical character recognition and computer interfaces are available, as are cameras that can be aimed at distant objects such as the blackboard in a classroom. Most provide features that allow users to reduce glare by reversing the polarity of print (i.e., displaying light characters on a dark background). Users can adjust the magnification, contrast, and (often) the colors displayed to meet personal preferences.

20.6.5 Pocket electronic magnifiers

In recent years, the advent of liquid-crystal displays has permitted the fabrication of handheld magnifiers incorporating the camera placed directly underneath a flat screen to form an electronic magnifier about six inches wide by three inches high and an inch thick. These devices offer a convenient means of magnification up to about 10–12 times.

20.6.6 Head-mounted electronic devices

Some versions of electronic magnifiers can be mounted on the head and used for reading text or viewing objects in the distance, such as the blackboard in a classroom or watching TV. An example of a more sophisticated version of this concept, the Orcam (Moisseiev and Mannis 2016), incorporates computer processing that analyzes the viewed image and can read it aloud to the user. The latter device can also be trained to read labels on commercial products such as food packaging.

20.6.7 Large print production

Many books are available in large print versions, and individuals can readily produce their own large print text using a computer and laser or inkjet printer. Some copy machines also allow the copied material to be magnified.

20.6.8 Low vision writing aids

CCTV magnifiers and some handheld optical and electronic magnifiers can be used as writing aids as well as for reading by placing the writing materials under the unit's camera.

20.6.9 Lighting

Good lighting is extremely important in low vision task performance since visual acuity declines rapidly in poor light. A strong reading light positioned behind the user to reduce glare, and focused on the reading material, may often improve conditions to the point where no other aid may be needed. In recent years, lighting technology has improved substantially with the introduction of halogen and LED lamps. Special reading lights are available from low vision clinics and catalogs.

20.7 Access to graphical and pictorial information

For blind individuals, access to pictorial and graphical information is still extremely difficult. However, there are a limited number of technologies and approaches that help reduce this major barrier to participation; a few examples are given in the following section.

20.7.1 Textual image description

Most website authoring software prompts the author to insert "alt text" descriptions of all images (see *Internet access*). This function can be overridden, however, so alt text is not universal.

20.7.2 Tactile and audio-tactile graphics

Although most tactile drawings are still hand-generated, there is increasing production of tactile images with computer-driven Braille embossers. For example, the View Plus "Tiger" embosser can produce dots of variable heights, placed closer together than standard Braille dot spacing. To help a blind user explore a tactile graphic, different hardware and software combinations have been developed with synthetic speech output. For example, the Talking Tactile Tablet from Touch Graphics combines a touch tablet with a tactile graphic overlay, interfaced to a computer to produce a talking map with programmed descriptions that are enunciated when the user presses any particular point on the map. Another example is the Smart Pen system from the same manufacturer, which allows a user to tap on any part of the graphic once, twice, or multiple times and hear several layers of pre-programmed information about the point being explored.

20.7.3 Active tactile displays

Active tactile arrays of modest sizes are now available in which an array of pins is set to the "up" or "down" position under computer control to form any desired image (or Braille character). KGS Corporation in Japan produces such a device known as the DotView, with a display size of 32 by 48 dots with a pitch of 2.4 mm. The American Printing House for the Blind (www.aph.org/) has a prototype "Gaphiti" 40×60 display.

20.7.4 Computer graphics access

Access to graphical information on computers and software packages is still a major problem. An exception is the availability of a free software package called "SKDATA Tools" that makes the graphics produced by MatLab accessible in either auditory or tactile formats. The auditory information display uses the pitch of a sound to represent the vertical axis of a graphed quantity while time represents the horizontal axis. (This pitch-based display of graphical information is also used in the Auditory Oscilloscope produced by Oehm Electronics.) Various tools to aid in accessing computer graphics are under development.

20.8 Access to computers and the internet

20.8.1 Screen readers

Screen readers are software packages used to access the contents of the screen and port them to speech or Braille output. Keyboard controls allow users to navigate the screen and specify what aspects of its information are read at any given time – for example, to read by lines, words, or characters, to select headings or specific forms of highlighting (e.g., underlined text). The advent of the Mac and Windows operating systems was a setback for this technology, but modern screen readers are able to access and display most information used in modern computer operating systems and office applications that are primarily text based. However, they are still largely incapable of displaying the information displayed in graphics. Apple provides a built-in basic screen reader ("VoiceOver"), and several third-party options are available for Windows, such as JAWS and the open-source NVDA screen reader.

20.8.2 Speech output

Synthetic speech can be implemented purely in software, so this is the most inexpensive and prevalent form of output for screen readers. Speed is controlled by keyboard commands, and a skilled user can utilize speech at several times the normal rate of production.

20.8.3 Braille output

"Refreshable" Braille displays (in which mechanical pins pop up under computer control) have long been available with one to three lines of output that can be interfaced to the computer and screen reader software. Many users prefer this form of output over speech, especially for checking spelling and formatting, although it is considerably more expensive.

20.8.4 Screen magnification software

Modern computer operating systems come with a number of screen magnification options built in. More powerful screen magnification packages are available such as Zoom Text, which can provide high magnification and more complete functionality with different software applications. An often-ignored option for low-vision computer access is simply to use a larger monitor.

20.8.5 Internet access

While text-based email communication and the textual components of social media present few barriers to the blind user, the increasing graphical and video content of the web and social media is another story. The Web Accessibility Initiative was launched with cooperation from the World Wide Web Consortium and many public and private entities to try and address such problems by developing guidelines that have been adopted by industry, including guidelines for web authoring software to help ensure that web pages contain features that make their content more accessible to a blind user with a regular screen reader. The commonly used web browsers include the ability to increase or decrease the displayed font size, and there are a small number of specially developed accessible web browsers designed to produce output for blind and visually impaired persons. For pictorial information, web authors are encouraged but not obliged to label pictures with "alt text" descriptors, so access is spotty. Facebook has developed "Automatic Alt Text" software intended to help blind users interpret its pictures, and research in computer vision, AI, and deep learning show future promise in assisting with this difficult problem.

20.8.6 Access to video information

Videos can be made accessible to a blind user by adding an audio description describing action and other features being displayed visually that are not obvious from the regular soundtrack (Packer, Vizenor, and Miele 2015). Interspersing the description with the regular audio track is an art, and professional video description is so expensive that the supply of videos with this feature is limited. However, a new technology called YouDescribe (youdescribe.org) utilizes crowd sourcing principles to allow any sighted viewer to record a description of any video available via YouTube, and any blind user to download the resulting described video. This has greatly increased the supply of accessible videos and makes it feasible for friends, family members, and teachers to record descriptions of videos that can subsequently be viewed by any blind user.

20.9 Access to communications and portable computing devices

20.9.1 Landline phones

The advent of phones with low contrast liquid-crystal displays (LCDs) and menus has meant that while basic placing and receiving of calls is not difficult, the advanced features of most of them cannot readily be accessed by a blind or severely visually impaired user.

20.9.2 Smartphones

The iPhone was the first "Smartphone" to address blind accessibility in its operating system (iOS), which includes the VoiceOver screen reader and a Zoom screen magnifier. Phones based on the Android operating system have traditionally been more difficult to access, but this situation has improved markedly in recent years with the advent of the built-in "TalkBack" system and the availability of third-party apps. For low vision phone users and older users wishing for simplified features, special cell phone and smartphone models are available with large buttons, numerals, and displays such as the "Jitterbug."

20.9.3 Smartphone apps

The advent of the smartphone app has been a boon for blind and sighted alike, since many of the apps are accessible, by accident or design, by blind users with the help of their phone's built-in accessibility features. The American Foundation of the Blind maintains a listing of such apps that is relatively accessible.

There are also apps that have been developed to solve specific problems faced by blind individuals, such as reading printed text, identifying currency bills, and pedestrian navigation, among a few examples. Some of these are detailed elsewhere in this chapter, and more are appearing over time.

20.10 Access to appliances, displays, and daily living activities

20.10.1 Appliances with mechanical controls

On the relatively small subset of appliances still using knobs for controls, tactile or large print labels can be applied to provide independent operation. Distinct dot patterns or actual Braille can serve equally well. This principle can also be applied to other devices such as insulin syringes to give a tactile indication of a setting or quantity.

20.10.2 Access to appliances with digital displays and controls

As more and more household and workplace devices and appliances use liquid crystal displays and require a user to page through menus for different settings, access has become very problematic. Most LCDs used on such devices are of low contrast making them hard to see by anyone with less than perfect vision. No opportunity should be lost to impress on manufacturers and salespeople the need for considering the visually impaired when products are designed. While research and development are ongoing to try and address these problems, a trial of appliances in the store before purchase is essential, and often reveals that some models can be set to certain modes by a blind user without using the feedback from the display.

20.10.3 Talking appliances

Companies marketing products to blind and visually impaired users have produced talking versions of certain commonplace devices and appliances such as clocks, calculators, scales, and thermostats. Blood-pressure monitors and sugar/insulin analyzers with speech displays are commercially available.

20.10.4 "Connected" appliances

Among mainstream products, it should be noted that just because a particular device "talks" for convenience to sighted users, it may not necessarily provide access to the information required to operate the device without vision. A possibly hopeful trend is the movement toward making appliances remotely controllable via the user's smartphone. To date, there are a limited number of examples of such "smart" and "connected" appliances with control apps that can be accessed by a user without sight, but more progress is hoped for in this field.

20.10.5 Lighting

For people with low vision, directing appropriate illumination to the task at hand or appliance being utilized is a fundamental step in easing daily living tasks. Providing appropriate magnification for the task is also important.

20.11 Jobsite, career, and STEM technology

20.11.1 Technologies for traditional professions

Many of the technologies mentioned earlier in this chapter can help make a job accessible for a blind or visually impaired worker. In addition, many other special adaptations can be made to facilitate the performance of specific job-related tasks. Examples include the use of jigs and fixtures for positioning and measurement or to facilitate the use of cutting tools, the provision of auditory tonal and speech feedback to read outputs of tools and instruments, and the provision of local lighting and magnification. In many cases, the job can be restructured with a redistribution of tasks. Through these means, blind individuals have been employed in a staggering array of jobs and professions. Accessible meters, oscilloscopes, vacuum gauges, machinist tools, and all manner of vocational tools and methods have been developed. If no commercially available device exists to assist with the specific task at hand, resources exist to guide the employee or rehabilitation professional through the exploration of the different possibilities and, if necessary, fabricate special purpose adaptive equipment. An excellent series of such examples is contained in the book "Business Owners who are Blind or Visually Impaired" by Deborah Kendrick.

20.11.2 Technology for STEM careers and pastimes

Although there are many barriers to participation in STEM (science, technology, engineering, and math) occupations and hobbies, there are also many examples of successes, and new tools emerging all the time. For example, the Blind Arduino Project (blarbl.blogspot.com) is making the popular Arduino modular robotic/ electronic technologies accessible to blind users who can employ it to fabricate a vast array of useful devices, assistive and otherwise. In the wider context of the Maker Movement, there are encouraging efforts to make tools such as 3D printing more accessible to blind users. Technologies mentioned elsewhere in this chapter, including new methods for graphics and computer access, are also important in this regard.

20.12 Technology for independent travel

20.12.1 Canes and guide dogs

The most common tool used by blind travelers is the long cane – normally long enough to allow the user to reach two steps in front while striding forward. The best long canes are lightweight, well-balanced, sturdy, flexible, and produce high-frequency sounds from the metal tip tapping on the ground. These sounds are reflected off nearby surfaces and the returning echoes can be interpreted by the user to assist perception of the surrounding environment. In addition to its use by blind individuals, the cane can be beneficial to many people with low vision as an extra safety measure. The other common "low tech" travel aid is the guide dog – a service animal that is professionally trained to aid blind pedestrians to avoid obstacles and detect curbs and steps. The guide dog user needs to be comfortable living with and caring for the dog, and the dog largely relies on the user to maintain orientation and to know the directions to desired destinations.

20.12.2 Obstacle detectors and environmental sensors

Electronic travel aids (ETAs) developed to assist blind pedestrians include obstacle detection devices that detect echoes from ultrasonic or infrared signals emitted by the device as they reflect off environmental surfaces. This information may be displayed as audio or vibration. Numerous manifestations of this approach have come and gone over the years, so no attempt at a current listing is made here.

20.12.3 Accessible GPS

GPS is an excellent outdoor navigation aid for blind and visually impaired travelers. Accuracy is limited in the vicinity of tall buildings, and the system cannot be used indoors or in underground transit systems, but in relatively open outdoor areas, very good positioning accuracy can be obtained. Specialized GPS aids for blind travelers are available, such as the Braille Note GPS and Trekker. Now that GPS receivers are incorporated into smartphones, apps are available to help blind users take advantage of its navigational capabilities. For example, "Over There" is a free iPhone app that simulates the Talking Signs system mentioned below – allowing a user to scan around the environment and hear what shops (and other environmental landmarks represented on Google Maps) are present in any direction.

20.12.4 Accessible signage

Sighted individuals take the ability to see signs and landmarks for granted. Braille signage can provide valuable assistance in personal orientation but have to be found before it can be read. New printing methods can allow combined visual and tactile signs to be made. Various forms of remotely accessible signage have been developed (the most well-known being Talking Signs, which used infrared transmitters and user-carried receivers with directional beam patterns; see Crandall et al. 2001). Audible pedestrian signals (Barlow, Scott, and Bentzen 2009) are becoming more widespread and improve safety at intersections where they are installed. Currently, several studies and demonstrations of the use of Bluetooth beacons as signs (for navigation within limited areas such as an airport) are underway.

20.12.5 Travel with low vision

Independent travel skills of people with low vision differ depending on different aspects of their vision loss. Many people with low vision are highly susceptible to glare and find seeing signs and other cues against the sky or in bright light problematic. Filtered glasses or photochromic lenses can help cope with very bright light. Individuals who retain a wide visual field generally find independent travel easier than those with tunnel vision (like looking through a narrow tube, common to people with retinitis pigmentosa). Retention of peripheral vision (even when the central vision is significantly reduced, as with macular degeneration) frequently permits good independent pedestrian skills to be retained.

Diseases such as age-related maculopathy and retinitis pigmentosa produce poorer performance in reduced light, making travel at night difficult. Night vision telescopes or goggles, derived from defense technology, are available, although expensive. A bright handheld or head-mounted flashlight can also be an effective mobility aid.

Reductions in contrast sensitivity (associated with most visual impairments) make it hard to see objects that do not contrast well with the background – such as curbs and steps. Simple environmental modifications such as painting the edges of steps in a contrasting color can greatly aid visibility and safety.

Visually impaired pedestrians traveling in unfamiliar areas can use pocket-sized handheld telescopes to read signs in the distance or read items on a menu behind a counter. Spectacle-mounted telescopes are also available, such as an autofocus model from Ocutech, while available electronic versions include the VisAble 40× handheld zoom video telescope from Artic Technologies.

20.12.6 Tactile, audio-tactile, and large print maps

Historically, the types of maps that sighted people take for granted for planning and executing travel have been largely unavailable to blind users. Limited audio maps are available in conjunction with the various accessible GPS systems mentioned previously, but do not provide all the functionality of a regular map. For low vision travelers, a limited number of enhanced large print maps exist but there is no widespread availability. A new development in this field is the Tactile Map Automated Production (TMAP) system, which now makes it possible for a blind or sighted individual to request a tactile street map centered on any address he or she specifies via the system website. The resulting map can be downloaded and printed on the user's own Braille embosser. If the user does not have one, they can have the map sent to a Braille embossing service for production and have it mailed to him.

Audio-tactile systems such as the Talking Tactile Tablet from Touch Graphics combine a touch tablet with a tactile map or graphic overlay, interfaced to a computer to produce a talking map with programmed descriptions that are enunciated when the user presses any particular point on the map. This approach obviously requires the individual map to be produced and custom programming of the software for each map, but it can also be generalized to help access other tactile graphics (see Section 20.7).

20.13 Recreational technology

20.13.1 Physical recreation

Many sports are popular with blind people, including skiing, sailing, and kayaking. Braille and auditory compasses are available, as are kayak and canoe paddles with tactile grips that help orient them correctly. Bowling is aided by a "bowling rail" that is placed prior to the spot for releasing the ball, giving orientation to the bowling lane. "Goal Ball" is a game akin to soccer for blind or blindfolded players, in which the ball emits auditory signals to help localize its position.

20.13.2 Indoor recreational activities

Many popular board games are available with Braille and/or tactile markings. Large print playing cards are also available. Interactive text-based computer games are available from many software and internet sites. Electronics, including amateur radio, is a popular hobby for blind people, and as mentioned previously, accessible audio and audio-tactile electrical meter readouts are available as well as methods for electronic circuit construction. (See also the Blind Arduino Project mentioned earlier.)

20.13.3 Music

Home sound systems are mixed in their accessibility and need to be tested in the store before buying. Many portable digital music players (iPods, MP3 players, etc.) can be difficult to access, although some, such as the Zen Stone have no display and use buttons instead of touch pads, and can be operated without vision, with uploads from a suitably equipped accessible computer.

20.13.4 Television and movies

Audio descriptions of visual scenes and actions are available in very few theaters for live performances. For movies, TV, and video entertainment, recorded descriptions are the preferred mode of access. For current programming, these have limited but increasing availability – for example, the FCC has recently (July 2017) mandated an increase in the quantity of television material required to be described. A limited number of PBS and cable television series and documentaries are available with descriptions. The WGBH MoPix system provides captioning and audio description of many new release movies and is available in about 350 theaters in the United States including many IMAX theaters.

20.13.5 Low vision aids

Large-print books, magazines, and games are available from many sources. Watching television and live performances can be aided with head-mounted monocular or binocular viewers, including electronic magnifying systems with head-mounted displays.

20.14 General purpose remote assistance technology

The advent of the internet, smartphone, and fast remote data services have made possible the practical implementation of the "Remote Sighted Guide" concept that has been experimented with since the early 1990s. As a result, there are smartphone apps such as "Be My Eyes" that allow a blind user to transmit an image or live video of the problem in front of him or her and have it analyzed by a sighted individual at some remote location who can provide the information. Automated versions of such a service such as "Tap Tap See" bypass the human assistant and use computer vision technology instead to attempt recognition of the image, scene, or desired information. A variety of these types of services is now available.

20.15 Hearing loss: Prevalence and types of loss

Hearing loss (HL) is one of the most common impairments. Approximately 15% of American adults (37.5 million) aged 18 and over report some trouble hearing (National Institute on Deafness and Other Communication Disorders 2016). The prevalence of HL increases with age. Approximately 30% of adults over 60 years of age have HL and approximately 0.5% of children under the age of 18 have HL. The percentage of children in the United States born with HL is about 0.25%. One in ten of these children has a parent with congenital HL.

20.15.1 Causes of hearing loss

Causes of HL can be classified into three broad categories; age-related HL, adventitious HL that is independent of the aging process, and congenital HL. The categories are broad with some overlap between categories.

Age-related HL is the largest of the three categories. It is caused by a combination of the aging process and the cumulative effect of a lifetime of minor insults to the ear such as exposure to very loud sounds or the use of mildly ototoxic medication. For many, the first evidence of an emerging age-related HL is a reduction of auditory sensitivity (e.g., not hearing a telephone ring in a nearby room) beginning at about 30 years of age. The loss in sensitivity increases with age, the loss being greater at high frequencies. From age 60, the increase in HL increases more rapidly so that names or words out of context become harder to recognize. As the aging process continues, older adults have increasing difficulty understanding rapid speech as well as speech sounds with significant high-frequency content. Rapid, high-pitched children's speech becomes increasingly more difficult to understand for aging grandparents.

Adventitious HL is usually caused by a major insult to the ear (e.g., a bomb explosion), or a series of lesser insults over an extended period, such as exposure to high sound levels in a noisy work environment without hearing protection. Loud rock music listened to over long periods using ear inserts is a growing cause of adventitious HL in teenagers. The prevalence of adventitious HL is dependent on human activity and can be reduced substantially by taking appropriate hearing-health precautions. The proportion of the population with adventitious HL is usually much smaller than that for people with age-related HL, except in wartime. At the end of World War II, large numbers of veterans returned with battlefield-acquired adventitious HL. The USA, UK, and Australia set up major rehabilitation programs to address this problem resulting in historic advances in rehabilitation engineering for hearing loss.

Congenital HL (including HL resulting from birth defects) has the lowest prevalence among the three major categories of HL, but the investment in (re)habilitation for people in this category is far greater for each individual than for any other category. Children born with HL, or who acquire HL in the earliest years of life, have difficulty acquiring speech, language, and related communication skills.

20.15.2 Types of hearing loss

Types of HL can be classified into the following three broad categories: conductive, sensorineural, and central HL. These categories are orthogonal to the above set of categories identifying the three main causes of HL.

Conductive HL is the result of attenuated sound transmission through the outer and middle ear. Possible causes are as follows; fluid in the middle ear (a common problem in children); ossification of the tiny bones in the middle ear (a common problem in adults); constriction of the ear canal; perforation of the eardrum; and other injuries/diseases involving components of the outer and middle ear. Attenuation of the acoustic signal traveling through the outer and middle ear raises the threshold of hearing but does not alter the dynamic range of hearing.

Acoustic amplification compensating for the attenuation resulting from a conductive HL is an effective treatment. In the 1950s, advances in medical/surgical intervention became the preferred treatment for most forms of conductive HL. Prior to this development, most candidates for acoustic amplification had significant conductive HL with some sensorineural HL. Today, most candidates for acoustic amplification have significant sensorineural HL and possibly some conductive HL that does not require, or has not been resolved completely by, medical/surgical intervention. This is an important development to bear in mind when reviewing hearing-aid research prior to the 1950s; major advances were made in the medical/surgical treatment of conductive hearing loss during this decade.

Sensorineural HL, in contrast to conductive HL, not only raises the threshold of hearing, it also reduces the dynamic range of hearing; that is, low-level sounds are not audible or have significantly reduced loudness, while high-level sounds are similar in loudness to that of an ear without sensorineural HL. Reduced dynamic range is a major problem in acoustic amplification for sensorineural HL. If acoustic amplification is used to make low-level sounds audible, high-level sounds will be painfully loud with a high probability of further damage to the auditory system. The reduction in dynamic range in sensorineural HL is also frequency dependent, the reduction usually being most severe at high frequencies.

The neural component of sensorineural HL introduces another complicating factor in that temporal resolution in the neural processing of sound beyond the cochlea is reduced, resulting in less reliable neural firings in the transmission of sound from the cochlea to the auditory cortex. Reduced temporal resolution is common in the normal aging process and older adults with normal hearing for their age have reduced temporal processing of sound. Background noise also reduces the reliability of neural processing in the auditory system, the decrement in neural processing increasing with increasing sensorineural HL (Levitt, Oden, and Simon 2012).

Normal age-related reduction in cognitive processing is another factor reducing speech understanding, particularly rapid speech, in older adults. Research on normal age-related reductions in cognitive processing has provided new insights with respect to methods for dealing with reduced cognitive processing in age-related HL. Cognitive processing involving memory for names, dates, and events is more susceptible to age-related decline in cognitive processing than top-down global processing of incomplete information, an important consideration in the development of hearing rehabilitation methods and instrumentation for older adults (Peters 2006).

Central HL can occur with or without a concomitant conductive or sensorineural HL. It involves high-level central processing and is not well understood. Recent research using powerful measurement techniques such as MRI and other brain scanning tools are providing new insights. A common form of hearing impairment involving a central component is that of tinnitus, often referred to in lay terms as "ringing in the ears." Training programs provide some relief from tinnitus but are not a cure. Experimental treatments involving stimulation of the vagus nerve have shown short-term reductions in tinnitus, but it is too early to say whether this approach can provide a practical long-term solution (Tyler et al. 2017).

20.16 Evolution of the hearing aid

20.16.1 The pre-electronic era

The ear trumpet was the first engineering device to help people with hearing loss. It was invented in the 17th century and became the sensory aid of choice for HL until it was replaced by the electronic hearing aid. The ear trumpet captures sound passing through a large cross-sectional area at the entrance to the trumpet and then concentrates the sound as it travels through the trumpet and then exits through an opening with a small cross-sectional area. The sound pressure per unit area at the exit of the ear trumpet is substantially higher than that at the entrance to the trumpet. The gain in sound level provided by an ear trumpet is on the order of 10 to 15 dB.

The carbon microphone invented in 1878 was a turning point in the development of a practical telephone, resulting in exponential growth of the telephone system. It was also a starting point for the development of an electric hearing aid. Prior to 1878, methods for converting pressure variations in air-borne sound into electrical signals were complicated, inefficient, and unreliable, while the newly invented carbon microphone did not have any of these problems. A variation of the carbon microphone was also used to amplify electric signals.

The first electric hearing aid was invented by Miller Reese Hutchinson in 1885 and the manufacture of hearing aids began at the turn of the century (Wikipedia 2018). Although electric hearing aids provided more gain than ear trumpets, most people with HL did not take to the use of electric hearing aids. There were several reasons for the slow growth of the emerging hearing-aid industry. Early electric hearing aids were large, unwieldy, and difficult to use. They also introduced two new problems: internally generated noise and non-linear distortion. The ear trumpet, in contrast, is a passive, linear device that does not generate internal noise or introduce non-linear distortion.

20.16.2 The electronic era

In 1906, Lee De Forest invented the Audion, a three-electrode thermionic vacuum tube that could amplify electric signals. Several years later, a practical electronic amplifier was developed. This development was a game changer. Initially, the electronic amplifier found applications in the telephone industry and the military.

As new applications of electronics were discovered, the electronics industry grew substantially, introducing the benefits and problems of mass production. A key development for rehabilitation engineering for HL took place in the early 1920s when mass production of electronic hearing aids began in both the United States and Europe. The manufacture of a related electronic device, the audiometer, also began at the time.

The electronic hearing aid soon replaced both the ear trumpet and electric hearing aid as the sensory aid of choice for HL. The audiometer was developed as a clinical tool for evaluating hearing and fitting hearing aids. It also proved to be a valuable research tool. It provided the first complete mapping of the intensity and frequency range of human hearing.

The earliest hearing aids were large instruments and the dominant driving force in hearing aid engineering for more than 50 years was miniaturization to make hearing aids less conspicuous and cosmetically acceptable. The miniaturization of hearing aids depended on the miniaturization of electronic components. A major step in the miniaturization process was the invention of miniature vacuum tubes in the mid-1930s, leading to the development of wearable hearing aids. Wearability and convenience are important considerations for the acceptance of hearing aids by people who need acoustic amplification. The introduction of body-worn hearing aids in the 1930s led to a substantial increase in the use of hearing aids. Although the sale of wearable hearing aids was substantial, the number of people who could benefit from acoustic amplification but did not use hearing aids was even more substantial by a wide margin. The low use of hearing aids by people who could benefit from acoustic amplification is an ongoing hearing health problem.

The invention of the transistor in 1947 was another technological game changer. The telecommunications industry was the first industry to use transistors, followed closely by the hearing-aid industry. By the 1960s, transistor hearing aids could be made small enough to fit on or in the ear. Ear-level hearing aids soon replaced the body-worn instruments as the preferred method of acoustic amplification.

Moore's Law predicts that processing speed in solid-state circuits doubles every two years with a concomitant halving of component size (Moore 1965). The law held sway with respect to the miniaturization of hearing aids until the mid-1980s when hearing aids small enough to fit entirely in the ear canal were developed. These hearing aids were virtually invisible and there was little additional cosmetic advantage in continuing the miniaturization process. At this point in time, the focus on hearing-aid development broadened to include advanced signal processing techniques in the space available in a cosmetically acceptable hearing aid.

Villchur's classic paper on multichannel compression amplification was a straw in the wind of the coming changes in hearing-aid research and development

(Villchur 1973). Multichannel hearing aids addressed the problem of frequency-dependent reduction in dynamic range in sensorineural HL by splitting the incoming signal into contiguous frequency bands. Amplitude compression is used in each band to reduce the dynamic range of the incoming audio signal to match the reduced dynamic range of the impaired ear. Multichannel hearing aids spearheaded the introduction of advanced signal processing in hearing aids. In a later development, multichannel hearing aids were also used to reduce background noise, a major problem limiting hearing aid benefits. Whereas multiband compression hearing aids are effective in compensating for a frequency-dependent reduction in dynamic range, they provide only a marginal improvement in effective noise reduction (approximately 1 dB) for a single microphone input.

20.16.3 The digital era

The next game-changing technological development was the introduction of digital signal processing. In the early 1960s, Bell Laboratories developed methods of simulating complex speech processing systems in a large digital computer. The Block Diagram Compiler (BLODI) developed by Kelly et al. was used in the first offline digital simulation of an experimental hearing aid in the mid-1960s (Kelly, Lochbaum, and Vyssotsky 1961). The use of computers to simulate complex analog systems required a change in mindset. The researchers who pioneered digital simulation of analog systems had acquired their engineering skills in analog technology and their first attempts using digital methods to improve analog signal processing simulated improved versions of analog technology. The outcome was improved signal processing, but only by a small margin. On the next attempt, significantly improved signal processing was achieved using digital techniques well beyond the capabilities of analog technology.

The introduction of small laboratory computers in the 1960s opened the door for smaller, less well-endowed research laboratories to use computers as research tools and acquire the mindset for developing methods and devices using the unique advantages of digital technology. Initially, these laboratory computers were not fast enough for digital signal processing of audio signals in real time, but they could be used for controlling analog equipment in real time, thereby creating a means for investigating experimental methods of signal processing using hybrid digital-analog equipment.

The computer industry continued to make rapid progress during this period. New types of special-purpose computers were developed, such as a reduced instruction set computer (RISC), dedicated signal processors for specific applications, and high-speed array processors for parallel processing. The speed of array processors in the early 1980s was fast enough to process speech in virtual in real time; that is, processing speech within 10 or 20 msec such that there is no perceptible loss of synchrony between the auditory and visual components of speech in face-to-face conversation. This was an important breakthrough for hearing-aid research.

In 1982, the first all-digital hearing aid configured around an array processor was developed at the City University of New York (Levitt 2007). Computations were performed by a desk-mounted array processor controlled by a small minicomputer. The user of the hearing aid wore a behind-the-ear (BTE) hearing-aid case containing a microphone and a hearing-aid output transducer. The two transducers were connected by wire to a small body-worn two-channel FM transmitter-receiver providing a wireless link to the input and output, respectively, of the high-speed array processor. From the user's perspective, the digital hearing aid appeared to be a conventional BTE hearing aid connected to a body-worn FM unit of the type used at schools for the deaf. At about the same time, a prototype wearable digital hearing aid was developed by Nunley et al. (1983). It was a body-worn unit somewhat larger than a conventional body-worn hearing aid. These two developments initiated a race among major hearing-aid manufacturers and several high-tech companies to produce a practical wearable digital hearing aid.

The array-processor hearing aid was designed to be a research tool for investigating the potential of digital signal processing in hearing aids. The resulting research focused on the use of advanced digital signal processing to improve speech understanding in noise, a problem that has eluded a satisfactory solution despite decades of research. The main findings were that major improvements in speech understanding are possible if more than one input microphone is used. The multimicrophone methods showing the largest improvements were adaptive beamforming, adaptive noise cancelation, and dichotic signal processing utilizing the unique properties of human binaural hearing (Dillon 2012). Digital noise reduction with single and multimicrophone inputs was evaluated, the multimicrophone methods being far superior except in highly reverberant rooms. A general method of frequency-dependent amplitude compression was also developed that reduced internal masking in amplitude compressed speech as well as reducing between-channel distortion in conventional multichannel amplitude compression (Levitt and Neuman 1991). The array processor hearing aid was also used in developing efficient multivariate adaptive strategies in hearing aid evaluation and fitting (Preminger et al. 2000). The transition from a large, unwieldy body-worn digital hearing aid to a practical, cosmetically acceptable hearing aid that could be worn on or in the ear was long and arduous. Two major obstacles had to be overcome. (1) Digital chips had to be developed that were considerably smaller and drew considerably less power than the digital chips in the experimental prototype. (2) Analog chips used in hearing aids at that time had been miniaturized over many years of development and were technologically far more advanced than miniaturized digital chips developed for the first prototype wearable digital hearing aid. There was a lot of catching up to do. Predictions based on Moore's

Law indicated that it would take more than a decade for micro-digital technology to catch up with micro-analog technology that would allow for the many advantages of digital signal processing to be implemented in a practical, cosmetically acceptable hearing aid. The predictions turned out to be correct.

The first generation of so-called "digital hearing aids" was developed in the late 1980s. These hearing aids were not true digital hearing aids; they were hybrid digital-analog instruments in which a small digital unit controlled analog components that amplified the audio signal. The digital controller in these hearing aids allowed for several innovative features to be introduced. These included the following: (1) programmability (a new world for most clinicians who had to learn about both software and hardware capabilities of hearing aids); (2) memory capabilities (for storing several frequency-gain characteristics for use in different acoustic environments); (3) improved fitting procedures (such as storing audiological test data digitally and then using these data for programming the hearing aid for improved, more efficient individualized fitting); (4) adaptive control of hearing aid variables (such as adaptive frequency-gain characteristics for improved time-varying frequency-dependent amplitude compression); and (5) adaptive noise reduction (such as adaptive control of directional input, and adaptive attenuation of frequency regions in which high noise levels mask the speech signal).

Societal factors also spurred the development of digital hearing aids. At that time, public figures hid the fact that they had hearing loss. When President Reagan made it known that he wore a hearing aid there was a sudden large increase in the sale of hearing aids. Wall Street mavens spotted the new trend and several large companies with substantial high-tech capabilities entered the hearing-aid market or invested in research for a better hearing aid with intent to enter the market – 3m, Nicolet, AT&T, Panasonic, and several other large companies, which were careful to maintain anonymity, and many small startups. The result was a surge in productivity in developing high-tech hearing aids. When the rate of increase in hearing aid sales fell back to that of the pre-Reagan bubble, most of the large high-tech companies terminated their involvement in hearing-aid development.

The hearing-aid industry by then had undergone an irreversible shakeup. Several established hearing-aid manufacturers ceased to exist and several new startup companies with high-tech capabilities had become major players. The traditional hearing-aid companies, which survived the shakeup, had also substantially improved their high-tech capabilities to survive. The net result was a sleeker high-tech industry with the initiative to develop innovative new ways of improving the communication capabilities of people with HL. The previous narrow focus on miniaturization had given way to a broader vision of the hearing aid as a communication tool.

The race to develop a wearable, cosmetically acceptable, digital hearing aid was on and the competition was keen. The Nicolet Instrumentation Company, a

517

high-tech company with no previous experience in hearing aids was the first to develop and market a wearable all-digital hearing aid in 1989 (Heide 1994). Their first product, the Phoenix, was a body-worn instrument. This was a mistake in that it was not cosmetically acceptable for most of the intended market. Nicolet went on to develop a much smaller behind-the-ear digital hearing aid, but the company went bankrupt before it could be marketed. In 1996, two established Danish hearing-aid companies, Oticon and Widex, began marketing the first commercially viable, wearable ear-level all-digital hearing aids. Although these digital hearing aids were superior to competing hybrid digital-analog hearing aids, they were not substantially better. The first generation of digital hearing aids was essentially improved replications of existing hybrid digital-analog hearing aids. It was only when the next generation of all-digital hearing aids introduced innovative new features that were beyond the capabilities of hybrid digital-analog hearing aids that the inherent advantages of an all-digital hearing aid were recognized.

The introduction of adaptive feedback cancelation in digital hearing aids is a case in point. The necessary signal processing for adaptive feedback cancelation is far too difficult to be implemented in a hearing aid using analog technology, but it can be implemented digitally. A digital hearing aid with adaptive feedback cancelation is substantially better than an analog hearing aid without the capability of canceling acoustic feedback. It not only eliminates howling in high gain hearing aids, it also allows for the use of more comfortable open earmolds as well as increasing the allowable gain at high frequencies, thereby increasing the effective bandwidth of hearing aids for people with substantial high-frequency HL. Although methods for adaptive feedback cancelation had been developed well over a decade before, it was only after the necessary advanced signal processing could be implemented digitally in a wearable, cosmetically acceptable instrument that the digital hearing aid became the instrument of choice for acoustic amplification in the 21st century (Levitt, Dugot, and Kopper 1988).

20.17 The hearing aid as a personal communication aid

The original purpose of a hearing aid was to amplify sound. In the 1930s, a serendipitous discovery introduced a second useful function for a hearing aid – that of wireless links with telephones and other devices. The handsets of early telephones produced a stray electromagnetic (EM) field strong enough to induce an electrical signal in a coil within the field. In 1937, Joseph Poliakoff made use of this stray electric field to transmit electric signals from a telephone directly to the electric input of the hearing-aid amplifier. A small coil (telecoil, T-coil) was mounted in a hearing aid such that frequency fluctuations in the stray EM field induced electric current fluctuations in the telecoil. A telephone signal transmitted by wireless means to a hearing aid is much clearer than the signal transmitted acoustically to the hearing aid. The acoustic transmission path includes non-linear distortion introduced by the electric-to-acoustic output transducer in the telephone, non-linear distortion introduced by the hearing-aid microphone in transducing the acoustic signal back to an electric signal, and the addition of ambient noise in the acoustic pathway from telephone output to hearing-aid microphone.

Some 30 years later when telephone engineers refined the design of telephone handsets to eliminate the stray EM field, the outcry from hearing-aid users was immediate, angry, and influential. The Federal Communication Commission (FCC) responded by requiring telephones to be hearing aid compatible (HAC) by maintaining a stray EM field powerful enough to induce usable signals in the telecoil of a hearing aid.

Inductive coupling to a hearing aid can also be used with devices other than a telephone. One such application is to create an EM field in a room within which one or more hearing-aid users can receive audio signals via the telecoil in their hearing aids. The method of creating the EM field is quite simple. The room is encircled by a multi-turn wire loop and the two ends of the wire loop are connected to the output of an audio amplifier. The fluctuating electric current flowing through the wire loop induces fluctuations in the EM field, which are picked up by the telecoil in each user's hearing aids. An acoustic signal generated within the room, such as a speech produced by a talker, will be partially masked by room reverberation and ambient room noise. In contrast, an audio signal delivered electrically to the inductive loop will be received by the hearing-aid user free of reverberation and room noise. Inductive loop systems of this type are inexpensive, simple to install, and of benefit to hearing-aid users. Inductive loop systems are widely used in classrooms, auditoria, churches, museums, and other public spaces.

Inductive loop systems are useful, but there are practical problems limiting their use. When the telecoil was invented, hearing aids were relatively large and early telecoils were also relatively large. Today's hearing aids and their telecoils are much smaller. Signals induced in smaller coils are correspondingly weaker. Telecoils are also directional. The coil needs to lie in a plane corresponding to the directional characteristics of the EM field. The optimal angle of a telecoil for a telephone is often different from that of an inductive loop and is a source of confusion. Many older hearing-aid users have difficulty holding the telephone in exactly the right position for the telecoil to pick up the EM signal efficiently.

A fundamental limitation of inductive loop systems is that the audio signal in a telecoil is induced by audio-frequency fluctuations of the EM field. This is not the most reliable method of wireless signal transmission. Other methods of wireless communication use a high-frequency carrier signal that is modulated by the low-frequency audio signal. Radio broadcasting began with amplitude modulated

(AM) carrier signals. Distortions of the EM field by sunspots, static electricity in the atmosphere, and other sources of EM distortion caused fading, static interference, and other distortions of AM radio signals. Wideband frequency modulation (FM) was invented by Edwin Armstrong in the 1930s. A wideband FM transmission not only transmits wideband audio signals with high fidelity, but it is also much less susceptible to distortions of the EM medium. Although Armstrong patented his invention in 1933, legal challenges to his patent delayed the implementation of FM radio transmissions for many years. Hearing aids with FM wireless links were developed in the 1950s. These were body-worn instruments because of the relatively large size of FM transmitters/receivers at the time. They were used primarily at schools for the deaf where cosmetic acceptability is not of overriding importance.

With time, the ongoing process of miniaturization in digital electronics resulted in the development of ear-worn hearing aid FM wireless links, but by this time newer methods of wireless communication were being developed. In 1989, a digital wireless protocol, Bluetooth (named after a medieval Danish king) was introduced. It was designed for short-distance, low-power transmissions. It was an ideal protocol for hearing-aid applications and it soon became a de facto standard for wireless links between digital hearing aids and other devices, including mobile telephones, computers, and the internet.

Another method of wireless communication was developed during this period using infrared light, which is also an EM signal, but viewed in a different light (pun intended). Infrared systems are like loop systems in concept in that they are designed for one-way transmissions, such as television viewing in the home and for very large auditoria, theaters, and churches. Infrared systems are designed for use by anyone who has difficulty understanding speech in large reverberant spaces, or by family members who wish to watch television without an audible output that may disturb others. Infrared communications are limited to line-of-sight links and are more secure than other forms of EM transmissions. The market for infrared systems includes people with normal hearing as well as people with HL.

Digital wireless transmission of signals has important advantages over analog wireless transmission. Digital signal transmission is not only more efficient and more flexible than analog signal transmission, it also provides new insights on how to transmit speech efficiently for hearing-aid applications. For example, two important variables control the quality of speech signals transmitted using analog technology: the bandwidth and the precision with which the waveform is processed. In practice, precision may be determined by the internal noise of the analog transmission system divided by its dynamic range. In analog engineering, bandwidth and precision are separate concepts. In digital engineering, they are different facets of a single, more general concept.

The product of sampling rate (the digital analog of bandwidth) and the number of bits needed to specify each sample (the digital analog of waveform precision) determines the information rate at which the signal is transmitted. This method of deriving information rate is quite general and applies to all types of signals including speech, music, alerting signals, and video, which are of great importance to people with HL.

There have been several novel applications of digital wireless transmission in hearing aids. One method uses a digital wireless link between the hearing aids at each ear to implement directional beam forming for improving speech understanding in noise. Another application uses a wireless link to a remote hand-held microphone used by the person talking to the hearing-aid user. An inverse inversion of this method places a remote microphone close to a noise source. The noise signal is transmitted by wireless means to the hearing aid worn by the listener with HL. The noise signal also travels acoustically to the microphone of the hearing aid, as does the acoustic speech signal. The noise signal received by wireless means is adjusted adaptively and subtracted from the acoustic speech-plus-noise signal. When the acoustic speech-plus-noise signal is minimized, the noise component has been canceled. Perfect cancelation is seldom achieved in practice, but improvements in the speech-to-noise ratio on the order of 10 to 20 dB are achievable.

Modern digital hearing aids have many variables that need to be adjusted. A third application uses an automated multivariate search strategy to find the parameter set that maximizes speech intelligibility. The wireless link between the hearing aid and the computer allows control signals from the computer to adjust the hearing aid. These adjustments can also be carried out by a cloud computer via the internet while the user is wearing the hearing aid. This method adjusts a hearing aid for maximum intelligibility under conditions of actual use.

Another application using a wireless link to a powerful computer is as follows. The computer uses automatic speech recognition (ASR) to first recognize the speech and then synthesizes the speech to be more easily recognized by the user considering audiological information characteristics of the user's residual hearing. A very useful application of this method is to recognize speech in noise and then synthesize the speech in quiet. This method of noise reduction was demonstrated in 1993 (Levitt, Bakke, and Kates 1993). The method showed some benefits for a person with a profound hearing loss. There were two major limitations of the method that rendered it impractical at the time: the relatively high rate of ASR errors and the time taken for the computer to recognize the speech. ASR technology today is quite practical and is offered as a service by wireless telephone companies for missed calls. ASR computation times are not a problem for messaging services but may be a problem for face-to-face conversations.

521

20.18 Future vision

Prediction is very difficult, especially if it involves the future (Chinese proverb).

Although prediction is difficult, the identification of trends is not. But trends are notoriously transient. The following observations, rather than predictions, refer to the near future only.

Trend 1. The hearing-aid industry is an offspring of the telephone industry. Major advances in telephony are followed by corresponding advances in hearing aids. The synergistic merger of digital and wireless technologies is another game changer, which has had an enormous impact on the telephone industry. The worldwide expansion of landline telephones, which took more than a century, has been replaced by an even greater expansion of wireless telephony within a decade. The smartphone of today is in reality a portable computer with a telephone as an app.

Observation 1. The hearing aid is likely to be replaced by a "smartaid," that is, a general-purpose audio communication device that also amplifies sound as needed for people with HL.

Trend 2. The internet began as an information-sharing system in a nation-wide military project. It expanded to include information sharing with universities and then with industry. The enormous information sharing capabilities of the internet have continued to grow exponentially and have expanded to include activities other than information sharing, including entertainment, new forms of commerce, political activities, and so on, affecting virtually every aspect of modern society.

Observation 2. The smart hearing-aid/communication device will expand to include activities other than speech communication by wireless links to the internet with its enormous reach and access to cloud computing, thereby involving people with HL more actively in everyday societal activities.

Trend 3. The internet has given birth to new scientific and medical methods that address the limitations imposed by large physical distances, such as international studies including remote locations and the delivery of medical services to remote locations.

Observation 3. The internet will play an important role in advancing the new field of tele-audiology and improving the delivery of hearing health services to people with HL who have difficulty accessing clinics and other audiologic facilities.

Trend 4. A major problem for people with HL is the growing use of movies, television broadcasts, and video games requiring good listening skills. Examples include rapid speech in news broadcasts and movies with realistic background sounds and exciting soundtracks that are hard to understand even for people with normal hearing.

Observation 4. The wireless links that allow modern hearing aids to access audio-video material on the internet or via smartphones can be designed to include signal processing to improve the audio of these audio-poor movies, videos, and internet videophones such as Skype.

Bibliography

Barlow, J. M., A. C. Scott, and B. L. Bentzen. 2009. "Audible Beaconing with Accessible Pedestrian Signals." *AER Journal: Research and Practice in Visual Impairment and Blindness* 2 (4): 149–58.

Brabyn, John, Marilyn Schneck, Gunilla Haegerstrom-Portnoy, and Lori Lott. 2004. "Functional Vision: 'Real World' Impairment Examples from the SKI Study." *Visual Impairment Research* 6 (1): 35–44.

Brabyn, John A., Marilyn E. Schneck, Gunilla Haegerstrom-Portnoy, and Lori A. Lott. 2007. "Dual Sensory Loss: Overview of Problems, Visual Assessment, and Rehabilitation." *Trends in Amplification* 11 (4): 219–26.

Congdon, N., B. O'Colmain, C. C. Klaver, R. Klein, B. Munoz, D. S. Friedman, J. Kempen, H. R. Taylor, P. Mitchell, and Eye Diseases Prevalence Research Group. 2004. "Causes and Prevalence of Visual Impairment among Adults in the United States." *Archives of Ophthalmology (Chicago, Ill.: 1960)* 122 (4): 477–85. https://doi.org/10.1001/archopht.122.4.477.

Crandall, William, Billie Louise Bentzen, Linda Myers, and John Brabyn. 2001. "New Orientation and Accessibility Option for Persons with Visual Impairment: Transportation Applications for Remote Infrared Audible Signage." *Clinical and Experimental OPTOMETRY* 84 (3): 120–31.

Dillon, H. 2012. "Directional Microphones and Arrays." In *Hearing Aids*, edited by H. Dillon, 2nd ed. New York: Thieme.

Erickson, W., C. Lee, and S. Von Schrader. 2017. *2015 Disability Status Report: United States.* Ithaca, NY: Cornell University.

Good, William V. 2007. "The Spectrum of Vision Impairment Caused by Pediatric Neurological Injury." *Journal of American Association for Pediatric Ophthalmology and Strabismus* 11 (5): 424–25.

Heide, V. 1994. "Project Phoenix, Inc., 1984–1989: The Development of a Wearable Digital Signal Processing Hearing Aid." In *Understanding Digitally Programmable Hearing Aids*, edited by R. E. Sandlin, 123–50. Boston, MA: Allyn and Bacon, 1994.

Kelly, John L., Carol Lochbaum, and Victor A. Vyssotsky. 1961. "A Block Diagram Compiler." *The Bell System Technical Journal* 40 (3): 669–78.

Levitt, H., M. Bakke, and J. Kates. 1993. "Advanced Signal Processing Hearing Aids; Subsection A Speech-Recognition Hearing Aid." In *Recent Developments in Hearing Instrument Technology*, edited by J Beilin and G. R. Jensen, 347–50. 15th Danavax Symposium, Denmark.

Levitt, H., C. Oden, C. Noack, H. Simon, and A. Lotze. 2012. "Chapter 30 in Auditory Processing Disorders: Assessment, Management and Treatment." In *Computer-Based Training Methods for Age-Related APD: Past, Present, and Future*, edited by D Geffner and D Swain, 2nd ed. San Diego: Plural Press.

Levitt, Harry. 2007. "A Historical Perspective on Digital Hearing Aids: How Digital Technology Has Changed Modern Hearing Aids." *Trends in Amplification* 11 (1): 7–24.

Levitt, Harry, Richard S. Dugot, and Kenneth W. Kopper. 1988. *Programmable Digital Hearing Aid System.* 4,731,850, issued 1988.

Levitt, Harry, and Arlene C. Neuman. 1991. "Evaluation of Orthogonal Polynomial Compression." *The Journal of the Acoustical Society of America* 90 (1): 241–52.

Mills, J. O., A. Jalil, and P. E. Stanga. 2017. "Electronic Retinal Implants and Artificial Vision: Journey and Present." *Eye* 31 (10): 1383.

Moisseiev, Elad, and Mark J. Mannis. 2016. "Evaluation of a Portable Artificial Vision Device among Patients with Low Vision." *JAMA Ophthalmology* 134 (7): 748–52.

Moore, Gordon E. 1965. "Cramming More Components onto Integrated Circuits." *Electronics*, pp. 114–117.

National Institute on Deafness and Other Communication Disorders. 2016. "Statistics and Epidemiology." https://www.nidcd.nih.gov/health/statistics.

Nunley, J., W. Staab, J. Steadman, P. Wechsler, and B. Spenser. 1983. "A Wearable Digital Hearing Aid." *Hearing Journal* 36 (10): 29–31.

Packer, Jaclyn, Katie Vizenor, and Joshua A. Miele. 2015. "An Overview of Video Description: History, Benefits, and Guidelines." *Journal of Visual Impairment & Blindness* 109 (2): 83–93.

Peters, R. 2006. "Ageing and the Brain." *Postgraduate Medical Journal* 82 (964): 84–88.

Preminger, J. E., A. C. Neuman, M. H. Bakke, D. Walters, and H. Levitt. 2000. "An Examination of the Practicality of the Simplex Procedure." *Ear and Hearing* 21 (3): 177–93. https://doi.org/10.1097/00003446-200006000-00001.

Ryles, Ruby. 1996. "The Impact of Braille Reading Skills on Employment, Income, Education, and Reading Habits." *Journal of Visual Impairment and Blindness* 90: 219–26.

Ryskulova, Asel, Kathleen Turczyn, Diane M. Makuc, Mary Frances Cotch, Richard J. Klein, and Rosemary Janiszewski. 2008. "Self-Reported Age-Related Eye Diseases and Visual Impairment in the United States: Results of the 2002 National Health Interview Survey." *American Journal of Public Health* 98 (3): 454–61.

Spooner, Kimberly, Thomas Hong, Samantha Fraser-Bell, and Andrew A. Chang. 2019. "Current Outcomes of Anti-VEGF Therapy in the Treatment of Macular Oedema Secondary to Branch Retinal Vein Occlusions: A Meta-Analysis." *Ophthalmologica* 8 (3): 236–246.

Tyler, Richard, Anthony Cacace, Christina Stocking, Brent Tarver, Navzer Engineer, Jeffrey Martin, Aniruddha Deshpande, Nancy Stecker, Melissa Pereira, and Michael Kilgard. 2017. "Vagus Nerve Stimulation Paired with Tones for the Treatment of Tinnitus: A Prospective Randomized Double-Blind Controlled Pilot Study in Humans." *Scientific Reports* 7 (1): 11960.

Varma, Rohit, Thasarat S. Vajaranant, Bruce Burkemper, Shuang Wu, Mina Torres, Chunyi Hsu, Farzana Choudhury, and Roberta McKean-Cowdin. 2016. "Visual Impairment and Blindness in Adults in the United States: Demographic and Geographic Variations from 2015 to 2050." *JAMA Ophthalmology* 134 (7): 802–9.

Villchur, Edgar. 1973. "Signal Processing to Improve Speech Intelligibility in Perceptive Deafness." *The Journal of the Acoustical Society of America* 53 (6): 1646–57.

Wikipedia. 2018. "History of Hearing Aids." https://en.wikipedia.org/wiki/History_of_hearing_aids.

Chapter 21 Prosthetic and orthotic devices

Joel Kempfer, Renee Lewis,
Goeran Fiedler, and
Barbara Silver-Thorn

Contents

DOI: 10.1201/b21964-24

21.1 Chapter overview

This chapter will present an overview of amputation surgery and the history of prosthetic and orthotic design to set the stage for current and future technology. Amputation causes and incidence rates will be summarized. Lower and upper limb prostheses, both preparatory and definitive, will be presented, as well as common options regarding prosthetic socket, foot, and knee components. The typical progression and rehabilitation, from amputation surgery through prosthetic prescription, fabrication, and fitting, will be described. Lower limb prosthetic alignment and upper limb prosthetic control will also be discussed. Similarly, medical conditions and functional losses warranting orthotic treatment will be described. Orthotic designs, fabrication, and fitting will be presented. The corresponding biomechanical loading in terms of both three-point and four-point designs will be described. Both static and dynamic orthotic designs will be presented, as well as various joint components and control options. Finally, modern technology advances and device designs under development will be introduced.

21.2 Prosthetic devices

21.2.1 History of limb prostheses

The earliest prosthetic device was found in ancient Egypt where a prosthetic toe was exhumed from the tomb of the warrior queen, Vishpala (Michael and Bowker 2004). While other devices from the Middle Ages have been found, the beginnings of a prosthetics industry can be traced to the years following the American Civil War. The human carnage of this conflict included multitudes of amputees as medical advances, including the use of tourniquets, ligatures, anesthesia, and antiseptics, greatly improved post-operative amputation survival rates. Common battlefield medicine included the practice of joint disarticulations, the surgical procedure with the highest survival potential for wounded soldiers. Numerous prosthetic appliance companies were founded in both the South and North including J.E. Hanger in Atlanta and A.A. Marks in New York City.

526

Early "scientific" approaches to prosthetic design are largely attributed to the formation of the Veteran's Administration following World War II. Federally funded prosthetic research supported the development of socket technology and advances in prosthetic components. Similar investment and development were occurring in Europe, especially in Germany, where industrial fabrication of components had started with the establishment of the Otto Bock Corporation after World War I.

War has always been the impetus for prosthetic advances as the increased population of young amputees necessitated increased federal funding to service the veterans' needs. Progress in rehabilitative practices, in both physical and occupational therapy, also developed post-conflict. Some of these historic prosthetic design innovations include the development of modular (exoskeletal) prosthesis design in the 1910s, endoskeletal components in the late 1960s, myoelectric control of upper extremity prosthetic devices in the late 1970s, and microprocessor control of prosthetic knees in the late 1990s (Michael and Bowker 2004). Current fabrication technology includes computer-aided design and manufacturing, 3D printing, and the use of carbon fiber and other new materials.

21.2.2 Amputation levels and etiology

It is estimated that more than 2.2 million Americans are living with limb loss (Ziegler-Graham et al. 2008) and approximately 185,000 amputation surgeries are performed each year in the United States alone (Owings and Kozak 1998). Globally, it is estimated that 0.5% of the population, 35–40 million individuals, require prostheses or orthoses (World Health Organization & USAID 2017). Many of the differences in incidence rates across the globe are attributable to differences in life expectancy, obesity rates, and recency of armed conflict. It is a misconception that the most common cause of amputation is trauma, such as vehicular or industrial accidents. Although trauma is a predominant cause of upper extremity amputation, the most common cause of lower limb amputation in high-income countries is gangrenous infection secondary to a wound or pressure ulcer in elderly individuals with diabetes (Dillingham, Pezzin, and MacKenzie 2002; Chaturvedi et al. 2001). Diabetes mellitus commonly affects the geriatric population and often results in an ulcer on the foot due to poor fit or inappropriate footwear, or poor toenail care. As diabetes also causes peripheral neuropathy and impairs vision, the detection and subsequent treatment of these wounds may be delayed. The concomitant development of peripheral vascular disease hinders healthy blood flow in the lower extremity, retarding healing.

A chronic ulcer may result in infection, ultimately requiring lower limb amputation, most commonly at the trans-tibial level. The second most common level of amputation is above-the-knee (trans-femoral). Proximal amputation levels pose increasing functional challenges as the incorporation of additional prosthetic

527

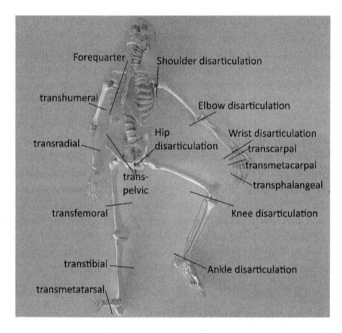

Figure 21.1 Upper and lower extremity amputation levels.

componentry (e.g., a knee joint), in combination with the more substantial loss of body segments, requires increased physical stamina to ambulate. Other less common lower limb amputation levels warranting a prosthetic device include partial foot (trans-metatarsal), ankle disarticulation (Symes), knee and hip disarticulation, and hemipelvectomy (trans-pelvic) (Figure 21.1). Factors like end-weight bearing capacity and/or the bulbous shape of some of these lower limb amputation types make them less likely to warrant prosthetic intervention (e.g., partial foot).

Upper extremity amputations are less common (approximately 10–20% relative incidence; Dillingham, Pezzin, and MacKenzie 2002) than lower limb amputations; their primary cause is trauma. Upper limb amputation levels (Figure 21.1) warranting prosthetic replacement include partial hand, wrist disarticulation, below-elbow (trans-radial), above-elbow (trans-humeral), shoulder disarticulation, and forequarter (disarticulation of the scapula and clavicle).

21.2.3 Rehabilitation and prosthetic design for lower extremity amputees

Regardless of the lower extremity amputation level or etiology, the goal of the rehabilitation team is to return the patient to their pre-amputation level of independence. Realistically, factors such as progression of underlying diseases and comorbidities or weakened physical state and prolonged convalescence may adversely affect this goal. The energy cost of ambulation influences functional outcomes as well: more proximal amputation levels increase energy expenditure. In general, amputation at the trans-tibial and trans-femoral levels require approximately 10% to 35% more energy cost, respectively, than for age-matched able-bodied individuals (Waters and Mulroy 1999). Prosthetic design and componentry may help minimize this increased energy demand during ambulation (Kaufman et al. 2008; Schmalz, Blumentritt, and Jarasch 2002). Ultimately, however, current prosthetic limbs remain to be merely assistive devices used by patients to perform their activities of daily living.

21.2.3.1 Rehabilitation   A successful functional outcome for a patient with limb loss requires the cooperation and communication of the rehabilitation team. This collaborative effort may begin before amputation. For example, the amputation surgeon (e.g., vascular or orthopedic surgeon) may confer with a prosthetist or therapist regarding the amputation level. The patient may also meet with a prosthetist or therapist prior to surgery for pre-prosthetic education to alleviate fears or ambiguity regarding post-surgical and rehabilitation procedures, prosthetic options, and future function. Such consultation is less common when amputation is performed as an emergency measure or is the last recourse to other vascular procedures. Interestingly, amputation surgery may differ based on the surgeon's training. Vascular surgeons review the level of vascular impairment and commonly select the amputation level based on the location of healthy tissue and blood supply that will yield the greatest potential for healing. Conversely, an orthopedic surgeon will choose the amputation level based on biomechanical principles that will result in improved prosthetic functional outcomes.

Although individual procedures differ, amputation surgery typically incorporates myoplasty or myodesis. Myoplasty, which entails connecting the severed opposing muscles over the distal bone, aims to provide distal soft tissue padding to enhance comfort in the prosthetic socket and secure the muscles at functional lengths such that they can generate force. In contrast, myodesis attaches the severed muscles directly to the bone with the goal of improving the effectiveness of muscle work and control of limb motion. The surgical procedure is more time intensive and thus more taxing for the patient than myoplasty, making it contraindicated for many elderly or frail amputation candidates. Common post-surgical problems include phantom limb pain and the formation of bone spurs and neuromas. Phantom limb pain typically diminishes with wound healing and compression therapy but can develop into a chronic issue for a considerable portion of patients. Bone spurs result from the calcification of cut bone ends attempting to attach to other bone. Neuromas, small nerve end bundles at the severed nerve site, are perceived as "electric shock" when palpated. If severe, bone spurs and neuromas may necessitate revision surgery.

The rehabilitation team may also include peer support counselors and fellow amputees who have received training to educate new amputees in post-surgical care and rehabilitation expectations. Of course, nursing staff (and therapists) play an integral role throughout the process, during both inpatient and outpatient care. A rehabilitation engineer may help provide access to assistive technology to support seating and positioning, mobility, and independent performance of activities of daily living as well as vocational activities.

Rehabilitation care includes the involvement of physical therapists immediately following the surgery. Activities include the application of an immediate post-surgical dressing (see below), as well as education and assistance with transfers, personal hygiene tasks, and ambulating with a walker.

The prosthetist's activities may involve fabricating an immediate post-surgical cast to prevent post-operative edema and incidental contact and pain. If not contra-indicated by the patient's overall health condition or potential vascular impairment, the prosthetist may also fabricate a device to facilitate early weight-bearing and ambulation. This can help mitigate the risk of joint contractures and other sequelae of prolonged immobilization. After the removal of sutures or staples, approximately five weeks post-operatively, the prosthetist fits the patient with a compression garment or "shrinker." Shrinkers should be worn constantly and removed only to bathe. Even after prosthetic use is initiated, the shrinker should still be donned whenever the prosthesis is removed; regular shrinker use will prevent significant volume fluctuations of the residual limb. Depending on the amount of post-operative edema, the prosthetist will cast the patient's residual limb approximately one week after the shrinker fitting; this cast is used to fabricate a socket for the preparatory prosthesis.

The preparatory prosthesis is a temporary endoskeletal device that typically consists of a thermoplastic socket, suction suspension with liner and lock, and flexible keel foot (Figure 21.2). This temporary prosthesis is initially worn solely during physical therapy. In addition to the therapy itself, these sessions include education regarding how to properly don and doff the prosthesis. Prosthetic training and activities include weight transfer to and from the prosthetic limb, ambulation (initially within parallel bars, advancing to ambulation with an assistive device, and finally independent ambulation), and safe negotiation on environmental obstacles such as ramps, curbs, and stairs. The patient then begins a wearing schedule for their prosthesis, gradually increasing weight bearing on the non-traditionally weighted tissues of their residual limb. Prosthetic use is progressively increased in one- to two-hour increments twice a day, gradually increasing time as tolerated.

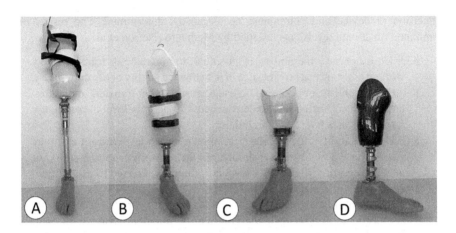

Figure 21.2 Examples of preparatory prostheses with an adjustable socket. (A) Trans-femoral; (B) trans-tibial, trial prosthesis with check socket; (C) trans-tibial, and definitive prosthesis; (D) trans-tibial. Common components are the foot/ankle modules, pylon adapters for static alignment, and (in trans-femoral prosthetics) the knee component.

This preparatory phase of the patient's prosthetic rehabilitation is often the most difficult due to surgical healing, pain, edema, and potential complications, as well as naivety regarding prosthetic use. The residual limb volume changes as the post-operative edema subsides and the muscles severed during the amputation surgery atrophy. Continued use of shrinkers, replaced to maintain consistent fit with the varying residual limb volume, is necessary. The body normally expels interstitial fluid via muscular contraction, as due to reduced muscular activity, the residual limb tissues may fill with fluid. Prosthetic use and ambulation will assist fluid expulsion and result in further limb atrophy. To maintain socket fit while the limb volume is decreasing, the patient must add prosthetic socks of varying thickness or ply. When the residual limb volume has stabilized, usually after three to six months of prosthetic use for most of the day, every day, the rehabilitation physician will prescribe a definitive prosthesis.

21.2.3.2 Prosthetic prescription Reimbursement criteria for prosthetic devices via both federal and private insurance in the United States typically adhere to Medicare policies and guidelines. These guidelines are based on functional level definitions that ultimately determine prosthetic component selection and reimbursement based on the anticipated abilities of the amputee. These functional levels are jointly determined by the physician, therapist, and prosthetist on an individual basis. A common assessment tool is the Amputee Mobility Predictor (Gailey et al. 2002), which measures the patient's abilities such that an informed decision of device and component needs can be determined. The respective amputee functional levels, as classified by Medicare (Nelson et al. 2006), are:

K-0: Does not have the ability, or potential, to ambulate or transfer safely without assistance; a prosthesis will not enhance quality of life or mobility.

K-1: Has the ability, or potential, to use a prosthesis for transfers and ambulation on level surfaces at fixed cadence; this activity level is commonly referred to as a household ambulator.

K-2: Has the ability, or potential, for ambulation on level terrain and may also traverse low level environmental barriers such as curbs, stairs, or uneven surfaces; this activity level is commonly referred to as a limited community ambulator.

K-3: Has the ability, or potential, for ambulation with variable cadence; this activity level is typical of the community ambulator with vocational, therapeutic, or exercise activities that demand prosthetic utilization *beyond* simple locomotion (e.g., unlimited community ambulator).

K-4: Has the ability, or potential, for prosthetic mobility that exceeds basic ambulation skills, exhibiting high impact, stress, or energy levels of an active user or athlete.

Adoption of these criteria and definitions facilitates reimbursement for appropriate prosthetic components for each patient, which with increasing K-level, tend to be more complex, and typically more expensive, such as dynamic response feet, hydraulic ankles and knees, microprocessor-controlled knees, and/or elevated vacuum systems (see Section 23.2.3.3).

Technological advances continue to provide new options that may enhance the capabilities and quality of life for many amputees. However, realistic expectations must be made to fully utilize technology and afford reimbursement. A recent encounter illustrates the potential for misinterpretation: an 87-year-old lower limb amputee who viewed a TV commercial depicting a bilateral transtibial amputee playing basketball requested the same shock absorbing dynamic response feet so that he might play basketball again. This particular client was essentially wheelchair bound with limited ambulation potential (e.g., K-0 to K-1 functional level). His misconception was that the technology would enable him to perform well above his capabilities. No matter what the technology, even today's most advanced prosthesis is simply a tool that enables patients to perform at *their* physical capabilities.

21.2.3.3 Prosthetic components and design Various prosthetic components are available, from many manufacturers, to meet the different functional needs of the individual. New components are frequently introduced to address unmet needs, reduce prosthesis mass, enhance joint range of motion, and/or incorporate new technology and materials.

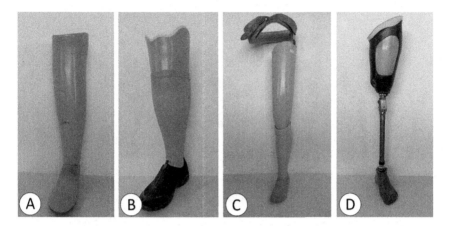

Figure 21.3 Endoskeletal versus exoskeletal prosthetic design. (A) Trans-tibial prosthesis with crustacean "hard cosmesis" exoskeleton from laminate; (B) trans-tibial prosthesis with laminated socket and foam cosmesis covering the endoskeletal pylon; (C) trans-femoral exoskeletal prosthesis from wood with outer lamination for strength; (D) Trans-femoral endoskeletal design. A cosmesis cover can affect knee motion and is often omitted.

Lower limb prostheses can be categorized as exoskeletal or endoskeletal (Figure 21.3). Exoskeletal or crustacean designs transfer load through the exterior structures. These designs are durable, but are often heavy (e.g., carved from wood), more difficult to modify, and incompatible with much of modern prosthetic componentry. As such, these designs are seldom used today. Endoskeletal designs incorporate an internal structure and may include an external, cosmetic cover that matches the shape of the contralateral limb. Endoskeletal designs provide facile changes in components, as well as variation in the alignment of the respective componentry, maximizing function as the patient's needs change.

Lower limb prostheses include a prosthetic socket that serves as the mechanical interface providing load transfer from the distal prosthesis to the residual limb. The remaining components include a prosthetic foot, a knee joint (if trans-femoral or more proximal level of amputation), and a hip joint (if hip disarticulation or more proximal amputation). The length of the shank or leg and thigh is established by internal pylons and various connective hardware (Figure 21.4).

21.2.3.3.1 Socket design As the prosthetic socket connects the prosthesis to the residual limb, its geometry varies based on the level of amputation, the dimensions of the residual limb, the strength of the remnant musculature, and sensitive regions of the limb for which soft tissue pressures must be minimized. The typical socket design for a Symes amputation includes a medial opening "door" to

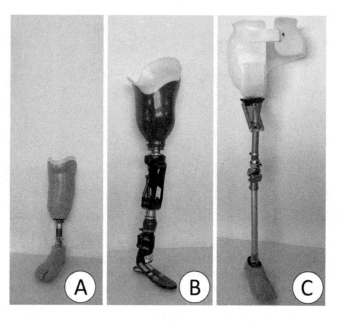

Figure 21.4 Endoskeletal prostheses for (A) trans-tibial, (B) trans-femoral, and (C) hip disarticulation limb loss levels

allow the bulbous distal residual limb to pass when donning. This socket may allow end bearing as Symes amputation often retains the heel pad tissues. For trans-tibial amputees, there are two primary socket designs: patella tendon bearing (PTB) and total surface bearing (TSB). The PTB socket design preferentially weights the residual limb tissues based on their ability to tolerate load (i.e., predominantly load the patellar tendon, posterior calf, and pre-tibial muscle group; minimally load the fibular head and distal bone ends). The TSB or total surface weight bearing (TSWB) design distributes load evenly over the *entire* limb surface; it is the most common socket design used today. For the trans-femoral amputation level, the prosthetic socket either employs some variation of ischial containment or, in sub-ischial designs, hydrostatic soft tissue compression. The historically popular quadrilateral socket incorporated an ischial seat to facilitate skeletal loading through the ischium that resulted in compromised biomechanics and, to retain the ischium's position on the seat, required the proximal anterior wall to provide unhealthy counter pressure. The ischial containment socket is the standard of care today, encompassing the ischium to provide a skeletal lock to keep the residual femur in an adducted position and to assist with rotational control. For the more proximal hip disarticulation and trans-pelvic amputation levels, the prosthetic sockets provide weight bearing, as well as suspension, through the pelvis and iliac crests, respectively. As trans-pelvic amputation results in loss

534

of the ipsilateral pelvic structures, the socket for these individuals often extends more superiorly, enclosing the chest wall, taking care not to adversely affect deep breathing.

The classical process of prosthetic socket fabrication is typically conducted by (1) casting the residual limb, (2) filling the cast with plaster to create a positive model of the limb geometry, (3) modifying the plaster model, as needed, to preferentially distribute or relieve load, and (4) vacuum forming a socket over the plaster positive model. Prior to fabrication of the definitive socket, "test" or "check" sockets may be utilized. The purpose of these clear sockets is to observe both the position of the limb and skin loading during weight bearing and gait. Simple modifications may be made to ensure optimal fit before fabricating a definitive socket using laminated carbon fiber and acrylic resin. For geriatric or low activity patients, lightweight thermoplastic sockets are used.

The fabrication process may be modified to incorporate computer-aided design and manufacturing technology. For example, residual limb geometry can be acquired using cameras, lasers, or various scanning technology; modifications can be performed digitally on a virtual model; the limb model can be carved using a milling machine; or the socket can be generated directly from the data file using additive manufacturing. Central fabrication sites can also be used to minimize equipment resources needed at the prosthetist's office.

The fit of the socket is critical to a successful prosthetic outcome. If the socket is not comfortable, the prosthesis will not be worn; poor fit may also contribute to instability and potential damage to the residual limb tissues. Socket fit is assessed by visual inspection of the limb tissues after donning a clear test socket. For trans-tibial amputees, it is important that the socket fully encapsulates the residuum, with load transfer creating uniform pressure over the entire residual limb (e.g., blanched skin with loading). No areas of high pressure or discomfort should be observed. For trans-femoral sockets, the ischial tuberosity should be properly "seated" on the ischial seat (quadrilateral socket) or within the socket pocket (ischial containment socket). The adjacent joint should be unencumbered in its useful range of motion and the residuum should be free from discomfort or brim pressure. Total contact is imperative as gaps may result in blister formation.

21.2.3.3.2 Prosthetic feet There are hundreds of different prosthetic feet commercially available today (Figure 21.5). These feet can be broadly categorized in terms of their respective functional levels. For household (K-1) and community (K-2) ambulators, the most basic (and least expensive) variety, either the single-axis or the solid-ankle-cushioned-heel (SACH) foot, is indicated. The SACH foot provides shock absorption at heel strike via compression of the soft foam heel, as well as roll-over and stability during mid-stance via the wooden or plastic keel. Community ambulators may also benefit from single-axis or flexible keel

535

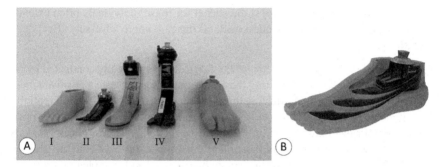

Figure 21.5 Selection of prosthetic feet. (A) Modern energy storage and return (ESAR) feet commonly have a removable cosmetic shell (I) to conform to the shoe without inhibiting the motion of the spring elements. These elements are traditionally made from carbon fiber laminate (II and IV), although other materials (e.g., fiberglass, III) have also proven effective. More traditional designs that are compatible with endoskeletal prosthesis design such as the single-axis foot (V) are by trend lower in cost and functional performance. (B) The cut-away shows the inner workings of an early generation ESAR foot, where several spring elastic carbon elements are embedded in a rubber material.

feet that provide enhanced heel shock absorption and roll-over; flexible keel feet also permit minor inversion and eversion to further accommodate uneven terrain. More active amputees at the K-3 through K-4 levels are often prescribed dynamic response or energy storage and return (ESAR) feet. These feet typically incorporate leaf spring structures that are compressed during early and mid-stance, storing energy that is released during late stance at the initiation of the swing phase. Other options for these active amputees include multiaxial ankle-feet for individuals who frequently traverse uneven terrain or hydraulic ankles to control plantar and dorsiflexion. Powered ankle-feet are also available at a substantially greater cost (see Section 23.2.3.7).

21.2.3.3.3 Knee units There is also a wide variety of knee designs (Figure 21.6) to accommodate the limb loss levels of the knee-disarticulation, trans-femoral amputation, and hip disarticulation (individuals with trans-pelvic amputation are largely non-ambulatory due to excessive energy cost). Household ambulators are frequently prescribed a locked knee that prevents knee flexion or buckling, facilitating safe, albeit very slow, ambulation and transfers; this knee may be manually unlocked for sitting. Alternative knee units that provide enhanced safety, while permitting flexion during swing, are weight-activated stance-controlled designs with a braking mechanism that engages during weight-bearing to prevent inadvertent buckling. More active amputees might be prescribed polycentric knee designs for which the knee center of rotation varies,

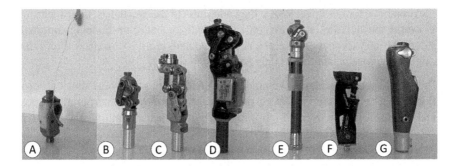

Figure 21.6 Selection of prosthetic knee joint components. (A) Lock knee, the user can unlock the knee by pulling on a cable when sitting down; (B) polycentric knee, provides stance stability by its axis geometry; (C) advanced polycentric, the additional axes facilitate some degree of knee flexion in stance phase to resemble natural biomechanics; (D) polycentric with microprocessor-controlled swing phase pneumatic, allows variable gait speeds; (E) single-axis knee with weight-activated friction brake to prevent buckling during weight bearing; (F) single-axis knee with stance-and-swing (SnS) hydraulic to control flexion resistance in the stance phase and both flexion and extension resistance in the swing phase; (G) single-axis hydraulic with microprocessor control optimizes safety and dynamic efficiency by continuously adopting to gait phase and speed.

thereby proving good stability and the potential for stance flexion for shock absorption at heel strike. These designs essentially fold on themselves, better approximating the complex gliding and rotation of the femur on the tibial plateau in an intact, healthy knee.

In addition to stability in stance, prosthetic knees also incorporate some degree of swing phase control. Most prosthetic knees provide some form of extension assistance to assure the knee is in full extension at the point of weight acceptance during heel strike. In addition to a simple spring mechanism, fluid control (e.g., hydraulic or pneumatic) can be used to accommodate walking at a varied cadence. The fluid flow and resistance vary with flexion and extension speed; settings also permit the flexion and extension resistance to be independently adjusted. In the most advanced devices for active amputees, microprocessors control these functions. These designs are typically hydraulic, with multiple sensors to provide precise, variable resistance and cadence control; many designs also support multiple modes of ambulation such that walking, stair ascent/descent, roller-blading, and so on might be accommodated.

21.2.3.3.4 Rotators and shock absorbers While prosthetic feet may provide some frontal and coronal plane mobility, additional axial rotators are indicated for some users. These are typically separate units that can be incorporated near the prosthetic foot or knee. While they add mass to the prosthesis, their inclusion is useful for activities such as golf, basketball, or ballroom dancing; internal/external rotary torques are thereby accommodated, minimizing shear forces that might otherwise be applied to the residual limb tissues.

Prosthetic feet, particularly dynamic and ESAR feet provide some shock absorption at heel strike. Additionally, vertical shock pylons may be incorporated to protect the residual limb during high-impact activities such as running and jumping.

21.2.3.3.5 Hip joints Prostheses for hip disarticulation and trans-pelvic amputees must incorporate a prosthetic hip joint for ambulation and sitting. These designs permit hip flexion, often with springs or elastic straps for flexion assistance, to facilitate the forward progression of the prosthetic limb. As with the prosthetic knee, alignment is critical to prevent inadvertent buckling during stance.

21.2.3.3.6 Prosthetic suspension For both trans-tibial and trans-femoral amputees, the most common suspension method is a soft liner worn inside the prosthetic socket. These liners, usually made from a silicone or polyurethane gel material help provide a very effective force coupling while also cushioning the residual limb. Liners may incorporate pin or lanyard locking mechanisms to attach to the rigid outer socket. Supplemental suspension options, specifically for trans-tibial amputees, include sleeves and supra-condylar cuffs (Figure 21.7). Most recently, elevated and passive vacuum systems have been developed to use in conjunction with liners. These systems incorporate a sealing sleeve with either an expulsion valve or (gravity- or battery-powered) suction pump to create a vacuum between the liner and socket.

One of the challenges that affects both prosthetic socket fit and suspension is volume fluctuations of the residual limb. The residual limb undergoes the largest volume changes during the initial 3–12 months post-amputation. More modest, but still clinically significant, changes occur daily, particularly for individuals with diabetes who may take diuretics due to impaired kidney function. To accommodate these changes, amputees don socks of varying ply. Since most prosthetic sockets cannot adjust for changes in residual limb volume, it is important that patients understand the need for adjustment and use of prosthetic socks to prevent socket movement relative to the limb, which may cause skin damage.

21.2.3.4 Sports/running prostheses Other technologies include activity-specific prostheses such as "running blades" (Figure 21.8), swim legs, modified feet for rock climbing, and rotators to facilitate golfing and dancing. The running feet incorporate carbon fiber leaf spring designs that store energy during loading or impact and return energy when off-loaded. These designs typically do not incorporate a heel

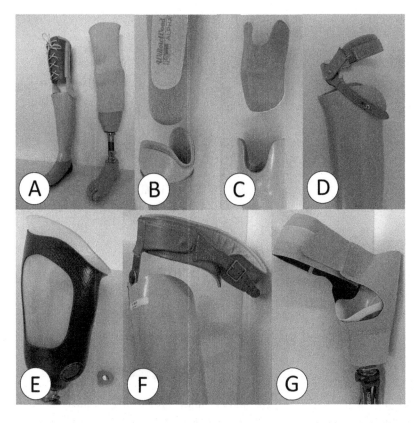

Figure 21.7 Prosthesis suspension methods. (A) Thigh corset (left) and elastic knee sleeve (right); (B) liner suspension; (C) supracondylar suspension, the flexible inner socket contains wedges to utilize the geometry proximal of the knee; (D) cuff strap, following a similar principle and may be combined with an additional waist belt for extra secure suspension (e.g., in athletes); (E) suction suspension, the valve (pictured next to the socket) helps maintain a vacuum in the socket; (F) pelvic band may be designed with (pictured) or without hip joint; (G) total elastic suspension (TES) belt.

and are aligned to promote forefoot loading and spring compression during running. They are not appropriate for daily use and are therefore seldom covered by insurance. Other sports prostheses include swimming or beach limbs that enable access to water without sacrificing componentry. Most amputees find using a prosthesis for swimming difficult without a flipper to assist propulsion.

21.2.3.5 Prosthetic fit, volume adjustment, and alignment While the fit and comfort of the prosthetic socket are critical to prosthesis use, the stability and

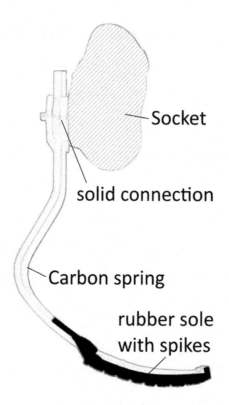

Figure 21.8 Illustration of lower limb prosthesis design considerations for sprinting/running. Unlike a prosthetic foot for everyday use, the sprint foot does not have a heel element, making stable standing or slow walking challenging.

function of the prosthesis are also dependent on the alignment of the various prosthetic components. As is the case for component selection and adjustment as well, the alignment optimization aims at a compromise between static stability and dynamic (gait) efficiency – objectives that are not easily reconcilable. Prior to initial walking within parallel bars, the prosthetist will perform a basic or "bench" alignment. Specific guidelines for this vary depending on the type of foot, knee, and socket design. For trans-tibial prostheses, the socket is centered over the foot in the sagittal plane and over the middle third of the foot in the coronal plane. This initial alignment provides medial-lateral stability at mid-stance and a smooth roll over the prosthetic foot. For trans-femoral prostheses, the classical alignment is referred to as the trochanter-knee-ankle (TKA) alignment. The socket is aligned such that the weight line (i.e., a visualized plumb line from the assumed body center of mass just anterior to the second sacral vertebra) is through or slightly anterior to the knee center of rotation. This is needed in knee joints without hydraulic stance control to prevent knee buckling. The socket is centered over the foot in the sagittal plane, with slight adduction and flexion (approximately 5° plus any contracture) to help position the hip abductors and extensors in a stretched state and facilitate muscle force generation, thereby controlling knee flexion and providing even step length.

After socket fit and static bench alignment have been achieved, dynamic alignment is conducted. The prosthetist assesses the stability of the device as the patient walks. Adjustments are made to "fine-tune" the alignment, based on observation of gait in both the frontal and sagittal planes. In the frontal plane, weight transitions between the limbs should be smooth, without excessive pelvic shifting to one side or the other. In the sagittal plane, a harmonic roll-over of the prosthetic foot should be seen. For trans-tibial amputees, common gait deviations include excessive varus or lateral shifting; this can be corrected by out-setting the foot to improve lateral stability. For trans-femoral amputees, alignment problems may include knee buckling if the knee is too far anterior, lateral pelvic displacement if the foot is too far inset, and vaulting or circumduction if the knee flexion resistance is too stiff or the prosthetic limb is too long.

21.2.3.6 Functional outcomes   In addition to the qualitative assessment of socket fit and static/dynamic prosthetic alignment, quantitative evaluation of functional outcomes is imperative in demonstrating the medical necessity for the prescribed prosthesis and components. Validated clinical tools are often used for such evaluation. Common tools include the six-minute or ten-meter walk test (Dean, Richards, and Malouin 2001; Troosters, Gosselink, and Decramer 1999), the timed up and go test (Bohannon 2006), the Amputee Mobility Predictor (with and without a prosthesis; Gailey et al. 2002), the Locomotor Capabilities Index (Franchignoni et al. 2004), the Prosthesis Evaluation Questionnaire (Legro et al. 1998), the Prosthetic Limb Users Survey-Mobility (PLUS-M) (Hafner et al. 2017), and the Comprehensive High-Level Activity Mobility Predictor (Gailey et al. 2013). These tools are often modified by clinicians due to space and/or time constraints.

21.2.3.7 Emerging technologies in lower extremity prosthetic devices and amputation surgery   Emerging technologies include recent advances in prosthetic power and control. Until recently, all lower limb prostheses were passive, relying on the remnant musculature of the patient's residual limb and potential energy return via leaf spring designs (e.g., Flex foot, Össur) for ambulation. Active, externally powered components include the EmPower (Otto Bock) and Odyssey (SpringActive) ankle-feet, and the adaptive orientation Proprio Foot (Össur). Other active ankles (Hitt et al. 2010; Bergelin and Voglewede 2012; Grimmer et al. 2016; Gao, Liu, and Liao 2018; Cempini, Hargrove, and Lenzi 2017) and knees (Varol, Sup, and Goldfarb 2009; Lawson et al. 2012; Young et al. 2014;

Elery et al. 2018; Tran et al. 2019; Azocar et al. 2018) are in development. Various control options, including state classifiers and intent recognition of intrinsic prosthetic sensors, as well as neural control using the electromyogram of residual limb muscles (Ha, Varol, and Goldfarb 2010; Huang et al. 2011; Hargrove et al. 2013; Farmer et al. 2014; Windrich et al. 2016), are also being investigated.

In addition, advances in amputation surgery including osseointegration and targeted muscle reinnervation (TMR) are being investigated for both the lower and upper limbs. Osseointegration, or direct skeletal attachment, has been used in Sweden since the 1980s (Branemark et al. 2001; Hagberg and Brånemark 2009). Due to challenges with respect to infection and regulatory issues, this procedure has only recently been adopted in the United States (Knox 2016). Osseointegration involves implanting a "post" into the remnant bone of the amputee's residual limb. An abutment is then attached, extending through the distal skin, to provide direct skeletal attachment to the prosthesis. The direct skeleton-prosthesis attachment eliminates the need for a prosthetic socket, thereby reducing the potential for pistoning or rotation of the socket relative to the residual limb soft tissues. Prerequisites currently exclude patients with certain vascular conditions as well as patients with high activity levels as candidates for this procedure. Further advances to minimize infection risk, develop rehabilitation protocols, and prevent potential excessive loading that might damage the abutment, the implant, and/or the osseointegration of the implant itself are necessary.

21.2.4 Upper extremity amputation, rehabilitation, and prosthetic devices

Similar to lower limb prostheses, upper extremity prosthetic devices have also been used as early as medieval times. Technological improvements in recent decades include the incorporation of externally powered components, myoelectric control, and various materials that have resulted in improved cosmesis. Enhanced industrial safety regulations, improved prenatal care, and regulatory practices regarding pharmaceutical testing have reduced the incidence of both traumatic upper limb amputation and congenital upper limb deficiencies.

Upper extremity prosthetic devices can be classified as: (1) passive, (2) body-powered (Figure 21.9), or (3) externally powered. Passive prostheses are typically cosmetic devices that perform little to no function but fulfill the need for a life-like appearance. Body-powered prosthetic devices, the most common type of upper extremity prosthesis due to their lower cost, high durability, and high function, utilize the mobility of a patient's remnant upper extremity joints to operate the prosthesis using harness and cable systems. With practice, patients can become extremely adept at operating body-powered terminal devices and/or elbows with ease. In contrast, externally powered upper extremity prosthetic components are

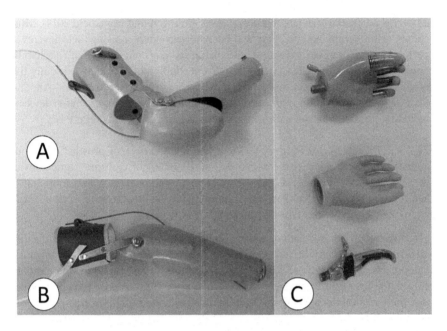

Figure 21.9 Upper extremity prostheses and components. (A) body-powered trans-radial prosthesis with step-up hinges; (B) body-powered, trans-radial prosthesis without a terminal device attached; (C) selection of passive and body-powered terminal devices: spring-fingered hand, cosmetic cover for mechanical hand, active opening hook.

powered by a rechargeable battery and are typically controlled by switches or myoelectric control. Myoelectric control utilizes surface electrodes placed on the residual limb musculature (e.g., wrist flexors/extensors, elbow flexors/extensors; Fougner et al. 2012). If the patient demonstrates independent control of muscle agonist-antagonist pairs, the respective prosthetic device may incorporate proportional control such that the speed or torque of the terminal device or elbow is regulated by the strength of the muscle signal. Other approaches to increasing the functionality (e.g., the degrees of freedom in controlling the prosthetic device) include pattern recognition and TMR (detailed below).

21.2.4.1 Rehabilitation In contrast to lower limb amputees for whom physical therapy is critical for successful prosthetic outcomes, both physical and occupational therapy are important for upper extremity amputees. Many activities of daily living require bilateral upper limb use. In addition, body-powered prostheses require a full range of motion and strength of the proximal upper extremity joints. Physical therapy, both pre- and post-amputation surgery, is therefore important. Post-prosthetic fitting, occupational therapy is important to achieve prosthetic dexterity, particularly during bimanual tasks (Johnson and Mansfield 2014). Most clients, with therapy and practice, will become very adept at using their devices to perform activities of daily living. These therapists may collaborate with a rehabilitation engineer to provide access to assistive technology for activities of daily living, including bathing, dressing, meal preparation, dining, and transfers. Another focus of the rehabilitation engineer is the use of alternative communication devices, including modifications to technologies such as computers and cell phones.

21.2.4.2 Prosthetic prescription   There is a wide variety of prosthetic components available to address the functional needs of upper extremity amputees at the various amputation levels. As the most common upper extremity amputation levels are at the trans-radial and trans-humeral levels, prosthetic prescription and components will be discussed for these levels only.

Trans-radial prostheses include a socket with a forearm section, inclusive of a distal wrist unit to secure the terminal device. Body-powered prostheses incorporate a figure-of-eight harness and cable system that use biscapular abduction to apply tension to the control cable and open (voluntary opening) or close (voluntary closing) the terminal device (Figure 21.9). In contrast, externally powered prostheses do not need a harness and cable system for prosthetic control and suspension (Figure 21.10). The prosthetic socket itself provides suspension; the embedded

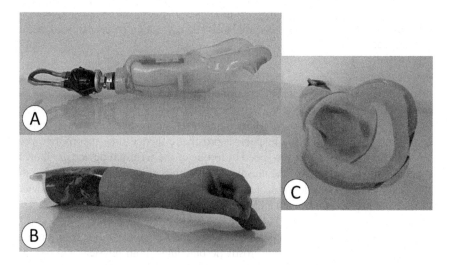

Figure 21.10 Externally powered prosthesis for trans-radial amputee with myoelectric control. (A) prosthesis with powered hook without cover and exposed electronics; (B) externally powered hand without cosmetic/protective cover; (C) inside socket view of externally powered, myoelectric control trans-radial prosthesis, showing the position of the skin electrodes.

surface electrodes over the wrist flexors/extensors are then used for myoelectric control of the terminal device. The forearm section houses the rechargeable battery and control unit for the externally powered terminal device, which is again connected via a wrist unit. The selection of body-powered versus externally powered prostheses is dependent on the patient's desired comfort, durability, and functional needs, as well as cost constraints.

Prostheses for trans-humeral amputees include a socket and an elbow unit to lengthen/shorten the arm and position the forearm and terminal device in a position for function. If body-powered, the prosthesis again incorporates a harness/cable system to control the elbow and terminal device. This harness includes a second cable that functions as a switching mechanism using shoulder elevation and/or extension to transfer control to/from the elbow from/to the terminal device. If the elbow is locked, the harness/cable operates the terminal device; if the elbow is unlocked, the harness/cable controls elbow flexion and the terminal device is locked. While externally powered prostheses may be used for trans-humeral amputees to operate the elbow and terminal device independently, or serially with a switching mechanism, the combined weight of externally powered elbow and terminal devices often dictates the use of a hybrid design (Ohnishi, Weir, and Kuiken 2007). For example, the elbow may be body-powered with an externally powered terminal device to provide greater grip force. Alternatively, a body-powered terminal device might be used in concert with an externally powered elbow, minimizing the perceived mass of the prosthesis by keeping the weight more proximal.

21.2.4.3 Prosthetic components   Similar to lower limb prostheses, upper limb prostheses vary based on amputation level, proximal joint mobility, functional needs, desired reliability, comfort, cosmesis, and cost constraints. These factors influence the selection of power and control (e.g., body versus externally powered, myoelectric control), which, in turn, affects the prosthetic component options.

21.2.4.3.1 Sockets and suspension   Upper extremity prosthetic sockets are often laminated and again fabricated from a cast and plaster model of the residual limb. For body-powered prostheses, the harness system provides suspension to minimize the motion of the socket relative to the residual limb. For externally powered prostheses, the sockets are self-suspending, securing the socket via proximal trim lines. For example, trans-radial sockets are suspended over the medial and lateral humeral epicondyles, and may also incorporate suction; trans-humeral sockets often incorporate anterior-posterior "wings" that stabilize the socket on the thorax and scapula. Liner suspension is less common in upper than lower limb prosthetics, mostly due to limited compatibility with surface electrodes and the ready availability of effective harness suspension as a durable alternative.

21.2.4.3.2 Terminal devices: Hands and non-hands Although less cosmetic, non-hands or "hooks" are generally more functional. These non-hands might be stainless steel or aluminum and may include lined "fingers" to resist slipping of grasped objects. Non-hands support hook, tip, and cylindrical grasp. The "fingers" are canted to improve sight lines for picking up various objects. In contrast, hands, whether body-powered or externally powered, provide palmar (e.g., three-jaw chuck) and cylindrical grasp only, unless the design includes motors for the fingers themselves (see Section 21.2.4.4). Most prosthetic hands are covered with a cosmetic glove. The pinch force of a body-powered, voluntary opening, non-hand is determined by the number of rubber bands as the typical means to provide closing force; the pinch force of externally powered, myoelectric controlled hands is based on the motor design and muscle signal magnitude (in proportional control).

21.2.4.3.3 Wrist units The most common types of wrist units can be classified into constant friction, quick disconnect, and wrist flexion designs. These devices support pre-positioning and stability of the terminal device. The quick disconnect option provides facile changing of terminal devices, from hand to non-hand or vocational tools. Wrist flexion units are indicated for bilateral amputees to assist in performing personal hygiene tasks. Most wrist units are passive, although externally powered wrist rotators are available for bilateral or high-level amputees. Externally powered designs are most commonly controlled by a switch.

21.2.4.3.4 Elbow units While elbow components are incorporated in trans-humeral prostheses, elbow joints are also required for body-powered trans-radial prostheses. These designs link the socket to the harness/cable system and also support the remnant elbow. For body-powered trans-humeral prostheses, the most common elbow unit is the positive locking elbow. This design provides passive humeral rotation and permits elbow flexion with locks in multiple positions (via shoulder extension or elevation with the dual control cable that switches control from the elbow to the terminal device). Prosthetic elbows may also incorporate a lift assist for patients with very short residual limbs and/or limited motion of the proximal joints and cable excursion. Finally, externally powered elbows are available for use with myoelectric control. If dual independent muscle sites are used for control, the elbow flexion/extension speed or torque is proportional to the biceps/triceps signal magnitude.

21.2.4.3.5 Shoulder units For shoulder disarticulation and forequarter amputees, a prosthetic shoulder unit is necessary. These units are typically passive, providing flexion/extension to preposition the prosthetic arm, as well as abduction to facilitate donning/doffing clothing.

21.2.4.4 Emerging technology in upper extremity prosthetic devices and amputation surgery Recent advances in upper extremity componentry include externally powered prosthetic hands that incorporate independent finger movement and variable grasp patterns, with proportional myoelectric control (Segil 2013; Al-Timemy et al. 2015). These devices include the i-Limb (Touch Bionics), Bebionic (RSL Steeper), and Michelangelo (Otto Bock) hands. Recent versions may also be fitted on partial hand amputees.

In contrast to these very complex designs, designs are also available via shareware to support the fabrication of articulated prosthetic hands for pediatric and adult amputees using 3D printer technology, both in the United States and in the developing world. The resultant designs can be fabricated at a low cost, but are not as durable as commercial designs. Such designs also are not supported clinically and they do not address the need for a well-fitting custom socket.

Finally, there have been surgical advances that affect upper limb amputees and prosthetic design. Current commercially available externally powered prostheses for high-level upper limb amputees require asynchronous, serial control as there are limited control sources (e.g., single agonist-antagonist muscle pair and switching mechanism). TMR has now been performed on several trans-humeral and shoulder disarticulation amputees (Kuiken et al. 2004; 2007; 2009). The TMR surgery is conducted post-amputation; it involves deinnervating the target muscles (e.g., pectoralis) and transferring the severed, but functional, nerves that normally control the elbow, wrist, and hand to different segments of the target muscle. The reinnervated target muscle thus provides multiple new muscle sites for a more intuitive and synchronous myoelectric control of the externally prosthetic elbow, wrist, and/or hand. In addition to refined myoelectric control algorithms for TMR amputees, this work has recently been extrapolated to trans-femoral amputation (Hargrove et al. 2011; 2013).

21.3 Orthotic devices

While prostheses refer to interventions and devices designed to *replace* body segments, orthoses *support* body segments through splinting or bracing. Prosthetic and orthotic practices are close partners, often incorporating similar materials, fabrication methods, assessment, reimbursement, and educational models. Until recently, educational programs supported prosthetic and/or orthotic training. Now, however, students complete joint training programs prior to seeking certification in one or both professions.

21.3.1 History of orthotics

Orthotic devices have changed over the years to incorporate technological advancements and adapt to changing needs. Disease outbreaks, but also reduced mortality rates of various debilitating conditions, necessitated developments in orthotic designs. The polio epidemic in the late 1940s and early 1950s, for example, left thousands of survivors with lower limb paralysis. Various metal and leather orthotic designs emerged to address the resultant deformities and weaknesses. In recent decades, medical advances have improved survival rates from cerebrovascular accidents (CVAs) or strokes and traumatic brain injuries (TBIs). Many of these patients subsequently require orthotic interventions to improve function during activities of daily living.

Orthotic designs also changed due to advances in materials technology, providing alternatives to leather and metal to better reconcile strength requirements and mass constraints. The incorporation of thermoplastics, carbon fiber, and titanium have improved the capabilities of many orthotic designs. Today, most orthoses are fabricated from thermoplastics rather than metal and leather.

21.3.2 Types of orthoses

Orthoses are primarily classified into lower extremity, upper extremity, and spinal devices. While some specific designs have common use names such as foot drop splint or Jewitt back brace, most orthoses are described in terms of the encompassed body segments and joints.

21.3.3 Lower limb orthoses

The clinical objective of lower limb orthoses is to support, constrain, or enhance the lower extremity joints (ankle, knee, hip) and segments (foot, leg, thigh). These orthoses (Figure 21.11) include foot orthoses (FOs) or pedorthic designs, ankle-foot orthoses (AFOs), knee orthoses (KOs), knee-ankle-foot orthoses (KAFOs), hip orthoses (HOs), and hip-knee-ankle-foot orthoses (HKAFOs). Pedorthics refer to shoes and foot orthoses designed to treat conditions of the foot, including management of the diabetic foot. They can be corrective, in that a foot deformity is being rectified (usually in children), or accommodative, to alleviate symptoms of an uncorrectable deformity (e.g., pain). Custom FOs are used to treat pain such as that associated with plantar fasciitis and posterior tibial tendon dysfunction (PTTD).

21.3.4 Upper limb orthoses

Upper limb orthoses are used to treat pain, weakness, and mobility impairment of the shoulder, elbow, wrist, hands, and/or fingers. Most designs are positional and intended to hold the respective body segment(s) in a specific position to promote healing or manage joint contractures. These orthoses (Figure 21.12) include wrist-hand orthoses (WHOs), wrist-hand-finger orthoses (WHFOs), and elbow-wrist-finger orthoses (EWFOs). Less common designs include an active component to

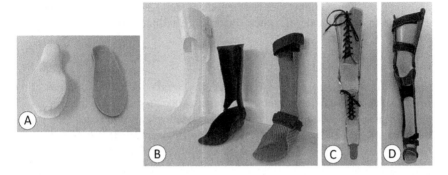

Figure 21.11 Lower extremity orthoses. (A) Custom foot orthosis (right) with plaster positive used for fabrication (left); (B) ankle-foot orthosis (AFO) variants (from left): ground-reaction AFO to stabilize ankle and knee, articulating AFO may be combined with spring elements to support joint motion, solid AFO; (C) knee-ankle-foot orthosis (KAFO) in traditional leather/steel design. The footplate is intended to be solidly attached to the shoe; (D) carbon fiber KAFO provides a superior weight/strength ratio at the expense of adjustability

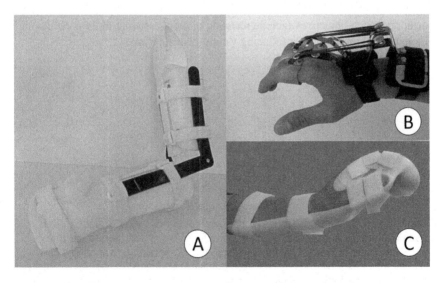

Figure 21.12 Upper extremity orthoses. (A) Elbow-wrist-hand orthosis; (B) dynamic wrist-hand orthosis; (C) static wrist-hand orthosis.

assist motion. For example, the wrist tenodesis splint uses a patient's active wrist extension to mechanically flex their fingers and facilitate grasp.

21.3.5 Spinal orthoses

Spinal orthoses are designed to treat instability, weakness, and deformities of the trunk and spine (e.g., after vertebral fractures). Idiopathic spinal deformities, such as scoliosis, often require spinal bracing during adolescence to reduce the risk of the deformity progressing and eventually requiring surgery. In rehabilitation settings, orthotic devices are often used for positioning and supporting a weak core. For example, a child with neuromuscular scoliosis attributed to cerebral palsy with instability when seated might be fitted with a spinal orthosis. Spinal orthoses are also utilized to safely maintain the trunk in an upright position and reduce the load on internal organs. This more upright position also helps the child see and interact with the world in front of them. As with lower and upper limb orthoses, spinal orthoses are referenced in terms of the spinal vertebra supported, for example, cervical orthosis (CO), cervical-thoracic orthosis (CTO), cervical-thoracic-lumbar-sacral orthosis (CTLSO), and lumbar-sacral orthosis (LSO) (Figure 21.13).

21.3.6 Orthotic design and treatment objectives

The treatment objectives of orthoses vary, affecting orthotic design. Joint impairment due to disease or injury might require orthotic intervention to assist motion or hold the body segment in a specific position to promote healing. Specific orthotic design objectives include resisting motion, assisting motion, achieving a more neutral alignment, or reducing weight-bearing forces.

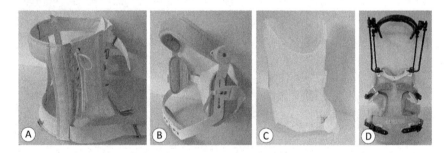

Figure 21.13 Spinal orthoses. (A) Lumbo-sacral orthoses (LSO) made in the traditional metal/leather design; (B) hyperextension orthosis utilizes the three-forces principle to support spine extension; (C) thoraco-lumbo-sacral orthosis (TLSO) made as a two-piece shell from padded thermoplastic; (D) cervico-thoraco-lumbo-sacral orthoses (CTLSO) with a halo to stabilize the cervical spine by fixating the patient's head. The typically long and uninterrupted wear times make effective padding important to prevent skin damage.

550

Resisting motion is often a goal when weak musculature can no longer support a person during standing or ambulation. For example, an AFO may be designed to resist foot drop due to dorsiflexor weakness. Similarly, a KO may be designed to enhance knee stability and prevent knee flexion when the quadriceps or knee extensors are weak. A KO may also be designed to prevent anterior motion of the tibia relative to the femur in the absence of an intact anterior cruciate ligament. Resisting motion may also be an orthotic treatment objective to prevent contractures when muscle spasticity is a concern.

While muscle weakness is frequently treated by resisting motion due to unopposed, or modestly opposed, antagonistic muscle group activity, some orthoses are designed to assist motion of the weakened agonist muscle. For example, an AFO may incorporate a mechanical joint with spring tension to actively pull the foot into dorsiflexion. Orthotic joints that assist knee extension may similarly be integrated into KO or KAFO designs.

Both lower and upper limb orthoses may be designed to hold a joint in a more neutral alignment to promote healing due to an acute injury or prevent further injury. Examples include fracture orthoses and KOs.

Chronic diabetic foot ulcers or foot injuries may require orthotic treatment to reduce weight-bearing pressures. For example, a FO may be utilized to relieve or remove pressure over plantar tissues affected by chronic ulcers. In the case of a foot injury, an AFO may be utilized to increase pressure in the patellar tendon area, similar to that for a PTB socket for a trans-tibial amputee, to reduce load on the injured foot.

Unique to lower limb orthoses is the need to consider design effects during both the swing and stance phases of gait. For example, an AFO designed to resist plantarflexion during the swing phase and facilitate foot clearance will also resist plantarflexion during stance, thereby preventing active push-off during late stance.

21.3.7 Medical conditions benefiting from orthotic intervention

Orthoses may be used to treat symptoms or problems caused by congenital conditions, diseases, traumatic injuries, or overuse injuries. Any condition that affects the skeletal or neuromuscular system can potentially benefit from orthotic intervention. Congenital conditions that frequently warrant orthotic treatment include spina bifida, cerebral palsy, clubfoot, muscular dystrophy, Charcot-Marie-Tooth disease, and hip dysplasia. Orthotic intervention for individuals affected by such diseases often begins at an early age and sometimes continues throughout the patient's life. Diseases such as stroke, multiple sclerosis, arthritis, and diabetes may result in muscle weakness, hypertonia, and joint contractures, and therefore may warrant orthotic interventions. Aftereffects of traumatic injuries including fractures, ligamentous tears, spinal cord injury, and brain injury have also been managed with orthoses. Acute injuries may be treated with orthoses for a brief time to stabilize and/or immobilize the joint to promote healing or may require ongoing orthotic treatment for neuromuscular weakness or malfunction in the long term. Traumatic injuries may also result in arthritis, weakness, or recurring pain many years post-injury, warranting orthotic intervention later in life. Finally, repetitive motions, perhaps with poor biomechanics, may stretch or tear ligaments or tendons. Examples of these overuse (e.g., repetitive stress) injuries or cumulative trauma disorders include lateral epicondylitis, often referred to as "tennis elbow," and carpal tunnel syndrome. These conditions are treated with orthoses that relieve the affected section either by providing compression or reducing motion. Chronic ankle and knee instability are other overuse injuries often attributed to years of wear and tear on the joints; these conditions are treated with orthoses that support the weakened joint in a neutral alignment.

21.3.8 Orthotic prescription and fitting

A physician specializing in physical medicine and rehabilitation, neurology, or orthopedics may initiate orthotic treatment in consultation with a physical therapist, occupational therapist, and orthotist. This coordinated care to evaluate, prescribe, implement, and train a patient in the utilization of an orthosis may be achieved in either an inpatient or outpatient setting.

The goal of many therapists is to correct weakness or deformity *before* attempting an orthotic intervention. However, if a patient is at risk of falling or sustaining further injury, orthotic intervention may be recommended earlier in the process. If, as in inpatient settings, safety is not a factor, strengthening, stretching, and other therapy modalities are generally implemented prior to seeking orthotic intervention. In some cases, a physician will evaluate a patient, recommend a specific orthosis, and refer that patient directly to an orthotist for care. Alternatively, a physician may refer a patient to physical or occupational therapy; the therapist may then involve the orthotist at the appropriate time to recommend an orthosis as needed.

Both approaches ultimately require an orthotic prescription. State statutes differ regarding who can write a prescription; insurance companies may also dictate that the prescription be written by physicians with a certain specialty. The prescribing physician must note whether a custom, custom-fitted, or prefabricated device is necessary based on criteria set forth by Medicare or other reimbursing insurance companies.

21.3.8.1 Prefabricated versus custom orthoses   Orthoses may be classified as prefabricated or "off-the-shelf" (OTS), custom-fitted, and custom-fabricated. Prefabricated orthoses are available in a variety of sizes and require minimal adjustments to fit an individual patient. A custom-fitted device is prefabricated, but requires substantial modifications (e.g., trimming, bending, molding) by a trained therapist or orthotist to achieve a customized fit. There may be no physical difference between the prefabricated and custom-fitted orthoses; the same device may qualify for a different designation based solely on the respective modifications (Render et al. 2003). In contrast, custom-fabricated orthoses are fabricated for a specific individual. These orthoses use impressions, detailed measurements, or digital images and scans to create a positive model of the patient's anatomy. The orthosis is then molded using this positive model.

The prescription of a prefabricated, custom-fitted versus custom-fabricated orthosis is often dictated by the insurance company. One Medicare criterion (Render et al. 2003), for example, states:

> AFOs and KAFOs that are custom-fabricated are covered for ambulatory beneficiaries when the basic coverage criteria listed above and one of the following criteria are met:The beneficiary could not be fit with a prefabricated AFO; or,
>
> 1. The condition necessitating the orthosis is expected to be permanent or of longstanding duration (more than 6 months); or,
> 2. There is a need to control the knee, ankle, or foot in more than one plane; or,
> 3. The beneficiary has a documented neurological, circulatory, or orthopedic status that requires custom fabricating over a model to prevent tissue injury; or,
> 4. The beneficiary has a healing fracture which lacks normal anatomical integrity or anthropometric proportions.

Medicare regularly updates its standards, and many insurance providers use these standards to establish their guidelines for orthotic reimbursements.

21.3.9 Orthotic design

Many orthotic designs incorporate three- or four-point loading systems (Figure 21.14). For example, a knee orthosis designed to prevent varus deformity will apply a corrective valgus moment in the frontal plane via three-point loading with a medially directed force applied at the knee with laterally directed forces proximal and distal to the joint. Note that an orthosis need not encompass a specific joint to have a biomechanical effect on that joint. For example, a ground- reaction AFO does not directly apply force to the knee. However, the restricted ankle motion transfers the ground-reaction force to the knee, resisting knee flexion.

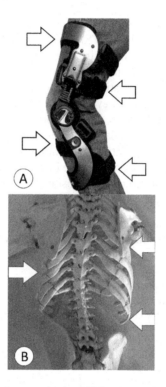

Figure 21.14 Illustration of corrective/stabilizing forces in orthotics. (A) Four-point principle in knee orthosis. The forces applied by the straps prevent the "anterior drawer" symptom, typical for ACL injuries. (B) Three-point principle in scoliosis orthoses. The major scoliotic curve is countered by corrective forces applied by a custom-fitted rigid trunk orthosis.

Static orthoses are typically designed to resist motion. For example, an AFO may resist plantarflexion, thereby minimizing foot drop. In contrast, dynamic designs often assist motion. An AFO may incorporate a dorsiflexion assist, lifting the foot to increase dorsiflexion during swing. Similarly, a static KAFO may include a locked knee joint to resist both knee extension and flexion; a dynamic KAFO may include a knee extension assist, via rubber bands or springs, applying forces to assist extension of the knee joint.

Some orthotic designs are both static and dynamic. For example, an AFO may incorporate a carbon-fiber, leaf spring design. Statically, the solid AFO resists excessive dorsiflexion; deformation of the carbon-fiber leaf spring stores energy during stance as it is compressed, dynamically providing plantarflexion force when unloading during swing.

Designing an orthosis for an individual requires understanding current motion to be corrected or assisted. An effective orthosis must accommodate the joint's passive and active range of motion, as well as the desired motion. The orthosis must then apply forces to the encompassed limb segment(s) and joint(s) to resist or assist motion, as needed. The location of the orthotic forces and their magnitude affect the efficacy of the orthotic design, and whether it meets the desired treatment objectives. Challenges include the joint's range of motion, the potential for excessive loading of the skin and soft tissue due to orthotic loading, the effects of the orthotic forces and moments on the proximal and distal joints, and the potential for out-of-plane loading as the segment(s) move (e.g., sagittal plane loading may induce moments in the transverse or frontal planes).

21.3.10 Functional outcomes

A goal for many lower extremity orthoses is to minimize gait deviations and energy expenditure. Simple clinical tests to assess the effects of an orthosis on mobility and gait include timed walking (e.g., six-minute or 10 m walk; Dean, Richards, and Malouin 2001; Troosters, Gosselink, and Decramer 1999) or the timed up and go test (Bohannon 2006). These tests are performed with and without the orthosis, using an assistive device if necessary.

If the treatment objective of an orthosis is to resist contracture or stretch a muscle/muscle group, a range of motion tests are performed pre- and post-orthotic treatment for a specific duration. These ranges of motion, for example, peak flexion/extension, are measured with a goniometer and contrasted to objectively assess the impact of the orthotic treatment.

An orthotic patient may also benefit from the services of a rehabilitation engineer to evaluate the benefits of assistive technologies for activities of daily living as well as activities related to a vocation. These assistive technologies might include vehicle modifications and modified computer access technologies.

21.4 Future vision

While prosthetic advances are often perceived as more high-tech, orthotic designs have the additional complexity that the design must accommodate the pathologic musculoskeletal physiology of the respective limb segments and joints. A prosthetic limb can simply replace the full system. For example, the battery, controllers, hydraulics, motors, and/or sensors of externally powered and microprocessor-controlled devices are difficult to integrate into an orthosis – but may more easily be housed in a prosthesis. Weight distribution, interference with the environment and other body segments, and aesthetics must all be considered with such components.

Several of the technological advances developed for lower limb prostheses have recently been incorporated into lower limb orthoses. The Intrepid Dynamic Exoskeleton Orthosis (IDEO, Hanger Clinic) incorporates carbon-fiber leaf spring technology of ESAR prosthetic feet. This orthosis has been shown to dramatically improve functional outcomes for patients with severe ankle-foot injuries (e.g., limb salvage). A number of KAFO designs now incorporate stance flexion (e.g., Becker Orthopedic, Horton, Fillauer), preventing the knee from buckling during early stance, even if flexed. These designs permit knee flexion during swing, thereby minimizing gait deviations adopted to provide foot clearance with a locked knee. While most of these designs are purely mechanical, at least one stance flexion KAFO design incorporates microprocessor control (e.g., C-brace, Otto Bock). Similar technology has been incorporated into full lower extremity exoskeletons (ReWalk and Ekso Bionics), enabling those with lower extremity paralysis to walk.

Neurocontrol has also been incorporated into orthotic designs. The two most common commercially available systems include the WalkAide (Innovative Neurotronics) and L300 (Bioness) which stimulate the peroneal nerve to dorsiflex the ankle and lift the foot, a treatment option for individuals with foot drop due to stroke, multiple sclerosis, incomplete spinal cord injury, and cerebral palsy. Bioness' H200 uses similar technology to assist with grasp for individuals with hand paralysis. Unlike more traditional functional electrical stimulation (FES; Peckham and Knutson 2005) used in research environments, these systems are non-invasive.

While some research has been conducted on both hydraulic and pneumatic AFOs, recent work has investigated powered AFOs (Cain, Gordon, and Ferris 2007; Shorter et al. 2011; Arazpour, Hutchins, and Ahmadi Bani 2015). To date, these systems have not yet been commercialized.

21.5 Discussion questions

1. Discuss key medical advances that improved survival from amputation surgery. Contrast the amputation level, cause, age, and gender of these early amputees with those in the world today.
2. Discuss technological advances that influenced early prosthetic and orthotic design. Discuss recent technological advances in amputation surgery, as well as prosthetic and orthotic design. Discuss the clinical potential of these advances.
3. Case study analysis:
   a. Describe a hypothetical lower and upper extremity amputee. Discuss potential prosthetic prescriptions, including the rationale for your selections.

    b. Describe a hypothetical gait deviation (e.g., excessive, or minimal knee flexion during loading support or swing, knee valgus during mid-stance, vaulting, circumduction) for a trans-tibial and trans-femoral amputee. Discuss potential prosthetic causes and relevant prosthetic socket or alignment modifications.

    c. Describe a hypothetical patient requiring lower or upper limb orthotic treatment. Discuss potential orthotic prescriptions, including the rationale for your selections.

4. For various lower and upper extremity orthoses to correct a hypothetical deformity, sketch the relevant free body diagram and corresponding shear and bending moment diagrams. Discuss orthotic design factors that might influence the respective three- or four-point design(s).

Bibliography

Al-Timemy, Ali H., Rami N. Khushaba, Guido Bugmann, and Javier Escudero. 2015. "Improving the Performance against Force Variation of EMG Controlled Multifunctional Upper-Limb Prostheses for Transradial Amputees." *IEEE Transactions on Neural Systems and Rehabilitation Engineering* 24 (6): 650–61.

Arazpour, Mokhtar, Stephen William Hutchins, and Monireh Ahmadi Bani. 2015. "The Efficacy of Powered Orthoses on Walking in Persons with Paraplegia." *Prosthetics and Orthotics International* 39 (2): 90–99.

Azocar, Alejandro F., Luke M. Mooney, Levi J. Hargrove, and Elliott J. Rouse. 2018. "Design and Characterization of an Open-Source Robotic Leg Prosthesis." In *2018 7th IEEE International Conference on Biomedical Robotics and Biomechatronics (Biorob)*, 111–18. IEEE.

Bergelin, Bryan J., and Philip A. Voglewede. 2012. "Design of an Active Ankle-Foot Prosthesis Utilizing a Four-Bar Mechanism." *Journal of Mechanical Design* 134 (6): 061004.

Bohannon, Richard W. 2006. "Reference Values for the Timed Up and Go Test: A Descriptive Meta-Analysis." *Journal of Geriatric Physical Therapy* 29 (2): 64–68.

Branemark, Rickard, PI Branemark, Björn Rydevik, and Robert R. Myers. 2001. "Osseointegration in Skeletal Reconstruction and Rehabilitation: A Review." *Journal of Rehabilitation Research and Development* 38 (2): 175–82.

Cain, Stephen M., Keith E. Gordon, and Daniel P. Ferris. 2007. "Locomotor Adaptation to a Powered Ankle-Foot Orthosis Depends on Control Method." *Journal of Neuroengineering and Rehabilitation* 4 (1): 48.

Cempini, Marco, Levi J. Hargrove, and Tommaso Lenzi. 2017. "Design, Development, and Bench-Top Testing of a Powered Polycentric Ankle Prosthesis." In *2017 IEEE/RSJ International Conference on Intelligent Robots and Systems (IROS)*, 1064–69. IEEE.

Chaturvedi, N., L. K. Stevens, J. H Fuller, E. T. Lee, M. Lu, and WHO Multinational Study Group. 2001. "Risk Factors, Ethnic Differences and Mortality Associated with Lower-Extremity Gangrene and Amputation in Diabetes. The WHO Multinational Study of Vascular Disease in Diabetes." *Diabetologia* 44 (2): S65.

Dean, Catherine M., Carol L. Richards, and Francine Malouin. 2001. "Walking Speed over 10 Metres Overestimates Locomotor Capacity after Stroke." *Clinical Rehabilitation* 15 (4): 415–21.

Dillingham, Timothy R., Liliana E. Pezzin, and Ellen J. MacKenzie. 2002. "Limb Amputation and Limb Deficiency: Epidemiology and Recent Trends in the United States." *Southern Medical Journal* 95 (8): 875–84.

Elery, Toby, Siavash Rezazadeh, Christopher Nesler, Jack Doan, Hanqi Zhu, and Robert D. Gregg. 2018. "Design and Benchtop Validation of a Powered Knee-Ankle Prosthesis with High-Torque, Low-Impedance Actuators." In *2018 IEEE International Conference on Robotics and Automation (ICRA)*, 2788–95. IEEE.

Farmer, Samuel, Barbara Silver-Thorn, Philip Voglewede, and Scott A. Beardsley. 2014. "Within-Socket Myoelectric Prediction of Continuous Ankle Kinematics for Control of a Powered Transtibial Prosthesis." *Journal of Neural Engineering* 11 (5): 056027.

Fougner, Anders, Øyvind Stavdahl, Peter J. Kyberd, Yves G. Losier, and Philip A. Parker. 2012. "Control of Upper Limb Prostheses: Terminology and Proportional Myoelectric Control—A Review." *IEEE Transactions on Neural Systems and Rehabilitation Engineering* 20 (5): 663–77.

Franchignoni, Franco, Duccio Orlandini, Giorgio Ferriero, and Tancredi A. Moscato. 2004. "Reliability, Validity, and Responsiveness of the Locomotor Capabilities Index in Adults with Lower-Limb Amputation Undergoing Prosthetic Training." *Archives of Physical Medicine and Rehabilitation* 85 (5): 743–48.

Gailey, Robert S., Kathryn E. Roach, E. Brooks Applegate, Brandon Cho, Bridgid Cunniffe, Stephanie Licht, Melanie Maguire, and Mark S. Nash. 2002. "The Amputee Mobility Predictor: An Instrument to Assess Determinants of the Lower-Limb Amputee's Ability to Ambulate." *Archives of Physical Medicine and Rehabilitation* 83 (5): 613–27.

Gailey, Robert S., Charles Scoville, Ignacio A. Gaunaurd, Michele A. Raya, Alison A. Linberg, Paul D. Stoneman, Stuart M. Campbell, and Kathryn E. Roach. 2013. "Construct Validity of Comprehensive High-Level Activity Mobility Predictor (CHAMP) for Male Servicemembers with Traumatic Lowerlimb Loss." *Journal of Rehabilitation Research and Development* 50 (7): 919.

Gao, Fei, Yannan Liu, and Wei-Hsin Liao. 2018. "Design of Powered Ankle-Foot Prosthesis with Nonlinear Parallel Spring Mechanism." *Journal of Mechanical Design* 140 (5): 055001.

Grimmer, Martin, Matthew Holgate, Robert Holgate, Alexander Boehler, Jeffrey Ward, Kevin Hollander, Thomas Sugar, and André Seyfarth. 2016. "A Powered Prosthetic Ankle Joint for Walking and Running." *Biomedical Engineering Online* 15 (3): 37–52.

Ha, Kevin H., Huseyin Atakan Varol, and Michael Goldfarb. 2010. "Volitional Control of a Prosthetic Knee Using Surface Electromyography." *IEEE Transactions on Biomedical Engineering* 58 (1): 144–51.

Hafner, Brian J., Ignacio A. Gaunaurd, Sara J. Morgan, Dagmar Amtmann, Rana Salem, and Robert S. Gailey. 2017. "Construct Validity of the Prosthetic Limb Users Survey of Mobility (PLUS-M) in Adults with Lower Limb Amputation." *Archives of Physical Medicine and Rehabilitation* 98 (2): 277–85.

Hagberg, Kerstin, and Rickard Brånemark. 2009. "One Hundred Patients Treated with Osseointegrated Transfemoral Amputation Prostheses--Rehabilitation Perspective." *Journal of Rehabilitation Research & Development* 46 (3): 331–44.

Hargrove, Levi J., Ann M. Simon, Robert D. Lipschutz, Suzanne B. Finucane, and Todd A. Kuiken. 2011. "Real-Time Myoelectric Control of Knee and Ankle Motions for Transfemoral Amputees." *JAMA* 305 (15): 1542–44.

Hargrove, Levi J., Ann M. Simon, Aaron J. Young, Robert D. Lipschutz, Suzanne B. Finucane, Douglas G. Smith, and Todd A. Kuiken. 2013. "Robotic Leg Control with EMG Decoding in an Amputee with Nerve Transfers." *New England Journal of Medicine* 369 (13): 1237–42.

558

Hitt, Joseph K., Thomas G. Sugar, Matthew Holgate, and Ryan Bellman. 2010. "An Active Foot-Ankle Prosthesis with Biomechanical Energy Regeneration." *Journal of Medical Devices* 4 (1): 011003.

Huang, He, Fan Zhang, Levi J. Hargrove, Zhi Dou, Daniel R. Rogers, and Kevin B. Englehart. 2011. "Continuous Locomotion-Mode Identification for Prosthetic Legs Based on Neuromuscular–Mechanical Fusion." *IEEE Transactions on Biomedical Engineering* 58 (10): 2867–75.

Johnson, S. S., and E. Mansfield. 2014. "Prosthetic Training: Upper Limb." *Physical Medicine and Rehabilitation Clinics of North America* 25 (1): 133–51. https://doi.org/10.1016/j.pmr. 2013.09.012.

Kaufman, Kenton R., James A. Levine, Robert H. Brey, Shelly K. McCrady, Denny J. Padgett, and Michael J. Joyner. 2008. "Energy Expenditure and Activity of Transfemoral Amputees Using Mechanical and Microprocessor-Controlled Prosthetic Knees." *Archives of Physical Medicine and Rehabilitation* 89 (7): 1380–85.

Knox, Annie. 2016. "Veterans Stand and Walk after First-of-Its-Kind Prosthesis Surgery in Utah." *The Salt Lake Tribune*, 2016. http://www.sltrib.com/home/3577365-155/veterans-stand-and-walk-after-first-of-its.

Kuiken, Todd A., Gregory Ara Dumanian, Robert D. Lipschutz, Laura A. Miller, and K. A. Stubblefield. 2004. "The Use of Targeted Muscle Reinnervation for Improved Myoelectric Prosthesis Control in a Bilateral Shoulder Disarticulation Amputee." *Prosthetics and Orthotics International* 28 (3): 245–53.

Kuiken, Todd A., Guanglin Li, Blair A. Lock, Robert D. Lipschutz, Laura A. Miller, Kathy A. Stubblefield, and Kevin B. Englehart. 2009. "Targeted Muscle Reinnervation for Real-Time Myoelectric Control of Multifunction Artificial Arms." *JAMA* 301 (6): 619–28.

Kuiken, Todd A., Laura A. Miller, Robert D. Lipschutz, Blair A. Lock, Kathy Stubblefield, Paul D. Marasco, Ping Zhou, and Gregory A. Dumanian. 2007. "Targeted Reinnervation for Enhanced Prosthetic Arm Function in a Woman with a Proximal Amputation: A Case Study." *The Lancet* 369 (9559): 371–80.

Lawson, Brian Edward, Huseyin Atakan Varol, Amanda Huff, Erdem Erdemir, and Michael Goldfarb. 2012. "Control of Stair Ascent and Descent with a Powered Transfemoral Prosthesis." *IEEE Transactions on Neural Systems and Rehabilitation Engineering* 21 (3): 466–73.

Legro, Marcia W., Gayle D. Reiber, Douglas G. Smith, Michael del Aguila, Jerrie Larsen, and David Boone. 1998. "Prosthesis Evaluation Questionnaire for Persons with Lower Limb Amputations: Assessing Prosthesis-Related Quality of Life." *Archives of Physical Medicine and Rehabilitation* 79 (8): 931–38.

Michael, John W., and John H. Bowker. 2004. *Atlas of Amputations and Limb Deficiencies: Surgical, Prosthetic, and Rehabilitation Principles*. Rosemont, IL: American Academy of Orthopaedic Surgeons.

Nelson, Virginia S., Katherine M. Flood, Phillip R. Bryant, Mark E. Huang, Paul F. Pasquina, and Toni L. Roberts. 2006. "Limb Deficiency and Prosthetic Management. 1. Decision Making in Prosthetic Prescription and Management." *Archives of Physical Medicine and Rehabilitation* 87 (3) Supplement 1: 3–9.

Ohnishi, Kengo, Richard F. Weir, and Todd A. Kuiken. 2007. "Neural Machine Interfaces for Controlling Multifunctional Powered Upper-Limb Prostheses." *Expert Review of Medical Devices* 4 (1): 43–53.

Owings, M. F., and L. J. Kozak. 1998. "Ambulatory and Inpatient Procedures in the United States, 1996." *Vital and Health Statistics. Series 13, Data from the National Health Survey* 139: 1–119.

559

Peckham, P. Hunter, and Jayme S. Knutson. 2005. "Functional Electrical Stimulation for Neuromuscular Applications." *Annual Review of Biomedical Engineering* 7: 327–60.

Render, Marta L., Patrick Taylor, James Plunkett, and Gary N. Nugent. 2003. "Methods to Estimate and Compare VA Expenditures for Assistive Devices to Medicare Payments." *Medical Care* 41 (6 Suppl): II70–9.

Schmalz, Thomas, Siegmar Blumentritt, and Rolf Jarasch. 2002. "Energy Expenditure and Biomechanical Characteristics of Lower Limb Amputee Gait: The Influence of Prosthetic Alignment and Different Prosthetic Components." *Gait & Posture* 16 (3): 255–63.

Segil, Jacob L. 2013. "Design and Validation of a Morphing Myoelectric Hand Posture Controller Based on Principal Component Analysis of Human Grasping." *IEEE Transactions on Neural Systems and Rehabilitation Engineering* 22 (2): 249–57.

Shorter, K. Alex, Géza F. Kogler, Eric Loth, William K. Durfee, and Elizabeth T. Hsiao-Wecksler. 2011. "A Portable Powered Ankle-Foot Orthosis for Rehabilitation." *Journal of Rehabilitation Research & Development* 48 (4): 459–72.

Tran, Minh, Lukas Gabert, Marco Cempini, and Tommaso Lenzi. 2019. "A Lightweight, Efficient Fully Powered Knee Prosthesis with Actively Variable Transmission." *IEEE Robotics and Automation Letters* 4 (2): 1186–93.

Troosters, Thierry, Rik Gosselink, and Marc Decramer. 1999. "Six Minute Walking Distance in Healthy Elderly Subjects." *European Respiratory Journal* 14 (2): 270–74.

Varol, Huseyin Atakan, Frank Sup, and Michael Goldfarb. 2009. "Multiclass Real-Time Intent Recognition of a Powered Lower Limb Prosthesis." *IEEE Transactions on Biomedical Engineering* 57 (3): 542–51.

Waters, Robert L., and Sara Mulroy. 1999. "The Energy Expenditure of Normal and Pathologic Gait." *Gait & Posture* 9 (3): 207–31.

Windrich, Michael, Martin Grimmer, Oliver Christ, Stephan Rinderknecht, and Philipp Beckerle. 2016. "Active Lower Limb Prosthetics: A Systematic Review of Design Issues and Solutions." *Biomedical Engineering Online* 15 (3): 5–19.

World Health Organization and USAID. 2017. "WHO Standards for Prosthetics and Orthotics." https://apps.who.int/iris/handle/10665/259209.

Young, Aaron J., Ann M. Simon, Nicholas P. Fey, and Levi J. Hargrove. 2014. "Intent Recognition in a Powered Lower Limb Prosthesis Using Time History Information." *Annals of Biomedical Engineering* 42 (3): 631–41.

Ziegler-Graham, Kathryn, Ellen J. MacKenzie, Patti L. Ephraim, Thomas G. Travison, and Ron Brookmeyer. 2008. "Estimating the Prevalence of Limb Loss in the United States: 2005 to 2050." *Archives of Physical Medicine and Rehabilitation* 89 (3): 422–29.

Chapter 22 Neural engineering

Kei Masani and Paul Yoo

Contents

22.1 Chapter overview

Information transmission within a body relies on electrical signals that are characterized as nerve action potentials. These signals travel throughout the nervous system and mediate all forms of function such as limb movement, sensation, autonomic control of visceral organs, and cognition. It has long been established that electrical stimulation can initiate action potentials, which in turn are capable of artificially eliciting one or more forms of physiological or even psychological functions. Neural engineering aims to take advantage of this simple input-output relationship by strategically applying electrical pulses at various anatomical locations to restore or markedly improve lost or deteriorated functions in individuals impacted by neurological impairments such as spinal cord injury (SCI) and stroke. One of the oldest and most widely studied applications in neural engineering is called functional electrical stimulation (FES), where electrical stimulation is used to restore motor functions by directly/indirectly activating motor nerves.

Over the past several decades, the field of neural engineering has evolved to include the "indirect" use of electrical nerve stimulation to treat chronic neurological

DOI: 10.1201/b21964-25

disorders, such as urinary dysfunction, movement disorders, epilepsy, and depression. This clinical tool is called electrical neuromodulation and is defined as the process by which altered neural activity caused by electrical stimulation in one part of the nervous system modulates the ongoing activity of a targeted neural circuit. For example, electrical stimulation of peripheral nerves in the lower leg can inhibit bladder contractility via neural pathways that connect through the brainstem and also the lumbosacral spinal cord. There are numerous clinically effective therapies based on electrical neuromodulation that can suppress disease symptoms and significantly improve quality of life.

This chapter will focus on peripheral nerve stimulation, where we will provide a broad overview of FES applications and also a detailed example of electrical neuromodulation applied to restoring and/or treating symptoms of urinary dysfunction. For the sake of brevity, we will not cover FES systems used with fitness exercises that are aimed at improving cardiovascular function or preventing muscle atrophy (e.g., FES cycling and muscle strength training), nor will we be able to cover the myriad of electrical neuromodulation systems used to treat movement disorders, epilepsy, and depression (e.g., deep brain stimulation, vagus nerve stimulation, and transcranial direct-current stimulation).

22.2 Functional electrical stimulation

22.2.1 Introduction to functional electrical stimulation

Electrical stimulation that is used to activate motor nerves is called neuromuscular electrical stimulation (NMES). When NMES is applied to specifically induce an organized, patterned, and functional action, it is called FES. An NMES or an FES system requires an electrical stimulator and a pair of electrodes per stimulation channel (Figure 22.1). The electrical stimulation will be delivered by a series of current or voltage-regulated electrical pulses. The current regulated pulse has an advantage in that changes in the tissue resistance do not affect the amount of charge delivered to the nerves when using the current regulated pulse, indicating that the current regulated pulse consistently delivers the same amount of charge to the targeted tissue, that is, consistent and accurate nerve activation.

On the electrical stimulator, three pulse parameters are specified, that is, the pulse intensity (electrical current/voltage), the pulse duration, and the pulse frequency (Figure 22.1). A popular set of parameters often used for an NMES using transcutaneous electrodes (regarding the electrodes, more details in the following sections) are 30–100 mA, 200–400 micro-seconds, and 30–40 Hz for the pulse current, duration, and frequency, respectively. The stimulation pulses can be either monophasic or biphasic. In the monophasic pulse, it delivers the charge to the tissue without removing the charge from the tissue. In the biphasic pulse,

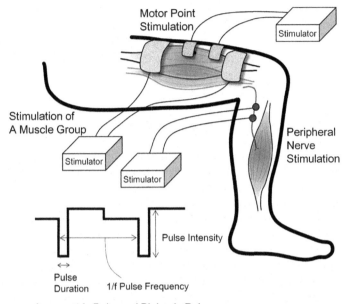

Asymmetric Balanced Biphasic Pulse

Figure 22.1 Transcutaneous electrical stimulation. Schemes on three styles of transcutaneous electrical stimulation, and the asymmetric biphasic balanced pulse and its parameters (waiting on permission).

the charge is delivered to the tissue with the removal of the charge. Usually, the biphasic pulse is balanced so that the amount of charge delivered to the tissue is removed from it within a pulse. The balanced biphasic pulse can be symmetric or asymmetric. In the asymmetric balanced biphasic pulse, the muscle contraction occurs only in the muscle over which the anode electrode is placed.

A device or system that achieves FES is often called a neuroprosthesis. FES can be used as an orthotic tool or as a therapeutic tool. Initially, FES was developed for orthotic purposes. That is, FES is used when a user needs to achieve or restore a target function such as walking. However, researchers have discovered that prolonged and repeated use of FES can induce the recovery of lost motor function, for example, going beyond the direct activation of the target muscle groups. More recently, therapeutic applications are gaining in popularity, and they have also been proven to be clinically successful (Popovic, Masani, and Micera 2016, 513–532).

The peripheral nerve can be stimulated either non-invasively using (1) transcutaneous/surface electrodes or invasively using (2) percutaneous or (3) implanted electrodes. The transcutaneous electrode can be placed on the skin surface above a nerve branch, a muscle belly, or a group of muscle bellies (Figure 22.1). The size of the transcutaneous electrode should be selected depending on the target. The electrodes have traditionally been connected with flexible leads to a stimulator that may be worn on the body trunk or a limb. However, several manufacturers now have designs resembling large band-aids, where the stimulator is mounted onto the surface electrodes and controlled wirelessly with hand-held devices such as a smartphone or tablet computer. Some systems require the transcutaneous electrodes placed above a nerve branch aiming to activate the whole nerve branch, such as a foot drop stimulator. Other systems are designed to place transcutaneous electrodes on a specific point of a muscle belly, that is, the motor point. The motor point is the site that produces the strongest contraction with the lowest level of stimulation. When the transcutaneous electrode is placed over the motor point of the target muscle, we can expect to induce muscle contraction efficiently. However, to do so, the location of the motor point must be identified manually using a probe electrode, which requires skill, time, and specialized devices. Therefore, in clinical settings, motor point stimulation is not used very often. Instead, FES is achieved by electrically stimulating a group of muscles with a pair of large electrodes covering the entire muscle group. For example, in the case of activating quadriceps femoris, a pair of large electrodes located at the proximal and distal ends of the thigh is often used instead of locating multiple electrodes over specific motor points of each muscle head. Since the transcutaneous FES is a non-invasive treatment method, it can be easily applied to patients and is relatively inexpensive, which is beneficial for therapeutic applications. However, the transcutaneous FES requires knowledge and skillsets to place electrodes at appropriate locations to induce isolated, ideal limb movements, while it is also difficult to activate deep muscles. In addition, the transcutaneous FES can be significantly limited by discomfort/pain caused by the electrical activation of cutaneous sensory receptors.

Although not widely used, FES can be achieved by electrically stimulating muscles with percutaneous electrodes, which consist of thin wires inserted through the skin and into muscular tissue close to the targeted nerve. Similar to transcutaneous FES, the electrical stimulator is an external device. More advanced versions of percutaneous electrodes can consist of flexible multifilament leads that are inserted through the skin and implanted in a muscle using a hypodermic needle. Given that the lead wire is electrically insulated, percutaneous electrodes can be used to induce selective electrical recruitment of deep muscle fibers, leading to a significantly lower incidence of painful cutaneous sensation during stimulation. Percutaneous systems can serve as precursors to fully implanted systems, and they can provide function for years in some cases (Peckham and Knutson 2005, 327–360).

In the case of implanted systems, both the electrode(s) and electrical stimulator are permanently implanted within the body. The implanted, thin-wire electrodes are connected by leads under the skin to the implanted stimulator, which is often placed subcutaneously in the chest or abdominal regions. The stimulator may have a self-contained battery or it can receive power and command signals via wireless connections from an external control unit. Obviously, implanted systems are designed for long-term use, unlike transcutaneous and percutaneous systems, and are intended for orthotic use. The implanted system is free from cumbersome wiring and troubles related to transcutaneous/percutaneous electrodes such as pain or infections at the skin surface where percutaneous electrodes might exit. However, since the power demand for electrically activating muscles is large, an implanted system requires recharging of batteries much more often than systems, for example, used for cardiac pacing (Peckham and Knutson 2005).

22.2.2 Drop foot stimulator

Drop foot is a common symptom among individuals with stroke and is characterized by a lack of dorsiflexion/ankle flexion during gait. Individuals lacking dorsiflexion tend to drag their foot at the beginning of the swing phase, which results in a very unstable gait and increased incidence of falls. It has been shown that electrical stimulation-induced dorsiflexion can be used to effectively compensate for the drop foot during the swing phase of gait. For that purpose, electrical stimulation must be delivered at a precise timing to induce the dorsiflexion right at the beginning of the swing phase. Therefore, the drop foot stimulator system requires a sensor that can detect the phase of gait, such as a tilt sensor (WalkAide; Stein et al. 2010) and heel switch (Bioness L300; Hausdorff and Ring 2008) (Figure 22.2). The tilt sensor or the heel switch detects the heel off moment of gait, which triggers the electrical stimulation of the common peroneal nerve via a surface electrode, which, in turn, activates muscles (e.g., tibialis anterior) that result in dorsiflexion.

Drop foot stimulators are one of the most successful neuroprostheses to date, both clinically and commercially. The overall perception of drop foot stimulators by patients/consumers is superior to that of the ankle-foot orthosis (Van Swigchem et al. 2010). Both orthotic and therapeutic effects of drop foot stimulators have been shown in individuals with both progressive (multiple sclerosis) and nonprogressive (stroke) disorders, such as indicated by significant increases in walking speed (Stein et al. 2010). Although the actual mechanism of therapeutic effect is not completely understood, an increase in corticomuscular excitation has been reported after the use of a drop foot stimulator for three to 12 months (Everaert et al. 2010). The corticomuscular excitation can be evaluated by measuring the motor evoked potential (MEP) induced by transcranial magnetic stimulation (TMS). MEP is measured using an electromyogram (EMG) when TMS activates neurons at the motor cortex. The activation of neurons at the motor cortex is

565

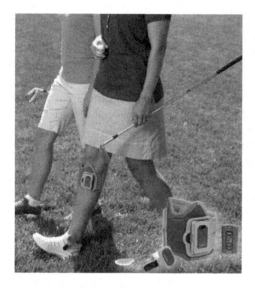
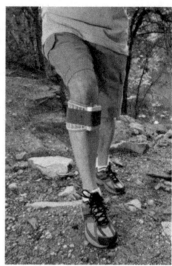

a   b

Figure 22.2 (A) Bioness L300 Foot Drop System; (B) WalkAid System (waiting on permission).

transmitted to the motor neurons at the spinal cord, which activates the innervated muscle and is then measured as MEP. Therefore, the magnitude of the MEP indicates the strength of connection between the neurons within the motor cortex and those innervating the distal muscle. The increase of MEP after the use of a drop foot stimulator for three to 12 months indicates that the connection between the motor cortex and the tibialis anterior muscle is increased. This, in turn, suggests that the repetitive use of FES induces neuroplasticity within the central nervous system, resulting in the therapeutic effect. The precise location at which neuroplasticity occurs has not yet been identified.

22.2.3 FES for standing

Upright standing posture is to be achieved as a basis for walking using FES. Further, the upright posture itself is beneficial for improving blood circulation and muscle atrophy as well as providing face-to-face interactions with other people for individuals with SCI. Several early studies have shown that standing posture is somewhat achievable by stimulating the quadriceps femoris muscles and glutei muscles via surface electrodes, but only for individuals with partial paralysis such as incomplete SCI (Peckham and Knutson 2005). For individuals with complete

SCI, an implantable system with eight to 16 channels has been developed at Case Western Reserve University (CWRU) and the Department of Veterans Affairs (VA; the CWRU/VA neuroprosthesis). It consists of an implanted stimulator, in-line connectors, and epimysial and intramuscular electrodes with an external control unit (Davis et al. 2001). The CWRU/VA neuroprosthesis activates the hip, knee, and trunk extensor muscles to make the upright standing posture in an open-loop manner, with foot-ankle orthoses stabilizing the ankle joints, to make the body stiff in an upright posture against gravity. The CWRU/VA neuroprosthesis can achieve more than ten minutes of uninterrupted upright stance (Kobetic et al. 1999). However, this system does not provide balance control and the consumer has to rely on a walker or a similar device to maintain balance, which limits users' usage of the arms during standing.

It is often misunderstood that constant activation of anti-gravity muscles and stiffening of the legs is sufficient for maintaining upright standing. However, we know that the activation of anti-gravity muscles is continuously modified based on the leaning angle of the body (Masani 2003). The abovementioned systems with surface or implanted electrodes in an open-loop controlled FES require the use of the arms for balance. On the contrary, a closed-loop controlled FES has the potential to achieve arm-free upright standing. Therefore, multiple attempts have been made with the intention of allowing individuals with paralysis in the lower extremities to maintain balance and stand freely without the use of their arms. Jaime et al. proposed a strategy that allowed an individual with complete SCI to maintain balance in a constricting multipurpose rehabilitation frame (Jaime, Matjačić, and Hunt 2002). Their control strategy implemented voluntary and reflex activity of the upper body while a closed-loop FES system regulated the stiffness of the ankle joints. Gollee et al. developed and evaluated a series of nested feedback systems that used FES to control the ankle torque of an individual with complete SCI (Gollee, Hunt, and Wood 2004). During the experiments, the individual stood in an apparatus that acted as a full body cast, solely allowing the ankle joints to move in the anterior–posterior direction. Vette et al. applied a linear feedback controller mimicking a physiological controller and succeeded in better stabilizing an individual with incomplete SCI (Vette, Masani, and Popovic 2007). Recently, CWRU/VA neuroprosthesis has been also incorporated with a closed-loop controller to stabilize externally perturbed posture (Audu, Odle, and Triolo 2018).

22.2.4 FES for walking

Enabling walking is one of the priorities of individuals with SCI (Anderson 2004). The flexor withdrawal reflex has been used to substitute for the stepping movement during walking. When one receives noxious stimulus at the foot, leg flexors at the hip, knee, and ankle joints are reflexly activated, inducing an immediate leg flexion. This is called the flexor withdrawal reflex. As this movement is similar to the stepping movement during the swing phase of gait, the flexor withdrawal reflex can be used as a substitute for the stepping movement if it is induced in a timely fashion. As electrical stimulation of cutaneous sensors on the foot can serve as the noxious stimulus, it was proposed that FES can be used to induce the flexor withdrawal reflex for walking (Kralj, Bajd, and Turk 1980). Parastep was developed to help individuals with SCI to walk by taking advantage of the flexor withdrawal reflex (Graupe and Kohn 1998). Six pairs of electrodes are located at the quadriceps femoris muscles, common peroneal nerves, and the paraspinals or the gluteus maximum muscles bilaterally. The quadriceps femoris and the paraspinals or the gluteus maximum muscles contribute to induce anti-gravity muscle contractions, helping upright standing posture, although the gluteus maximum muscles may not be used depending on the clients. The user needs to utilize a walker for balance using the arms. A manual switch is attached to the walker frame, which is used for changing the stimulation modes, including stand-up, sit-down, left step, right step, increase stimulation, and decrease stimulation. The user controls the manual switch to stand up, make a left/right step, sit down, or modify the stimulation strength. When the stand-up mode is turned on, both quadriceps muscles and paraspinals or gluteus muscles are stimulated to provide standing posture. Then the left step mode initiates the swing phase in the left leg by briefly stopping stimulation of the left quadriceps and stimulating the common peroneal nerve, triggering the flexor withdrawal reflex, resulting in simultaneous hip and knee flexion, as well as dorsiflexion. After a fixed period of time, the common peroneal nerve stimulation is stopped and quadriceps stimulation is initiated while the reflex is still active to complete the stride. Similarly, the right step mode initiates the swing phase of the right leg. A major limitation of this neuroprosthesis is that the resulting gait is slow, awkward, and unnatural looking. Users exhibit poor stance phase posture due to hip flexion induced by rectus femoris activity during stimulation of the quadriceps. Further, the flexor withdrawal reflex is subject to rapid habituation and can also be highly variable.

As an alternative to eliciting the flexor withdrawal reflex, Thrasher et al. applied neuromuscular electrical stimulation in a manner that mimics how the central nervous system would engage these muscles during walking (Thrasher, Flett, and Popovic 2006). They stimulated eight major leg muscle groups involving knee extensors/flexors and ankle extensors/flexors. The stimulation pattern was developed using previous reports on muscle activation patterns in able-bodied individuals. Thrasher et al. tested their system with five individuals with motor incomplete SCI. They used this system for therapeutic purposes. That is, the participants received ten weeks of repeated therapeutic sessions using this neuroprosthesis. They reported improvements in walking function such as an increase in their walking speed. This surface stimulation system can be a good therapeutic tool for individuals with partial paralysis, but there are difficulties associated with donning the device, and therefore, it may be impractical for daily use. Further, the functional limitations of the surface stimulation system may not provide sufficiently strong muscle contractions for individuals with complete paralysis to stand and walk.

Percutaneous systems have been proposed to selectively activate muscles for ambulation in individuals with complete paralysis. Kobetic et al. proposed a percutaneous system with eight to 16 channel stimulations (Kobetic, Triolo, and Marsolais 1997). Three individuals with complete SCI tested their system and they reported successful improvements in gait, increase in walking speed, stride length, and cadence for a short distance, independent, walker-support walking. The percutaneous system is beneficial in inducing ambulation for individuals with complete paralysis.

The abovementioned CWRU/VA neuroprosthesis has also been used for walking. An individual with complete SCI tested the CWRU/VA neuroprosthesis with 16 channels implanted for over a year (Kobetic et al. 1999). It was found that their system is feasible for use in daily exercise, standing, and walking. There were no adverse physiologic effects due to the implant and the subject reported health benefits as a result of using the FES system.

To overcome challenges in FES for walking, such as weak hip flexion during the swing phase and hip extension during the stance phase, hybrid systems combining FES with orthotic braces or robotic exoskeletons have been proposed. For example, Stauffer et al. (2009) developed a hybrid robotic and FES system (WalkTrainer). The robotic device consisted of leg and pelvic orthoses, active bodyweight support, and a mobile frame that allowed the user to perform walking therapy during overground walking. The system also incorporated a closed-loop controlled FES mechanism. This WalkTrainer system was tested in six individuals with SCI, and its feasibility as a therapeutic tool was confirmed. CWRU/VA neuroprosthesis has been also tested with an exoskeleton (Chang et al. 2017). Three individuals with complete SCI participated in the study, and it was reported that the hybrid system successfully supported the participants' walking performance. These hybrid systems, consisting of an orthotics or a robotic device and an FES system, are not a new idea. However, this approach has become a more attractive and realistic solution in recent years due to drastic progress in exoskeleton technology. It is likely that in the near future we will see more devices that combine FES and robotic technologies to develop advanced neurorehabilitation tools and interventions.

22.2.5 Spinal cord stimulation

The spinal cord involves multiple neural circuits that are partially responsible for standing and walking, such as the rhythmicity and activation patterns of multiple muscles. By activating those neural circuits invasively or non-invasively, individuals with SCI can partially regain standing and walking functions.

It has been shown that using epidural spinal cord stimulation (ESCS), rhythmic or sustained muscle activations responsible for stepping and standing can be reproduced (Dimitrijevic, Gerasimenko, and Pinter 1998; Jilge et al. 2004). ESCS can actually assist individuals with complete SCI to stand and walk (Harkema et al. 2011). Harkema et al. applied ESCS to an individual with complete SCI with minimum mechanical support for balance. A 16-electrode array was implanted at T11–L1, over the midline of the exposed dura. After systematic assessment, the optimal electrodes were identified. ESCS enabled the participant to achieve full weight-bearing standing for over four minutes. ESCS also induced locomotor-like movement patterns when stimulation parameters were optimized for stepping over a moving treadmill belt. Although these results were achieved after months of training, Grahn et al. showed that the same outcomes can be obtained in the first two weeks of training (Grahn et al. 2017). Thus, ESCS potentiates the spinal neural circuit, which results in generating sustained muscle contraction of anti-gravity muscles helping the standing posture, and additional proprioceptive inputs induced by treadmill belt movement induced rhythmic muscle activation patterns in those anti-gravity muscles, leading to a coordinated stepping movement of the lower extremities.

Instead of invasive ESCS, recent studies have shown that non-invasive transcutaneous spinal cord stimulation (TSCS) has the potential for assisting standing and walking in individuals with complete SCI. Gerasimenko et al. applied TSCS in five individuals with complete SCI who were lying down with mechanical support of their legs. They placed an electrode midline on the skin between T11 and T12 as a cathode and two electrodes placed on the skin over the iliac crests as anodes. They showed that locomotor-like stepping was induced by TSCS when the leg was in a gravity-free condition due to the support. They also found that there was some therapeutic effect after 18 weeks of weekly interventions, suggesting that the participants' residual functions were improved, although the participants were clinically complete SCI.

ESCS and TSCS dominantly activate the dorsal root in the spinal cord, which secondarily activates the spinal neural circuit responsible for standing and walking. By inserting electrodes into the spinal cord, direct stimulation of the spinal neural circuit has been proposed, which is called intraspinal microstimulation (ISMS). ISMS directly targets specific motor neurons or interneurons responsible for muscle activations during standing and walking. ISMS of the lumbosacral spinal cord has been shown to restore standing and walking in animals with spinal cord injury (Mushahwar et al. 2007). The use of ISMS in humans for restoring standing and walking is expected in the future.

22.2.6 FES for upper limb function

FES has been used to restore or improve grasping and reaching function in individuals with stroke or SCI. Some example FES systems specifically designed for grasping and/or reaching neuroprostheses are the Freehand system (Smith et al. 1998; the Bioness H200, which used to be called NESS; Hendricks et al. 2001), and the Bionic Glove (Prochazka et al. 1997). The Freehand system is an implantable system; whereas all other devices use surface FES technology.

The key element for achieving the synergistic activity of muscles, which results in reaching and/or grasping, is the appropriate sequencing of the stimulation pulses. The available neuroprostheses for grasping can restore the most frequently used postures: power, lateral pinch, and precision grasps. The power grasp is used for grasping bigger and heavier objects such as water bottles and coffee mugs. The lateral pinch is used for grasping smaller and thinner objects such as keys and paper. The precision grip is used for grasping smaller objects such as dice and popcorn. Power grasp is generated by partly flexing the fingers and the thumb in flexion and slight opposition. Lateral pinch is generated by fully flexing the fingers followed by the thumb flexion. And precision grip is generated by first forming opposition between the thumb and the palm, which is followed by index finger and thumb flexion.

The Freehand system (Smith et al. 1998) consists of eight implanted epimysial stimulation electrodes that stimulate flexion and extension of the fingers and the thumb in order to provide lateral and palmar grasp. Commands are provided by an external position sensor placed on the shoulder of the subject's opposite arm. An additional external switch allows the user to choose between palmar and lateral grasp. This sequence is then sent, via a radio frequency coil, to the implanted unit, which generates the stimulation sequences for each channel. The electrode leads are tunneled subcutaneously to the implanted stimulator located in the pectoral region. Surgical procedures to enhance both voluntary and stimulated hand functions are often performed in conjunction with stimulator implantation. The main advantage of the Freehand system is that it uses an implanted system, and thus the time needed to don and doff the system is shorter compared with most other surface FES systems.

The Bioness H200 consists of an orthosis that has built-in flexibility to enhance and control freedom of movement within the forearm and hand while supporting the wrist joint at a functional angle of extension (Hendricks et al. 2001). The Bioness H200 multiplexes a single channel of stimulation through a selected combination of surface electrodes on the inner surface of the orthosis; this effectively transforms the device into a three-channel neuroprosthesis. One stimulation channel is used to stimulate the extensor pollicis brevis. The second channel stimulates the flexor digitorum superficialis. The third channel stimulates the flexor pollicis longus and thenar muscle groups. The Bioness H200 is controlled with an array of push buttons that allow the subject to select the operating mode and trigger pre-programmed movement sequences. Using buttons, the subject can also control stimulation intensity and thumb posture, thereby adjusting the grasp to the size and shape of the target object. One of the major advantages of the NESS H200 is that it is very easy to don and doff.

Bionic Glove is a neuroprosthesis designed to enhance the tenodesis grasp (by extending their wrist, users can cause passive finger flexion due to the limited length of the finger flexors) in subjects who have good voluntary control over wrist flexion and extension (Prochazka et al. 1997). Bionic Glove stimulates finger flexors and extensors, significantly enhancing the strength of the tenodesis grasp. Four self-adhesive surface stimulation electrodes provide stimulation, with both the stimulator and wrist position sensor located on the forearm of the glove. An easy-to-use interface, with three push buttons on the stimulator, is used to set the stimulation parameters, while optional audio feedback facilitates faster learning.

The abovementioned systems were developed primarily for orthotic use. However, it has been shown that neuroprostheses for grasping and reaching also have higher potential as a therapeutic tool. For example, Popovic et al. recently demonstrated that individuals with incomplete SCI achieved significant recovery of their voluntary grasping functions compared with conventional therapy after 40 hours of therapy using FES (Popovic et al. 2011). This is a new avenue of research and development that holds great promise for individuals with stroke or SCI. This proposed therapy is currently available in a clinical setting (Figure 22.3).

22.3 Electrical neuromodulation

In contrast to the FES approach, electrical neuromodulation aims to achieve therapeutic outcomes in patients by indirectly modulating one or more circuits within the central nervous system (CNS). Electrical stimulation of sensory nerve fibers is tuned to specific input parameters – such as amplitude, frequency, and duration – that elicit desired changes in physiological function. Depending on the location and anatomical characteristics of the target nerve, various types of neural interfaces have been developed and clinically tested for use in patients. In the following section, we will introduce neuroprostheses that have been clinically developed for electrically modulating bladder function in patients.

22.3.1 Restoring bladder function

The urinary bladder performs two simple tasks. The first is urine storage (continence), which is achieved by maintaining low intra-vesical pressure and high

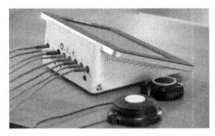
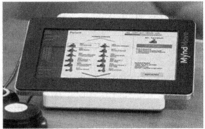
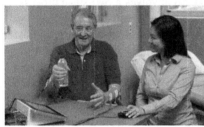

Figure 22.3 MyndMove System (waiting on permission).

mechanical compliance of the bladder wall. Urine excretion (micturition), on the other hand, is achieved by a rapid and sustained increase in bladder pressure coupled with inhibition of the urethral sphincter muscle. Surprisingly, the loss of normal urinary function is a rather common medical problem within the general population. Idiopathic overactive bladder (OAB) affects approximately 18% of adults and over 30% of the elderly population. The symptoms of OAB include urinary frequency (> 8 bathroom trips per 24 hours), urgency (uncontrolled urge to urinate), nocturia (> 1 bathroom trip during sleep at night), and urge incontinence (leaks associated with urgency). Individuals with neurological disorders (e.g., SCI, multiple sclerosis, Parkinson's disease) can also suffer from urinary incontinence. More commonly known as detrusor overactivity in persons with SCI, hyperactivity of the urinary bladder not only causes repeated urinary leaks but it can also lead to severe episodes of autonomic dysreflexia. It has been shown that restoring bladder function is a high priority for persons with SCI (Anderson 2004), but the problem remains a significant clinical challenge.

22.3.2 Neuroprostheses for urinary incontinence

Electrical neuromodulation is an established therapeutic alternative for patients with OAB symptoms who are refractory to bladder medication. Electrical stimulation of the dorsal sacral roots, better known as sacral neuromodulation, has particularly gained acceptance among clinicians and patients as a viable long-term therapy. Originally developed by researchers at the University of California

573

at San Francisco (Tanagho and Schmidt 1988), sacral neuromodulation therapy aims to reduce overactive symptoms by reflexively inhibiting any ongoing activity of the urinary bladder and/or suppressing the sensation of needing to urinate (i.e., urgency). Although the therapeutic mechanism remains unclear, electrical activation of pudendal nerve afferents is thought to play a significant role (Snellings and Grill 2012; Spinelli et al. 2005). Commercially available as the InterStim system (Medtronic Corporation, USA), therapy is achieved by delivering trains of electrical pulses to the posterior S3 nerve roots through surgically implanted electrodes (Figure 22.4). The implant procedure typically involves a two-stage process. An initial screening stage uses a temporarily implanted percutaneous electrode to stimulate the sacral roots. If this is found to be effective after several days of stimulation, the electrode is surgically replaced with the complete InterStim system (electrode and pulse generator). In over 250,000 implants worldwide, sacral neuromodulation has been shown to significantly reduce OAB symptoms (Jonas et al. 2001; Chartier-Kastler et al. 2000; Peeren, Hoebeke, and Everaert 2005).

A second alternative involves the electrical stimulation of pudendal nerve afferents, which unlike sacral neuromodulation targets a single nerve target. The primary advantage is that there are minimal side effects caused by electrical stimulation. As demonstrated in recent clinical studies (Peters et al. 2010; Goldman et al. 2008), long-term electrical activation of the dorsal genital nerve (DGN, derived from S2 to S4 spinal roots) achieves therapeutic effects comparable to that of the InterStim system. These findings corroborate the robust bladder-inhibitory effects of DGN stimulation that have been demonstrated in spinal intact

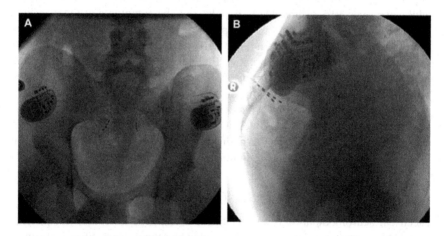

Figure 22.4 Images of a bilaterally implanted sacral neuromodulation (InterStim) system obtained from x-ray images of (A) abdominal and (B) lateral views. Each lead consists of four stimulation sites that deliver electrical pulses from the implanted pulse generator. (Permission obtained from John Wiley and Sons).

or chronic spinal cord injured animals (Woock, Yoo, and Grill 2008; Tai et al. 2007), and also in persons with chronic SCI (Kirkham et al. 2001). Interestingly, the stimulation parameters (amplitude = at least twice the bulbocavernosus reflex, frequency = 5–20 Hz) used to evoke this inhibitory reflex are remarkably similar among various mammalian species. Moreover, the presence of this stimulation-evoked reflex following spinal cord injury suggests that this reflex is mediated at the level of the sacral spinal cord.

Another alternative involves the electrical activation of the posterior tibial nerve (derived from L5 to S3 spinal roots). This treatment approach was first investigated by McGuire et al. (1983), where significant improvements in urinary function were demonstrated across a wide range of patients that included idiopathic OAB to chronic SCI. It was commercialized as the Stoller afferent nerve stimulator (SANS) and is now clinically available as Urgent PC (Laborie Inc, Canada). Also referred to as PTNS therapy, it is clinically implemented as weekly stimulation sessions during which the clinician inserts a percutaneous needle electrode in close proximity to the posterior tibial nerve and uses a hand-held pulse generator to deliver 30 minutes of continuous electrical stimulation (pulse width = 200 μs, frequency = 20 Hz, and amplitude = maximum 9 mA). Each session is repeated weekly over a period of three months, at which time patients achieve at least a 50% decrease in urgency and/or urge-incontinence episodes (Vandoninck et al. 2003; van Balken 2007). The therapeutic effects of PTNS therapy have also been validated in randomized, double-blind studies that compare electrical neuromodulation with pharmacological treatment and even sham nerve stimulation (Kenneth M. Peters et al. 2009; Kenneth M. Peters et al. 2010; Finazzi-Agrò et al. 2010). However, a recent meta-analysis shows that the overall success rate of PTNS therapy is limited to approximately 60% of patients (Burton et al. 2012).

As an alternative to all of these therapies, electrical stimulation of the saphenous nerve (SAFN) is being investigated as a means of modulating bladder function. The SAFN is a purely sensory nerve that branches off the femoral nerve trunk. It innervates the medial skin surface of the lower leg and projects proximally to the lumbar spinal cord (L2–L3 in humans). The projection of the SAFN to the lumbar nerve roots is notably different from that of the pudendal nerve and the tibial nerve. And while the precise mechanism is not yet known, it is hypothesized that the SAFN electrically activates a different bladder-inhibitory reflex than those evoked by pudendal, sacral, and tibial nerve stimulation. Evidence of an inhibitory SAFN-to-bladder reflex has been shown in urethane anesthetized rats (Moazzam and Yoo 2018), where low-amplitude electrical pulses applied between 10 Hz and 20 Hz resulted in significant increases in bladder capacity and also the interval between successive bladder contractions. The effects of SAFN stimulation were also demonstrated in a pilot clinical study involving OAB patients (Macdiarmid, John, and Yoo 2018). This recently published study showed that 87.5% of patients responded positively to percutaneous SAFN stimulation, which was applied weekly for 12 weeks. Patients showed significant improvements in every quality-of-life measure (OAB-q survey) and showed particularly notable reductions in nighttime symptoms (nocturia and urge incontinence). This novel therapeutic approach is being further clinically validated and commercialized.

22.3.3 Neuroprosthesis for bladder voiding

The loss of normal voiding function following a neurological lesion (neurogenic bladder) – such as spinal cord injury (SCI), multiple sclerosis, or stroke – poses a significant clinical challenge for providing effective long-term management of urinary function. This can manifest as either the inability to generate sufficient bladder pressure (common in sub-thoracic SCI) or as the simultaneous activation of the bladder and EUS muscles (detrusor sphincter dyssynergia, DSD), which occurs in SCI above the sacral spinal cord. This leads to large residual bladder volumes, persistent urinary tract infections, excessively high bladder pressures, vesicoureteral reflux, and kidney damage. The current gold standard for managing bladder function is clean intermittent or indwelling catheterization. While very effective, this approach is prone to recurrent urinary tract infections and urethral damage. In addition, catheterization also requires a high degree of dexterity, which may preclude some patients (e.g., quadriplegic patients) from performing self-catheterization. Given the physical and psychological burden associated with many of these therapies, it is not surprising that restoring urinary function remains a high priority for improving the quality of life in both paraplegics and quadriplegics (Anderson 2004).

Some of the earliest attempts involved direct electrical stimulation of the bladder wall, which targeted the parasympathetic nerve fibers innervating the detrusor muscles. This approach was implemented by wires surgically threaded into the detrusor muscle (Merrill and Conway 1974) or by disk electrodes implanted onto the outer surface of the bladder wall (Magasi and Simon 1986). Clinical success was reported but with careful selection of patients (e.g., preclusion of upper motor neuron lesions) and/or surgical denervation of the urethral sphincter. In many cases, direct electrical stimulation of the bladder wall resulted in stimulation-evoked side effects (e.g., stimulus spillover into pelvic muscles causing pain or DSD), frequent device failure (e.g., electrode migration), and even damage to the bladder wall. This approach is not used clinically.

The ventral (or anterior) nerve roots of the sacral spinal cord (S3 and S4 in humans) provide an alternative anatomical location for directly activating the efferent parasympathetic nerves that innervate the urinary bladder. The utility of this approach was recognized by Sir Giles Brindley and colleagues, who were the first to successfully develop this technology and commercialize it as the Finetech-Brindley Bladder System (Finetech Medical Ltd.). The implant procedure consists of a laminectomy that provides direct access to the spinal

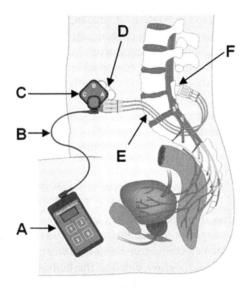

Figure 22.5 Diagram of the Finetech-Brindley system used for restoring micturition.

nerve roots (Figure 22.5). Nerve cuff electrodes (i.e., book electrodes) are implanted around each nerve root and connected to an implanted pulse generator (Brindley 1994).

The Finetech-Brindley system has thus far been successfully implanted in over 2500 patients worldwide (N. J. M. Rijkhoff 2004), but unfortunately, commercialization of this therapy in North America was not successful. The highly complex and invasive nature of the surgical implant procedure and the unintended effects (e.g., loss of reflex sexual function) resulting from bilateral dorsal rhizotomies are cited as the main reasons. Nevertheless, many innovative technologies are being developed to circumvent the need for the requisite transection of the dorsal roots, which minimizes reflex activation of the urethral sphincter. They include novel designs of nerve cuff electrodes aimed at selectively activating small-diameter sacral nerve fibers (instead of large-diameter myelinated fibers), which predominantly correspond to axons innervating the bladder (N. J. Rijkhoff et al. 1998), or high frequency (>2 kHz, sinusoid or square pulses) electrical stimulation of the pudendal nerve, which can block sphincter muscle activity (Bhadra et al. 2002).

Since the first successful reports of electrically restoring micturition function by intraspinal microstimulation (Nashold Jr. et al. 1971), advances in implantable microelectrode technology and their applications in neural engineering have supported this approach as a potential long-term therapy for restoring urinary function. Microstimulation in both spinal-intact and chronically injured animals has demonstrated selective activation of preganglionic sacral parasympathetic and somatic (i.e., Onuf's nucleus) motor neurons, resulting in contraction of the urinary bladder and EUS muscles, respectively (Grill, Bhadra, and Wang 1999; Pikov, Bullara, and McCreery 2007). Electrical microstimulation of spinal interneurons has even been shown to inhibit reflexively the urinary sphincter muscle. However, this approach is still in the preclinical stage of development due to various factors: limited long-term reliability of microelectrodes implanted within the spinal cord (e.g., electrode damage or movement), difficulties associated with the precise placement of electrodes within the spinal cord, and the highly invasive surgical implant procedure.

Electrical stimulation of the pudendal nerve provides a comparatively less-invasive means of restoring micturition function. This is a form of electrical neuromodulation that is based on the notion of electrically engaging reflex pathways that can significantly augment the excitability of the urinary bladder. Preclinical studies in cats show that electrical stimulation of the pudendal nerve – at amplitudes at or above the threshold for eliciting the bulbospongiosus reflex in cats and using stimulation frequencies between 20 Hz and 40 Hz – can elicit reflex contractions of the urinary bladder (Boggs et al. 2006). A closer examination of this reflex has led to the identification of two sensory pathways that can independently elicit reflex bladder contractions within different stimulation frequency ranges (P. Yoo, Woock, and Grill 2008; P. B. Yoo, Woock, and Grill 2008): the cranial urethral sensory (CSN, 2 Hz to 5 Hz) and dorsal genital (DGN, 20 Hz to 50 Hz) nerves. Each nerve branch innervates the proximal (prostatic) and the distal (penile) segments of the urethra, respectively. Subsequent investigation of pudendal nerve stimulation in persons with chronic SCI has demonstrated promising results (Gustafson, Creasey, and Grill 2004; P. Yoo et al. 2007; Kennelly et al. 2011), whether the electrical pulses were applied to the nerve trunk or via intra-urethral electrodes (P. B. Yoo et al. 2011). However, further work is needed to refine the method by which the electrical pulses are used to reflexively activate the urinary bladder (e.g., biomimetic stimulation of pudendal afferent nerves).

22.4 Concluding remarks

Since the earliest implantable stimulators were used to restore lost function (e.g., upper extremity function) in disabled persons, the field of functional electrical nerve stimulation has rapidly evolved into multiple sub-specialties that span various disease states, types of neural interfaces/devices, and therapeutic approaches. As briefly outlined in this chapter, we introduced several examples, including FES used for restoring standing, walking, and upper limb functions, as well as spinal stimulation and electrical neuromodulation technologies applied to address chronic bladder dysfunctions. There have been a few failures along the way, but there have also been many success stories that have significantly improved the lives of individuals with previously untreatable conditions.

However, it is important to note that the field of neural engineering is on the verge of experiencing another era of rapid expansion. Countless new clinical indications are positioned to take advantage of neurostimulation technologies, which are either commercially available for clinical use or are expected to receive regulatory approval in the near future. In addition to peripheral and spinal targets for electrical nerve stimulation, electrical neuromodulation of the brain (e.g., deep brain stimulation or cortical stimulation – not discussed in this chapter) is another clinical tool that can be used to treat intractable neurological disorders safely and effectively. At this point in time, the foreseeable future of neural engineering points to the need for innovations that enable long-term and stable use of implantable devices in patients, control strategies aimed at optimizing therapeutic efficacy (e.g., open-loop vs. closed-loop controlled systems), and a better understanding of the neurophysiological mechanisms that mediate treatment outcomes. We point readers to the following references for further examples or more general discussions of the topics covered in this chapter: Popovic, Masani, and Micera (2016) and Masani and Popovic (2011).

22.5 Discussion questions

1. What are the conditions required for orthotic and therapeutic FES? What kind of device would be ideal for patients who need orthotic or therapeutic FES?
2. In developing an FES controller that induces a functional movement, how would you design the required muscle activation pattern?
3. What other future therapeutic strategies involving neuromodulation could be investigated for restoring continence and/or micturition function in patients?
4. Despite the clinical efficacy and commercial success of sacral neuromodulation, why is there continued interest in developing new electrical neuromodulation therapies?

Bibliography

Anderson, Kim D. 2004. "Targeting Recovery: Priorities of the Spinal Cord-Injured Population." *Journal of Neurotrauma* 21 (10): 1371–83. doi:10.1089/neu.2004.21.1371.

Audu, Musa L., Brooke M. Odle, and Ronald J. Triolo. 2018. "Control of Standing Balance at Leaning Postures with Functional Neuromuscular Stimulation Following Spinal Cord Injury." *Medical and Biological Engineering and Computing* 56 (2): 317–30. doi:10.1007/s11517-017-1687-x.

Balken, Michael Rogier van. 2007. "Percutaneous Tibial Nerve Stimulation: The Urgent PC Device." *Expert Review of Medical Devices* 4 (5): 693–98. doi:10.1586/17434440.4.5.693.

Bhadra, N., V. Grunewald, G. Creasey, and J. T. Mortimer. 2002. "Selective Suppression of Sphincter Activation during Sacral Anterior Nerve Root Stimulation." *Neurourology and Urodynamics* 21 (1): 55–64. doi:10.1002/nau.2068.

Boggs, J. W., B. J. Wenzel, K. J. Gustafson, and W. M. Grill. 2006. "Frequency-Dependent Selection of Reflexes by Pudendal Afferents in the Cat." *The Journal of Physiology* 577 (Pt 1): 115–26. doi:10.1113/jphysiol.2006.111815.

Brindley, G. S. 1994. "The First 500 Patients with Sacral Anterior Root Stimulator Implants: General Description." *Paraplegia* 32 (12): 795–805. doi:10.1038/sc.1994.126.

Burton, C., A. Sajja, P. M. Latthe, A. Sajja, and P. M. Latthe. 2012. "Effectiveness of Percutaneous Posterior Tibial Nerve Stimulation for Overactive Bladder: A Systematic Review and Meta-analysis." *Neurourology and Urodynamics* 31 (8): 1206–16. doi:10.1002/nau.

Chang, Sarah R., Mark J. Nandor, Lu Li, Rudi Kobetic, Kevin M. Foglyano, John R. Schnellenberger, Musa L. Audu, Gilles Pinault, Roger D. Quinn, and Ronald J. Triolo. 2017. "A Muscle-Driven Approach to Restore Stepping with an Exoskeleton for Individuals with Paraplegia." *Journal of NeuroEngineering and Rehabilitation* 14 (1): 48. doi:10.1186/s12984-017-0258-6.

Chartier-Kastler, E. J., J. L. Ruud Bosch, M. Perrigot, M. B. Chancellor, F. Richard, and P. Denys. 2000. "Long-Term Results of Sacral Nerve Stimulation (S3) for the Treatment of Neurogenic Refractory Urge Incontinence Related to Detrusor Hyperreflexia." *Journal of Urology* 164 (5): 1476–80. doi:10.1016/S0022-5347(05)67010-3.

Davis, J. A., R. J. Triolo, J. Uhlir, C. Bieri, L. Rohde, D. Lissy, and S. Kukke. 2001. "Preliminary Performance of a Surgically Implanted Neuroprosthesis for Standing and Transfers-- Where Do We Stand?" *Journal of Rehabilitation Research and Development* 38 (6): 609–17.

Dimitrijevic, Milan R., Yuri Gerasimenko, and Michaela M. Pinter. 1998. "Evidence for a Spinal Central Pattern Generator in Humans." *Annals of the New York Academy of Sciences* 860: 360–76. doi:10.1111/j.1749-6632.1998.tb09062.x.

Everaert, Dirk G., Aiko K. Thompson, Su Ling Chong, and Richard B. Stein. 2010. "Does Functional Electrical Stimulation for Foot Drop Strengthen Corticospinal Connections?" *Neurorehabilitation and Neural Repair* 24 (2): 168–77. doi:10.1177/1545968309349939.

Finazzi-Agrò, Enrico, Filomena Petta, Francesco Sciobica, Patrizio Pasqualetti, Stefania Musco, Pierluigi Bove, E. Finazzi-Agro, et al. 2010. "Percutaneous Tibial Nerve Stimulation Effects on Detrusor Overactivity Incontinence Are Not Due to a Placebo Effect: A Randomized, Double-Blind, Placebo Controlled Trial." *Journal of Urology* 184 (5): 2001–6. doi:10.1016/j.juro.2010.06.113.

Gerasimenko, Y., R. Gorodnichev, A. Puhov, T. Moshonkina, A. Savochin, V. Selionov, R. R. Roy, et al. 2015. "Initiation and Modulation of Locomotor Circuitry Output with Multisite Transcutaneous Electrical Stimulation of the Spinal Cord in Noninjured Humans." *Journal of Neurophysiology* 113: 834–42. doi: 10.1152/jn.00609.2014.

Goldman, H. B., C. L. Amundsen, J. Mangel, J. Grill, M. Bennett, K. J. Gustafson, and W. M. Grill. 2008. "Dorsal Genital Nerve Stimulation for the Treatment of Overactive Bladder Symptoms." *Neurourology and Urodynamics* 27 (6): 499–503. doi:10.1002/nau.20544.

Gollee, Henrik, Ken J. Hunt, and Duncan E. Wood. 2004. "New Results in Feedback Control of Unsupported Standing in Paraplegia." *IEEE Transactions on Neural Systems and Rehabilitation Engineering* 12 (1): 73–80. doi:10.1109/TNSRE.2003.822765.

Grahn, Peter J., Igor A. Lavrov, Dimitry G. Sayenko, Meegan G. Van Straaten, Megan L. Gill, Jeffrey A. Strommen, Jonathan S. Calvert, et al. 2017. "Enabling Task-Specific Volitional Motor Functions via Spinal Cord Neuromodulation in a Human with Paraplegia." *Mayo Clinic Proceedings* 92 (4): 544–54. doi:10.1016/j.mayocp.2017.02.014.

Graupe, Daniel, and Kate H. Kohn. 1998. "Functional Neuromuscular Stimulator for Short-Distance Ambulation by Certain Thoracic-Level Spinal-Cord-Injured Paraplegics." *Surgical Neurology* 50 (3): 202–7. doi:10.1016/S0090-3019(98)00074-3.

Grill, W. M., N. Bhadra, and B. Wang. 1999. "Bladder and Urethral Pressures Evoked by Microstimulation of the Sacral Spinal Cord in Cats." *Brain Research* 836 (1–2): 19–30. doi:10.1016/S0006-8993(99)01581-4.

Gustafson, K. J., G. H. Creasey, and W. M. Grill. 2004. "A Urethral Afferent Mediated Excitatory Bladder Reflex Exists in Humans." *Neuroscience Letters* 360 (1–2): 9–12. doi:10.1016/j.neulet.2004.01.001.

Harkema, Susan, Yury Gerasimenko, Jonathan Hodes, Joel Burdick, Claudia Angeli, Yangsheng Chen, Christie Ferreira, et al. 2011. "Effect of Epidural Stimulation of the Lumbosacral Spinal Cord on Voluntary Movement, Standing, and Assisted Stepping after Motor Complete Paraplegia: A Case Study." *The Lancet* 377 (9781): 1938–47. doi:10.1016/S0140-6736(11)60547-3.

Hausdorff, Jeffrey M., and Haim Ring. 2008. "Effects of a New Radio Frequency-Controlled Neuroprosthesis on Gait Symmetry and Rhythmicity in Patients with Chronic Hemiparesis." *American Journal of Physical Medicine and Rehabilitation* 87 (1): 4–13. doi:10.1097/PHM.0b013e31815e6680.

Hendricks, H. T., M. J. Ijzerman, J. R. De Kroon, F. A. in 't Groen, and G. Zilvold. 2001. "Functional Electrical Stimulation by Means of the 'Ness Handmaster Orthosis' in Chronic Stroke Patients: An Exploratory Study." *Clinical Rehabilitation* 15 (2): 217–20. doi:10.1191/026921501672937235.

Jaime, Ralf Peter, Zlatko Matjačić, and Kenneth J. Hunt. 2002. "Paraplegic Standing Supported by FES-Controlled Ankle Stiffness." *IEEE Transactions on Neural Systems and Rehabilitation Engineering* 10 (4): 239–48. doi:10.1109/TNSRE.2002.806830.

Jilge, B., K. Minassian, F. Rattay, M. M. Pinter, F. Gerstenbrand, H. Binder, and M. R. Dimitrijevic. 2004. "Initiating Extension of the Lower Limbs in Subjects with Complete Spinal Cord Injury by Epidural Lumbar Cord Stimulation." *Experimental Brain Research* 154 (3): 308–26. doi:10.1007/s00221-003-1666-3.

Jonas, U., C. J. Fowler, M. B. Chancellor, M. M. Elhilali, M. Fall, J. B. Gajewski, V. Grunewald, et al. 2001. "Efficacy of Sacral Nerve Stimulation for Urinary Retention: Results 18 Months after Implantation." *Journal of Urology* 165 (1): 15–19.

Kennelly, M. J., M. E. Bennett, W. M. Grill, J. H. Grill, and J. W. Boggs. 2011. "Electrical Stimulation of the Urethra Evokes Bladder Contractions and Emptying in Spinal Cord Injury Men: Case Studies." *Journal of Spinal Cord Medicine* 34 (3): 315–21. doi:10.1179/2045772311Y.0000000012.

Kirkham, A. P., N. C. Shah, S. L. Knight, P. J. Shah, and M. D. Craggs. 2001. "The Acute Effects of Continuous and Conditional Neuromodulation on the Bladder in Spinal Cord Injury." *Spinal Cord* 39 (8): 420–28.

Kobetic, R., R. J. Triolo, and E. B. Marsolais. 1997. "Muscle Selection and Walking Performance of Multichannel FES Systems for Ambulation in Paraplegia." *IEEE Transactions on Rehabilitation Engineering* 5 (1): 23–9. doi:10.1109/86.559346.

Kobetic, R., R. J. Triolo, J. P. Uhlir, C. Bieri, M. Wibowo, G. Polando, E. B. Marsolais, J. A. Davis Jr., K. A. Ferguson, and M. Sharma. 1999. "Implanted Functional Electrical Stimulation System for Mobility in Paraplegia: A Follow-Up Case Report." *IEEE Transactions on Rehabilitation Engineering* 7 (4): 390–8. doi:10.1109/86.808942.

Kralj, A., T. Bajd, and R. Turk. 1980. "Electrical Stimulation Providing Functional Use of Paraplegic Patient Muscles." *Medical Progress Technology* 7 (1): 3–9.

Macdiarmid, S. A., M. S. John, and P. B. Yoo. 2018. "A Pilot Feasibility Study of Treating Overactive Bladder Patients with Percutaneous Saphenous Nerve Stimulation." *Neurourology and Urodynamics* 37 (5): 1815–20. doi:10.1002/nau.23531.

Magasi, P., and Z. Simon. 1986. "Electrical Stimulation of the Bladder and Gravidity." *Urologia Internationalis* 41 (4): 241–45.

Masani, K. 2003. "Importance of Body Sway Velocity Information in Controlling Ankle Extensor Activities during Quiet Stance." *Journal of Neurophysiology* 90 (6): 3774–82. doi:10.1152/jn.00730.2002.

Masani, K., and M. R. Popovic. 2011. "Functional Electrical Stimulation in Rehabilitation and Neurorehabilitation." In *Handbook of Medical Technology*, edited by K.-P. Hoffman, R. S. Pozos and R. Kramme, 877–96. New York: Springer.

McGuire, Edward J., S. C. Zhang, Elwood R. Horwinski, Bernard Lytton, Zhang Shi-chun, Elwood R. Horwinski, Bernard Lytton, et al. 1983. "Treatment of Motor and Sensory Detrusor Instability by Electrical Stimulation." *Journal of Urology* 129 (1): 78–79.

Merrill, D. C., and C. J. Conway. 1974. "Clinical Experience with the Mentor Bladder Stimulator. I. Patients with Upper Motor Neuron Lesions." *Journal of Urology* 112 (2): 52–6. doi:10.1016/S0022-5347(17)59640-8.

Moazzam, Zainab, and Paul B. Yoo. 2018. "Frequency-Dependent Inhibition of Bladder Function by Saphenous Nerve Stimulation in Anesthetized Rats." *Neurourology and Urodynamics* 37 (2): 592–9. doi:10.1002/nau.23323.

Mushahwar, Vivian K., Patrick L. Jacobs, Richard A. Normann, Ronald J. Triolo, and Naomi Kleitman. 2007. "New Functional Electrical Stimulation Approaches to Standing and Walking." *Journal of Neural Engineering* 4 (3): S181–97. doi:10.1088/1741-2560/4/3/S05.

Nashold Jr., B. S., H. Friedman, and S. Boyarsky. 1971. "Electrical Activation of Micturition by Spinal Cord Stimulation." *Journal of Surgical Research* 11 (3): 144–47. doi:10.1016/0022-4804(71)90039-4.

Peckham, P. Hunter, and Jayme S. Knutson. 2005. "Functional Electrical Stimulation for Neuromuscular Applications." *Annual Review of Biomedical Engineering* 7: 327–360.

Peeren, F., P. Hoebeke, and K. Everaert. 2005. "Sacral Nerve Stimulation: Interstim Therapy." *Expert Review of Medical Devices* 2 (3): 253–58. doi:10.1586/17434440.2.3.253.

Peters, K. M., K. A. Killinger, B. M. Boguslawski, and J. A. Boura. 2010. "Chronic Pudendal Neuromodulation: Expanding Available Treatment Options for Refractory Urologic Symptoms." *Neurourol Urodyn* 29 (7): 1267–71. doi:10.1002/nau.20823.

Peters, Kenneth M., Donna J. Carrico, Ramon A. Perez-Marrero, Ansar U. Khan, Leslie S. Wooldridge, Gregory L. Davis, and Scott A. MacDiarmid. 2010. "Randomized Trial of Percutaneous Tibial Nerve Stimulation versus Sham Efficacy in the Treatment of Overactive Bladder Syndrome: Results from the SUmiT Trial." *Journal of Urology* 183 (4): 1438–43. doi:10.1016/j.juro.2009.12.036.

Peters, Kenneth M., Scott A. Macdiarmid, Leslie S. Wooldridge, Fah Che Leong, S. Abbas Shobeiri, Eric S. Rovner, Steven W. Siegel, et al. 2009. "Randomized Trial of Percutaneous Tibial Nerve Stimulation versus Extended-Release Tolterodine: Results from the Overactive Bladder Innovative Therapy Trial." *Journal of Urology* 182 (3): 1055–61. doi:10.1016/j.juro.2009.05.045.

Pikov, V., L. Bullara, and D. B. McCreery. 2007. "Intraspinal Stimulation for Bladder Voiding in Cats before and after Chronic Spinal Cord Injury." *Journal of Neural Engineering* 4 (4): 356–68. doi:10.1088/1741-2560/4/4/002.

Popovic, M. R., K. Masani, and S. Micera. 2016. "Functional Electrical Stimulation Therapy: Recovery of Function Following Spinal Cord Injury and Stroke." In *Neurorehabilitation Technology*, 2nd ed., edited by D. Reinkensmeyer and V. Dietz, 513–32. New York: Springer.

Popovic, Milos R., Naaz Kapadia, Vera Zivanovic, Julio C. Furlan, B. Cathy Craven, and Colleen McGillivray. 2011. "Functional Electrical Stimulation Therapy of Voluntary Grasping versus Only Conventional Rehabilitation for Patients with Subacute Incomplete Tetraplegia: A Randomized Clinical Trial." *Neurorehabilitation and Neural Repair* 25 (5): 433–42. doi:10.1177/1545968310392924.

Prochazka, Arthur, Michel Gauthier, Marguerite Wieler, and Zoltan Kenwell. 1997. "The Bionic Glove: An Electrical Stimulator Garment that Provides Controlled Grasp and Hand Opening in Quadriplegia." *Archives of Physical Medicine and Rehabilitation* 78 (6): 608–14. doi:10.1016/S0003-9993(97)90426-3.

Rijkhoff, N. J., H. Wijkstra, P. E. van Kerrebroeck, and F. M. Debruyne. 1998. "Selective Detrusor Activation by Sacral Ventral Nerve-Root Stimulation: Results of Intraoperative Testing in Humans during Implantation of a Finetech-Brindley System." *World Journal of Urology* 16 (5): 337–41.

Rijkhoff, Nico J. M. 2004. "Neuroprostheses to Treat Neurogenic Bladder Dysfunction: Current Status and Future Perspectives." *Child's Nervous System: ChNS : Official Journal of the International Society for Pediatric Neurosurgery* 20 (2): 75–86. doi:10.1007/s00381-003-0859-1.

Smith, Brian, Zhengnian Tang, Mark W. Johnson, Soheyl Pourmehdi, Martha M. Gazdik, James R. Buckett, and P. Hunter Peckham. 1998. "An Externally Powered, Multichannel, Implantable Stimulator-Telemeter for Control of Paralyzed Muscle." *IEEE Transactions on Biomedical Engineering* 45 (4): 463–75. doi:10.1109/10.664202.

Snellings, Andre' E., and Warren M. Grill. 2012. "Effects of Stimulation Site and Stimulation Parameters on Bladder Inhibition by Electrical Nerve Stimulation." *BJU* International 110 (1): 136–43. doi:10.1111/j.1464-410X.2011.10789.x.

Spinelli, M., S. Malaguti, G. Giardiello, M. Lazzeri, J. Tarantola, and U. Van Den Hombergh. 2005. "A New Minimally Invasive Procedure for Pudendal Nerve Stimulation to Treat Neurogenic Bladder: Description of the Method and Preliminary Data." *Neurourol Urodyn* 24 (4): 305–9.

Stauffer, Y., Y. Allemand, M. Bouri, J. Fournier, R. Clavel, P. Metrailler, R. Brodard, and F. Reynard. 2009. "The WalkTrainer - A New Generation of Walking Reeducation Device Combining Orthoses and Muscle Stimulation." *IEEE Transactions on Neural Systems and Rehabilitation Engineering* 17 (1): 38–45. doi:10.1109/TNSRE.2008.2008288.

Stein, Richard B., Dirk G. Everaert, Aiko K. Thompson, Su Ling Chong, Maura Whittaker, Jenny Robertson, and Gerald Kuether. 2010. "Long-Term Therapeutic and Orthotic Effects of a Foot Drop Stimulator on Walking Performance in Progressive and Nonprogressive Neurological Disorders." *Neurorehabilitation and Neural Repair* 24 (2): 152–67. doi:10.1177/1545968309347681.

Swigchem, Roos Van, Judith Vloothuis, Jasper Den Boer, Vivian Weerdesteyn, and Alexander C. H. Geurts. 2010. "Is Transcutaneous Peroneal Stimulation Beneficial to Patients with Chronic Stroke Using an Ankle-Foot Orthosis? A Within-Subjects Study of Patients' Satisfaction, Walking Speed and Physical Activity Level." *Journal of Rehabilitation Medicine* 42 (2): 117–21. doi:10.2340/16501977-0489.

Tai, Changfeng, Jicheng Wang, Xianchun Wang, William C. de Groat, and James R. Roppolo. 2007. "Bladder Inhibition or Voiding Induced by Pudendal Nerve Stimulation in Chronic Spinal Cord Injured Cats." *Neurourol Urodyn* 26 (4): 570–77. doi:10.1002/nau.20374.

Tanagho, E. A., and R. A. Schmidt. 1988. "Electrical Stimulation in the Clinical Management of the Neurogenic Bladder." *Journal of Urology* 140 (6): 1331–39.

Thrasher, T. A., H. M. Flett, and M. R. Popovic. 2006. "Gait Training Regimen for Incomplete Spinal Cord Injury Using Functional Electrical Stimulation." *Spinal Cord: The Official Journal of the International Medical Society of Paraplegia* 44 (6): 357–61. doi:10.1038/sj.sc.3101864.

Vandoninck, V., M. R. Van Balken, E. Finazzi Agro, F. Petta, C. Caltagirone, J. P. Heesakkers, L. A. Kiemeney, F. M. Debruyne, and B. L. Bemelmans. 2003. "Posterior Tibial Nerve Stimulation in the Treatment of Urge Incontinence." *Neurourol Urodyn* 22 (1): 17–23. doi:10.1002/nau.10036.

583

Vette, Albert H., Kei Masani, and Milos R. Popovic. 2007. "Implementation of a Physiologically Identified PD Feedback Controller for Regulating the Active Ankle Torque during Quiet Stance." *IEEE Transactions on Neural Systems and Rehabilitation Engineering* 15 (2): 235–43. doi:10.1109/TNSRE.2007.897016.

Woock, J. P., P. B. Yoo, and W. M. Grill. 2008. "Activation and Inhibition of the Micturition Reflex by Penile Afferents in the Cat." *American Journal of Physiology-Regulatory, Integrative and Comparative Physiology* 294 (6): R1880–9. doi:10.1152/ajpregu.00029.2008.

Yoo, P. B., E. E. Horvath, C. L. Amundsen, G. D. Webster, and W. M. Grill. 2011. "Multiple Pudendal Sensory Pathways Reflexly Modulate Bladder and Urethral Activity in Patients with Spinal Cord Injury." *Journal of Urology* 185 (2): 737–43. doi:10.1016/j.juro.2010.09.079.

Yoo, P. B., J. P. Woock, and W. M. Grill. 2008a. "Bladder Activation by Selective Stimulation of Pudendal Nerve Afferents in the Cat." *Experimental Neurology* 212 (1): 218–25. doi:10.1016/j.expneurol.2008.04.010.

Yoo, P. B., J. P. Woock, and W. M. Grill. 2008b. "Somatic Innervation of the Feline Lower Urinary Tract." *Brain Research* 1246: 80–87. doi:10.1016/j.brainres.2008.09.053.

Yoo, P. B., S. M. Klein, N. H. Grafstein, E. E. Horvath, C. L. Amundsen, G. D. Webster, and W. M. Grill. 2007. "Pudendal Nerve Stimulation Evokes Reflex Bladder Contractions in Persons with Chronic Spinal Cord Injury." *Neurourology and Urodynamics* 26 (7): 1020–23. doi:10.1002/nau.20441.

Section IV
Outcomes and assessments

Chapter 23 Assessment approaches in rehabilitation engineering

M. Donahue and P. Schwartz

Contents

DOI: 10.1201/b21964-27

23.1 Chapter overview

Having a breadth and depth of knowledge of human function and an extensive acquaintance of specific assistive technology (AT) devices does not provide enough background to recommend AT devices. Understanding the AT assessment process provides the practitioner with a framework to conduct assessments in a systematic way, thereby ensuring that the AT meets the goals of the individual.

This chapter provides an overview of AT assessment protocols, describing three important models in the field including the international classification of functioning, disability and health (ICF), matching person and technology (MPT) and human activity assistive technology (HAAT). The chapter also highlights the steps of the assessment process including presenting the commonalities of assessment protocols studied in the literature. We also explain six key components of high-quality AT assessments: centering the assessment around the individual, including the family and support system, goal setting, consideration of the environment and task, developing a transdisciplinary team and considering culture. Additionally, we detail nine assessment process steps, including recognizing the need, collecting information, assessing abilities, developing specifications, determining potential solutions, selecting a preferred solution, communicating the plan, implementing the plan and continuing service. Best practices for AT assessments are also discussed. Finally, we ponder our future vision of AT assessments.

However, this chapter is not exhaustive. It does not detail every AT assessment model, framework, protocol or instrument detailed in the literature. The reader is encouraged to read the suggested readings and documents listed in the bibliography for more background. Further, this chapter is not prescriptive of particular AT devices or strategies. Rather, the AT assessment process described in this chapter is purposefully broad in nature to address the wide variety of settings and situations that the rehabilitation engineering professional (REP) may encounter in practice.

23.2 The rehabilitation engineering assessment methodology

The rehabilitation engineering (RE) assessment process is a continuation or modification of the scientific method, developed over the ages by Aristotle, Ibn al-Haytham, Bacon, Galileo, Newton and others, and applied to the field of AT

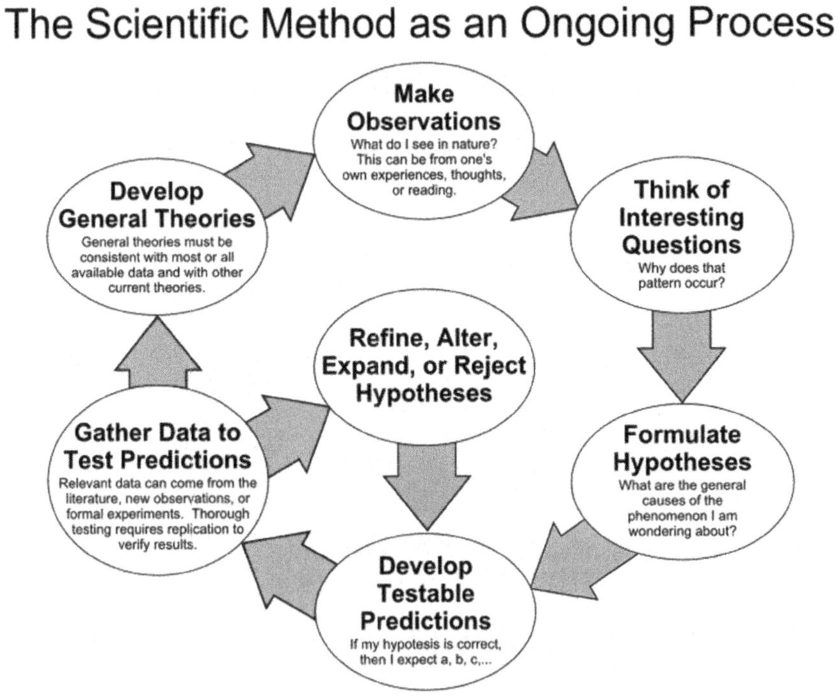

The Scientific Method as an Ongoing Process

Figure 23.1 The scientific method (https://commons.wikimedia.org/wiki/File:The_ Scientific_Method_as_an_Ongoing_Process.svg, https://commons.wikimedia.org/ wiki/File:The_Scientific_Method_as_an_Ongoing_Process.svg).

and RE. An illustration of the ongoing process of the scientific method is shown in Figure 23.1. Although the specific language is different, the REP conducting an AT assessment makes observations, develops questions and continues through the cycle of the scientific method shown in Figure 23.1.

The AT assessment process also relates closely to the engineering design process: defining a problem or identifying a need, conducting background research, specifying requirements, brainstorming, evaluating and choosing a solution as illustrated in Figure 23.2. To select the best computer access method for an AT user, the REP identifies a need (i.e., the individual cannot use a standard keyboard), researches the individual's abilities (i.e., conducts background research), specifies keyboard requirements and together with the individual, determines the best keyboard system (i.e., selecting the best solution). This also is an iterative process, where the keyboard is tested during the assessment or trials (test solution), with refinements to the keyboard type, positioning and environment in each iteration. Applying the systematic scientific method and engineering design process to the AT assessment process ensures that the process is comprehensive, minimizing the risk of AT abandonment.

589

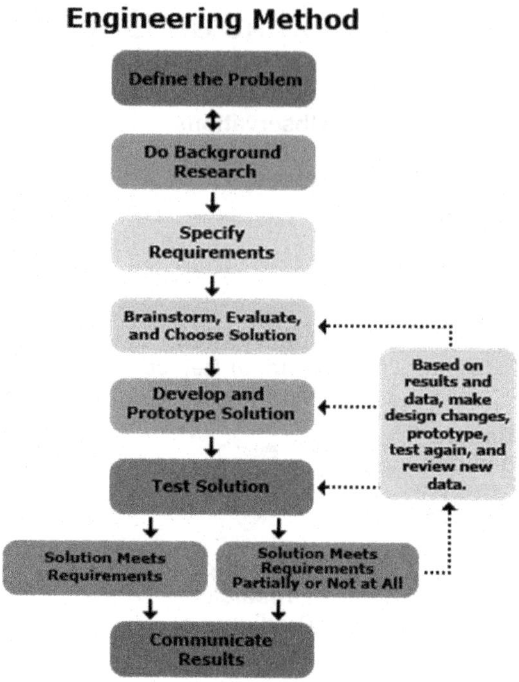

Engineering Method

Figure 23.2 Engineering process "Comparing the Engineering Design Process and the Scientific Method" (Science Buddies.org 2017).

23.3 Models and instruments contribute to a systematic approach of the assessment process

While the scientific method and engineering design process are important models in understanding the RE assessment process, they are not enough to develop a functional framework or model for this process. Many researchers have developed models to aid in this understanding.

Many assessment models, frameworks and processes that REPs use are published. Multiple researchers have cataloged assessment strategies. Bromley describes five models of AT assessments, including MPT; lifespace access profile; student, environments, tasks and tools (SETT); education tech points and Wisconsin assistive technology initiative (WATI). She found four similarities among the models: (1) all emphasize the process of AT assessment and goal setting; (2) all assess person, environment and task with an ecological function; (3) all emphasize a multidisciplinary collaborative approach to AT assessment and (4) all share the goal of facilitating an effective match between the individual and the AT for the environment used (Bromley 2001). Lenker and Paquet reviewed a sample of conceptual models of AT outcomes research and practice. They noted that these models should include descriptive and/or predictive functions that support AT that positively impacts the individual. They reviewed six models including HAAT, ICF and MPT (Lenker and Paquet 2003). Edyburn reviewed 12 models of special education technology and Wissick and Gardner reviewed seven models (Edyburn 2001; Wissick and Gardner 2008). The ATOMS website lists over fifty assessment instruments "ID-AT-Assessments – All Instruments – ATOMS Project – UW-Milwaukee" and 52 models for assessment (Smith et al. 2017). Bernd reviews seven models and concludes that AT is a poorly developed field resulting in lack of evidence-based procedures for AT selection and calls for future research in the field (Bernd, Van Der Pijl and De Witte 2009).

Although there are many models proposed in AT, the three models that are consistently cited in the literature are the ICF, the MPT and HAAT. Many of the other models described in literature have little testing for external validity and reliability or are narrow in their focus. The ICF, the MPT and HAAT are briefly described here.

ICF: The World Health Organization's International Classification of Functioning, Disability and Health (WHO 2001) is a model that classifies individuals based on the components of categories: (1) body functions, (2) body structures, (3) activities and participation, (4) environmental factors and (5) personal factors. Its purpose is to provide a framework for assessment, diagnosis, intervention and outcome measurement, regardless of health or ability level. The ICF model is helpful in changing the idea in rehabilitation research from a "problem in person" to "problem in system" (Lenker and Paquet 2003).

MPT: Matching person and technology is an assessment model developed to provide a personal approach to the AT assessment process "Matching Person and Technology Home Page" (MPT 2017). The MPT model is shown in Figure 23.3 (MPT 2017). Using MPT, the user of the technology is a collaborative partner in the selection process. The model focuses on three primary components. These include: 1) the milieu or environment in which the person will interact with the technology, 2) the person using the technology and 3) the technology itself. The interaction between these three characteristics influences the success or failure of the AT. The MPT process has four different instruments that guide selection of 1) technology, 2) technology for education, 3) technology for the workplace and 4) technology for health maintenance or pain relief.

HAAT: The human activity assistive technology model was first proposed by Cook and Hussey (1995) and was designed to provide assessment and prescription, as well as to evaluate the result. The performance of the entire system, rather than evaluation of the human performance, was considered paramount. The model describes someone (human) doing something (activity) in a context using AT. The HAAT model has evolved over time to include the physical, social,

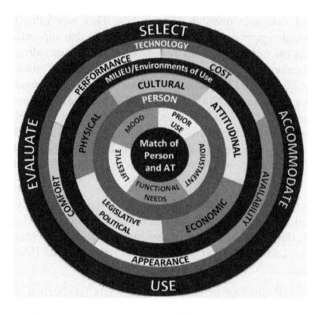

Figure 23.3 MPT Model (Institute for Matching Person & Technology, 1995 http://matchingpersonandtechnology.com).

cultural and environmental aspects, but the four key components of user, activity, AT and context have remained the same. Giesbrecht provides an extensive review of design and evolution of HAAT and proposes a new graphical representation of the model in Figure 23.4.

23.4 Best practices and commonalities

A common and primary goal of the AT assessment is to find the best fit of technology (including strategies) for the individual and the environment of use (Lenker and Paquet 2003). A systematic approach to the assessment process that incorporates these best practices will ensure they are followed during the assessment. Many of the models, frameworks and instruments are intended to provide structure to the assessment (Copley and Ziviani 2005; Lenker and Paquet 2003; Mumford et al. 2014).

Regardless of the model, it is generally agreed that a high-quality AT assessment is centered around the individual with the disability and considers the task (or goal) and the context/environment in which the technology is used (Desideri et al. 2014; Mirza and Hammel 2009; Lenker and Paquet 2003; Mumford et al. 2014). It is also crucial that the individual's and family's goals are considered and that they are included in the transdisciplinary team. This will increase the individual's ownership of the AT (Copley and Ziviani 2005; Desideri et al. 2014; Mirza and

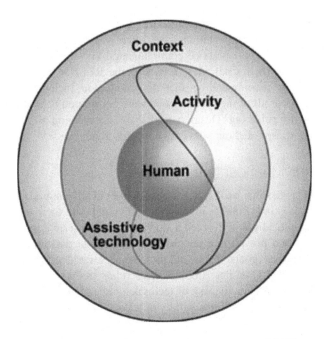

Figure 23.4 Giesbrecht's proposed HAAT model (Giesbrecht 2013).

Hammel 2009; Mumford et al. 2014). In addition to including them on the transdisciplinary team, the process should consider the individual's support system and culture (Desideri et al. 2014; Mirza and Hammel 2009; Mumford et al. 2014). A collaboration between the individual and professional produces the best results in obtaining the appropriate AT (Johnston et al. 2014).

The assessment needs to gather enough information to allow the team to make informed recommendations. To do this, you must identify clear goals, collect sufficient medical and educational background information and complete a functional assessment and task analysis that characterizes the individual's sensory function, motor performance, cognitive skills, social/emotional development and communication needs (Copley and Ziviani 2005; Desideri et al. 2014; Mumford et al. 2014). With this information, the REP can determine an access method and then identify characteristics of an AT system to guide the search for an individualized AT solution (Copley and Ziviani 2005; Mumford et al. 2014).

Once the assessment is complete, it is important to communicate results clearly. It should include a description of the assessment process, the recommendations, a plan for implementation and resources for acquisition of the AT system (Copley and Ziviani 2005; Desideri et al. 2014; Mirza and Hammel 2009; Wissick and Gardner 2008). Desideri completed a study to develop a method of assuring quality of the documentation communicating the assessment process and results. Quality assurance in documentation drives quality assessments because the REP can incorporate each best practice communicated into the assessment process. In preparation for their study, they reference the RESNA *Wheelchair Service Provision Guide*, recommending that documentation includes solutions and reports findings for all of the products that were considered or evaluated, including those that are ruled out (Desideri et al. 2014). Describing all options considered including those ruled out alleviates concerns about bias.

23.4.1 Individual centered

The RE field agrees that an AT assessment is individual centered. Regardless of the disability, it is important to involve the individual (and their support system) in the assessment. Mirza performed a study on AT long term advocacy and support (ATLAS) and proved that people with intellectual disabilities have better outcomes when their goals, needs and preferences are valued in the assessment process (Mirza and Hammel 2009). Several other studies emphasize this and suggest that it will reduce the risk of technology abandonment. The assessment should include the individual in a variety of ways, as much as possible.

Include the individual with the disability at the beginning when the goals and priorities are determined. Give the individual's goals significant weight, recognizing they may differ from the goals of their family, support system or referring/hiring agency. Ultimately, the end user of the technology is the individual. If they are provided AT to help them perform an activity that they don't find valuable, they won't use it to its capacity, or not to use it at all.

After goals are determined, involve the individual in both the functional assessment and determination of features that are important to their solution. Specify low-tech or familiar technology on the system feature list if the individual does not like to learn new technology. Solicit input from the transdisciplinary team, including the family, but do not diminish the individual's preferences.

Using technology that meets the feature list, the individual participates in device trials and provides feedback. This helps with the decision-making process. It is important for the REP to remain unbiased and not ask leading questions when soliciting feedback. After the trials are complete, the individual participates in device selection. After the device is selected, involve the individual in planning the implementation and training.

23.4.2 Family/support system inclusion

Include the family or support system of the individual. This includes the people who know the individual well, provide care for the individual and either advocate for the individual or assist them with self-advocacy. Often it includes parents, guardians, siblings, caregivers and friends. All these people have different perspectives and roles relating to assessment goals. There are many details, challenges and strengths regarding how the individual accomplishes their activity pre-intervention that they may not notice within their frame of reference, where people observing them accomplish the task pre-intervention can each add a different perspective. Additionally, these people are often the ones who provide support with setup and troubleshooting of the technology, so their preferences may influence development of the feature and specification list when all things are equal with respect to the individual. For example, if the application being recommended is used on all operating systems, but all the support people use brand A's operating system, then a brand A device should be recommended because the support team has the familiarity with the operating system to provide troubleshooting assistance.

23.4.3 Goal setting

The assessment process is typically triggered through the recognition of a need, but the development of measurable goals within the assessment process is often more complex. Often during discussion of AT, there are various areas where AT could assist that are important to the individual with the disability. The referral source may only identify one goal or use broad language. It is important to include the transdisciplinary team in the development of measurable goals, but the individual's goals have greater precedence, to empower them through the process. Copley suggests inclusion of a facilitator to promote discussion among the team (Copley and Ziviani 2005).

23.4.4 Consideration of environment and task

Consider all the environments and contexts throughout the assessment process. If the individual will use their technology at home, what are the circumstances that they will use it? Are there other people/animals around and how might they affect the solution (e.g., are they going to increase the risk of damage, does the individual have a pet who will damage any device with cords, will the loud noise of the environment such as the TV, pet parrots or playing children affect the efficacy of a voice recognition system or the output of a communication system)?

It is also important to consider all perspectives of the environments and contexts that the device is used. It is the location of the AT and the physical environment (e.g., lighting, ambient sound, workstation layout, temperature). It is also the cultural aspects of the individual and their family. It includes the social context ranging from the most immediate level within which the individual interacts directly and frequently to the largest scale where policy affects the use of the AT. Consider and discuss all these intrinsic aspects that affect the use of the AT throughout the assessment process to fully address the individual's needs.

23.4.5 Transdisciplinary

Most literature agrees that the incorporation of a transdisciplinary team in the assessment is crucial (Copley and Ziviani 2005; Desideri et al. 2014; Mirza and Hammel 2009; Mumford et al. 2014). This helps ensure that all the AT works together, and one aspect is not missed. It creates a comprehensive approach, reducing the likelihood that the recommendations interfere with each other that could lead to device abandonment. The team includes all the professionals and specialists who work with the individual, including but not limited to, individual occupational therapists, physical therapists, speech and language pathologists, special education teachers, rehabilitation technologists, rehabilitation engineers, physicians, neuropsychologists, vocational rehabilitation counselors, job developers, complex rehabilitation technology vendors, employers, caregivers and family/support system. An REP typically leads the team to coordinate the assessment.

Sometimes AT is implemented in stages. This is common when a person's "career" changes and they are a previous AT user. Although it is not best practice, resources may limit the number of participants in the assessment. When this happens, it is the responsibility of the REP leading the assessment to obtain as much background information from reports that other professionals (who are typically on the team) have provided through their individual services. When possible, contact and consult them remotely. It is best if the REP understands the common roles of the transdisciplinary team members so they can recommend and refer the individual for services needed to enable the full comprehensive approach desired through the transdisciplinary model. For example, an REP is hired to conduct a workstation assessment for an individual with hemiplegia who plans to work out of his home. The individual is working with a vocational rehabilitation counselor. The vocational rehabilitation counselor provided medical background information in the form of a functional assessment rating that subjectively discusses mobility, communication, self-care, self-direction, interpersonal skills, work tolerance and work skills. This provides limited information, so the REP requests medical records pertaining to rehabilitation therapies and learns that the individual has not received therapy in several years. During the assessment, the REP notices that the individual's wheelchair is not providing adequate support for long-term use. It is the responsibility of the REP to recognize that there are seating and mobility needs outside of their expertise and recommends that the individual work with a physical therapist and complex rehabilitation technology supplier to address this concern.

23.4.6 Consideration of culture

Culture includes a group's common set of beliefs, values, behaviors and communication patterns, but it is also the way individuals see themselves as part of the world and in relation to other people. It has a large impact on the interactions between the people on the transdisciplinary team, and in particular how the individual and their family relate to the professionals, ultimately affecting the decision-making process (stigma may be attached to a specific device, or training preferences) (Parette, Huer and Scherer 2004). Sensitivity to the culture is important for the REP to help increase the synergy of the transdisciplinary team. As a professional, it is important to avoid making assumptions and to keep an open mind. It is helpful to conduct background research and have a general awareness of common typecasts, without applying the stereotypes to the individual. This will help the REP to have a foundation to help build rapport with the individual and help them to recognize that they are a valuable member of the team and their input is crucial.

23.5 Following best practices in lieu of REP environment or referral source constraints

The different settings the REP works in will also affect the assessment of the individual. Cook and Polgar describe eight settings where direct consumer service takes place and AT assessments may occur. These settings include rehabilitation programs, university programs, state agency programs (including K–12 schools), private practice, rehabilitation technology supplier/durable medical equipment supplier, Department of Veterans Affairs, local affiliate of a national nonprofit disability organization and volunteer organizations (Cook and Polgar 2014). A comprehensive, high-quality assessment encourages consideration of all aspects of the individual's life through the inclusion of all the environments and contexts. Often the funding source's intention for the assessment, or constraints of the REP's setting, will limit the assessment to the focus of their mission, contradicting the best practices. If the vocational rehabilitation agency is funding the services for the assessment, they may not have the flexibility to address components focusing on non-vocational activities of daily living. A school system may not have the freedom to explore components of the assessment focusing on recreation.

This creates a challenging paradox. To serve the individual well, comprehensive assessment is desired, but to serve the customer paying for their work, they need to primarily address the goals of that agency. Often, there are recommended practices within the referring agency that incorporate motivational interviewing or another technique that includes and empowers the individual to pursue an AT assessment and with the development of the referral goals. Additionally, a comprehensive assessment is often overwhelming in the amount of AT that is addressed, particularly if the individual is not a previous user of AT. When possible, the REP can recognize other areas and goals where AT is useful, recommending further assessments to address those areas and suggest alternative funding sources for the goals outside of the mission of the current funding agency. This documents the need and provides a starting point to move forward in those streams when they are ready.

Regardless of the setting that the REP works in, they can still incorporate best practices into their technique. The REP's assessment should include the individual's goals, objectives and preferences, and a transdisciplinary approach is still the best approach. The context and all the environments should also have significant weight in the development of a feature list or specifications for the AT solution. When the REP enters the decision-making process, it is important to keep the big picture (all environments and contexts) in view even when the lens of the assessment is focused on a specific situation (employment, home, school). If possible, the REP should recommend a device or system that is compatible across systems. If that is not possible (often due to conflicting needs) then the REP may consider two systems; possibly only one is funded by the specified funding source and the other acquired through alternative funding. For example, if a computer with voice recognition software is required for communication at work, it is often not possible for the work computer to leave the premises and be used at home. In that situation, a vocational rehabilitation provider or the employer may purchase the voice recognition software for use at work. However, if the individual needs it to access the computer at home they may need to seek alternative funding methods to acquire a second copy that can be used on the home computer.

23.6 Conducting a high-quality assistive technology assessment

A systematic and organized approach enables the REP to coordinate and conduct the AT assessment to follow the best practices. An assessment process is an adaptation of the scientific method or engineering design process. The consortium model describes the AT service delivery process to include recognition of the problem, evaluation identification of outcomes, assess barriers/identify AT and AT services, develop an AT menu, match intervention to need, select an AT device and identify training need, identify supplier, identify funding source, implement plan, and follow-up (Long et al. 2003). Cook and Polgar describe the service delivery process to include referral and intake, initial evaluation (skills, device characteristics), recommendations and report, implementation (order and setup, delivery and fitting, training), follow-up (maintenance, repair as needed) and follow-along (maintenance, repair as needed). There are additional processes and frameworks that have their own language and approach (Cook and Polgar 2014). A generalization of the different assessment processes is illustrated in Figure 23.5. This contains all the essential components outlined in the literature. Although implementation, delivery, training, follow-up/follow-along and outcome measurement are important parts of service delivery, they are discussed separately because they are not part of the assessment. It is important to note that although this is a process, it is not necessarily linear. Often information is learned during later stages in the process that require the team to move back a few steps and restart.

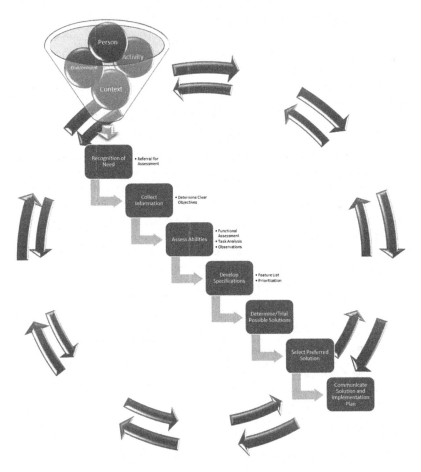

Figure 23.5 General components of an assistive technology assessment regardless of model.

23.6.1 Recognition of need

The assessment process begins with the recognition of a need. Typically, there is an area where the individual unduly struggles and wants to improve an aspect of the process. The individual or someone who works with them (e.g., teacher, vocational rehabilitation counselor, parent, caregiver or doctor) recognizes the need. Common needs include improving the activity to reduce pain, increase efficiency, or reduce fatigue, sometimes with a specific task identified, other times with a combination of different activities that all have a similar struggle. These needs can be phrased into measurable goals for the assessment.

Once the need is identified, someone must determine if an AT assessment is appropriate. This process varies significantly with each service environment and service provider. Sometimes a physician referral is necessary, other times the individual can seek help independently, or an agency such as a school or vocational rehabilitation agency may facilitate the initiation of services. The payer for AT services also varies depending on the service environment, in some situations, the REP is only paid if services are implemented, in other situations the REP is paid for the assessment service, other places are funded through alternative means and provide assessments to the consumer free of charge.

When the services are paid for by a funding source separate from the individual, then there are two customers: the payer and the individual with a disability. In these situations, differing goals from the payer and individual can lead to miscommunication. To help mitigate this, Wisconsin's Technology Act Program (WisTech) developed a list of best practices for AT assessments. A result of these best practices is the components that lead to a good referral with enough clear information that the REP provides services matching what the payer desires. Table 23.1 is a list of information that referring agencies are encouraged to provide at the time of referral (WisTech 2017). This encourages the payer to include

Table 23.1 WisTech Best Practices: Payer's Responsibilities for a Quality Referral

Before the Assessment is Requested – Payer's Responsibilities

The referral source should supply the following information to the assessment provider:
- What are the consumer's goals?
- Why are you referring this person?
- What is the functional outcome desired?
- What is the consumer's disability or disabilities?
- What is the impact of the disability or disabilities on functional skills?
- What are the relevant environmental concerns?
- Have appropriate releases of information been signed and has any relevant documentation been included with the referral?

the individual with preliminary goal development and increases the likelihood that the goals are between both parties.

> Sophie's assessment – recognition of need: Sophie has an interest in working but has never had a job before. She is a 28-year-old with cerebral palsy. She isn't sure what she could do, or how to go about gaining employment. Sophie went to the local job center and learned about the state vocational rehabilitation agency. She completed the enrollment process and was accepted into the program. Sophie met with her rehabilitation counselor, Karen, to start the process and develop an individualized plan for employment (IPE).
>
> Together, Karen and Sophie decided to pursue part-time office-based employment. Sophie's ability to use the computer is slow and tedious because her gross motor control is limited, and it takes a long time to initiate and execute movement. They are concerned that Sophie won't be able to reach the productivity requirements of a position with her current computer access techniques.
>
> Karen contacts you, the RE technologist, and requests that you provide an AT assessment for Sophie to improve her use and endurance with the computer so she can develop skills to become ready for a job.

23.6.2 Collect information

Sufficient background information is required prior to starting the assessment. The background information can include medical records, therapy updates, previous AT assessment reports, individualized education plans (IEP), self-reported information from the individual and their family/support system and neuropsychologist reports. Collecting background from a variety of sources will allow the transdisciplinary team to have a comprehensive picture of the situation. Often there are details mentioned in the background information that may not present themselves during the assessment. For example, if the only background information collected is what is self-reported by the individual and the goal of the assessment is to reduce pain, the REP will likely only address pain. If background information was collected from other people who have worked with her and included a report from the neuropsychologist, it would have been apparent that she also has mental health challenges and struggles with anxiety. From her perspective, her mental health and anxiety are not relevant because they aren't related to the physical pain. However, if it had been disclosed, the REP would have considered different training methods and a different strategy/plan for implementation that would have been tailored to her needs and reduced her anxiety about the change in how she completes the task. The more background information that is available and provided, the more the team will have a comprehensive picture of the situation. In turn, this will help with ensuring all aspects of the human and environment/context are considered throughout the assessment.

Although a substantial amount of the information is collected prior to the assessment, additional information during the assessment that might require follow-up. For example, during the assessment, it is mentioned that the individual has chosen what college they will be attending, and it is located far from their family/support system. Resources available at the chosen college help in final determination of the product and development of the implementation plan (e.g., the college may be a training resource or provide information that impacts the device selection, such as prior experience revealed that the preferred AT software conflicts with their security software).

During information collection, it is important to clarify goals and objectives. Perhaps they were provided at the time of referral and were vague. In this process, all the goals should be phrased in measurable terms. Through gathering and sharing of background information within the transdisciplinary team, the objectives are clarified so that everyone knows the expectations of the assessment and their roles during and after the assessment. Long describes two different approaches to decision making which directly reflect on the goals and assessment approach. The REP can use the impairment-oriented method where the purpose of the assessment is to determine what skills are needed and the impairments to overcome. The result of the assessment is remediation of the impairment or acquisition of a new skill. An outcome-driven assessment is designed to promote the attainment of the desired outcome or to maximize skills, recommending AT and strategies used at any time and not specifically for remediation or skill acquisition (Long et al. 2003).

Sophie's assessment – collect information: prior to meeting with Sophie, we called her and discussed her goals and abilities. Sophie explained that she uses a powered wheelchair for mobility and drives it with a joystick on her left side. She currently uses the computer by typing with one finger on a laptop, but it can take an hour to type one sentence. Sophie has a high school diploma but has not gone to college. She relies on public transportation (a combination of paratransit and accessible buses) for community mobility.

Sophie reports that she doesn't have a job yet and isn't sure what she can do. She wants to work with us to figure out what technology will make her better at working at an office job. She will work to practice her skills so she can demonstrate solutions to barriers her future employer might envision. After developing these skills, she expects to participate in a couple of short-term work experiences to further develop skills while she seeks employment.

After the phone call, Sophie's goals are:

- Increase her typing speed and accuracy by 50%
- Use the computer for up to four hours per day
- Require zero assistance while using the computer

Sophie reports that she hasn't had any difficulty with depression or anxiety. She lives alone with her husband who also has a disability. They live in an accessible apartment. Sophie is also close with her family who lives in the same town. She has two cats. When Sophie is not working, she seeks opportunities to perform advocacy and to work in the community as a volunteer. Sophie identifies as a Christian and her faith is important to her. She is an active participant in her local church.

Sophie's IPE was reviewed. It indicated that her primary disability is cerebral palsy and when described, mentioned that she requires a wheelchair for mobility and her limited motor control is the biggest barrier to independence with work. The plan for her is to have an AT assessment to determine what technology would open employment opportunities for work in an office, complete job shadows to further explore her aptitudes and other areas where she may need employment support and provide training on using Microsoft Office.

Using this information and Sophie's preferences, we planned the assessment to take place in our lab. Sophie took pictures of her home setup to help include the environment where she will first use her equipment while developing her skills. These pictures will provide additional insight of things she may not have thought to share with us or that we didn't think to ask.

23.6.3 Assess abilities

Once the transdisciplinary team and individual clearly define the goals and expectations of the assessment (remember, often assessments can include many phases) and the "problem" is fully understood, then a functional assessment of the individual's abilities is needed. This is comprehensive and considers the individual's motor, sensory and cognitive capabilities. Motor capabilities include motor movement, strength and endurance related to gross and fine motor coordination of the extremities. They also include postural control and other control areas such as the voice, lips or tongue. Sensory is not only seeing and hearing but includes proprioception and tactile sensation. Cognitive capabilities relate to executive function, memory and processing speed, but it also relates to emotional control. This is going to affect the individual's ability to adapt to new techniques, the training method and degree of training required. Often this is difficult to assess in a single meeting, and if Sophie copes well, limitations may not become apparent until after several meetings or a significant stressor is placed on the individual. Medical reports and observations from the trans-disciplinary team's collective observations can help proactively plan for these limitations. The method, formality and systematic process for the functional assessment can and often does vary depending on the composition of the trans-disciplinary team, time permitted for the assessment, environment where the assessment occurs, instruments used and the model followed. The crucial part is that all aspects are considered regardless of the severity of the disability. For example, if you are working with a student with dyslexia, don't assume that they don't have any motor impairments and although it may not be necessary to ask them to conduct a test to examine this area, this should be verified at a minimum through questioning or observation.

Observations of the individual interacting with others, and how they currently complete tasks that are part of the goal can give the transdisciplinary team perspective of the individual's capabilities in a different context than may have arisen from the functional assessment. Additionally, it may bring additional perspective to the goal that was not previously recognized by the team in the interview. For example, when collecting background information, the individual reports that he is a touch typist, and the goal is to improve his efficiency by 30%. During the functional assessment, it is determined that he has the motor capabilities to touch type. Without observation, the REP may launch into trying different size keyboards and encouraging the use of keyboard shortcuts. During observation of him replying to an email, it is revealed that his touch-typing style is atypical, doesn't use the home-row and primarily uses six fingers. If the goal of the assessment is to increase text entry efficiency, this information could lead to the consideration of learning a new typing strategy or it could be decided that employing keyboard shortcuts won't be more efficient because he doesn't type in the traditional fashion and the use of them would slow him down.

An analysis of the steps to accomplish the tasks related to the goal is also important. The key to completing this is to use broad terms that won't constrain development, and brainstorming of possible solutions. As a different example, if the referring source, individual and family determine that the objective is to have a cart which engages the individual and facilitates interpersonal interaction to maintain motivation, the task analysis might be described as:

1. Deliver snacks to students in classroom
   a. Individual moves next to student
   b. Individual retrieves snack from its holding location
   c. Individual places snack on desk

2. Deliver cards to people in nursing home
   a. Individual moves next to patient

604

    b.   Individual retrieves card from its holding location

    c.   Individual places card in hands of patient

This task analysis may indicate that a method of moving materials is necessary to accommodate the individual, but it doesn't constrain the solution to a cart. A cart should be considered because it is something the family has suggested, and it is important to include their ideas and preferences into the process with a value equal to that of any other member on the transdisciplinary team.

Sophie's assessment – assess abilities: at the lab, Sophie demonstrated how she currently uses her laptop computer. She demonstrated her reach and wheelchair driving abilities. Next, Sophie's typing speed and accuracy were measured using her laptop keyboard. We also measured her speed and accuracy with the trackpad mouse that was on her computer.

Sophie has no limits to her range of motion in the lateral plane for her right arm but has essentially no control of her left arm or hand. She can reach above her head but has difficulty feeling what she is doing and relies on her sight. Sophie can reach down, but her trunk control makes it difficult to correct her posture if she does. Therefore, she doesn't reach down. It was noticed that Sophie's hair was clipped back. This could be an indicator of her motor control. However, Sophie reported that she had assistance doing her hair. Primarily, Sophie can control her right index finger. She has difficulty gripping/grasping with her hands and isolating movement of her other fingers. Sophie's resolution of movement is small; she can activate small targets that are close together without error.

Sophie reported that she wears glasses and brought them with her. This corrects her vision, but many keyboards were on display in the lab and one with large print letters in a color contrast was a lot easier to see. While being asked to complete tasks on the computer, it was apparent that she sometimes had difficulty locating the mouse cursor.

Sophie is able to speak verbally, but she has dysarthria. She often coughs while speaking and only has the breath to support a couple of words at a time. Her speech can be understood by another person, but it is questionable whether a computer would understand her speech.

During the assessment, spasms and reflex patterns were not observed. Sophie reported that she does not have difficulty with these interfering with her life. It was noticed that initiation of movement was slow, and all movements were slow and deliberate. Sophie mentioned she sometimes gets sore in her shoulders on active days.

23.6.4 Develop specifications

23.6.4.1 Determination of access method Next, determine an access method. An access method is how the individual is going to interface with the technology. There are two components, one is input and one is feedback. How does the person know that their input was effective? A person who has full use of their hands and arms and is trained in keyboard use may access a computer through a keyboard and ten fingers. His feedback is the movement of the keys and output on the monitor (or through the speaker if it is voice feedback). Someone else may access it with their voice, head, toes, eyes or mouth. The access method should be reliable, low effort and comfortable (Mumford et al. 2014). Someone with a disability who does not have motor impairments still needs to have their access method identified, particularly because their access method may include non-traditional feedback (voice output).

The access method starts from the results of the functional assessment. Motor control is often considered first, and control sites with reliable movement are considered. In addition to control reliability, strength and endurance play a role in selection. Sensory function will influence the feedback and cognition may exclude some options. Mumford describes this selection process as the method that takes the least amount of activation effort and is the best method, but effort includes the physical and cognitive effort as well as the response effectiveness of the technology (Mumford et al. 2014). Potential control sites are identified from the functional assessment and then when there are multiple feasible control sites; trials to determine the individual's preference for control site are conducted. Each access method may generate different specifications, feature list and device trials.

23.6.4.2 Development and prioritization of a feature list After possible access methods are determined, the next step is the development of a feature list (also called a specification list or characteristic list). This helps the REP and transdisciplinary team choose the most appropriate device to fully meet the individual's needs. It also helps prevent the trial and consideration of inappropriate devices. Features are characteristics of the AT system and specifications are features with specified parameters. Examples of features may include lightweight, durable, easy to learn, text to speech, large targets and speech to text. Examples of specifications include the requirement of an activation force of less than 100 mm Hg, targets spaced at least 10 mm apart, accommodation of 20 targets and reach of 40 cm. Notice that none of these features refer to a specific device or model. Instead, they are characteristics of a possible model or system. The most helpful feature list is one that has specifications for the most important characteristics (ideally all the characteristics).

Prioritize the feature list after it is developed. Similar to the engineering design process, sometimes the features may conflict with each other and one of them is compromised. The transdisciplinary team should prioritize the feature list to prepare for compromises during device selection. Trying devices is a great way to experience features and develop the list. It is important to remember when using this technique that you aren't selecting a device yet and are only exploring possible features in the final device/system.

Sophie's assessment – develop specifications: Sophie's access methods are her right index finger and her voice.

First the workstation was considered. To aid in development of specifications, various AT devices were tried to determine the features on each device that would be useful. Forearm supports would help Sophie divert her strength and energy to the activity instead of supporting the arm against gravity. An articulating forearm support that pivots and allows her arm to move freely in her range provided greater speed of movement than a fixed forearm support. It was determined that her workstation needed to accommodate her wheelchair and allow her to get close enough to it. To do this, either Sophie will need to retract her wheelchair joystick back and to the side, or the surface needs to be taller than her joystick. A large screen monitor is necessary to allow Sophie to have multiple program windows open at once and reduce effort to switch between them. It will also be easier for Sophie to see without her glasses.

After identifying the arm supports and approximate workstation height, we considered methods of controlling the mouse. The mouse emulator should be positioned close to where Sophie's wheelchair joystick is. She will be using multiple computers in her future and their capabilities are unknown, therefore the mouse should connect to the computer through a USB plug because that is the most common interface (e.g., not every computer has Bluetooth). A wireless mouse is preferable to reduce the risk of cord entanglement and her cats chewing on them. The mouse emulator should also separate cursor control movement from item selection movements. This will allow Sophie to navigate her cursor to the isolated location and then while activating the "click" she won't accidentally move her cursor.

A keyboard that requires low force for activation is going to be useful because of Sophie's limited finger strength. A typing splint that allows the entire arm to generate the force to activate keys is also appropriate. This typing splint should not obstruct Sophie's view of the keys. The keyboard should have large print/ high contrast key labels to make it easier for Sophie to identify keys. Sophie also would benefit from a smaller keyboard so she can reach all parts of the keyboard with less movement, and conserve effort and time.

Voice is also appropriate for text entry and, when tried, it had many errors, but after correcting errors was still two times faster than using the keyboard. The

---

errors could be too frustrating for some users, but Sophie didn't mind them. Voice recognition software, with an efficient computer and high-quality microphone would be ideal in the system. The software should be forgiving of errors and improve with use. Donning and doffing the microphone will be challenging, so it should be wireless so as not to impact mobility.

23.6.5 Determine/trial possible solutions

The next step in the process is trialing possible solutions. Trial the devices that have the desired set of features (or can be modified to match the features) to assist with selection and confidence in the decision of the most appropriate device. The best approach is to conduct a device trial long enough to use the device in all the individual's environments. Often there are constraints that prevent this (e.g., device availability, support available for the trial period). If a long trial period is not possible, use the device during the assessment or a device that is similar. For example, when determining the access method, it is decided that the best way to access a computer is with the mouth. The feature list was developed, and it includes low effort, single device for mouse and keyboard control, independent setup, oral motor control and sip/puff for clicking the mouse (not dwell). A head-operated mouse might be ruled out because of the setup to apply the reflective dot to her forehead and to don/doff the sip/puff headset switch. There are wireless options, and creativity could overcome these barriers, but for simplicity this would initially be ruled out and other options explored. A viable option that meets the feature list is an oral joystick. There are a few styles on the market including pressure sensitive, displacement sensitive, wireless, ability to pair with multiple devices on the workstation, Morse Code text entry and additional gaming controls. The feature list may help rule out some of the options, then the different oral joystick models that meet her needs should be trialed.

Throughout the trials, revise the feature specification list and add in new features or adjust the parameters of some of the specifications as needed. The ability to revisit those iterations in the process through device experience helps to convert the feature list from abstract ideas to concrete ones that resonate with the individual. Adjust it after some of the device trials if the individual realizes through experience that something that was high priority conceptually wasn't a barrier during the trials. The individual in the example above may find through oral joystick trials that she does not like something in front of her face and adds "device can't be in front of the face during use" and the setup restriction may be adjusted so it can be worn all day, so that donning and doffing assistance is only required once each throughout the day.

Sophie's assessment – determine trial/possible solutions: with the specification list, various devices that meet the criteria were trialed or considered to determine what would be best when looking at all the needs together. Mouse options could be a joystick mouse or a trackball mouse. The keyboard options could be mini or compact. High visibility keyboards are available, but we could also consider placing stickers on the computer. Dragon voice recognition software could be considered and so could Windows built-in software. A variety of typing splints were also considered and trialed. The articulating, mobile forearm rests have different lengths and the options needed to be trialed for comfort.

Through these trials all the possibilities can be narrowed down into a shortlist of what should be recommended, based on what Sophie found to work the best, what was observed to work the best (towards the goals), what is easy for setup, what gives Sophie the most independence and efficiency. When all things are equal for the other criteria (such as efficiency, accuracy and ease) then cost is also considered.

23.6.6 Select preferred solution

After devices are trialed and the feature list is finalized, the team must decide what to recommend and acquire for the individual. Decision making is easier when there is more data, such as the individual having the opportunity to trial the exact devices considered or long-term trials in a variety of environments and contexts. There are multiple ways to make a decision, but it is important to recognize that the decision maker has a finite amount of information that they can process with their working memory. To assist decision making, it is helpful to collect data (subjective and or objective) throughout the trials. It is recommended to start with an empty set and only consider devices that meet the specifications and preferences of the feature list, this will create a smaller set than if all devices are considered and inappropriate ones are excluded and then subjectively picking the device that best meets the specifications. This strategy is often used when there is not enough time to employ a compensatory decision-making strategy, such as a decision matrix (Simpson 2008).

The lack of feedback from the effectiveness of decisions can lead to the REP thinking they are making good decisions when, in actuality, the decisions aren't adequately meeting the needs of the individual. To improve decision making over time the REP should invest their time in learning about decision-making biases and how to overcome them, developing a means to receive immediate feedback on decision outcomes such as a quality assurance plan, employing a formal decision-making process that is used for all decisions and by using tools to support automated decision assistance (e.g., data collection or displaying data in graphs or charts) (Simpson 2008).

Sophie's assessment – select preferred solution: Sophie is using this equipment to develop job skills and plans to work in the community; therefore we decided to use her existing desk and recommend workstation access equipment. Recommended items included:

- One ErgoRest articulating arm support with a long rest for easier movement within workspace
- One compact keyboard with high contrast stickers added to keys
- One utensil cuff style typing splint with cutoff upside-down pencil
- One wireless Kensington Expert Mouse trackball
- Dragon Professional Individual voice recognition software
- A laptop computer with a high-speed processor, 8GB RAM, Bluetooth and three USB ports
- An adjustable height, adjustable angle large screen monitor (22″)
- An OfficeRunner wireless headset to control the computer and landline phone (this leaves phone control to be an option in the future if needed)

23.6.7 Communicate solution and implementation plan

Communication of the results of the assessment is crucial, as it provides information to the funding source to help them make the decision as to whether they will fund the recommended technology, implementation services and training. It also assists with the transition of services if the person implementing the technology is not one of the people who provided the assessment. An assessment report should explain the need for the assessment, how the assessment was conducted, the recommendation of the AT system and the recommended plan to acquire, implement and train the individual of the AT system (Desideri et al. 2014; Long et al. 2003). Make the report clear and relevant to the people who are making the decision to fund the recommended technology (Simpson 2008).

Clear communication helps the reader understand the considerations and decision-making process that lead to the recommendations. It will also alleviate concerns about bias. There are many formats that the report can assume, but there are key components of what it should include. Desideri et al. developed a method of measuring quality of their AT reports, particularly because in their model the REP providing the assessment was not the same person who performed the implementation. Through focus groups and discussions, it was determined that a report should communicate interdisciplinarity, user-centeredness, initial request, functional assessment, environmental factors, solutions explored, goal setting, information, monitoring and readability (Desideri et al. 2014). In a school setting, the

IEP is often the form of the report. Provide details in the IEP pertaining to desired outcomes, expected behaviors and proficiency levels and detailed descriptions of the AT environments and activities. The detailed descriptions should include AT usage, including when and where, how long on each occasion and who is responsible for facilitating the use of the AT (Copley and Ziviani 2005). Incorporate these features into reports for other service environments.

WisTech had concerns about communication of the AT assessment and how to ensure that the individual is receiving a quality, comprehensive assessment. How does the individual and funding source (for both services and AT) receive assurance that the technology considered and recommended is truly an optimal solution, versus something that a vendor recommended because they receive a large profit margin, or a practitioner recommended because they didn't want to learn a new technology? To address this, they developed a list of best practices for AT assessments. These provide guidelines for a service provider when providing AT recommendations to consider the entire range of options and the exhibition of transparency. Overall, these best practices reflect the trends in the literature of what makes a high-quality assessment. Although they don't reflect a specific model, they incorporate the strengths of all models (Copley and Ziviani 2005; Desideri et al. 2014). They are presented as a checklist document that the REP can refer to when writing their report. Table 23.2 is a list of the information that REPs are encouraged to include when they write their report to communicate their recommendations (WisTech 2017).

> Sophie's assessment – communicate solution and implementation plan: a report of the recommended equipment that explains the reasons each device is needed and how we came to that conclusion was sent to Sophie's vocational rehabilitation counselor, Karen. The report also included a plan for acquiring the equipment, which in our service model means that we purchase the equipment for Sophie and then deliver it, set it up for Sophie and train her on how to use it along with a quote for this process.
>
> Multiple training sessions were recommended for Sophie to advance her skills with voice recognition software. Three additional training sessions in the use of Dragon were included in the report. Submission of this report ends the assessment phase.

23.7 Continuing service delivery process – implementation and training

In most cases the work of the REP is not done when the REP submits her report to the referring agency. Meetings and dialog with the referring agency, individual

Table 23.2 WisTech Best Practices: Components of a Comprehensive Assessment

Evaluating the AT Assessment – Components of a Comprehensive Assessment

An AT assessment should inform the payer about how the consumer can benefit from assistive technology, including:

- A description of the consumer's disability as it relates to the assessment and relevant background information
- The specific type(s) of assistive technology solutions that were assessed and the pros/cons of each
- Identification of any variables that should be considered if the assessment did not occur in the setting where the technology will be used
- The specific type(s) of assistive technology being recommended
- How and why the equipment will specifically meet the consumer's needs
- How the decision was reached (e.g., physical assessment with a variety of options, funding options available, etc.)
- Where or from which vendor the appropriate equipment can be purchased
- Potential funding alternatives for the equipment
- The availability of a maintenance agreement, warranty or other safeguard, and whether this is included in the purchase price or available at an additional cost
- The anticipated cost of the equipment, training and maintenance
- Description of the repair procedures (e.g., shipped, in-home, remote service, etc.)
- The availability of loaner equipment prior to purchase or during repair services
- Identification of training needs for the recommended device(s), who is able to provide that training (i.e., the vendor, manufacturer, or an outside provider) and training related expenses

and team members often occur, reviewing recommendations, confirming specifications and developing a plan for implementation. In some settings, the REP may implement the AT and in others, another party will complete the technology purchases, installation and training. The possibility of another party implementing the technology is another important reason for clear, concise communication in documenting the AT needs for the individual.

When the REP is purchasing and implementing the technology, it is helpful to inspect, configure and test the equipment prior to the installation at the individual's home or workplace. This greatly increases success on the day of implementation and reduces lost time and frustration of resolving errors from missing parts, software crashes and other mishaps that may occur during valuable time with the individual. Additionally, it reduces apprehension of the individual as some people may see the expert struggling and become wary of the technology. If custom or fabricated AT devices are part of the solution, the engineering design process shown earlier in Figure 23.2 is needed. Attention to detail in custom-designed products is important, because the REP will commonly become the "warranty service" person, as they are the designers and fabricators of the device.

Training is a vital aspect of any successful AT implementation. Effective training can maximize the AT user's potential to reach the original goal of the assessment, increase the individual's capacity to use all the features relevant in a particular AT device and minimize the abandonment of the device. Depending on the complexity of the technology and the individual's learning style, consider a variety of training modalities and options, including one versus several sessions, remote versus in-person and the amount of time per session. Often it is beneficial for family and support members or caregivers to participate in the training. Develop specific training goals and include them in the report. They should include training on the use of the technology, troubleshooting strategies, how to service the technology and warranty information.

Regardless of the AT setup with the individual, the AT service delivery process is not completed without follow-up and follow-along communications or visits. This will ensure the technology meets the needs of the individual as intended and provides the opportunity to answer any questions on use of the technology that arise after spending time and practicing with the technology.

Sophie's assessment – implementation, training and future iterations: it was our hope that every piece of equipment recommended would be purchased by the state vocational rehabilitation agency. In Sophie's case, it was decided that the articulating arm rests (ErgoRest) and back-up keyboard were not necessary. After further conversations with Karen about why the laptop's keyboard won't work for Sophie because of positioning, that was added to the purchase list. The articulating arm rests weren't approved to be provided but could be considered after Sophie acquired a permanent position.

Implementation took one visit and there were three additional training visits for Dragon. At the conclusion of this, Sophie had met all of our training objectives and felt comfortable enough with her AT to start pursuing training in how to use Microsoft Office.

Several months later, Karen contacted us regarding Sophie. She had started a short-term job shadow and required assistance to use the office phone. This was important because independent phone use needed to be demonstrated prior to employment placement. This process was completed again to determine how to best allow Sophie to use the phone.

A few months later, Sophie started her new job and was having difficulty getting her phone system to work at the new office. We went in and determined what was necessary to connect the OfficeRunner that Sophie uses for Dragon onto the work phone. We also notified Sophie about a new version of Dragon and our experiences with it for Sophie to consider upgrading.

613

Once Sophie settled into her job, she asked for assistance with increasing her independence with the copy machine and in the mail room. After discussion and demonstration, we determined Sophie didn't need new AT, but instead she needed to adjust her strategies. We revised the strategies, and a few weeks later Sophie told us she was doing great and had settled well into her work.

23.8 Quality assurance and outcome measurement in the assessment process

Be sure to develop a quality assurance system for any AT assessment process. Depending on the service delivery setting, this may involve a paper, phone or electronic survey or other technique requesting feedback from the individual or referring agency. Another option is having another member of the REP's organization or outside agency provide a quality assurance call. This final check of the assessment gives another chance for the individual to let the REP know how the assessment process worked (or didn't work) for them. Using this feedback can be incorporated to continually improve the assessment process.

A quality assurance system may verify that the AT user is satisfied with the assessment process, but the REP may not truly know if the AT was effective in meeting the recognized need. Outcome measurements using both quantitative and qualitative measures can verify the extent to which the AT is helping the individual reach their goals. Outcome measurements are an important tool to help direct the field of AT from subjective practitioner experience influencing recommendations to an evidence-based decision-making process.

23.9 Future vision

Although many models exist, the perfect model that fits every situation does not exist. Each model has room for improvement in some form or another. Adding to the complication, technology is constantly changing and improving. A model is supposed to promote the advancement of the field (Lenker and Paquet 2003).

Current trends in technology reflect an increase in crowdsourcing data pools and easy methods of activity tracking. Society is shifting towards a world of information sharing instead of proprietary information. Research is often "open-source" to facilitate faster progress (Berg 2017). This presents opportunities for tracking the efficacy of AT interventions. The ideal AT assessment model is one that assists REPs in conducting assessments to make AT recommendations that enable the individual to reach their goals. The ideal model provides a way for the REP to predict the impact the AT system will make on the consumer. It provides a way for an REP working in research to develop a study that furthers the advancement of the field and can translate the knowledge to practice for the individual's benefit. It facilitates the comprehensive measurement of outcomes to drive the development of improved practice and evidence-based policy. Ultimately, this advances the field and has a direct impact on the individuals receiving the AT.

As science shifts from proprietary to open-source, there is an opportunity for greater collaboration across the field to develop an assessment model that suits our ideal. The model needs to be broadened to incorporate all the REPs' different needs, for all possible environments, while remaining customizable to each situation, and facilitate the tracking of outcomes. With this universal model, we could develop a dataset that exponentially increases the field's evidence-based practices. It would also mobilize the evidence-based practices more rapidly into the field.

Less invasive monitoring techniques will increase researchers' capabilities to develop more readily measurable feedback for productivity and energy expenditure of AT users. This will still likely remain the domain of RE researchers, not practitioners, due to the significant funding restraints that will remain in the delivery of AT services.

23.10 Discussion questions

1. How do the scientific method and the engineering design process relate to the AT assessment process?
2. What are three important AT models described in the chapter?
3. What are three common threads that are prevalent in the AT models described in the literature?
4. If you are the lead REP for an AT assessment, when you create your transdisciplinary team, how do you determine who should be included in the team?
5. What is the difference between creating a feature list, conducting device trials and selecting a device? Why are they considered distinct steps? How are they inter-related?
6. If you have the flexibility in your environment to develop your own report format, how would you structure your report to convey sufficient information while engaging the audience? How might you structure your report differently for the different environments and funding sources discussed in previous chapters?
7. What are two different situations where you would not follow a linear assessment process?
8. If you cannot work with other professionals during your assessment, what are four different ways that you could utilize to incorporate their input and opinion into your assessment?
9. Discuss how and why training should be conducted with AT devices. How would you decide on the best training method to provide an AT user?

Bibliography

Berg, Devin R. 2017. "Open Research, Open Engineering, and the Role of the University in Society."

Bernd, T., D. Van Der Pijl, and L. P. De Witte. 2009. "Existing Models and Instruments for the Selection of Assistive Technology in Rehabilitation Practice." *Scandinavian Journal of Occupational Therapy* 16 (3): 146–158.

Bromley, B. E. 2001. "Assistive Technology Assessment: A Comparative Analysis of Five Models." CSUN Conference, San Diego.

Cook, Albert M. and Susan M. Hussey. 1995. *Assistive Technologies: Principles and Practice.* Mosby Year Book.

Cook, Albert M. and Janice Miller Polgar. 2014. *Assistive Technologies-E-Book: Principles and Practice.* Elsevier Health Sciences.

Copley, Jodie and Jenny Ziviani. 2005. "Assistive Technology Assessment and Planning for Children with Multiple Disabilities in Educational Settings." *British Journal of Occupational Therapy* 68 (12): 559–566.

Desideri, Lorenzo, Francesca Marcella Ioele, Uta Roentgen, Gert-Jan Gelderblom, and Luc de Witte. 2014. "Development of a Team-Based Method for Assuring the Quality of Assistive Technology Documentation." *Assistive Technology* 26 (4): 175–183.

Edyburn, Dave L. 2001. "Models, Theories, and Frameworks: Contributions to Understanding Special Education Technology." *Special Education Technology Practice* 4 (2): 16–24.

Giesbrecht, Ed. 2013. "Application of the Human Activity Assistive Technology Model for Occupational Therapy Research." *Australian Occupational Therapy Journal* 60 (4): 230–240.

Johnston, Patricia, Leanne M. Currie, Donna Drynan, Tim Stainton, and Lyn Jongbloed. 2014. "Getting it "Right": How Collaborative Relationships between People with Disabilities and Professionals can Lead to the Acquisition of Needed Assistive Technology." *Disability and Rehabilitation: Assistive Technology* 9 (5): 421–431.

Lenker, James A. and Victor L. Paquet. 2003. "A Review of Conceptual Models for Assistive Technology Outcomes Research and Practice." *Assistive Technology* 15 (1): 1–15.

Long, Toby, Larke Huang, Michelle Woodbridge, Maria Woolverton, and Jean Minkel. 2003. "Integrating Assistive Technology into an Outcome-Driven Model of Service Delivery." *Infants & Young Children* 16 (4): 272–283.

Mirza, Mansha and Joy Hammel. 2009. "Consumer-Directed Goal Planning in the Delivery of Assistive Technology Services for People Who are Ageing with Intellectual Disabilities." *Journal of Applied Research in Intellectual Disabilities* 22 (5): 445–457.

MPT. 2017. "Matching Person and Technology." http://matchingpersonandtechnology.com.

Mumford, Leslie, Rachel Lam, Virginia Wright, and Tom Chau. 2014. "An Access Technology Delivery Protocol for Children with Severe and Multiple Disabilities: A Case Demonstration." *Developmental Neurorehabilitation* 17 (4): 232–242.

Parette, Howard P., Mary Blake Huer, and Marcia Scherer. 2004. "Effects of Acculturation on Assistive Technology Service Delivery." *Journal of Special Education Technology* 19 (2): 31–41.

Science Buddies.org. 2017. "Comparing the Engineering Design Process and the Scientific Method." http://www.sciencebuddies.org/engineering-design-process/engineering-design-compare-scientific-method.shtml.

Simpson, Richard. 2008. "Making Better Decisions [Modeling the Assistive Technology Assessment]." *IEEE Engineering in Medicine and Biology Magazine* 27 (2): 23–28.

Smith, R. O., J. Seitz, C. Jansen, and K. L. Rust. 2017. "ATOMS Project Technical Report: Models and Taxonomies Relating to Assistive Technology."

WHO. 2001. *World Health Organization: International Classification of Functioning, Disability and Health: ICF.* World Health Organization.

Wissick, Cheryl A. and J. Emmett Gardner. 2008. "Conducting Assessments in Technology Needs: From Assessment to Implementation." *Assessment for Effective Intervention* 33 (2): 78–93.

WisTech. 2017. "Wisconsin's Assistive Technology Program." https://www.dhs.wisconsin.gov/disabilities/wistech/index.htm.

Chapter 24 Product usability testing and outcomes
What works? for whom? and why?

Jon A. Sanford

Contents

DOI: 10.1201/b21964-28

24.1 Chapter overview

Once upon a time there were three bears who lived in a house in the forest. One morning, they went out for a walk having forgotten that they had an appointment with a researcher named Goldilocks. Shortly thereafter, Goldilocks knocked on their door. When there was no answer, she went in. In front of her was a table with three bowls of porridge. She randomly selected a bowl and tasted the porridge. On her data sheet she noted that "the porridge is too hot!" Then she randomly selected a second bowl and tasted the porridge, which she recorded as "too cold." So, she tasted the last bowl of porridge. She noted that "This porridge is just right," and she happily ate it all up.

Next, Goldilocks walked into the living room where she saw three chairs. Again, using random assignment of test order to avoid bias, she sat in one of the chairs. "This chair is too big!" she noted. So, she sat in the second chair. "This chair is too wide!" she marked in the proper column. Then she tried the last and smallest chair. "This chair is just right." But just as she started to record the data, the chair broke into pieces! Aching from this unanticipated adverse event, Goldilocks went upstairs to test the beds. She lay down in the first bed, but it was too hard. Then she lay in the second bed, but it was too soft. Then she lay down in the third bed and it was just right. In fact, it was so good that Goldilocks fell asleep.

You all know the rest of the story. The three bears came home. Irate that they had not consented (assented in Baby Bear's case), they chased Goldilocks off and immediately filed a protocol deviation with the Institutional Research Board (IRB).

Goldilocks and the Three Bears is a useful parable for product usability testing for several reasons. First, it demonstrates the three key research questions that drive all product usability testing – **what works**? **for whom**? and **why**? **What works** determines the *outcome measures* of interest (usually focused on performance and preference). **For whom** addresses the intended *target population and generalizability* to a broader audience. **Why** identifies the independent variables, including *product-specific attributes and contextual factors*, that influence what about the product works and **for whom** as well as the potential for replicating those outcomes in other products.

Second, it demonstrates how the relative importance of each of the three questions is driven by the purpose of the testing. Here Goldilocks's purpose was instant gratification – to satiate her hunger, to relax and to rest, in that order. To meet these goals, Goldilocks's testing focused, first and foremost, on the first two questions. She tested the porridge, chairs and beds with the intent of finding out **what worked** based on product performance and personal preference for what she considered "just right" for her (the third bowl of porridge, the smallest chair at least until it broke and the third bed). To a lesser extent, the testing addressed the question of **why** the products worked for her. The porridge was neither too hot nor too cold, the chair was neither too big nor too small and the bed was neither too hard nor too soft. Although the reasons **why** some products were just right, and others were not, did not address Goldilocks's immediate needs they did provide an evidence base that would enable her to replicate the experience in other bears' homes. In addition, these data provide some insights into what was probably just right for each of the three bears as well as what might be appropriate for human beings in general, and possibly other bears. Of course, this was an N of 1 study, so without any additional information about Goldilocks or testing of other people with a range of abilities, we would not expect Goldilocks to generalize her data to either the population as a whole or a specific cohort. Similarly, without additional anthropometric data on the bears, she cannot generalize to the bear population as a whole either.

Despite the acknowledged limitations of Goldilocks's methodology, it provides a good example of how the three research questions are integral to product usability testing. In addition, it illustrates how the relative importance of each question and the associated outcomes are based on the purpose of the testing. **This chapter will focus on how the intended goals and purpose of usability testing drives the specific emphasis of the three research questions and how those questions subsequently frame the test methods,** including target populations and sample, relevant outcome measures and salient design factors associated with those outcomes that are appropriate for different product usability testing scenarios.

It is important to note that the term usability, as used in the chapter, has a very narrow interpretation based on the fit between a product's functioning (as opposed to functionality) and users' functional abilities and needs (as opposed to wants and desires). As a result, **as used here, usability, is limited to performance and preference outcomes and excludes those related to utility** (i.e., useful functionality or desired features), is a related though mutually exclusive construct that is often included in the literature as a component of usability. The inclusion of utility and usefulness-related outcomes as a component of usability is likely derived from the International Organization for Standardization (ISO) definition of usability (ISO 9241-210 (2010), definition 2.13), which describes usability broadly as comprising effectiveness and efficiency, but also implicitly as including utility (Bevan 2001). Herein lies the quandary. Cannot a product that is totally useless or minimally useful in meeting a particular individual's specified goals be otherwise usable? While futility is not a preferred outcome, utility is a complementary and desirable outcome of product testing, although not a necessary condition for usability nor an outcome of usability testing that will be included in this chapter.

24.2 Background and problem

Today, the fit between product design and users' needs and abilities is well recognized as a key consideration in the development of all types of industrial, information technology and consumer products. For assistive technology (AT), however, that fit is not just important, it is (assuming the product has utility), the most critical design consideration. As described in Chapter 2, AT devices are designed to enable users to achieve the highest level of functioning (Cook and Hussey 2002). As a result, usability is the sole purpose of the product – either for enabling usability of existing products or replacing those products. For people with functional limitations, therefore, ATs are not just a means to overcome difficulties with product usability that can limit task performance, they are quite often the difference between being able to perform a task or not.

To ensure usability, the design processes for all types of products incorporate usability testing from the very beginning. Although different disciplines have proposed their own variations of the design process model, all models include an iterative design–test–redesign loop that evaluates product use against user needs and abilities to identify and resolve usability problems (Hersh 2010). This process of design, end user testing and redesign is repeated as often as required to minimize problems and maximize the usability of a product.

24.2.1 Literature on usability testing

Among the hundreds of recent articles on usability and usability testing, most focus on either describing the methods or the measures that are believed to reflect product usability. These include descriptions of the wide variety of usability evaluation methods that have been developed, how usability is measured objectively (i.e., user performance such as task completion time and error rate) and subjectively (i.e., user preferences) and whether the methods and measures meet ISO standards on measuring usability. In contrast, less attention has been given to understanding the purposes and underlying questions that should drive the selection of appropriate test methods and measures. As a result, it not surprising that many of the documented studies had to wrestle with reconciling contradictory outcome data, particularly in relation to objective performance and subjective preference outcomes. The challenge is to identify and employ situationally appropriate test methods and measures that enable an empirical comparison of subjective and objective usability measures (Hornbaek 2006) for a product as a whole, its component features and/or its design characteristics, within or outside the context of use, as defined by the purpose of the testing. This necessitates an understanding of **what works, for whom** and **why**.

By its very nature, rehabilitation engineering is engaged in developing AT products that are usable by people with various functional limitations. As such, usability testing has always been an integral part of the development process. Interestingly, despite its long history of usability testing, the majority of the recent rehabilitation engineering literature focuses on practical application of usability testing, while there is little attention given to the debate about conceptual models and frameworks, outcome measures and design factors that should be considered in the testing process. Perhaps because the field is sufficiently applied and usability testing is, necessarily, an integral part of the AT development process, that conceptual models and frameworks to drive its testing are unnecessary; or perhaps because the sole purpose of AT is usability, that testing processes (e.g., target populations, outcome and independent variables and procedures) are deemed self-evident. Alternatively, the lack of recent literature may reflect a field that is sufficiently mature to have resolved these issues.

623

Like rehabilitation engineering, usability and human-centered design have long been recognized as an important component of industrial design, although its history of product usability testing as an important factor in making successful products (Anna 2000; Rubin 1994; Rudy 1997) is somewhat more recent. As a result, usability testing has become more widely adopted as an essential part of the mainstream product development process. Despite its recognition as an integral part of the iterative design process, other than consumer electronics products (see below), little has been published in the design literature related to usability testing processes.

In contrast, the vast majority of literature on usability testing comes from the literature on human–computer interaction (HCI), which is coincidentally the youngest of the design professions. The reasons for the emergence of usability testing in HCI can be traced to three factors. First, as a young but maturing profession, HCI needed a foundational basis with which to gain ideological and academic legitimacy. Second, while software (as well as electronic) interfaces can add many new product functions, it can also make them increasingly complex, less intuitive and much more difficult to use compared to inanimate objects (a VCR vs a hammer), thus necessitating testing to ensure usability. Third, there are international standards for usability (ISO/TS 20282-1:2006 2006) and testing (ISO/TS 20282-2:2013 2013) that developers of mechanical and/or electrical consumer products with hardware and software interfaces (i.e., HCI and consumer electronics) are required to meet.

24.2.2 Usability standards

ISO/TS 20282 Part 1, "Design requirements for context of use and user characteristics" (ISO/TS 20282-1:2006 2006), standardizes the design process for developing consumer technology and leads into the test methods that comprise Part 2 of the standard. Part 2, "Summative test method" (ISO/TS 20282-2:2013 2013), specifies a user-based test method for the measurement of the usability and/or accessibility of consumer products to achieve a specified goal in a specified context of use.

Whereas Part 2 attempts to standardize usability testing, it is limited in scope and application. First, as the title of Part 2 indicates, it is a summative test method. More will be said about this in the next section of the chapter, but simply, summative testing involves testing to identify usability deficiencies in a complete product. As such, it is not useful in informing iterative design and is only intended to be used when there is a limited number of goals to be tested and it is possible to identify typical contexts of use and criteria for successful goal achievement (ISO/TS 20282-2:2013 2013). Further, the method cannot be reliably implemented with product inputs and outputs, or the contexts of use are highly variable and/or complex with variability or complexity (ISO/TS 20282-2:2013 2013).

Second, it treats accessibility as a special case of usability even though the test methods can be used interchangeably to assess either construct. This approach clearly reinforces accessibility as something different than usability, rather than advocating a more universal design approach where accessibility is embedded in product usability. It also begs the question of why it needs to be a special case when the only differences are based on who participates in testing. Further, the population is defined "people representing the extremes of the range of characteristics and capabilities within the general user population to achieve a specified goal in a specified context of use." Unfortunately, accessibility is not a one-size-fits-all proposition. People with different abilities not only have different accessibility needs but will also be differentially susceptible to usability demands in different contexts of use. Without clearly defined user characteristics and abilities, testing the extremes of ability only begs the questions of accessibility **for whom** and under what conditions.

Third, as described above, the standard only covers mechanical and/or electrical consumer products with hardware and software interfaces. It is not applicable to "purely physical products without an interactive user interface," such as a simple hammer. The argument for discipline-specific approaches to usability testing is not uncommon. In fact, until the most recent, 2013 revision of Part 2, software and hardware interfaces were considered as different products with their own standards (Parts 2 and 3), even though the language in the two was identical. Similarly, others (see Han and others 2000; Han et al. 1998; Han and others 1998) have argued that software usability testing is not applicable to consumer electronic products because user interfaces of consumer electronic products had both software-driven interactive features, as well as traditional hardware-oriented displays and controls to which dedicated functions were assigned.

24.2.3 Products, interfaces and usability

In contrast to the ISO, this chapter takes the approach that product usability criteria can be applied across all interface types, and that interfaces are the means by which end users interact with any product (Hersh 2010), not just those designated by the ISO. Even the current ISO definition of user interfaces identifies them as "elements of a product used to control it and receive information about its status" ((ISO/TS 20282-1:2006), definition 3.21). Clearly, all products with which end users interact have interfaces. They can be operable by mechanical hardware or digital software, or they can be inoperable inanimate physical objects. For complex interactive devices, such as those regulated by the ISO, interfaces will generally have both input and output components, whereas the interface on simple products like the lowly hammer, may be just a handle (Hersh 2010). Further, human–interface interactions can occur through any of the five senses or any body part. Thus, while test methods may vary slightly and some outcome measures may differ according to product type and interface design, **the basic questions that guide the process of usability testing – what works, for whom and why – is applicable across all products and interfaces, regardless of product type**.

24.3 Purpose of usability testing

24.3.1 Providing information to make informed decisions

Usability testing has only one goal – **to provide information at different points in the product production-to-consumption process** (i.e., design, production, service provision and consumption/use) **that will enable stakeholders** (i.e., designers, product manufacturers, service providers and consumers/users) **to make informed decisions about a product's design, production, user fit, distribution, acquisition and/or use**.

24.3.1.1 Informing design Designers are not generally representative of the range of users who will use the products they design and, even when they understand the needs of some users, users often use products or expect them to function in the ways that designers do not anticipate. Further, designers are often too close to a design and lose sight of its potential weaknesses. As a result, usability testing is an important component in informing design decisions at various stages of the design process to ensure that the right decisions and compromises are made at the right times.

24.3.1.2 Informing production Usability is a market separator. As a result, testing is used to enhance sales and get user buy-in for changes and updates. In addition, data that can be used to remedy usability problems prior to release can increase profitability by minimizing risk as well as service and support calls. Finally, testing provides a historical record of usability benchmarks for updates and future products.

24.3.1.3 Informing service provision Service providers, including rehabilitation specialists, clinicians, usability specialists, sales representatives, product support staff, third party payers and consumer organizations, among others, are responsible with recommending or making funding decisions about appropriate products (rehabilitation or otherwise) to their customers, clients or patients. Usability testing can provide important information about specific features of a product that would not otherwise be apparent that would enable these individuals to best match a specific product to an individual's needs, abilities and preferences.

24.3.1.4 Informing consumption/use Consumers, such as corporate buyers who purchase products for others, and actual users are most likely to know their own needs and abilities. As a result, usability information that will enable users to make their own decisions or to be able to advocate for themselves with service providers, employers or other decision makers are more likely to receive products that are most effective, efficient and satisfying.

24.3.2 Generating information to make informed decisions

Two different types of evaluations, formative and summative, are used to produce critical information to stakeholders. Each type has its own purpose and is effective at informing different stakeholder groups.

24.3.2.1 Formative evaluation Formative evaluation is a process that provides feedback to improve product usability during the design process. In practice, formative testing is a find-and-fix approach (Redish and others 2002) focused on problem diagnosis in order to inform designers how to correct those problems as part of the next iterative design. As such, results should be seamlessly integrated into the iterative design in order to be directly applied by designers. To do so, formative testing is focused on establishing usability of those elements of the interface about which design decisions have been or should be made. Specifically, this involves **evaluating the usability of specific design characteristics (e.g., size, shape, contrast) of both the product as a whole as well as each interface feature (e.g., handle, button, sequence) to identify what works, for whom and why.**

24.3.2.2 Summative evaluation **Summative evaluation is intended to establish the usability of a complete product rather than its specific characteristics.** It can be used to inform each of the four types of decisions described above, although it is most useful in informing post-design decision making. Summative evaluation is specifically defined by the ISO as presenting conclusions about the merit or worth of the object of evaluation ((ISO/TS 18152:2010), definition 4.1). Specifically, it is used to validate a product against usability requirements, to provide a comparison of usability among several products, establish a usability benchmark or to provide a basis for comparison of different products. Summative testing is most useful in describing **what works** and to a lesser extent **for whom**. It is most helpful in informing manufacturers about the merits (or deficiencies) of their products, and secondarily to inform service providers and consumers/users about overall product effectiveness, efficiency and satisfaction. However, when post-test interviews are conducted with participants to obtain a better understanding of specific usability problems, such information can be useful in providing insights about **why** that are useful to designers in refining the design prior to distribution.

24.3.2.3 Formative vs summative evaluation   Formative testing can be a quick-and-dirty process to quickly identify **what works at the level of the product and interface features, for whom and why**. As a result, it identifies the broadest range of potential usability problems with sufficient depth of information to change the design prior to retesting. In contrast, summative usability testing tells us **what works and for whom at the product level**. As a result, it typically includes less breadth and more depth than formative testing. ISO suggests that summative testing should focus on the most frequent and/or important user goals that the product is intended to support. This means that participants will be asked to complete a more limited number of distinct tasks than formative testing, but more information will be collected about those tasks.

24.4 What works, for whom and why

24.4.1 Models for understanding what works, for whom and why

Usability is not an inherent quality of a product in and of itself. Rather, it is the result of the interaction of the product and the user within the context of use (i.e., task and environment). Therefore, usability is not only based on the characteristics, functions and features of the product, but also on the user's activity needs and abilities within the context of use (Arthanat and others 2007).

In defining the concept of usability in the field of computing, Shackel (1984) presented a model of usability based on the interaction of the user, task, tool and environment. This understanding of person–environment fit is, terminology notwithstanding, consistent across all disciplines and ecological models (Sanford 2012; Stark and Sanford 2005; Stark, Sanford and Keglovits 2014). Although ecological models differ slightly on the articulation of the relationship among person (user), environment (including physical spaces, products and technologies, as well as social influences) and task they are always dynamic, complex and interdependent (Rigby and Letts 2003).

Among the various models, there are five rehabilitation-focused models of person–environment (P–E) interaction that are fundamental to an understanding of **what works, for whom and why**. The environmental press model (Lawton and Nahemow 1973), which provides the foundation for most other models, is a gerontological psychology concept that explains how adaptive behavior is an expression of the fit or **misfit** (i.e., usability) between an individual and his/her environment. All occupational therapy (OT) models are a variation on the environmental press theme, beginning with the model of human occupation (Kielhofner and Burke 1980; Kielhofner 1995). However, among those models, the **person–environment-occupation** (PEO) model (Law et al. 1996) is perhaps the most relevant as it specifically articulates task performance (i.e., usability) as an outcome of the interaction among P–E and occupation (e.g., activity and task). Similarly, the rehabilitation engineering model of human activity assistive technology (HAAT) (Cook and Hussey 2002) provide a conceptual understanding of how AT works through the interaction among person, activity and AT. The enabling–disabling process model (Brandt and Pope 1997) is a medical rehabilitation model developed by the Institute of Medicine that clearly identifies the environment as a pathway for both disability and rehabilitation intervention. Finally, the most recent model, the international classification of functioning, disability and health (ICF) (WHO 2001), is a health-based paradigm that not only defines disability as the interaction of body function and structure with contextual (that is, environmental and personal) factors, but extends that interaction to include health, as well as activity and participation outcomes.

Regardless of which ecological model of P–E fit one subscribes to, it is clear that **the interacting components of user, product/device/technology, environment and activity/task/occupation form the conceptual framework for product usability testing**. As such, product usability testing is a process by which the fit or misfit between user and product within any context of task performance can be both maximized or minimized, respectively, through an understanding of **what works, for whom and why**.

24.4.2 Methods for understanding what works, for whom and why

Usability testing can be accomplished through both expert and user evaluations of proposed or existing products. Most methods can be used for both summative and formative evaluations, although each is typically better suited to one evaluation type or the other. Formative methods are typically implemented sequentially, with expert input being incorporated early in the design process to refine a prototype prior to obtaining user feedback and user input at the middle or later stages. All methods can explicitly answer the questions of **what works** and **for whom**, although the latter is dependent on user samples and generalizability. In contrast, to inform design decisions, the primary goal of formative expert and user testing methods is an in-depth and objective understanding of **why** specific product features work. However, it is also possible to use post-test probing interview techniques in summative evaluation user testing methods to gain a general, subjective understanding of **why**.

24.4.2.1 Usability expert reviews   Expert reviews are formative evaluations that occur early in the design process (i.e., at the conceptual stage) to provide feedback that will either guide or refine initial design concepts. Expert reviews are useful in providing preliminary feedback about **expectations for what design features and characteristics will/won't work, for whom it will/won't work and why it will/won't work**.

24.4.2.1.1 Cognitive walkthroughs The cognitive walkthrough technique is conducted at the conceptual or storyboard phase to determine how well the product works at the cognitive level. To accomplish this requires a detailed description of the user interface, a set of tasks, the demographics of the end user population, the context in which the use would occur, and a successful sequence of actions that should be performed. For each task, the participating expert walks through the set of actions to suggest whether the user will be able to select the one that is most appropriate and will see progress towards the solution.

24.4.2.1.2 Heuristic evaluation Heuristic evaluation uses a small set of evaluators to assess a prototype product for compliance with usability design principles and any applicable usability standards specific to the target audience. Experts work independently to evaluate the usability of the prototype design. Five evaluators are typically recommended, although no fewer than three evaluators should be used for any heuristic review (Scholtz 2004). While heuristic evaluation is a quick-and-dirty technique that provides a proxy for user testing, it can only anticipate potential usability problems. As a result, the accuracy with which this method predicts problems that real users would encounter is of less importance than identifying usability problems that are most obvious in order to eliminate or change the design features prior to user testing.

24.4.2.2 Focus group reviews (subject matter experts or users) Group discussions are used to provide formative evaluation of one or more prototype designs at the middle stages of the design process. It is typically effective in comparing several initial design concepts as well as evaluating the usability of the final concept. While focus groups are typically most often used as a user-based methodology, they can also provide a platform to involve subject matter experts (SMEs) who are professionals in fields related to needs and abilities of the target audience. Like other expert reviews, focus groups with SMEs (e.g., rehabilitation engineers or therapists), are most useful for providing what is **expected** to work for that target group and why. In contrast, focus groups with users, who are experts about themselves, can address what will **actually** work and why.

Focus groups are carefully planned discussions, designed to obtain perceptions of a group of individuals on a defined area of interest (Langford and McDonagh 2003). Focus groups are a qualitative research tool that is useful in identifying potential interface issues, understanding end user needs and abilities as well as the target market (which may not be the end users), informing design decision making and generating new concepts. They work best when group participants can react to an actual product that they can hold, manipulate and use. It is useful for gaining an understanding and insights about existing products and proposed products that are at the prototype stage. The more realistic the prototype, the more usability feedback will be produced. As such, paper or physical mockups would be the minimal levels of a new product that would be useful in a focus group discussion. For example, watching a demonstration video of a product is fundamentally different than actually using a product (Nielsen 1997). As a result, it may be effective in producing data on the potential usefulness of the product (i.e., utility), but it cannot produce actual usability information. In contrast, a paper mockup will mostly produce feedback about cognitive usability. Similarly, a physical mockup will produce cognitive data and, depending on how realistic the prototype is, physical and sensory usability data. In contrast, a working prototype will provide feedback about product usability across the broadest range of needs and abilities.

While the literature varies in terms of the recommended number of focus group participants it is consistently 5–10 individuals (e.g., Nielsen (1997) recommends 6–9, whereas Langford and McDonagh (2003) recommend 8–10). Nonetheless, a key advantage of focus groups is that group leaders, such as designers, manufacturers, researchers or human factors consultants, are able to directly observe and interact with participants. As a result, they can observe spontaneous individual verbal and non-verbal (e.g., facial expressions) reactions and feedback as well as group dynamics. In addition, they can respond with probing questions to understand more about **why** something does or does not work.

While focus groups do provide a powerful tool for informing design decisions, particularly at the prototype stages, Nielsen (1997) maintains that no amount of subjective preference will make a product viable without actual use data. As a result, focus groups are a poor method for evaluating tangible interface usability and should not be used as the only source of usability data. To assess whether users can use a product, the only proper methodology is to have them use the actual product, or at a minimum, a highly functional prototype.

24.4.2.3 User testing Testing with actual product users is the most effective method of conducting both formative and summative evaluations. The former is most often implemented in a controlled laboratory setting to inform the design process. Although laboratory testing is also used as a summative evaluation of the entire product, that process is best served by user field testing when a product is in its final stage of design. Like user focus groups, user testing is designed to answer all three research questions.

24.4.2.3.1 Controlled laboratory testing Observation of performance and subjective feedback of user preferences during and after a series of defined tasks using the test product(s) in a controlled laboratory environment is the most effective method of obtaining an understanding of users' abilities, needs and preferences. As a result, it is the most useful method of identifying usability problems at all stages of the design process. **Laboratory testing provides an opportunity for all test participants to use the same products to perform the same tasks under the same conditions**. The intent is to minimize the influence of confounding external factors (i.e., unpredictable and variable real-world conditions) that can affect outcome measures. As a result, laboratory testing is a valuable methodology not only for problem identification, but also for competitive evaluations and collecting quantitative data about a product's usability (Rosenbaum and Kantner 2007).

User testing is accomplished with representative samples of the target audience performing a series of tasks with one or more test products that simulate real-world use. The more realistic the tasks simulate real-world use, the more useful the usability data will be. As a result, the closer that the laboratory environment simulates a real-world setting (e.g., an actual house with working fixtures and appliances), the more likely the results of the testing will represent real-world performance.

During testing, all participants are asked to perform the same series of tasks that will make use of the specific product features that are of interest to the design research team. Fully developed, final prototypes or existing products will most closely approximate real-world applications and will therefore provide the most reliable data. A test session might include evaluation of all of the interface features of the product(s), just those features about which design decisions have been made (e.g., an updated version of an existing product) or a subset of the design features based on use criteria such as frequency of use or how mission-critical the tasks are to overall successful use of the product (Rosenbaum and Kantner 2007). Testing subsets of design features is particularly useful if multiple sessions are required due to the length of testing or the amount of fatigue it might induce among the participants. Product testing might also be iterative, beginning with one or a small number of tasks that will test a few design features, refining those features and then testing them as well as additional ones in subsequent test sessions.

Task performance typically generates both quantitative observational performance data (through either direct observation or archival videotape or both) about **what works** and **for whom** as well as qualitative subjective user feedback (through "talk-aloud" techniques or directed questions) about **why** it works. However, while subjective feedback during task performance provides richer, real-time data, it is also more intrusive and disruptive of the real-world use simulation. As a result, less intrusive, but potentially less reliable, retroactive post-test subjective feedback through questionnaires and semi-structured interviews is often used

632

to address the question of **why** in formative evaluations. Nonetheless, post-test feedback does provide a rich source for obtaining subject preference and satisfaction data. Similar methods can be used in summative evaluations, although in that case the emphasis is on usability of a product as a whole. Because there is less variation in evaluating the usability of products as a whole in contrast to the usability of specific design features that comprise the product, summative evaluations lend themselves more readily to the use of standardized questionnaires, such as the Software Usability Measurement Inventory (SUMI) (Kirakowski and Corbett 1993) and System Usability Scale (SUS) (Brooke 1996), as usability evaluation tools.

24.4.2.3.2 Field testing Obviously, product use does not take place in a contrived laboratory; it occurs in the messy real world that has a myriad of uncontrolled factors. Nonetheless, despite the contextual confounds, usability testing in vivo is the preferred method of testing. Unfortunately, rather than utilize the unique aspects of a field site to obtain information that would otherwise be unavailable through laboratory testing, the vast majority of the literature on field usability testing strongly resembles traditional laboratory testing transplanted into a contextual lab. The only difference is that a naturalistic contrived setting has been brazenly substituted for an artificial one. In doing so, the same arranged observer-based, rigid test session methodology with defined tasks (as described above) is employed. While such methods are useful for understanding the usefulness of a product in real-world environments (i.e., utility testing), other than taking the test to the participants, rather bringing the participants to the test, the advantages of understanding usability in naturalistic real-world situations (as distinct from occurring in real-world environments) is lost.

A more effective way to leverage naturalistic environments is to provide test products to participants or, in the case of environmental technologies, such as grab bars, install the products in participants' homes or places of work and then **monitor usability, unimpeded, in their actual contexts of use** – homes, workplaces and public places. Most importantly, it is up to the participant to use the product to perform the tasks for which that product was intended. As a result, the entire context of use, that is, the task and the environment are natural. Nothing is contrived. In this way **products can be tested over a period of time to assess the impact of factors that can only be assessed over time, including the effect of the social environment (e.g., other individuals who occupy the same environment) and product familiarity**.

Depending on the nature of the product, capturing real time data using direct observation methods may or may not be feasible in the context of use (e.g., mobility through the house versus toilet transfers). Nonetheless, using technology to capture either observational or other quantitative performance data may still be practical. In some cases, it may be possible to capture observational data using archival videotape or televideo technologies, although this is typically only achievable when the context of use is restricted, such as a home or workplace. When the test product is a personal technology, such as a wheelchair, it is difficult to obtain observational data as the user moves through the community. In such cases, other technologies, such as GPS, accelerometers, wheel revolution counters, heart rate monitors and seat sensors among others can provide quantitative performance data. Of course, these, as well as a host of other environmentally installed technologies, such as motion and force sensors, can provide quantitative data in homes and workplaces as well. In almost all cases, supporting subjective feedback is obtained through a diary and periodic follow-up calls. More recently, digital diaries have become common, enabling users to transmit subjective data to researchers as frequently as entries are made. In addition, while technology has created opportunities for researchers to monitor real-time data, mobile devices have created the opportunity to contact subjects in real time (and vice versa) to obtain a debrief.

The use of technology to gather real-time or near real-time quantitative and qualitative data has not only made field testing more viable, it has also made it the go-to method for summative testing. Nonetheless, while it is best suited to identifying **what works** or doesn't work and **for whom**, if structured creatively, this methodology can also provide valuable information about **why**.

24.5 What works: quantifying usability outcomes (dependent variables)

Although usability cannot be measured directly (Hornbaek 2006; Nielsen and Levy 1994), it can be operationally defined and measured by product-relevant and task-specific usability indicators that represent the dependent outcome variables of interest. For example, graspability may be of interest for measuring usability of grab bars or a cane, whereas volume and clarity are important for screen readers. As a result, it is not surprising that numerous outcome variables have been used to measure **what works**. In a review of 82 AT outcome studies, Lenker et al. (2005) reported that nearly 68% of outcome variables included a variety of usability outcome measures, including user satisfaction ease of use, comfort, environments of use, safety and task effectiveness.

Usability outcomes can be objective, such as task completion, task errors and completion time, which measure how capable users are at using the product or subjective, such as user preference and satisfaction, which measure how much users like the product (Nielsen and Levy 1994). The use of proxy outcomes to indirectly measure usability raises two interrelated concerns: 1) defining the appropriate domains of objective and subjective measures and 2) ensuring that those measures are valid indicators of usability (Hornbaek 2006). Clearly, the degree to which the measures are product-relevant and task-specific should maximize their probability of being valid. In addition, the concern of validity is, in large part, dependent on defining the domains of objective and subjective outcome measures that are appropriate for measuring usability across products and tasks. As such, this discussion will focus on the latter and leave the issue of product-relevant and task-specific measures to be determined on a case-by-case basis.

24.5.1 Outcome measure domains

While there is little disagreement that outcome measures are both objective and subjective, there is a number of competing taxonomies based on differences in the outcome domains that act as indicators of product usability. These domains, in turn, are decomposed into specific usability outcomes (Bevan 1995) that are direct measures of **what works** (see Table 24.1).

24.5.1.1 Types of outcome domains There are two types of outcome domains – those that identify key outcomes directly and those that do so indirectly. The former, as represented by the ISO and Nielsen's HCI domain models, directly identify performance and preference outcomes based on user-product interactions. The latter, as represented by Kim and Han's consumer electronics system, Arthanat, et al.'s usability scale for assistive technology and the principles of universal design, are written in the language of design criteria, which describe how a product should perform (e.g., simple, intuitive, predictable), rather than as the result of a user–product interaction (e.g., learnability, understandability, error minimization). In other words, design performance criteria that describe what a product should do must be reinterpreted to capture what that product actually did do during a user–product interaction (see Figure 24.1).

24.5.2 Direct outcome measures of user interaction

24.5.2.1 Usability outcomes for mechanical and consumer products (ISO 202082-2:2013) This standard classifies usability based on ISO 9241-11, which defines usability as product effectiveness, efficiency and satisfaction. This definition has remained intact since 1998 and provides the most commonly adopted usability criteria cited in the literature. Although these outcomes were originally applied to ergonomic requirements for office work with visual display terminals, they have been used to reconcile all references to product usability across the standards (see Table 24.1).

Effectiveness is the extent to which the intended goals of use of the product are achieved, such as accuracy and completeness of specified tasks. Efficiency is the

Table 24.1 ISO 9241-11 Outcome Domains and Examples of Usability Measures

Effectiveness

Task Completion
- Binary measure of task completion or not
- Extent of task completeness
- Number of incomplete tasks within a set time
- Number of tasks where users gave up
- Number of tasks completed in a given time

Understanding and Learning
- Recall – how much information is recalled
- Changes in task completion rates

Accuracy/Precision
- Number of errors made
- Accuracy of completed tasks
- Number of correct tasks
- Percent of correct responses to total number
- Ratio of successful interactions to errors
- Spatial accuracy (distance from a target)

Efficiency

Usage Patterns
Mental Effort/Cognitive Workload
- Number of references to help
- Number of deviations from optimal solution
- Amount of information requested

Physical Effort
- Physiological measures (heart rate, O_2 saturation)
- Expert ratings of difficulty
- Ratio distance traveled to shortest distance
- Number of target re-entries (e.g., mouse pointer enters area, leaves and re-enters)
- Number of times an action is performed (e.g., number of keystrokes or mouse clicks)

Time
Task Time
- Tasks completed per unit time
- Time spent using help or documentation
- Time to complete a task
- Time searching for correct response
- Task completion time
- Time spent in errors

Learning (changes due to familiarity vs effectiveness of interface)
- Changes in time to complete tasks
- Changes in errors
- Changes in usage patterns

Satisfaction

Individuals
- Ratings of preference
- Ratings of approval
- Ratings of pleasure
- Ratings of gratification
- Ratings of like/dislike
- Ratings of ease of use
- Number of complaints

Summary
- Proportion who say they would prefer using one product over another
- Proportion of positive to critical statements
- Frequency of complaints

amount of effort or resources that have to be expended to achieve the intended goals. Satisfaction is the extent to which users find the product acceptable and the level of comfort felt when using a product to achieve the intended goals. This includes quantifying the strength of a user's subjectively expressed reactions, feelings, perceptions, attitudes or opinions. In other words, effectiveness and efficiency measure functional outcomes, whereas satisfaction is derived on the basis

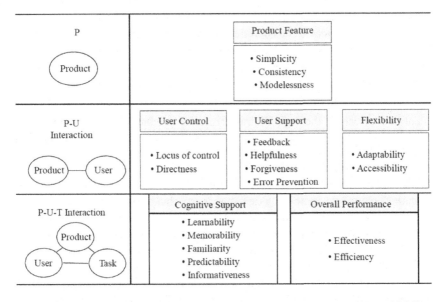

Figure 24.1 Usability dimensions classified by interactions (Kim and Han 2008).

of how effective and efficient the device is in permitting activity engagement and participation (Arthanat and others 2007).

24.5.2.2 Usability outcomes for quality in use and product quality (ISO/IEC 25010:2011) ISO/IEC 25010:2011 (2011) sets requirements for software and computer systems, although the standard recognizes that many of the character-istics are also relevant to wider systems and services. In contrast to ISO 2020082, which uses the usability outcome domains of EES, this standard includes two distinct domains of usability outcomes that correspond to different models of software and computer system quality.

The first, "quality in use" model applies to user–product interactions within a context of use. It is defined as the degree to which a product or system can be used by specific users to meet their needs to achieve specific goals with **effec-tiveness, efficiency, satisfaction, freedom from risk and in specific contexts of use**. Although the definition does not use the term usability, the first three domains of quality-related outcomes are clearly the same as those identified in ISO 9241-210 (2010). It further footnotes that consistency, usability (i.e., effective-ness, efficiency and satisfaction) is defined as a subset of quality in use. In addi-tion, while the standard does not identify outcome measures of effectiveness and efficiency, it identifies specific measurable characteristics of satisfaction, includ-ing usefulness, trust, pleasure and comfort. Here it should be noted that useful-ness is often used interchangeably with utility, although Nielsen (2012) attributes it to usability + utility. In either case, as described earlier in the chapter utility/ usefulness should not be considered a characteristic of usability, although it can be argued that usability is a characteristic of usefulness.

The second quality model, the "product quality model," is comprised of the characteristics that represent the static properties software and dynamic properties of computer systems (or other relevant products). Here, usability is specifically identified as one of the eight characteristics of product quality, which include functional suitability, reliability, performance efficiency, usability, security, compatibility, maintainability and portability. Further usability is further defined by the six outcome domains of appropriateness/recognizability, learnability, operability, user error protection, user interface aesthetics and accessibility. These domains comprise a completely different approach than the one of effectiveness, efficiency and satisfaction used in ISO 9241-210 (2010) and the ISO quality in use model. Interestingly, a note to the entry in the ISO states that usability can be measured either as a function of quality in use outcomes (i.e., effectiveness, efficiency and satisfaction) or as product quality outcomes (appropriateness/recognizability, learnability, operability, user error protection, user interface aesthetics and accessibility), even though the latter appears to be much more restrictive and prescriptive in terms of classifying usability outcome domains. For example, satisfaction is limited to esthetic impact and usefulness as defined by recognition of appropriateness; effectiveness is limited to ease of use, error protection and accessibility and efficiency is defined by learnability (see Table 24.2).

24.5.2.3 HCI outcomes (Nielsen 2012) Jakob Nielsen has long proposed a system for HCI that categorizes usability by **five domains: learnability, efficiency, memorability, errors and satisfaction.** In many ways these domains are a hybrid of the two ISO models. Learnability and errors are included in the product quality model, whereas efficiency and satisfaction are included in the quality in use model. However, Nielsen has added a new outcome in memorability, which replaces physical operability or ease of use at a single point in time, with cognitive operability or ease of use over time.

24.5.3 Indirect outcome measures of product performance

24.5.3.1 Usability dimensions for consumer electronic products (Kim and Han 2008) In an effort to develop an overall usability index for consumer electronic products, Kim and Han (2008) developed a comprehensive list of the usability outcomes that would be applicable to that category of products. Approximately 50 usability dimensions were identified and screened based on the relevance to consumer electronic products and conceptual discriminability. For example, portability and appropriate coding were excluded because they were specifically related to mobile and software products, not consumer electronics. The result was

Table 24.2 Domains of Direct Outcome Measures

Domains	Definition
ISO Quality in use model and ISO 9241-210	
Effectiveness	Extent to which the intended goals of use of the product are achieved, such as accuracy and completeness of specified tasks
Efficiency	The amount of effort or resources that have to be expended to achieve the intended goals
Satisfaction	Extent to which users finds the product acceptable and the level of comfort felt when using a product to achieve the intended goals
ISO Product quality model	
Appropriateness, recognizability	Degree to which users can recognize whether a product or system is appropriate for their needs
Learnability	Degree to which a product or system can be used by specified users to achieve specified goals of learning to use the product or system with effectiveness, efficiency, freedom from risk and satisfaction in a specified context of use
Operability	Degree to which a product or system has attributes that make it easy to operate and control
User error protection	Degree to which a system protects users against making errors
User interface aesthetics	Degree to which a user interface enables pleasing and satisfying interaction for the user
Accessibility	Degree to which a product can be used by people with the widest range of abilities to achieve a specified goal in a specified context of use [Note: accessibility for people with disabilities is either the extent to which a product can be used by users with specified disabilities to achieve specified goals or by the presence of product properties that support accessibility]
Nielsen HCI Model	
Learnability	Ease of accomplishing basic tasks the first time the design is used
Efficiency	How quickly tasks are performed, once they are learned
Memorability	How easily proficiency is reestablished after a period of nonuse
Errors	Number and severity of errors made and ease of recovery
Satisfaction	How pleasant the design is to use

a list of 18 usability dimensions (see Table 24.3). Further, based on the ecological models of P–E fit described above, those dimensions were categorized by whether they were specifically focused on the product only, the product–user interaction, or the product–user–task interaction (see Figure 24.1).

24.5.3.2 Usability scale for assistive technology (Arthanat and others 2007) To evaluate the usability of AT devices the usability scale for AT (USAT) was

639

Table 24.3 Performance Outcomes for Consumer Electronic Products (Kim and Han 2008)

Performance Outcome	Description
Simplicity	User interfaces and interaction methods should be simple, plain, and intuitively recognizable
Consistency	User interfaces and interaction methods should be consistent within a product and between the same product family
Modelessness	Each user interface and interaction method should have only one designated meaning and behavior
Locus of control	Authority to control all the functions and the appearance of user interfaces should be given to a user
Directness	Any operations should be designed to give a feeling of direct manipulation
Feedback	The status of a product and the consequences of any user operations should be immediately and clearly provided
Helpfulness	Any helpful information that a user may refer to should be provided whenever a user needs it
Forgiveness	When an error is recognized, ability for a user to take corrective actions should be given to a user
Error prevention	Interfaces and interaction methods should be designed to prevent a user from making any mistakes or errors
Adaptability	User interfaces should fit different users and conditions according to users' experience, knowledge and preference
Accessibility	Any functions and user interfaces should be accessible when a user wants them
Learnability	Efforts required to learn the user interfaces and the interaction methods should be small
Memorability	Interfaces and interaction methods should be easy to recall
Familiarity	Familiar user interfaces and interaction methods should be adopted to make users apply their previous experience
Predictability	The interaction method and the meanings of user interfaces should conform with user's expectations
Informativeness	Interfaces should be easy and clear to understand
Effectiveness	Every function that users want should be implemented
Efficiency	A product should be designed to allow a user to perform functions in a quick, easy, and economical way

conceptualized as a function of the individual's participation in activities with the AT device, the support provided by device functions and features to accomplish activities, the influence of the environment factors in usage of the device and the abilities and skills of the user in interacting with the device and environment (Arthanat and others 2007). Although the structure of the instrument was intended to be generic to all AT devices, the user-specific nature of any AT device required that the tool be developed as a series of modules (e.g., USAT-WM for wheeled mobility devices) to capture the activity specific user-AT interactions corresponding to each specific category of AT devices.

To develop the USAT-WM module, nearly 400 indicators pertaining to wheeled-mobility AT devices were derived from interviews with users of AT devices. A subsequent field test of the instrument with users established a 50-item version comprised of four sections with the section on device performance of direct relevance to usability outcome domains. Among the 17 items in this section, 11 product performance criteria (e.g., effectiveness, ease of use, suitability, comfort and adjustability) are translatable into generic domains of usability outcomes based on user-product interactions (see Table 24.4). The remaining six items (reliability, storage, portability, impact, durability and maintenance) are attributes of the device outside of any user–product interaction.

24.5.3.3 Principles of universal design (Connell and others 1997)   A decade before either Kim and Han's usability dimensions or the iPhone, a group of experts representing a range of design disciplines developed the seven principles

Table 24.4 Performance Outcomes for Assistive Technology (Arthanat and others 2007)

Performance Outcome	Description
Effectiveness*	The device must help in completing the activity
Efficiency*	The device must help in completing the activity sooner with less effort
Ease of use*	The device must be easy to use
Suitability*	The device must be suitable for you
Adjustability*	The device can be configured or adjusted to your abilities and needs
Comfort*	The device must be physically and mentally comfortable to use
Appearance*	The device must appear pleasing
Privacy & security*	The device must provide privacy and security of information
Safety*	The device must not endanger your or other's safety
Novelty*	The device must feel new to you
Value/Worthiness*	The device must feel valuable and worthy to you
Reliability	The device must be dependable and must always work well
Storage	The device must be easy to store away
Portability	The device must be easy to carry from one place to another
Environmental impact	The device must not cause any damage to the immediate environment
Durability	The device must resist wear and tear
Maintenance	The device must be easy to maintain

*indicates usability-relevant outcome

641

of universal design (UD). These include equitable use, flexibility in use, simple and intuitive use, perceptible information, tolerance for error, low physical effort and size and space for approach and use.

Although the principles were primarily intended to provide guidance for the design of physical products and spaces (i.e., they predated mobile software interfaces) that would be usable by all individuals (to the greatest extent possible), they have proven to be applicable to the design of all current products and technologies. Moreover, together with their accompanying guidelines (see Table 24.5), they not only encompass all domains of usability outcomes proposed in the other frameworks, they exceed them (see Table 24.6).

24.5.4 Performance and preference

Performance and preference are the broadest and least prescriptive ways to think about usability outcomes. Performance measures, capture how well users are able to use a product, whereas preference measures characterize subjective responses to how much the users like the product (Nielsen and Levy 1994). Although early work by Nielsen (1993) reported that there is a high correlation between the two types of measures, research has demonstrated that the two can be conflicting and may lead to different conclusions regarding the usability of an interface (Hornbaek 2006). To accommodate these differences, Bailey (1993) suggested that performance and preference be clearly separated, the limitations of each recognized, and design decisions made to optimize one or the other. However, he also argued that performance-oriented usability testing was the only way to ensure that products demonstrated acceptable performance. Regardless of the degree to which the two types of outcome measures are in agreement, the consensus in the literature (as well as common sense) suggests that using both measures of performance and preference outcomes provides a more complete and robust understanding of **what works**.

The most striking characteristic of the performance–preference dichotomy is that it does not distinguish between objective and subjective outcome domains. Although preference is clearly subjective, performance can be either objective and subjective, such as quantitative and perceived measures of task difficulty or safety using a certain interface. Among the domain models described above only the principles of UD do not make a distinction between objective and subjective domains. Notably, the adherence to quantitatively derived performance measures in lieu of those that are subjectively reported severely limits the range of performance data that are available to evaluate usability outcomes in those models. As a whole, the principles of UD not only provide the most comprehensive system of outcome measures, they do so in a way that provides flexibility to use those outcomes as either objective or subjective measures.

Table 24.5 Principles of Universal Design© (Copyright © 1997 NC State University, The Center for Universal Design).

Principle one: Equitable use: The design is useful and marketable to people with diverse abilities.

1a. Provide the same means of use for all users: identical whenever possible; equivalent when not.

1b. Avoid segregating or stigmatizing any users.

1c. Provisions for privacy, security and safety should be equally available to all users.

1d. Make the design appealing to all users.

Principle two: Flexibility in use: The design accommodates a wide range of individual preferences and abilities.

2a. Provide choice in methods of use.

2b. Accommodate right- or left-handed access and use.

2c. Facilitate the user's accuracy and precision.

2d. Provide adaptability to the user's pace.

Principle three: Simple and intuitive use: Use of the design is easy to understand, regardless of the user's experience, knowledge, language skills or current concentration level.

3a. Eliminate unnecessary complexity.

3b. Be consistent with user expectations and intuition.

3c. Accommodate a wide range of literacy and language skills.

3d. Arrange information consistent with its importance.

3e. Provide effective prompting and feedback during and after task completion.

Principle four: Perceptible information: The design communicates necessary information effectively to the user, regardless of ambient conditions or the user's sensory abilities.

4a. Use different modes (pictorial, verbal, tactile) for redundant presentation of essential information.

4b. Provide adequate contrast between essential information and its surroundings.

4c. Maximize "legibility" of essential information.

4d. Differentiate elements in ways that can be described (i.e., make it easy to give instructions or directions).

4e. Provide compatibility with a variety of techniques or devices used by people with sensory limitations.

Principle five: Tolerance for error: The design minimizes hazards and the adverse consequences of accidental or unintended actions.

5a. Arrange elements to minimize hazards and errors: most used elements, most accessible; hazardous elements eliminated, isolated, or shielded.

5b. Provide warnings of hazards and errors.

5c. Provide fail-safe features.

5d. Discourage unconscious action in tasks that require vigilance.

Principle six: Low physical effort: The design can be used efficiently and comfortably and with a minimum of fatigue.

6a. Allow user to maintain a neutral body position.

6b. Use reasonable operating forces.

6c. Minimize repetitive actions.

6d. Minimize sustained physical effort.

Principle seven: Size and space for approach and use: Appropriate size and space is provided for approach, reach, manipulation and use regardless of user's body size, posture or mobility.

7a. Provide a clear line of sight to important elements for any seated or standing user.

7b. Make reach to all components comfortable for any seated or standing user.

7c. Accommodate variations in hand and grip size.

7d. Provide adequate space for the use of assistive devices or personal assistance.

Table 24.6 Comparison of Outcome Domains across Usability Frameworks

		Usability Frameworks and Domains		
NCSU UD Principles	**ISO Product Quality**	**Nielsen HCI Model**	**Kim and Han Consumer Electronics**	**Arthanat et al. USAT**
Equitable Use	Esthetics	X	X	Appearance Privacy & security
Flexibility in Use	X	X	Adaptability Locus of control	Adjustability
Simple & Intuitive Use	Learnability	Memorability Learnability	Simplicity Consistency Modelessness Predictability Learnability Familiarity Memorability Informativeness	X
Perceptible Information	X	X	X	X
Tolerance for Error	User error protection	Errors	Feedback Error prevention Forgiveness Helpfulness	Safety
Low Physical Effort	Operability	Efficiency	Efficiency Directness	Ease of use Comfort Efficiency Effectiveness help
Size and Space	X		X	X
X	Accessibility	X	Accessibility	X
X	Appropriateness, recognizability	Satisfaction	Effectiveness	Value/Worthiness Suitability
X	X	X	X	Novelty

24.5.4.1 Subjective outcomes Although subjective response outcomes are identified in all four of the other frameworks, including ISO's domain of appropriateness recognizability, Nielsen's satisfaction, Kim and Han's effectiveness and USAT's suitability and novelty/worthiness, the constructs differ in intent. The subjective domains in both ISO and USAT represent an understanding on the user's part that the product meets one's needs. Nielsen defines satisfaction as being pleasant to use, whereas Kim and Han refer to effectiveness as what users want, not what they need. In contrast, the UD principles do not differentiate between objective performance and subjective preference outcomes. As a result, all of the UD outcome measures can be used as either objective or subjective measures.

24.5.4.2 Accessibility The UD principles are silent on the issue of accessibility for good reason. The first principle of equitable use includes a guideline that promotes the same means of use for all users, regardless of ability. Since this applies to all users, it preempts the need to provide accessibility for a specific set of users, which is included in the ISO principles (note that accessibility is also included in Kim and Han, but with a different meaning). In fact, the accessibility outcome in the ISO is unique in that it is the only measure among those that have been included in this discussion that distinguishes among users and addresses **what works** for a unique target audience. As a result, the accessibility outcomes actually address the question of **for whom** and does not belong in an outcome classification system that is intended to identify **what works**.

24.5.4.3 Breadth By virtue of their being design guidelines, the three indirectly derived outcome domain frameworks are more comprehensive compared to the domains in the two direct frameworks, with the UD principles being the most robust. Among those domains that are included in the UD principles, the other frameworks, with the exception of USAT, place a comparatively heavy emphasis, on cognitive functioning (i.e., principles of simple and intuitive use). This is particularly evident in the Kim and Han effort, which encompasses learning, memory, prediction and consistency. In addition, all of the frameworks include domains to minimize errors and the level of physical exertion. Surprisingly, UD is the only framework to include outcome measures related to sensory inputs or outputs (i.e., perceptible information) and to size and space allocation of design components. While the latter is not as surprising given that the principles were intended primarily for the design of the physical environment, this principle is, nonetheless, equally applicable to the design of physical hardware and software interfaces (e.g., size of buttons and space between them). Equitable use, and specifically esthetics (i.e., appealing for all) is only addressed in the ISO and USAT, while Kim and Han's outcomes of adaptability and locus of control and USAT's adjustability are the only frameworks to address the domain of flexibility in use. Finally, novelty, which is included in USAT is one domain that appears to be a complete outlier. Defined as feeling new, it is clearly a subjective response. However, why novelty is an outcome of AT use is not obvious. Moreover, it would seem to contradict other measures that promote predictability, familiarity and intuitiveness.

24.6 For whom: matching people to products

Product usability testing is intended to identify what does or does not work for specific groups of end users, based on their needs (not wants), abilities and preferences, including physical skills and cultural (e.g., language) factors. Where product features do not match the needs, abilities and/or preferences of targeted end users, that information can be used either to refine those features to improve usability for those users or to modify the target to those users **for whom** those features work.

Obviously, the wider the range of user needs, abilities and preferences that are met by product features, the more generalizable that information is to potential target audiences. For example, a UD product, which is intended to be usable by all people to the greatest extent possible, should match the widest range of needs, abilities and preferences and therefore should be generalizable to all individuals. In contrast, assistive products are intended for users with very specific needs, abilities and preferences resulting from a variety of limitations in vision, hearing, speech, dexterity and mobility. As a result, while assistive devices are rarely intended to be generalizable beyond the targeted end users, the degree of generalizability within the broad types of functional limitations will nonetheless depend on the range of needs, abilities and preferences included in the test participants. For example, testing people who have low vision or are hard of hearing, will not necessarily generalize to those who are blind or deaf, respectively. Similarly, people who use manual wheelchairs have fundamentally different needs and abilities compared to those who use scooters or powered wheelchairs.

24.6.1 Accessibility vs usability

Accessibility does not necessarily equate to usability. Accessibility is generally determined by either mandated (e.g., Americans with Disabilities Amendments Act Accessibility Standards) or accepted standards of practice (e.g., OT home modification guidelines). By design, an accessible product is intended to match the needs, abilities and preferences of the smallest groups of individuals. As a result, a product that is technically accessible might still be unusable for either the end users **for whom** the accessible features are intended or other users who have functional abilities and/or use AT that differs from the target users.

646

For example, a website may be accessible to people who use screen readers (typically those who are blind or have extremely low vision). However, user testing might discern that these individuals still have usability issues due to an interface that is not intuitive, understandable or learnable. Further, testing may identify problems encountered by other users, such as small font and poor contrast, which can limit usability by anyone with other types of vision loss (e.g., color blindness, contrast sensitivity or acuity problems); lack of protection from errors or too much information on a page, which can create usability problems for people with cognitive limitations; active buttons that require accuracy and precision, which can create usability issues for people with dexterity limitations or audio to provide key information, which can cause usability problems for people with hearing loss.

24.6.2 Identifying participants for usability testing

While end users are the only ones who fully understand what does and does not work for them, targeting end users should be based on those specific factors that are crucial for determining usability for the intended audience as well as generalizability of the data. However, to further complicate participant selection, products may have multiple end users, some of whom may not be the intended target audience.

Targeted users may be defined by a number of different factors, including demographics, such as age, socioeconomic status or education, or health or functional status, such as having a specific chronic condition or impairment. However, inclusion in usability testing should be based on those factors that might impact the usability of a product. For example, if age is a potential usability factor (e.g., it can impact optimal reaction times for a computer game), individuals across the age ranges should be included in the testing. On the other hand, if the target audience is a specific age group (e.g., the game is intended for college students), then testing should include only that specific age range. Alternatively, if age is not considered a usability factor, then testing can include people of any age. Regardless of inclusion criteria, the generalizability of usability testing is limited to those usability-relevant factors of the individuals who participate in testing.

Products often have several end users. For mainstream products, such as mobile applications, that are often used for different purposes by mutually exclusive user groups (e.g., practitioners and consumers), the usability-relevant factors that impact participant selection will also differ. Having multiple end users is particularly common with medical instrumentation and assistive devices. While the primary end users of medical products are clinical staff, it is not uncommon for consumers to utilize the same devices to monitor physiological status (e.g., blood pressure), particularly as more and more care occurs in the home. In contrast, the primary end users of assistive devices are consumers with functional limitations.

However, there are often secondary users, including informal and formal caregivers. as well as rehabilitation service providers.

Assistive devices exist for the sole purpose of compensating for otherwise unusable mainstream products and technologies. As a result, the usability of these products is crucial. To ensure usability, the population of individuals with the specific functional limitations (e.g., blind individuals) for which the devices (e.g., screen readers) are intended and SMEs with knowledge of that population should be included in the testing. It is also important to understand usability by secondary users as caregivers assisting the primary user, device users (e.g., a tub bench) facilitating their own activity and service providers training primary users and secondary caregivers to use the device. In addition, secondary users might act as SMEs to provide usability information on behalf of a primary user.

Ultimately, no matter how similar participants look based on the usability-relevant inclusion criteria, no two people are alike. The range of abilities, needs, preferences and experiences is diverse and factors that impact usability may be difficult to predict. Moreover, variability in abilities, needs and preferences even within identified cohorts of users, such as older adults, people with disabilities or even a specific type of disability (e.g., vision disability), or clinicians such as OTs, is significant in product design and evaluation. As a result, the more homogeneous the participants (i.e., the narrower the range of common usability-relevant factor), the more likely the information will produce a more usable design for that cohort, but at the same time limit the generalizability of that product's usability to a wider range of users.

24.6.3 Selecting the number of participants

The number of participants for a usability test has long been debated, particularly in the HCI literature. The long-held belief in HCI is that five is the magic number of participants for usability testing. This rationale for five participants is based on the cost-benefits of formative testing. Specifically, mathematical models by Nielsen (Landauer and Nielsen 1993; Nielsen 1993) suggest that five participants are sufficient to discover approximately 85% of the usability issues (see Figure 24.2). As a result, when the purpose of testing is to inform design, rather than demonstrate clinical and/or statistical significance, the cost in time and money to potentially identify the other 15% of the usability issues far outweighs the benefits. However, it is important to note that the five participant rule is applicable to testing that occurs in a controlled environment with participants that are fairly homogeneous in terms of usability-relevant factors. In other words, when participants represent multiple groups of target end users and/or have highly heterogeneous usability-relevant factors it is likely that more than five participants per usability test would be needed.

648

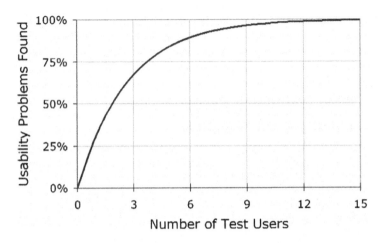

Figure 24.2 Usability problems per test participant (source: http://www.useit.com/ alertbox/20000319.html).

In contrast to Nielsen's work, a number of studies have demonstrated that five users reveal far less than 85% of the usability problems and that new users continue to identify new usability problems (e.g., Perfetti and Landesman 2017; Spool and Schroeder 2001; Woolrych and Cockton 2001). However, the purpose of the early efforts was to demonstrate that statistical rigor can be relaxed considerably in real-world usability testing, particularly when iterative testing is likely to eventually identify those other problems. The question is not whether five users are sufficient to identify 85% of the problems, but whether five users are sufficient to drive a useful iterative cycle. Nielsen advocates for less testing more often. He writes that "elaborate usability tests are a waste of resources. The best results come from testing no more than 5 users and running as many small tests as you can afford" (http://www.useit.com/alertbox/20000319.html).

This is not to say that greater numbers of participants are never required or will not generate new information. First, the greater the disparity among participants in usability-relevant factors, the greater the number of participants that should be included. Still, the optimal number of participants to include in real-world formative usability testing remains vague. Even in situations with high cohort homogeneity in "detailed and well-focused tests" (Hudson 2001) that would warrant small samples, there is a myriad of potential confounding factors that might not be anticipated or over which testing has little or no control. As a result, the best option to inform design is to test quickly and test often. Second, when the purpose of testing is summative, such as conducting clinical trials of a product, more rigorous research efforts with greater numbers of participants will be needed to demonstrate clinical and/or statistical significance. For summative evaluation of product usability, ISO 20282 stresses larger sample sizes of at least 50 participants. The larger sample is intended to ensure that the test includes a representative sample of users and that the results have sufficient predictive validity.

24.7 Why: identifying design measures (independent variables)

Understanding **why** a particular design works is crucial for informing design decisions for the current product being tested as well as for future products. For the product being tested, understanding **why** enables designers to change and refine those design features and/or characteristics that are associated with usability problems. For future products, it enables replicability without either duplicating existing designs or reinventing wheels.

Product usability is a function of the design features of a product, either as a whole, such as a hammer or a smartphone, or each of the component parts of its user interface(s), such as a hammer handle or a phone's icons. It is similarly a function of the unique characteristics that distinguish the design features of one product from those of another, such as the size and shape of a hammer handle or screen icons. Ultimately, it is the design characteristics that interact with an individual's needs, abilities and preferences to determine one's successful task performance and product usability. The size and shape of a handle affect one's ability to grasp it, whereas the same characteristics of a smartphone icon can affect one's ability to touch it accurately. As a result, identifying the relevant design measures associated with usability is rooted in understanding the difference between design features and design characteristics. Simply put, **design features are associated with task performance and preference; design characteristics are associated with performance and preference outcomes**.

24.7.1 Design features

A design **feature** (n.) is any identifiable design element at any scale of design, from spaces to products, devices and technologies to user interfaces. As categories of design elements, interface features, including both inputs and outputs, are identified by their names. Examples of interface features are knobs, buttons, switches, handles, transfer surfaces, visual displays and alarms. However, names are imprecise (i.e., what is the difference between a button and a knob?) and do not lend themselves to measurement. As a result, interface features, by any name, merely represent functionalities that are either present or absent. Nonetheless, not all interface features look or act alike. They possess characteristics about which design decisions are made. For example, buttons can be made of different materials and have different shapes, sizes, configurations and colors. Design characteristics differentiate one interface feature from other features with the same name.

24.7.2 Design characteristics

A design **characteristic** (n.) is an attribute of a design feature, such as height, length, width, color, texture and condition that defines the proportions, appearance and other qualities (e.g., acoustic) of that feature. Common product characteristics include orientation of use, sequencing of actions, structure and location and configuration (e.g., space between controls) of interfaces. Similarly, interface characteristics include dimensions (e.g., height, shape, width, diameter, length), weight, materials/finishes (type, texture, and color contrast), activation method (voice, grip required) and operational characteristics (direction and distance interfaces need to be moved, calibration, type of sensory feedback, activation forces, voice sensitivity). As adjectives, rather than nouns, design characteristics are not only variable within and across product and interface features, but also measurable in quantifiable and/or describable ways (see also Sanford and Bruce 2010; Stark and Sanford 2005; Stark, Sanford and Keglovits 2014). As measurable variables, specific design characteristics can be associated with specific tasks and usability outcomes to identify **why** a particular design works. For example, in the story of Goldilocks, the crucial interface characteristic of the bed was firmness. One bed was too hard, another was too soft. The one that worked was somewhere in between. Although an objective measure of firmness would provide a more specific criterion for replicability, the story does provide a comparative understanding of Goldilocks's subjective preference for bed firmness.

24.8 A case study of what works, for whom and why

The author recently reviewed a study of an interactive technology in a generic pediatric waiting room that was used by children with and without disabilities aged six months through 18 years. The review is reproduced below to illustrate the strengths and weaknesses of the paper based on **what worked, for whom and why**.

24.8.1 What works

The paper clearly focuses on a study designed to identify **what worked**, and provides a clear and well-written description to determine the effects of a hands-free interactive technology on child behavior in a pediatric waiting room. The study demonstrates that the primary intervention shows a statistically significant effect compared to a non-intervention control and a passive nature video intervention. However, there are no differences between the latter two. This finding is not at all

651

surprising given that the target population was a pediatric population, which is less likely to be engaged by a nature video. More importantly, it strongly suggests that comparing the intervention to one or more engaging interventions (e.g., cartoon, other interactive hands-free designs or hand-engaged technologies) would permit a more clinically generalizable conclusion. As it stands, the study shows that the interactive intervention is better than nothing (equating the passive condition to nothing), but there is no evidence to suggest that this particular intervention is any better than any other interactive or other engaging intervention.

A second issue with the interactive condition is exposure to the intervention. The study reported that 62/113 children actively engaged with the technology and 24/113 as onlookers for the majority of the ten-minute period. Somewhat concerning is the low percentage of children engaged, but the lack of specific detail about engagement time is a particular weakness. The difference between the lower and upper end of this spectrum (e.g., 5.1 minutes and 10 minutes) is quite remarkable, especially for children with short attention spans. A more precise outcome measure of how long children spent interacting with or watching the technology would have improved the study. Perhaps taking the lead from museum studies (e.g., art museums, zoos, children's museums, etc.), where engagement time (amount of time spent at an exhibit either as a whole or engaged in specific activities) is used as a measure of exhibit effectiveness would have been a more valid outcome measure.

24.8.2 For whom

Given the heterogeneous population (age, condition, ability, visit purpose) one would expect differential effects of the intervention. While the authors developed a statistical model that included age, media condition, and pre-exposure stress for purposes of demonstrating effectiveness, the model does not inform the question of who would be best suited for deployment of the technology. Among the three predictors, only age was an actual predictor or technology deployment, although the study did not have a large enough sample to determine what age group(s) would most benefit from the intervention. Thus, while the information is useful to a behavioral scientist, it is neither useful to designers nor to administrators who make decisions about what props to include for kids in a pediatric waiting room. Further, the purpose of visit/clinic attended (e.g., regular checkup vs surgery), which would seem to be a highly important factor in determining the effectiveness of the intervention, does not appear to be included in the analysis.

A second issue regarding target population was the mobility categories – independent/minimal limitations (I), independent with limitations (II–IV) and no mobility (V). First, it is unclear why children with no mobility were included in the analyses of child subjects as their ability to participate (presumably as onlookers) would be dependent on their parents, not themselves. Second, it would be helpful to describe the types of limitations in the category of independent with limitations (II–IV) for purpose of understanding whether limitation might have a differential effect on intervention effectiveness. Without more detailed information about the population **for whom** the intervention is effective, the intervention is not generalizable to waiting rooms that are used by specific groups of children.

24.8.3 Why

Finally, it is important to know **why** an intervention is effective in order to understand what specific factors are driving intervention effectiveness. For example, was the effect due to the hands-free interaction, colors, shapes on the wall, number of sensors in the floor, color of the floor, etc.? Without an analysis that examines effectiveness by its design attributes, the study is not generalizable to other hands-free interactive technologies. In other words, the study only tells us about the exact intervention tested. It is not possible to replicate the intervention (even the same intervention with different colors, for example) that may be equally effective or even better.

24.9 Chapter summary

Overall, this is an important study in documenting the potential for the use of interactive technologies to reduce patient stress in pediatric clinics. However, it is important to recognize that this is a summative study that is limited to an N of 1. In other words, the particular intervention studied was better than no intervention (including a non-comparable passive nature video). However, without a more valid outcome of effectiveness to identify **what works**, a better understanding of the population(s) characteristics **for whom** the intervention is effective and **why** certain design factors (i.e., design characteristics) are driving effectiveness, the intervention is neither generalizable to other applications nor replicable. As a result, the potential clinical application is limited to this particular intervention in general pediatric clinics.

24.10 Discussion questions

1. Why is understanding "why" important?
2. Why are summative evaluations not useful in understanding "why"?
3. Describe the relationships among the intended goals and purpose of usability testing, and the three basic research questions.
4. What determines usability?

5. What is the difference between design features and characteristics?
6. What are the factors that determine generalizability?
7. What data would enable Goldilocks to generalize her data to the bear population as a whole?
8. What factors should be considered in determining appropriate usability outcomes for a particular product?

Bibliography

Anna, M. W. 2000. "Usability Testing in 2000." *Ergonomics* 43 (7): 998–1006.

Arthanat, S., S. M. Bauer, J. A. Lenker, S. M. Nochajski, and Y. W. B. Wu. 2007. "Conceptualization and Measurement of Assistive Technology Usability." *Disability and Rehabilitation: Assistive Technology* 2 (4): 235–248.

Bailey, R. W. 1993. "Performance vs Preference." *Proceedings of the Human Factors and Ergonomics Society* 37(4).

Bevan, N. 2001. "International Standards for HCI and Usability." *International Journal of Human-Computer Studies* 55 (4): 533–552.

———. 1995. "Measuring Usability as Quality of Use." *Software Quality Journal* 4: 115–150.

Brandt, E. and A. M. Pope. 1997. *Enabling America: Assessing the Role of Rehabilitation Science and Engineering*. Washington, DC: National Academy Press.

Brooke, J. 1996. *SUS: A Quick and Dirty Usability Scale*. CRC Press.

Connell, B. R., M. L. Jones, R. Mace, J. Meuller, A. Mullick, E. Ostroff, J. A. Sanford, E. Steinfeld, M. Story, and G. Vanderheiden. 1997. *The Principles of Universal Design: Version 2*. Raleigh, NC: The Center for Universal Design.

Cook, A. and S. Hussey. 2002. *Assistive Technologies Principles and Practice*, 2nd ed. Toronto, Canada: Elsevier.

Han, S. H., E. S. Jung, M. Jung, J. Kwahk, and S. Park. 1998. "Psychophysical Methods and Passenger Preferences of Interior Designs." *Applied Ergonomics* 29 (6): 499.

Han, S. H., M. H. Yun, K. J. Kim, and J. Kwahk. 2000. "Evaluation of Product Usability: Development and Validation of Usability Dimensions and Design Elements Based on Empirical Models." *International Journal of Industrial Ergonomics* 26: 477–488.

Han, S. H., M. H. Yun, J. Kwahk, and S. W. Hong. 1998. "Usability of Consumer Electronic Products." In *Proceedings of the Fifth Pan-Pacific Conference on Occupational Ergonomics*, Kitakyushu, Japan.

Hersh, M. 2010. *The Design and Evaluation of Assistive Technology Products and Devices Part 1: Design*. Center for International Rehabilitation Research Information & Exchange (CIRRIE).

Hornbaek, K. 2006. "Current Practice in Measuring Usability: Challenges to Usability Studies and Research." *International Journal of Human-Computer Studies* 64: 79–102.

Hudson, William. 2001. "How Many Users Does it Take to Change a Web Site?" *ACM SIGCHI Bulletin-A Supplement to Interactions* 2001: 6–6.

ISO. 2010. ISO 9241-210. "Ergonomic Requirements for Office Work with Visual Display Terminals (VDTs)." International Organization for Standardization. https://www.iso.org/obp/ui/#iso:std:iso:9241:-210:ed-1:v1:en.

ISO/IEC 20510:2011. "Systems and Software Engineering – Systems and Software Quality Requirements and Evaluation (SQuaRE) – System and Software Quality Models." https://www.iso.org/standard/35733.html.

ISO/TS 18152:2010. "Ergonomics of Human-System Interaction – Specification for the Process Assessment of Human-System Issues." International Organization for Standardization. https://www.iso.org/standard/56174.html.

ISO/TS 20282-1:2006. "Ease of Operation of Everyday Products – Part 1: Design Requirements for Context of Use and User Characteristics." International Organization for Standardization. https://www.iso.org/standard/34122.html.

ISO/TS 20282-2:2013. "Usability of Consumer Products and Products for Public Use – Part 2: Summative Test Method." International Organization for Standardization. https://www.iso.org/standard/62733.html.

Kielhofner, G. 1995. *A Model of Human Occupation: Therapy and Application*, 2nd ed. Baltimore, MD: Williams & Wilkins.

Kielhofner, G. and J. P. Burke. 1980. "A Model of Human Occupation. Part 1. Conceptual Framework and Content." *American Journal of Occupational Therapy* 34: 572–581.

Kim, J. and S. H. Han. 2008. "A Methodology for Developing a Usability Index of Consumer Electronic Products." *International Journal of Industrial Ergonomics* 38: 333–345.

Kirakowski, J. and M. Corbett. 1993. "SUMI: The Software Usability Measurement Inventory." *British Journal of Educational Technology* 24: 210–212.

Landauer, T. K. and J. Nielsen. 1993. "A Mathematical Model of the Finding of Usability Problems." In *Interchi '93*, ACM, Computer-Human Interface Special Interest Group.

Langford, J. and D. McDonagh. 2003. *Focus Groups: Supporting Effective Product Development*. New York: Taylor and Francis.

Law, M., Cooper, B. A., S. Strong, D. Stewart, P. Rigby, and L. Letts. 1996. "The Person-Environment-Occupation Model: A Transactive Approach to Occupational Performance." *Canadian Journal of Occupational Therapy* 63: 186–192.

Lawton, M. P. and L. Nahemow. 1973. "Ecology and the Aging Process." In *The Psychology of Adult Development and Aging*, edited by C. Eisdorfer and M. P. Lawton, 619–674. Washington, DC: American Psychological Association.

Lenker, J. A., M. J. Scherer, M. J. Fuhrer, J. W. Jutai, and F. DeRuyter. 2005. "Psychometric and Administrative Properties of Measures Used in Assistive Technology Device Outcomes Research." *Assistive Technology* 17 (1): 7.

Nielsen, J. 1993. *Usability Engineering*. Boston, MA: AP Professional.

———. 1997. "The Use and Misuse of Focus Groups." *IEEE Software*. Paolo Alto, CA: IEEE.

———. 2012. *Usability 101*. https://www.nngroup.com/articles/usability-testing-101/.

Nielsen, J. and J. Levy. 1994. "Measuring Usability: Preference vs Performance." *Communications of the ACM* 37 (4): 66–75.

Perfetti, C. and L. Landesman. 2017. *Eight Is Not Enough*. Retrieved April 14 2022. ttps://articles.uie.com/eight_is_not_enough/.

Redish, J., R. G. Bias, R. Bailey, R. Molich, J. Dumas, and J. M. Spool. 2002. "Usability in Practice: Formative Usability Evaluations - Evolution and Revolution." In *CHI '02 Extended Abstracts on Human Factors in Computing Systems*. New York: ACM.

Rigby, P. and L. Letts. 2003. "Environment and Occupational Performance: Theoretical Considerations." In *Using Environments to Enable Occupational Performance*, edited by L. Letts, P. Rigby and D. Stewart, 17–32. Thorofare, NJ: Slack Inc.

Rosenbaum, S. and L. Kantner. 2007. "Field Usability Testing: Method, Not Compromise." In *IPCC 2007 Proceedings*, Seattle, WA: Institute of Electrical and Electronics Engineers, Inc.

Rubin, J. 1994. *Handbook of Usability Testing: How to Plan, Design, and Conduct Effective Tests*. Hoboken, NJ: Wiley Publishing.

Rudy, D. B. 1997. "User-Centered Design of Smart Product." *Ergonomics* 40 (10): 1159–1169.

Sanford, J. A. 2012. *Design for the Ages: Universal Design as a Rehabilitation Intervention*. New York: Springer Publishing.

Sanford, J. A. and C. Bruce. 2010. "Measuring the Impact of the Physical Environment." In *Rehabilitation and Health Assessment*, edited by T. Oakl and E. Mpofu, 207–228. New York: Springer.

Scholtz, Jean. 2004. "Usability Evaluation." National Institute of Standards and Technology. https://pdfs.semanticscholar.org/8dec/cec5ace9235878e6aab06c3cd54f7b33a2ce.pdf.

Shackel, B. 1984. "The Concept of Usability." In *Visual Display Terminals: Usability Issues and Health Concerns*, edited by J. L. Bennet, D. Case, J. Sandelin and M. Smith, 45. Englewood Cliffs, NJ: Prentice-Hall.

Spool, J. and W. Schroeder. 2001. "Testing Web Sites: Five Users is Nowhere Near Enough." In *CHI 2001 Extended Abstracts*, 285–286. New York: ACM Press.

Stark, S. and J. Sanford. 2005. "Environmental Enablers and Their Impact on Occupational Performance." In *Occupational Therapy: Performance Participation, and Well-Being*, edited by C. Christiansen and C. M. Baum, 298–337. Thorofare, NJ: Slack.

Stark, S., J. Sanford, and M. Keglovits. 2014. "Environmental Performance Enablers and Their Impact on Occupational Performance." In *Occupational Therapy, Performance, Participation and Well Being*, 4th ed., edited by C. Christianson, C. Baum, and J. D. Bass. Thorofare, NJ: Slack.

WHO. 2001. *World Health Organization: International Classification of Functioning, Disability and Health: ICF*. Geneva: World Health Organization.

Woolrych, A. and G. Cockton. 2001. "Why and When Five Test Users Aren't Enough." In *Proceedings of IHM-HCI 2001 Conference*, edited by J. Vanderdonckt, A. Blandford, and A. Derycke, Vol. 2, 105–108. Toulouse: Cépadèus.

Index

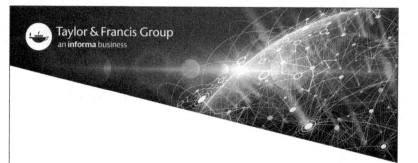

Printed in the United States
by Baker & Taylor Publisher Services